JO PETERS

RICHTIG ATMEN
KOMPAKT

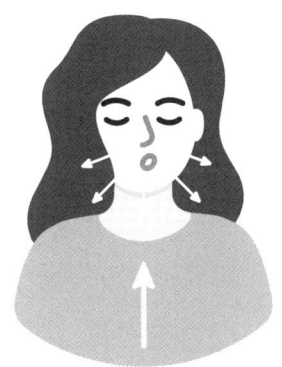

GESUNDHEIT UND KRAFT
DURCH DIE RICHTIGE ATMUNG

PETERSBERG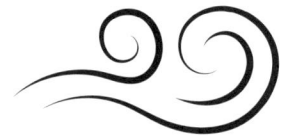

ist ein Imprint der

HEEL Verlag GmbH
Gut Pottscheidt
53639 Königswinter
Tel.: 02223 9230-0
Fax: 02223 9230-13
E-Mail: info@heel-verlag.de
www.heel-verlag.de

Deutsche Ausgabe:
© 2024 HEEL Verlag GmbH
Petersberg ist ein Imprint der HEEL Verlag GmbH

Published by arrangement with Summersdale Publishers.
© Summersdale Publishers, 2019
Part of Octopus Publishing Group Limited
www.summersdale.com

An Hachette UK Company
www.hachette.co.uk

Text © Olivia Coppin
Originaltitel: "The Little Book of Breathwork"
ISBN 978-1-80007-708-9

Deutsche Ausgabe:
Satz: Ralph Handmann, HEEL Verlag, GmbH

Alle Rechte, auch die des Nachdrucks, der Wiedergabe in jeder Form und der Übersetzung in andere Sprachen, behält sich der Herausgeber vor. Es ist ohne schriftliche Genehmigung des Verlags nicht erlaubt, das Buch und Teile daraus auf fotomechanischem Weg zu vervielfältigen oder unter Verwendung elektronischer bzw. mechanischer Systeme zu speichern, systematisch auszuwerten oder zu verbreiten. Ebenso untersagt ist die Erfassung und Nutzung auf Netzwerken, inklusive Internet, oder die Verbreitung des Werkes auf Portalen wie Google Books.

– Alle Rechte vorbehalten –

Printed in Czech Republic

ISBN 978-3-7553-0058-8

JO PETERS

RICHTIG ATMEN
KOMPAKT

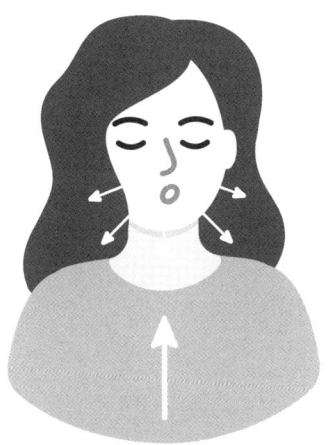

**GESUNDHEIT UND KRAFT
DURCH DIE RICHTIGE ATMUNG**

PETERSBERG

INHALT

Einführung 7

KAPITEL EINS:
Die Kraft der Atmung 8

KAPITEL ZWEI:
Eine kurze Geschichte der Atmung 28

KAPITEL DREI:
Atemtechniken für Anfänger 46

KAPITEL VIER:
Atemübungen 78

Fazit 123

Hilfreiche Links 124

ICH ATME EIN.

ICH ATME AUS.

Einführung

Willkommen zu diesem Kompaktratgeber über die Atmung, einem komplexen System, dessen Prozess in der Lunge sich auf den ganzen Körper auswirkt und von vielen Faktoren wie körperliche Aktivität, Stress oder Krankheiten beeinflusst wird.

Richtige und willentliche Atmung ist eine uralte Praxis, die seit Jahrhunderten zur Beruhigung, Erleuchtung und Reinigung von Körper und Geist eingesetzt wird. Aber erst in den letzten Jahren hat man begonnen, die Vorteile einer bewussten Atmungsarbeit allgemein anzuerkennen. Auf den folgenden Seiten werden wir gemeinsam erkunden, wie wichtig es ist, sich auf den Atem einzustimmen, und welche magischen Möglichkeiten es gibt, sich seine Kraft zunutze zu machen. Wir beginnen, die Wissenschaft hinter seinen beruhigenden Qualitäten zu verstehen und wie Sie Übungen leicht in Ihren Alltag einbauen können. Die Atmung ist das beste Werkzeug in unserem Arsenal, um Achtsamkeit zu erlangen, und Sie praktizieren sie bereits seit der Geburt. Mit Hilfe dieses Leitfadens werden Sie in der Lage sein, Ihre Verbindung zu ihr zu vertiefen und Ihre volle Kraft aufblühen zu sehen.

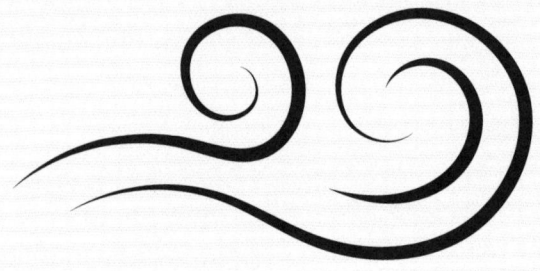

Kapitel Eins:

DIE KRAFT DER ATMUNG

Die Atemarbeit steht im Mittelpunkt vieler Selbsthilfepraktiken, ein Zeichen für ihre grundlegende Bedeutung für Ihr Wohlbefinden. Sie wird von den wissenschaftlichsten bis hin zu den spirituellsten Wohlfühlpraktikern als entscheidendes Instrument eingesetzt, da immer mehr Menschen ihre Kraft verstehen und schätzen.

In diesem Kapitel werden wir uns mit den zahlreichen Vorteilen befassen, die die Achtsamkeit auf den Atem haben kann, von der körperlichen über die geistige bis hin zur emotionalen Ebene, sowie mit den wissenschaftlichen Erkenntnissen dahinter. Wir werden lernen, was es eigentlich bedeutet, mit dem Atem zu arbeiten, und wie Sie es so gestalten können, dass es für Sie funktioniert. Dieses Kapitel wird den Grundstein für eine neue Denkweise legen, in der die Atmung mehr als nur ein funktioneller Mechanismus ist und stattdessen ein wertvolles Gut, das Ihnen hilft, Ihre körperliche und geistige Gesundheit zu verbessern.

ICH HABE DIE MACHT, MIT EINEM EINZIGEN ATEMZUG MEINE GESAMTE EINSTELLUNG ZU ÄNDERN.

Was ist Atmung?

Der durchschnittliche Mensch atmet 22.000-mal am Tag ein und aus, doch wie oft haben Sie heute schon auf ein Ein- oder Ausatmen geachtet? Meistens werden wir uns unseres Atems nur dann bewusst, wenn er uns schwerfällt – wenn wir eine verstopfte Nase bei einer Erkältung haben oder bei sportlicher Betätigung außer Atem sind. Aber er ist immer da, surrt leise vor sich hin und versorgt uns mit der Lebensquelle, die es uns ermöglicht, unseren Tag zu bewältigen.

Atemarbeit bezieht sich auf die Praxis, dieses tägliche Ein- und Ausatmen zu nutzen, um unsere geistige und körperliche Gesundheit zu verbessern. Manchmal besteht die Praxis einfach darin, dem natürlichen Rhythmus unseres Atems Aufmerksamkeit zu schenken, und ein anderes Mal kann es darum gehen, den Atem zu manipulieren, indem man ihn vertieft, anhält, seine Kraft erhöht oder nur die Nasenlöcher benutzt.

Atemarbeit ist einfach bewusstes, konzentriertes und zielgerichtetes Atmen mit Hilfe einer Vielzahl von Techniken und Übungen.

Die Ziele der Atmung

Es gibt eine Vielzahl von Gründen, warum jemand eine Atmungspraxis in sein Leben einführen könnte. Während wir in diesem Buch viele der Vorteile und Ziele des bewussten Atmens behandeln, sind die Möglichkeiten endlos und für jeden Menschen einzigartig.

Aufgrund der zahlreichen verschiedenen Techniken sind die angestrebten Ergebnisse vielfältig – von der Hilfe beim Einschlafen über das Gefühl, wach und energiegeladen zu sein, bis hin zur Förderung der Kreativität oder der Beruhigung des Geistes von Geschwätz. Das übergreifende Ziel ist jedoch oft dasselbe: Wir nutzen die uns bereits zur Verfügung stehenden Mittel, um Körper und Geist zu stärken und zu fokussieren.

Warum atmen wir?

Die Atmung ist der Prozess, bei dem Sauerstoff in den Körper gelangt und Kohlendioxid abtransportiert wird. Die Zellen in unserem Körper benötigen Sauerstoff, um alltägliche Funktionen zu erfüllen. Damit wir uns bewegen, essen und denken können, brauchen wir eine gesunde Menge an Sauerstoff in unseren Zellen. Wenn wir die Luft um uns herum einatmen, nehmen wir Sauerstoff auf.

Während die Zellen diese Aufgaben erfüllen, entsteht Kohlendioxid als Abfallprodukt. Dieses muss aus dem Blutkreislauf und dem Körper entfernt werden, was beim Ausatmen geschieht.

Das Gehirn empfängt ständig Signale über den Sauerstoff- und Kohlendioxidgehalt im Körper und passt die Atemfrequenz entsprechend an. Wenn Sie beispielsweise Sport treiben und Ihre Muskeln mit mehr Sauerstoff versorgen und Kohlendioxid schneller abtransportieren müssen, erhöht sich der Atemrhythmus.

Wie atmen wir?

Die Teile des Körpers, die am Atmungsprozess beteiligt sind, werden zusammen als Atmungssystem bezeichnet. Dazu gehören: die Nase, der Mund, der Rachen, die Luftröhre und die Lunge.

Außerdem sind viele Muskeln an der Atmung beteiligt. Das Zwerchfell ist der wichtigste Atemmuskel. Es ist ein großer Muskel, der den Brustkorb vom Bauchraum trennt. Bei vielen Atemübungen wird das Zwerchfell gespürt oder in den Mittelpunkt gestellt.

Die Bauchmuskeln und die Muskeln zwischen den Rippen, die Zwischenrippenmuskeln, unterstützen ebenfalls den Atmungsprozess.

Einatmen

Hier ist eine grundlegende Einführung in das, was beim Einatmen geschieht:

1. Das Atemzentrum im Gehirn gibt dem Zwerchfell und den anderen Muskeln das Signal, den Vorgang zu beginnen.
2. Das Zwerchfell bewegt sich nach unten, und der Brustkorb zieht sich nach oben und außen. Dadurch wird Platz für die Ausdehnung der Lunge geschaffen.
3. Die Luft wird über die Nase oder den Mund angesaugt und strömt die Luftröhre hinunter, die sich in zwei Atemwege teilt, die in den linken und rechten Lungenflügel führen.
4. Die Atemwege teilen sich weitere 15–25-mal und werden schließlich zu Tausenden von winzigen Atemwegen, die zu den Lungenbläschen führen.
5. Von diesen Bläschen geht der Sauerstoff in den Blutkreislauf über und wird über die Zellen dorthin transportiert, wo er benötigt wird.

Ausatmen

Hier eine grundlegende Einführung in das, was beim Ausatmen geschieht:

1. Kohlendioxid gelangt aus dem Blutkreislauf zurück in die Lungenbläschen.
2. Das Zwerchfell entspannt sich, kehrt in eine kuppelförmige Position zurück und verkleinert den Raum in der Lunge. Wenn die Luft schneller bewegt werden muss, wie z. B. bei sportlicher Betätigung, helfen auch die Bauchmuskeln, die Luft wieder nach außen zu drücken.
3. Dadurch wird die Luft durch die Luftröhre zurück nach oben und aus der Nase oder dem Mund gepresst.

ICH HALTE INNE.

ICH BIN HIER.

ICH ATME.

Die Fakten der Atmung

Das autonome Nervensystem des Körpers steuert alle unsere unwillkürlichen Funktionen, wie Herzschlag und Verdauung. Dieses Nervensystem ist in zwei Zweige unterteilt:

Sympathisches Nervensystem oder „Kampf- oder Flucht"-Modus

Dieser steuert, wann der Körper als Reaktion auf eine wahrgenommene Gefahr eine „Kampf- oder Flucht"-Reaktion aktivieren muss. Wenn der Körper gestresst ist, befindet er sich in diesem Zustand und kann unwillkürliche Funktionen beeinflussen, wie z. B. die Erhöhung der Herzfrequenz und die Unterbrechung von Prozessen, die nicht dringend sind.

Parasympathisches Nervensystem, oder „Ruhe- und Verdauungsmodus"

Wenn der Körper keinen Stress empfindet, wird der „Ruhe- und Verdauungszustand" aktiviert. Dadurch können die unwillkürlichen Funktionen, die für das unmittelbare Überleben weniger wichtig sind, wie z. B. die richtige Verdauung der Nahrung, ablaufen.

Die Atmung ist eine dieser unwillkürlichen Funktionen, die durch Atemübungen bewusst gesteuert werden kann. Daher kann eine gezielte Anpassung des Atemmusters bestimmen, welches Nervensystem aktiviert wird, was sich auf eine ganze Reihe von Körperfunktionen auswirkt.

Wenn bei einer Atemübung die Ausatmung verlängert oder der Atem verlangsamt wird, signalisiert dies dem Gehirn, dass der Körper nicht unter Stress steht, und das parasympathische Nervensystem kann aktiviert werden. Während dieser Entspannungsreaktion wird der Körper in einen ruhigeren Zustand versetzt und kann sich um alle lebenswichtigen Hintergrundfunktionen kümmern.

Ein Beispiel dafür kann man oft während einer Meditationssitzung sehen (oder hören), wenn die Mägen der Menschen zu gurgeln beginnen, weil das entspannte Nervensystem dem Verdauungsprozess grünes Licht gibt.

Körperliche Vorteile der Atmung

Es gibt viele potenzielle Vorteile der bewussten Atmung. Körperliche Vorteile können sein

- Senkung des Blutdrucks
- entspannte Schultern/Brustkorb
- erhöhte Energie
- gestärktes Immunsystem
- verbesserte Verdauung
- verbesserter Schlaf
- stärkere Atmungsfunktion
- reduzierte Gefühle von Posttraumatischen Belastungsstörungen (PTBS) und vergangenen Traumata

Emotionaler Nutzen von Atmung

Emotionale Vorteile können sein:

- verringerte Angstzustände
- verringerte Depression
- verbesserte Stimmung
- gesteigerte Produktivität/Fokus
- erhöhte Ruhe
- erhöhte Klarheit

Atmungsarbeit und andere Praktiken

Atemübungen sind eine zentrale Säule vieler Wellness-Praktiken, und oft gibt es Überschneidungen zwischen ihnen. Aufgrund der zahlreichen Vorteile und der beruhigenden Wirkung ist es nicht verwunderlich, dass sie ein wichtiger Bestandteil der meisten Wellness-Grundgedanken ist.

Kein ganzheitliches Wellnesskonzept ist vollständig, wenn man sich nicht auch mit der Atmung und deren Auswirkungen auf den gesamten Körper und Geist beschäftigt. Werfen wir einen Blick darauf, wie Atmung in andere Praktiken integriert werden kann.

Atmung und Meditation

Meditation ist eine Praxis, die dazu dient, den Geist zu beruhigen, zu besänftigen und sich zu fokussieren.

Wie auf den Seiten 18-19 beschrieben, kann eine kontrollierte Atmung den Körper in den Parasympathikus versetzen, den „Ruhe- und Verdauungszustand". Dieser Zustand ist der Schlüssel zum Meditieren, da er es dem Körper ermöglicht, sich zu verlangsamen und nicht in höchster Alarmbereitschaft für potenzielle Stressfaktoren zu sein.

Wenn es sich fast unmöglich anfühlt, sich einfach hinzusetzen und sich zu sagen: „Sei ruhig und mach den Kopf frei", kann die Atmung einen Fokuspunkt bieten, um dich aktiv in diesen ruhigeren Zustand zu ziehen. Insbesondere das verlängerte Ausatmen hilft Ihnen, Ihrem Gehirn zu signalisieren, dass Sie bereit sind, sich zu entspannen.

Atmung und Achtsamkeit

Achtsamkeit ist die Praxis des Gegenwärtigseins. Sie zielt darauf ab, den Fokus auf das Hier und Jetzt zu verlagern, das Gehirn vom Geplapper zu beruhigen und es Ihnen zu ermöglichen, im gegenwärtigen Moment zu existieren.

Da Ihr Atem nur in diesem Moment stattfindet – nicht in der Vergangenheit oder Zukunft –, verbindet Sie die Konzentration auf Ihre Atmung sofort mit der Gegenwart. Jedes Mal, wenn Sie sich auf das Einatmen oder Ausatmen konzentrieren, verlagern Sie Ihren Fokus auf die Gegenwart und vollziehen einen Akt der Achtsamkeit.

Andere Möglichkeiten, achtsam zu sein, bestehen darin, auf die Geräusche um Sie herum zu achten, wie sich Ihr Körper anfühlt, und sich umzuschauen, um wirklich wahrzunehmen, was Sie sehen.

Atmung und Selbstfürsorge

Selbstfürsorge umfasst eine ganze Reihe von Praktiken, die darauf abzielen, Ihr körperliches, geistiges und emotionales Wohlbefinden zu verbessern. Dazu kann es gehören, stimmungsaufhellende Musik zu hören, ein Bad zu nehmen oder joggen zu gehen.

Atmung kann ein wesentlicher Bestandteil der Selbstfürsorge sein. Wenn jemand zum Beispiel versucht, Ängste abzubauen oder die Produktivität in seiner Morgenroutine zu steigern, gibt es dafür entsprechende Atemübungen. Da sich die Ziele von Atmung und Selbstfürsorge weitgehend überschneiden, ist es nicht verwunderlich, dass Atmung häufig in Momenten der Selbstfürsorge eingesetzt wird. Wenn Sie das nächste Mal einen Akt der Selbstfürsorge durchführen, wie z. B. das Auflegen einer Gesichtsmaske, versuchen Sie, den Nutzen zu verdoppeln, indem Sie auch eine geeignete Atemtechnik einbeziehen, wie z. B. die einfache Beruhigungsübung, die auf den Seiten 58–59 beschrieben wird.

Wie man Atmung in den Alltag einbauen kann

Das Beste an der Atmung ist, dass sie keine zusätzlichen Hilfsmittel, komplizierte Ausrüstung oder finanzielle Investitionen erfordert. Sie haben buchstäblich alles, was Sie brauchen, um loszulegen.

Alles, was Sie brauchen, ist:

- das Wissen
- die Motivation
- die Zeit

Für die meisten Atemübungen benötigen Sie weniger als 5 Minuten, um eine ganze Reihe von Vorteilen zu spüren. Bei einigen können Sie die Vorteile sogar innerhalb einer Minute spüren. Auch wenn es gar nicht viel Zeit braucht, ist es vielleicht hilfreich, wenn Sie feste Zeiten oder bestimmte Methoden haben, um sie in Ihren Tag einzubauen.

Hier sind einige Beispiele dafür, wie Sie eine Atemtechnik in Ihren Tag einbauen können:

- Bleiben Sie nach dem Aufwachen, bevor Sie Ihren Tag beginnen, ein paar Minuten länger im Bett liegen und führen Sie eine Atemübung durch, um Ihren Tag bewusst und ruhig zu beginnen.
- Nutzen Sie eine gewöhnliche Tätigkeit wie das Zähneputzen oder Duschen als Zeit für eine entsprechende Übung.
- Stellen Sie einen Wecker für eine beliebige Tageszeit und nehmen Sie sich ein paar Minuten Zeit zum Atmen, sobald der Wecker klingelt, egal wo Sie sind.
- Nutzen Sie die Zeit vor einer Mahlzeit, um einen Moment innezuhalten und sich auf Ihren Atem zu konzentrieren.
- Nehmen Sie sich eine Auslösesituation vor, die in unregelmäßigen Abständen im Lauf des Tages auftaucht, z. B. jedes Mal, wenn Sie an einer roten Ampel anhalten oder eine SMS erhalten. Machen Sie eine Atemübung, die Sie immer dann anwenden können, wenn diese Situationen eintreten.
- Wenn Sie einschlafen, nutzen Sie die Stille und Ruhe, um eine entspannende Atemübung zu erkunden.

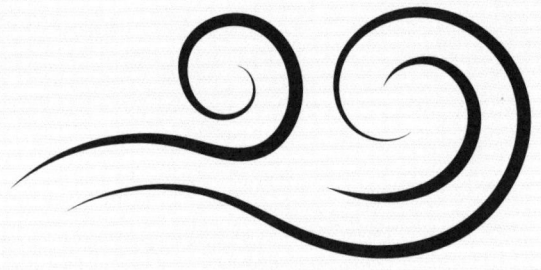

Kapitel Zwei:
EINE KURZE GESCHICHTE DER ATMUNG

Die Atemarbeit hat erst vor kurzem begonnen, in Wellness- und Wissenschaftskreisen weltweit an Bedeutung zu gewinnen, obwohl sie ihre Wurzeln in uralten Praktiken hat, die seit Tausenden von Jahren angewendet werden. In diesem Kapitel werden wir einen kurzen Blick darauf werfen, woher die Idee der Atmung stammt und wie sie sich im Lauf der modernen Geschichte entwickelt hat und gewachsen ist. Wenn Sie verstehen, wie die Atemarbeit entstanden ist und wie sie seit so vielen Jahren von den Menschen genutzt wird, und wie die Praxis für das heutige Leben verfeinert wurde, kann Ihnen das helfen, die vielen Vorteile dieses wunderbaren Zweigs des Wohlbefindens zu schätzen und zu nutzen.

Wenn der Atem unstetig ist, ist alles unruhig; wenn der Atem ruhig ist, ist alles ruhig.

Goraksha Shataka

Die Ursprünge der Atmungspraktiken

Das, was wir in der modernen westlichen Kultur als Atempraxis bezeichnen, hat seine Wurzeln in vielen traditionellen östlichen Religionen und kulturellen Praktiken, und wir können seine heutige Bedeutung nicht diskutieren, ohne diese Geschichte zu würdigen und anzuerkennen.

Auf den nächsten Seiten werden wir kurz darauf eingehen, wie Atemübungen im Buddhismus, im Tai-Chi und im Yoga tief verwurzelt sind. Diese traditionellen Praktiken und ihre Arbeit mit dem Atem werden zwar immer noch auf der ganzen Welt verehrt, aber sie wurden auch angepasst und modernisiert, um einer modernen Gesellschaft gerecht zu werden. Die Ziele der Atmung in diesen Praktiken sind jedoch dieselben geblieben: durch die Kontrolle des Atems Ruhe und Klarheit zu erlangen.

Buddhismus

Der Buddhismus ist eine Religion oder philosophische Tradition, die auf die ursprünglichen Lehren von Gautama Buddha aus dem sechsten bis vierten Jahrhundert vor Christus im alten Indien zurückgeht. Der Buddhismus ist derzeit die viertgrößte Religion der Welt.

Die Meditation ist ein zentraler Bestandteil des Buddhismus und des buddhistischen Strebens nach Befreiung und dem Erreichen des Nirwana. Von den verschiedenen Techniken der buddhistischen Meditation ist ānāpānasati wohl eine der wichtigsten. Ānāpāna bedeutet „Ein- und Ausatmen" und sati „Achtsamkeit", ānāpānasati bezieht sich auf die Achtsamkeit beim Atmen.

Ānāpānasati bedeutet, dem Atem Aufmerksamkeit zu schenken, und ist eine der wichtigsten Lehren des Buddha. Sie wird in mehreren buddhistischen Texten oder „Suttas" beschrieben. Insbesondere eine der Suttas, die ānāpāna Sutta, empfiehlt die Praxis, sich auf das Ein- und Ausatmen zu konzentrieren, um Achtsamkeit im Körper zu kultivieren und Befreiung vom Leiden zu finden.
Verschiedene Zweige des Buddhismus haben die Anapanasati-Praxis mit unterschiedlichen Techniken weiterentwickelt. Während einige den Schwerpunkt auf den natürlichen Rhythmus legen, setzen andere Schulen die Muskeln ein, um einen kräftigeren Atem zu erzeugen, und einige integrieren die Atmung in Gesänge und Gesänge.

Tai-Chi

Tai-Chi ist eine uralte chinesische Kampfkunst, die wegen ihrer gesundheitsfördernden Wirkung immer noch weltweit praktiziert wird. Sie basiert auf der Notwendigkeit, das natürliche Gleichgewicht in allen Dingen zu erhalten.

Im Mittelpunkt stehen Meditation und Bewegung, zu den fünf Schlüsselelementen gehören Neigong und Qigong, bei denen die Arbeit mit dem Atem im Vordergrund steht.

Ein hervorragendes Beispiel für die Atmung im Tai-Chi ist die als „Kranichatmung" bekannte Übung, bei der es darum geht, den Atem mit der Körperbewegung zu koordinieren. Obwohl die Kranichatmung für jeden geeignet ist, sollten Sie erst zu dieser Übung zurückkehren, sobald Sie Ihre Atemtechniken aufgebaut haben.

Kranich-Atmung

- Beginnen Sie im Stehen, die Füße hüftbreit oder breiter, und verteilen Sie das Gewicht gleichmäßig auf beide Beine.
- Halten Sie Ihren Körperschwerpunkt niedrig und Ihre Knie weich.
- Atmen Sie durch die Nase ein und aus. Hören Sie auf den Atem, wie er in Ihren Körper ein- und ausströmt.
- Legen Sie Ihre Hände auf Ihren Unterbauch. Entspannen Sie Ihre Schultern und Ellbogen.
- Verlagern Sie Ihr Gewicht auf die Vorderseite jedes Fußes und dann wieder auf die Rückseite jedes Fußes, während Sie die Füße flach auf dem Boden halten.
- Entwickeln Sie einen gleichmäßigen Rhythmus und achten Sie auf Ihr Ein- und Ausatmen. Können Sie die Schaukelbewegung und Ihren Atem miteinander verbinden?
- Behalten Sie diesen langsamen, gleichmäßigen Rhythmus bei. Einatmen, nach vorne schaukeln. Ausatmen, zurückwippen.
- Machen Sie so viele Wiederholungen, wie Sie möchten.

Yoga

Yoga ist eine uralte indische Praxis, die darauf abzielt, Körper, Geist und Seele in Einklang zu bringen. Yoga hat sich über Hunderte von Jahren weiterentwickelt und viele Zweige entwickelt und ist eine sehr beliebte Praxis für Gesundheit und Entspannung. Die verschiedenen Yogaschulen unterscheiden sich zwar in Bezug auf Körperlichkeit, Spiritualität und Meditation, doch die Bedeutung des Atems zieht sich wie ein roter Faden durch alle. Im Yoga wird die Praxis, sich auf den Atem zu konzentrieren, „Pranayama" genannt. Im Sanskrit bedeutet Prana „vitale Lebenskraft" und Yama „Kontrolle". In alten Schriften und Texten wie der Bhagavad Gita und den Yoga Sutras von Patanjali wird Pranayama und die Kontrolle des Atems als Schlüssel zur Beruhigung des Geistes und zum Erlangen eines höheren Bewusstseins bezeichnet.

In den modernen Praktiken, die sich oft um „Asanas" (Körperhaltungen) drehen, bleibt der Atem eine Schlüsselkomponente. Asanas werden oft für eine bestimmte Anzahl von Atemzügen gehalten, und Ausatmen und Einatmen werden zur Unterstützung der Bewegung und zur Vertiefung der Dehnungen eingesetzt.

Wir werden später einige grundlegende Pranayama-Techniken im Rahmen der Atemübungen erkunden, beginnend mit der yogischen Atmung auf den Seiten 66–67.

Wachsendes Interesse an der Atmung

Die Atmungsarbeit, die heute in der westlichen Gesellschaft am weitesten verbreitet ist, orientiert sich eher an den Techniken, die in den 1960er- und 1970er-Jahren entstanden sind. Einige entstanden aus der Erforschung von Bewusstseinszuständen und psychedelischen Effekten, während andere sich mehr auf Selbstbewusstsein und inneren Frieden konzentrierten.

Wir werden kurz auf die beiden ursprünglichen Zweige der modernen Atmung eingehen und darauf, wie sie sich in jüngerer Zeit im einundzwanzigsten Jahrhundert entwickelt hat

Die Atmung ist das größte Vergnügen im Leben.

Giovanni Papini

Holotrope Atmung

Holotrope Atmung bedeutet „sich zur Ganzheit bewegen". Sie wurde in den 1970er-Jahren von Stan und Christina Grof entwickelt, als sie als Psychotherapeuten arbeiteten und Forschungen über das Bewusstsein und die Auswirkungen psychedelischer Drogen durchführten.

Bevor LSD als illegale Droge eingestuft wurde, untersuchten sie Patienten, die unter dem Einfluss der Droge standen, und stellten ein bestimmtes Atemmuster fest, das bei denjenigen üblich war, die sich dem Ende eines Trips näherten, um die Wirkung der Droge zu verlängern. Dies veranlasste die Grofs, den Atem zu erforschen und herauszufinden, wie er kontrolliert werden kann, um nichtalltägliche Geisteszustände und schnelle Heilung zu erreichen.

Die Technik der holotropen Atmung besteht darin, 1 bis 2 Stunden lang in beschleunigtem Tempo zu atmen und dabei die Bauchmuskeln zu benutzen, um kräftig ein- und auszuatmen, oft begleitet von Musik. Sie wird als freiwillige Hyperventilation beschrieben und kann eine Vielzahl von Reaktionen hervorrufen, von Lachen und Weinen bis hin zu Visionen und Muskelkrämpfen.
Obwohl therapeutische Vorteile angenommen werden, ist es ratsam, sich gründlich zu informieren und ärztlichen Rat einzuholen, bevor man es ausprobiert, vor allem bei Personen mit Herzproblemen oder Nervenleiden. Sie sollte nur unter der Aufsicht eines ausgebildeten Ausbilders für holotrope Atmung durchgeführt werden.

Integrative Atemtherapie

„Rebirthing" oder „Verbundenes Atmen" entstand in den späten 1960er- bis 1970er-Jahren und wurde von Dr. Leonard Orr entwickelt und auch zur Heilung negativer frühkindlicher Erfahrungen eingesetzt.

Dr. Orr behauptet, er sei von einem Yogi namens Mahavatar Babaji inspiriert worden, als er sich in dessen Ashram im Himalaya aufhielt. Orr saß in der Badewanne und experimentierte mit verschiedenen Atemmustern, als sich sein Atem mit dem Zustand des warmen Wassers verband. Das Konzept, vergangenen Traumata zu entkommen und die Fähigkeit zur „Wiedergeburt" durch den Atem war geboren.

Die spirituelle Lehrerin Sondra Ray wird ebenfalls für den Aufstieg der Rebirthing-Atmung verantwortlich gemacht, nachdem sie direkt von Orr gelernt hatte und anschließend anderen dabei half, Geburtstraumata durch Rebirthing zu heilen.

Die Integrative Atemtherapie konzentriert sich auf einen zirkulären Atem, bei dem das Ein- und Ausatmen kontinuierlich und miteinander verbunden sind, um Sie in einen veränderten Zustand zu versetzen, in dem Sie Gedanken, Gefühle und Emotionen auf einer höheren Ebene verarbeiten. Anders als bei der holotropen Atmung gibt es bei der Rebirthing-Atmung keine Musik, und der Schwerpunkt liegt auf einem entspannten, volleren Einatmen im Gegensatz zu einem kraftvollen Ausatmen.

ICH BIN OFFEN, WOHIN AUCH IMMER MICH DIESE REISE FÜHREN WIRD UND ICH BIN DANKBAR FÜR ALLES, WAS SIE MICH LEHREN WIRD.

Atemtechniken im Einundzwanzigsten Jahrhundert

Die Popularität des Rebirthing und der holotropen Atmung hat nach den 1970er-Jahren etwas nachgelassen, erlebte aber im neuen Jahrhundert wieder einen Aufschwung.

Heutzutage gibt es Dutzende von verschiedenen Zweigen der Atmungstherapie, jeder mit seinen spezifischen Wegen und Zielen. Sie können unterschiedliche Stimuli (wie Musik oder Räucherstäbchen) verwenden, sie können sich auf Gruppen- oder Einzelsitzungen konzentrieren, und sie können in ihrer Dauer stark variieren, aber alle beinhalten eine bewusste Veränderung des Atemmusters, um den Geist, den Körper oder das emotionale Herz zu beeinflussen.

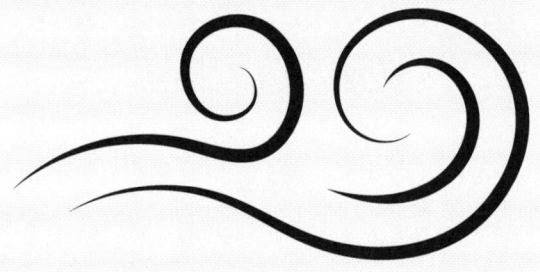

Kapitel Drei:

ATEMTECHNIKEN FÜR ANFÄNGER

Wir werden uns nun ansehen, wie Sie sich auf Ihre Atemübungen vorbereiten, was Sie erwarten können und wie Sie sie auf ein für Sie angenehmes Niveau einstellen. In diesem Kapitel werden auch einige einfache Atemübungen vorgestellt, die es ermöglichen, die Vorteile der richtigen Atmung zu entfalten. Diese legen auch den Grundstein für die fortgeschritteneren Übungen im nächsten Kapitel. Sobald Sie eine allgemeine Grundlage für das bewusste Atmen geschaffen haben, können Sie damit beginnen, es auf Ihre Bedürfnisse zuzuschneiden und sich ein Wissen über viele Techniken für verschiedene Zwecke aufzubauen.

ATME DIE ZUKUNFT EIN.

ATME DIE VERGANGENHEIT AUS.

Sicher atmen

Bevor Sie sich auf die Reise zu Ihrer Atmung begeben, sollten Sie einige wichtige Überlegungen anstellen, um Ihre Gesundheit und Sicherheit zu gewährleisten.

- Wenn Sie sich an irgendeinem Punkt benommen, schwindlig oder kurzatmig fühlen, beenden Sie die Atemübung und kehren Sie zu Ihrer natürlichen Atemtiefe und -geschwindigkeit zurück.
- Einige Atemübungen sind für Schwangere oder Menschen mit Herzproblemen nicht ratsam, daher sollten Sie vor der Durchführung einen Arzt aufsuchen.
- Wenn Sie eine unerwünschte Nebenwirkung spüren, wie z. B. erhöhte Angstgefühle, beenden Sie die Übung.
- Obwohl oft empfohlen wird, die Augen zu schließen, sollten Sie, wenn Sie sich dadurch klaustrophobisch fühlen, die Augen offenhalten und den Blick sanft schweifen lassen.

Allgemeine Tipps für Anfänger

Einige Dinge sollten Sie beachten, wenn Sie mit Ihrer persönlichen Atemtherapie beginnen:

- Obwohl viele der Übungen überall durchgeführt werden können, finden Sie sie zu Beginn vielleicht am nützlichsten, wenn Sie sich wirklich konzentrieren können. Versuchen Sie, Ablenkungen zu vermeiden, legen Sie Ihr Handy weg und setzen Sie sich an einen Ort, an dem Sie nicht gestört werden.
- Denken Sie daran, dass es völlig normal ist, dass Ihre Gedanken abschweifen. Haben Sie realistische Erwartungen und verurteilen Sie sich nicht, wenn es Ihnen nicht so leicht fällt, wie Sie es sich vorstellen. Denken Sie daran: Selbst, wenn Sie während Ihrer gesamten Praxis nur auf einen Atemzug achten, ist das vielleicht ein Atemzug mehr als an jedem anderen Tag.

- Es gibt keinen perfekten Weg, es zu tun. Wenn Sie sich im Liegen wohler fühlen, tun Sie es. Wenn Sie sich durch Kissen stützen wollen, dann tun Sie das. Lassen Sie sich nicht durch eine Vorstellung davon einschränken, wie Atmungsarbeit aussehen sollte; es geht darum, wie Sie sich dabei fühlen.
- Denken Sie daran, dass nicht alle Praktiken für Sie funktionieren, zu Ihnen passen oder für die Zwecke geeignet sind, die Sie brauchen. Dies ist eine allgemeine Anleitung und Einführung, aus der Sie sich das herauspicken können, was Sie benötigen.
- Auch wenn Ihnen alles zur Verfügung steht, um jederzeit zu üben, und Sie vielleicht wissen, wie gut Sie sich dabei fühlen, heißt das noch lange nicht, dass Sie sich immer motiviert fühlen. Genau wie beim Sport müssen Sie sich manchmal zwingen, den ersten Schritt zu tun.

Durch die Nase atmen

Wenn wir uns vorstellen, dass jemand tief einatmet, atmet er oft durch die Nase ein und durch den Mund aus. Dies kann zwar eine wirksame Atemtechnik sein, aber beachten Sie, dass viele Ausatmungen bei der Atmung auch durch die Nase erfolgen. Dies entspricht eher unserer natürlichen Atmung und verhindert Nebenwirkungen wie einen trockenen Mund und Halsschmerzen.

Sofern in den Übungen und Techniken in diesem Buch nicht anders angegeben, atmen Sie daher sowohl beim Ein- als auch beim Ausatmen immer durch die Nase.

Wie man die Übungen beginnt

Viele dieser Übungen enthalten kurze Ratschläge für den Aufbau und den Einstieg in die Praxis, wobei Sie sich oft ein paar Augenblicke Zeit nehmen, um sich einzuleben und Ihren Geist mit Ihrem Körper in Einklang zu bringen.

Mit zunehmender Vertrautheit mit den Techniken werden Sie wahrscheinlich bevorzugte Tageszeiten, Orte und Aufstellungen entdecken. Vielleicht stellen Sie fest, dass Sie die Atemübungen lieber auf nüchternen Magen praktizieren oder dass Sie am meisten davon profitieren, wenn sie mitten in einem geschäftigen Tag stattfindet.

Denken Sie daran, dass der Zweck vieler dieser Übungen darin besteht, Ruhe zu kultivieren, und Sie müssen sich nicht in einem bereits friedlichen Zustand befinden, um damit zu beginnen. Manchmal fühlen Sie sich vielleicht ängstlich, unruhig oder nicht in einem positiven Geisteszustand, aber das sollte Sie nur ermutigen, einen Schritt zu wagen und mit der Übung zu beginnen.

Ihren natürlichen Atem wahrnehmen

Die einfachste Übung für den Einstieg in die Atmung besteht darin, die Aufmerksamkeit auf Ihren natürlichen Atem zu richten. Indem Sie sich auf den Atem im gegenwärtigen Moment konzentrieren, vollziehen Sie einen Akt der Achtsamkeit.

Diese Übung eignet sich perfekt, wenn Sie in der Öffentlichkeit sind oder nur wenig Platz haben, da sie kaum wahrnehmbar ist und Sie sofort im Moment erdet.

1. Suchen Sie sich einen ruhigen, bequemen Platz, an dem Sie nicht gestört werden. Schließen Sie die Augen oder lassen Sie Ihren Blick schweifen.
2. Achten Sie auf jedes Ein- und Ausatmen, ohne zu versuchen, es zu verändern.
3. Achten Sie auf das Tempo, den Rhythmus. Ist er schnell oder langsam, konstant oder abwechslungsreich?
4. Beobachten Sie die Tiefe Ihres Atems. Ist er flach oder atmen Sie ganz ein und aus?
5. Spüren Sie, wo Ihr Atem Sie am meisten bewegt. Ist er in Ihrem Bauch, Ihrer Brust, Ihren Schultern?
6. Beobachten Sie Ihren natürlichen Atem so lange, wie es sich gut anfühlt. Wenn es Ihnen hilft, versuchen Sie sich vorzustellen, dass Sie sich ein vollständiges Bild davon machen, wie es sich anfühlt zu atmen – in Ihrem Körper in diesem Moment – als ob Sie es jemandem in allen Einzelheiten beschreiben würden.

Tagebuch

Denken Sie an zehn Wörter, die Sie mit dem Atmen verbinden, und schreiben Sie sie hier auf.

....

....

....

....

....

....

....

....

....

....

Beobachten Sie den ganzen Atem

Diese Übung klingt unglaublich einfach, aber es kann überraschend schwierig sein, die Konzentration aufrechtzuerhalten.

1. „Beobachten" oder spüren Sie Ihr gesamtes Einatmen, von Anfang bis Ende.
2. „Beobachten" Sie Ihr vollständiges Ausatmen, bis zum Ende.
3. Atmen Sie weiter und „beobachten" Sie dabei jeden Atemzug vollständig.

Können Sie die Konzentration für einen kompletten Atemzyklus aufrechterhalten?

Tipp

Geduld ist der Schlüssel. Auch wenn sich die ersten paar Zyklen schwer anfühlen durchzukommen, ohne dass Ihre Gedanken abschweifen, vertrauen Sie darauf, dass Sie es schaffen werden. Nehmen Sie sich Zeit, sich daran zu gewöhnen.

Vertiefung des Atems

Diese Übung ist unsere erste Einführung in die Veränderung oder Beeinflussung der natürlichen Atmung auf die einfachste Weise. Oft wird uns gesagt, wir sollen „tief einatmen", aber ohne eine echte Verbindung zu dem, wie sich das anfühlt und was es bedeutet, kann das ein überflüssiger Rat sein. Schon eine leichte Vertiefung des Atems kann helfen, Sie zu beruhigen und zu erden.

Probieren Sie diese Übung aus, um zu verstehen, wie Sie tiefer atmen können.

1. Konzentrieren Sie sich zunächst auf Ihren natürlichen Atem und achten Sie auf dessen Tempo und Tiefe.
2. Spüren Sie einige Augenblicke und einige Atemzyklen lang, wie sich Ihr Brustkorb ausdehnt und Ihr Brustkorb sich hebt.
3. Wenn Sie sich bereit fühlen, beginnen Sie, beim Ein- und Ausatmen sanft über Ihren natürlichen Haltepunkt hinauszugehen.

4. Führen Sie diese Ausdehnung langsam durch; Sie brauchen nur jedes Mal ein kleines bisschen tiefer zu atmen.

5. Setzen Sie diese Runden mit kontrollierten, tiefen Atemzügen fort, bis Sie einen Rhythmus gefunden haben, der sich angenehm anfühlt, aber über Ihren natürlichen Atemzustand hinausgeht.

Tipp

Versuchen Sie bei dieser Übung zu vermeiden, den Atem anzuhalten. Lasse Sie die Atmung in einem konstanten Rhythmus fließen.

Tagebuch

Beschreiben Sie, wie Sie sich vor Ihrer Atemübung gefühlt haben.

Beschreiben Sie nun, wie Sie sich danach gefühlt haben. Gab es eine Veränderung?

....

....

....

....

....

....

....

....

....

Den Atem ausdehnen

Nachdem Sie nun erforscht haben, wie Sie den Atem technisch vertiefen können, lässt sich dies durch Visualisierung verstärken. Mit dieser Methode können Sie vielleicht über das hinausgehen, was Sie für Ihre tiefsten Atemzüge hielten.

Die Visualisierung ist ein Schlüsselinstrument der Atemarbeit, die uns oft auffordert, den Atem auf bestimmte Weise zu „sehen". Es handelt sich dabei um eine sehr persönliche Technik, die es Ihnen ermöglicht, die Praxis so anzupassen, wie es für Ihren Geist und Ihre Vorstellungskraft am besten ist.

In dieser Praxis trifft die Visualisierung auf die Empfindung. Können Sie den Atem zu verschiedenen Teilen Ihres Körpers „schicken", indem Sie sich einfach auf sie konzentrieren?

1. Legen Sie sich zunächst hin, die Handflächen zeigen nach oben und die Finger sind leicht gespreizt. Knöchel und Füße können zur Seite fallen.
2. Richten Sie Ihre Aufmerksamkeit auf Ihren Atem und spüren Sie das sanfte Auf und Ab des Ein- und Ausatmens.
3. Stellen Sie sich vor, wie Ihr Atem in die Mitte Ihrer Brust, Ihr „Herzzentrum", fließt und bei jedem Einatmen Ihren Brustkorb füllt.

4. Stellen Sie sich beim nächsten Einatmen vor, wie sich der Raum, den der Atem füllt, leicht ausdehnt. Nach ein paar Atemzügen kannst du vielleicht sehen, wie er beide Lungenflügel füllt.
5. Mit jedem neuen Einatmen beginnen Sie sich vorzustellen, wie der Atem ein wenig weiterwandert, hinunter zum Bauch und hinauf zur Kehle.
6. Setzen Sie diese Visualisierung fort und weiten Sie die Reichweite Ihres Atems langsam aus, bis er den ganzen Weg über Ihre Arme und Beine zurücklegt. Schließlich wird es sich so anfühlen, als würden Ihre Einatmungen bis in die Spitzen Ihrer Finger und Zehen reichen.

Führen Sie diese Übung langsam durch und spüren Sie, wie sich der ganze Körper anfühlt, als wäre er mit Atem gefüllt.

Visualisierung des Atems

Diese Übung setzt die Arbeit mit der Visualisierung fort und beginnt mit der Erkundung fantasievoller Möglichkeiten. Sie ist ein nützliches Hilfsmittel, um eine Verbindung mit der Atmung herzustellen, wenn Sie einen eher visuellen oder kreativen Geist haben.

1. Schließen Sie die Augen und konzentrieren Sie sich auf Ihren Atem.
2. Beginnen Sie zu visualisieren, wie der Atem in Ihren Körper ein- und ausströmt. Dabei können Sie den tatsächlichen Atemwegen folgen oder Ihre eigene imaginäre Route wählen.
3. Stellen Sie sich die Farbe Ihres Atems vor. Stellen Sie sich vor, dass sich Ihr ganzer Körper bei jedem Einatmen mit dieser Farbe füllt.

Tipp

Konzentrieren Sie sich nicht zu sehr auf die Visualisierung der Atmung und machen Sie sich keine Sorgen um ein perfekt geformtes Bild. Erlauben Sie ihr, in welcher Form auch immer, zu Ihnen zu kommen.

Zählen des Atems

Das Zählen des Atems ist ein wichtiges Werkzeug in der Atmungsarbeit, sei es das Zählen der einzelnen Zyklen oder die Zeitmessung der Atemfrequenz.

Das Zählen ist eine besonders nützliche Methode, um sich auf den Atem zu konzentrieren, wenn es Ihnen schwerfällt, sich zu konzentrieren, ohne dass Ihr Geist abgelenkt wird. Es kann Ihnen helfen, sich in Ihrer Übungsphase zu erden.

Später werden wir erforschen, wie das Zählen dazu verwendet werden kann, den Atem zu verlängern, zu vertiefen oder zu kontrollieren, aber hier führen wir einfach die Idee des Zählens neben dem Ein- und Ausatmen ein.

1. Suchen Sie sich einen ruhigen Moment, um sich auf Ihre natürliche Atmung einzustellen. Erlauben Sie ihr, leicht und frei fließend zu sein.
2. Zählen Sie beim Einatmen in gleichmäßigem Tempo, bis Sie den höchsten Punkt Ihres Atems erreicht haben.
3. Wenn Sie ausatmen, beginnen Sie wieder mit der Eins zu zählen und halten Sie dabei einen konstanten Rhythmus ein.
4. Beginnen Sie die Zählung bei jedem Ein- und Ausatmen erneut und setzen Sie sie so lange fort, bis Sie mit Ihrem Atem in Einklang sind.

Tipp

Lassen Sie sich nicht von der Zählung den Atem diktieren. Mit dieser Übung zählen wir einfach die natürliche Atmung, versuchen Sie nicht, sie an eine Zahl anzupassen.

Yogische Atmung

Diese Übung kombiniert einige der bisher erlernten Hilfsmittel, darunter die Visualisierung und das Führen des Atems durch den Körper, zu einer Technik, die sowohl den Atem vertieft als auch die Konzentration steigert.

1. Beginnen Sie damit, aufrecht zu sitzen, die Schultern entspannt und den Scheitel nach oben gerichtet. Sie können sich gegen eine Wand oder einen Stuhl lehnen, wenn Ihnen das angenehmer ist, aber versuchen Sie, den Oberkörper lang zu halten.
2. Schließen Sie die Augen und nehmen Sie sich einen Moment Zeit, um sich mit Ihrem Atem zu verbinden.
3. Stellen Sie sich beim Einatmen vor, dass die Luft direkt in Ihren Bauch strömt.
4. Stellen Sie sich vor, dass sie zu Ihrer Brust aufsteigt.
5. Stellen Sie sich vor, dass sie zu Ihrer Kehle aufsteigt.

6. Stellen Sie sich vor, dass er zu Ihrem „dritten Auge" hinaufwandert – dem Raum zwischen Ihren Augenbrauen.
7. Stellen Sie sich beim Ausatmen vor, dass die Luft aus Ihrem „dritten Auge"" ausströmt, dann aus Ihrer Kehle, dann aus Ihrer Brust und dann aus Ihrem Bauch.
8. Fahren Sie fort, die Atemzüge auf diese Weise zu wiederholen. Einatmen durch den Magen, die Brust, die Kehle, das dritte Auge. Ausatmen durch das dritte Auge, Kehle, Brust und Magen.

Achten Sie nach dieser Übung darauf, wie Ihr Atem den gesamten Oberkörper ausfüllt und wie Sie in einen stetigen Rhythmus tiefer Atmung versunken sind.

ICH WEISS,
WANN ES
AN DER ZEIT IST
LOSZULASSEN,

UND ICH TUE ES.

Tagebuch

Schreiben Sie zehn Dinge auf, die Sie tun können, wenn Sie frei atmen können.

Atem und Körper miteinander verbinden

Einige der fortgeschritteneren Übungen verwenden körperliche Berührungen und Bewegungen, um den Atem zu kontrollieren und ihr Ziel zu erreichen. Diese einfache Übung soll Ihnen zeigen, wie Sie in Ihrer Praxis über den Einsatz der Atemmuskeln und des „geistigen Auges" (das, was Sie sich vorstellen oder visualisieren können) hinausgehen können.

1. Die Übung kann im Sitzen oder Stehen durchgeführt werden, solange Sie bequem sitzen und nicht abgelenkt sind.
2. Legen Sie zunächst eine Hand oder beide Hände sanft auf Ihre Brust. Folgen Sie dem Heben und Senken Ihrer Ein- und Ausatmung.
3. Bewegen Sie Ihre Hand auf Ihren Bauch und spüren Sie, wie er sich ausdehnt und zusammenzieht.
4. Bewegen Sie Ihre Hände zu Ihrem Brustkorb und beobachten Sie, wie er sich beim Einatmen hebt und ausdehnt und beim Ausatmen senkt.
5. Versuchen Sie nun, Ihre Hände auf zwei Bereiche zu legen, z. B. auf Brust und Bauch, um zu spüren, wie sie miteinander zusammenwirken.

Gleichmäßiges Atmen

Diese Übung eignet sich hervorragend für Momente großer Unruhe oder Stress, da sie den Geist mit sehr wenig Aufwand fokussiert. Sie ist außerdem unglaublich unauffällig und kann daher in der Öffentlichkeit durchgeführt werden, ohne Aufmerksamkeit zu erregen. Ihre Stärke liegt in ihrer Einfachheit.

1. Stimmen Sie sich auf Ihren natürlichen Atem ein und atmen Sie dann ganz aus.
2. Atmen Sie gleichmäßig ein und zählen Sie bis vier.
3. Atmen Sie gleichmäßig bis vier aus.
4. Wiederholen Sie den Zyklus und arbeiten Sie sich bis zu einer Zahl vor, die sich sowohl beim Ein- als auch beim Ausatmen angenehm anfühlt.

Probieren Sie diese Übung aus, bevor Sie vor Publikum sprechen oder wenn Sie sich in einer überfüllten Umgebung nervös fühlen oder nur eine Verschnaufpause an Ihrem Schreibtisch einlegen.

Resonanzatmung

Ein längerfristiger positiver Effekt einer starken Atemroutine und der Fähigkeit, Ihre Atmung zu kontrollieren, ist die Senkung Ihrer Ruheherzfrequenz. Indem Sie Ihre Atemzüge pro Minute verlangsamen, senken Sie Ihre Herzfrequenz und Ihren Blutdruck, was zu einer Vielzahl von Vorteilen für die Gesundheit insgesamt führt.

Diese Technik, die sich auf die Senkung der Atemfrequenz pro Minute konzentriert, senkt direkt die Herzfrequenz und entspannt das Nervensystem.

1. Nehmen Sie eine bequeme Position ein und stellen Sie sich auf Ihre natürliche Atemfrequenz ein.
2. Wenn Sie sich bereit fühlen, atmen Sie ganz aus.
3. Zählen Sie beim Einatmen gleichmäßig bis fünf.
4. Zählen Sie beim Ausatmen gleichmäßig bis fünf.
5. Passen Sie die Anzahl der Atemzüge an, wenn Sie sich wohler und entspannter fühlen, und streben Sie drei bis sieben volle Atemzüge pro Minute an.

Dies ist eine nützliche Übung, um Ihre anaerobe Ausdauer zu verbessern, z. B. beim Training für Ausdauersportarten. Insbesondere Schwimmer profitieren von der resonanten Atmung, da sie Ihre Fähigkeiten verbessert, Ihre Atemfrequenz zu verlangsamen und die Atemzüge außerhalb des Wassers zu reduzieren.

Tagebuch

Wie konzentriert haben Sie sich heute bei Ihrer Übung gefühlt? Wenn Ihre Gedanken abschweiften, wohin gingen sie dann? Schreiben Sie Ihre Antworten hier auf.

Atmen Sie.
Lassen Sie los.
Und erinneren Sie
sich daran, dass Sie
wissen, dass genau
dieser Moment der
einzige ist, den
Sie den Sie mit
Sicherheit haben.

Oprah Winfrey

Mit offenem Mund ausatmen

Wie oft seufzen Sie ganz automatisch und natürlich, wenn Sie sich von einem langen Tag erholen oder sich auf eine große Aufgabe vorbereiten? Das ist oft eine unwillkürliche Reaktion, wenn unser Körper (und unser Geist) einen Moment braucht, um „alles rauszulassen".

Diese Übung macht sich diese natürliche Reaktion zunutze, um das gleiche Gefühl der Erleichterung ganz bewusst zu kultivieren. Beobachten Sie, wie sich nicht nur aufgestaute emotionale oder mentale Spannungen lösen, sondern wie sich auch der Körper entspannt – vielleicht an Stellen, von denen Sie gar nicht wussten, dass Sie dort Spannungen haben, z. B. in Ihrem Kiefer, Ihren Schultern oder Ihrem Bauch.

1. Sobald Sie sich auf Ihren natürlichen Atem eingestellt haben, beginnen Sie, Ihre Einatmung zu vertiefen, Ihre Lungen bis zur vollen Kapazität aufzublasen und Ihren Brustkorb und Bauch auszudehnen.
2. Wenn Sie ausatmen, seufzen Sie durch den Mund aus. Erlauben Sie dem Seufzer, aus dem tiefste Herzen zu kommen. Er kann so laut sein, wie es sich gut und natürlich anfühlt.

Vielleicht ist es Ihnen zuerst zu unangenehm, laut auszuatmen. Daher wird diese Übung am besten an einem Ort durchgeführt, an dem Sie sich wohl und ungestört fühlen.

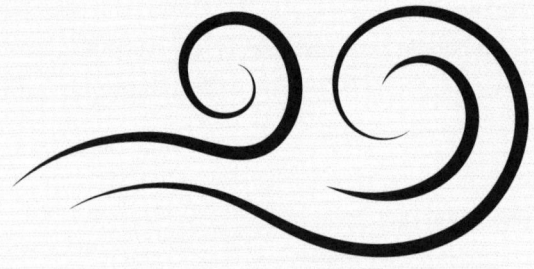

Kapitel Vier:

ATEMÜBUNGEN

Nachdem Sie nun kurz die Wissenschaft und die Geschichte hinter der Atmungsarbeit kennengelernt und die grundlegenden praktischen Grundlagen erworben haben, fühlen Sie sich hoffentlich bereit, Ihre Praxis zu vertiefen. In diesem Kapitel werden wir fortgeschrittenere Techniken und Übungen erforschen, jede mit ihrem eigenen einzigartigen Zweck. Diese sind nach Intentionen und Anwendungsbeispielen unterteilt – zum Beispiel für tieferen Schlaf oder energiereichere Trainingseinheiten.

Natürlich sind die beschriebenen Ziele nur ein Angebot und Sie könnten feststellen, dass die Übungen für Sie einen anderen Zweck erfüllen. Wenn Sie die Techniken durcharbeiten, werden Sie wahrscheinlich herausfinden, welche am besten zu Ihrem Körper, Ihrem Geist und Ihrer Stimmung passen.

Denken Sie daran: Je mehr Sie üben, desto mehr werden Sie sich mit Ihrem Atem verbinden und desto schneller werden Sie die Früchte ernten.

MEIN ATEM FÜLLT
MEINEN KÖRPER AUS
UND ICH BIN VOLL
VON LEBEN UND LICHT.

Zählen und Zeiteinteilung

Wie viel Zeit Sie für eine Atemübung aufwenden, hängt davon ab, wie viel Zeit Sie zur Verfügung haben. Ob Sie nun eine halbe Stunde für eine komplette Übungseinheit einplanen oder nur 5 Minuten in Ihren geschäftigen Tag einbauen, das Schöne an dieser Wellness-Praxis ist, dass sie sehr flexibel ist und für jeden Bedarf etwas bereithält.

Daher enthalten die folgenden Übungen keine Vorschläge für die Dauer oder Anzahl der Zyklen. Es könnte jedoch hilfreich sein, sich einen Timer zu setzen oder sich eine bestimmte Anzahl von Wiederholungen vorzuschreiben. Sie können diese Übungen als Einzelübungen durchführen oder einige Runden verschiedener Übungen als Teil derselben Atmungssitzung absolvieren.

Tipp

Um sich voll und ganz auf Ihre Technik zu konzentrieren, anstatt zu zählen, versuchen Sie, eine kleine Fingerzählmethode zu implementieren, z. B. indem Sie mit einer Fingerkuppe gegen Ihren Daumen tippen, um sanft den Überblick zu behalten, ohne Ihre Ausführung zu stören.

Übung für den Schlaf

Wie wir gelernt haben, hilft die Verlängerung der Ausatmung, das parasympathische Nervensystem des Körpers zu aktivieren, den „Ruhe- und Verdauungsmodus", den wir zum Einschlafen brauchen. Daher ist diese Technik ein perfektes Hilfsmittel, um in einen schläfrigen Zustand zu gleiten.

1. Atmen Sie ein und zählen Sie bis vier.
2. Zählen Sie beim Ausatmen bis sechs.
3. Wiederholen Sie die Übung so lange wie nötig.

Tipp

Die Anzahl dieser Übung kann an Ihre Bedürfnisse angepasst werden. Wenn Sie die Übung zum Einschlafen verwenden, vermeiden Sie aber zu stark auszuatmen, sodass es eine Anstrengung ist. Entscheiden Sie sich für Komfort und Beständigkeit statt für Anstrengung.

Tagebuch

Schreiben Sie alle Dinge auf, für die Sie heute dankbar sind. Warum nicht mit der Fähigkeit zu atmen beginnen?

....

....

....

....

....

....

....

....

....

....

Gleichmäßiges Dreiecksatmen

Diese Technik nutzt eine einfache Visualisierung, führt aber auch in das Anhalten des Atems ein.

Das Anhalten des Atems kann dazu beitragen, Ihre Technik zu vertiefen, und Sie werden sich mit der Zeit wahrscheinlich immer wohler dabei fühlen. Das Anhalten des Atems sollte sich niemals anstrengend oder angstauslösend anfühlen, und falls doch, lassen Sie die Übung sein und kehren Sie zu Ihrem natürlichen Atemmuster zurück.

1. Schließen Sie die Augen und stellen Sie sich vor Ihrem geistigen Auge ein Dreieck mit gleichen Seiten vor.
2. Zählen Sie beim Einatmen bis vier und folgen Sie im Geist der Linie des Dreiecks von der linken unteren Spitze zur oberen Spitze.
3. Halten Sie den Atem an und zählen Sie bis vier, während Sie zum rechten unteren Punkt zurückkreisen.
4. Folgen Sie der Unterseite des Dreiecks zurück zum Anfang und atmen Sie aus, zählen Sie dabei bis vier.
5. Beginnen Sie den Zyklus erneut: einatmen und bis vier zählen, halten und bis vier zählen und ausatmen und bis vier zählen, wobei Sie das Bild des Dreiecks nutzen, um Tempo und Konzentration beizubehalten.

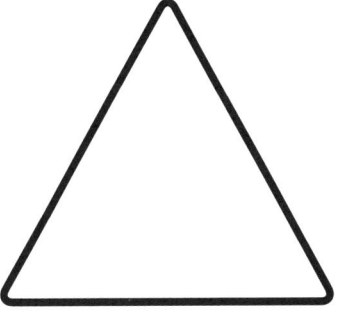

Tipp

Wenn es Ihnen schwerfällt, sich das Dreieck im Kopf vorzustellen, zeichnen Sie es auf ein Blatt Papier und zeichnen Sie es mit Ihrem Finger nach, während Sie die Zyklen durcharbeiten. Dies kann helfen, die Konzentration zu erhalten.

Box-Atmung

Zur Wiedererlangung der Kontrolle

Nachdem Sie nun das Anhalten des Atems kennengelernt haben, folgt diese Übung auf die gleiche Weise wie die gleichmäßige Dreiecksatmung auf den Seiten 84–85, nur mit einer weiteren Zählung beim Anhalten des Atems pro Zyklus.

Dadurch wird der Atem noch tiefer und die Fähigkeit, ihn zu kontrollieren, erhöht. Dies kann eine großartige Technik sein, um die mentale Kontrolle wiederzuerlangen, wenn Sie sich überwältigt oder verloren fühlen. Die Fähigkeit, die Kontrolle über den eigenen Atem zu erlangen, wirkt sich auf die gesamte Denkweise aus.

1. Schließen Sie die Augen und stellen Sie sich ein Quadrat vor.
2. Zählen Sie beim Einatmen bis vier und folgen Sie im Geiste der Linie auf dem Quadrat, von der linken unteren Ecke bis zur linken oberen Ecke.
3. Halten Sie den Atem bis zum vierten Mal an, während Sie an der Oberseite des Quadrats entlanggehen.
4. Wenn Sie ausatmen, folgen Sie dem Quadrat von rechts oben nach rechts unten und zählen Sie dabei bis vier.

5. Halten Sie den Atem für eine weitere Zählung von vier an, während Sie entlang der Unterseite des Quadrats zurück zum Anfang gehen.
6. Beginnen Sie den Zyklus erneut: einatmen, halten, ausatmen und halten und dabei jeweils bis vier zählen, wobei Sie das Bild des Quadrats nutzen, um Tempo und Konzentration beizubehalten.

Tipp

Nachdem Sie den Atem angehalten haben, neigen Sie möglicherweise dazu, scharf ein- oder auszuatmen. Versuchen Sie, dies zu vermeiden. Sorgen Sie für einen gleichmäßigen Luftstrom vom Anfang bis zum Ende eines Atemzugs. Denken Sie daran, dass es hier nur um Kontrolle geht.

Ungleiche Dreiecksatmung

Zur Entspannung

Wenn man die Techniken der Visualisierung eines Musters und der verlängerten Ausatmung kombiniert, erhält man die ungleiche Dreiecksatmung. Diese Methode ist ein eher proaktiver Ansatz zur Entspannung, da sie Konzentration und Kontrolle erfordert, aber der daraus resultierende Effekt ist eine starke Übung, die ein hohes Maß an Angst und Stress durchbrechen kann.

1. Schließen Sie die Augen und stellen Sie sich im Geiste ein gleichschenkliges Dreieck vor, bei dem die längste Seite die Unterseite ist.
2. Zählen Sie beim Einatmen bis vier und folgen Sie der Linie des Dreiecks von der linken unteren Spitze zur oberen Spitze.
3. Halten Sie den Atem an und zählen Sie bis vier, während Sie zum unteren rechten Punkt zurückgehen.
4. Beim Ausatmen zählen Sie entlang der Unterseite des Dreiecks zurück zum Anfang bis sechs.

5. Beginnen Sie den Zyklus erneut: einatmen bis vier zählen, anhalten und bis vier zählen, dann ausatmen und bis sechs zählen, wobei Sie das Bild des Dreiecks nutzen, um Tempo und Konzentration aufrechtzuerhalten.

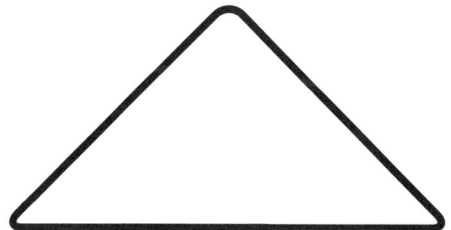

Ich atme ein, ich atme aus

Um gegenwärtig zu sein

Atmung ist eine der einfachsten und effektivsten Methoden, um gegenwärtig zu werden. Jedes Mal, wenn Sie sich auf einen Atemzug konzentrieren, sind Sie im Moment zugegen.

Manchmal kann es so leicht sein, sich in Gedanken an die Vergangenheit und Erwartungen an die Zukunft zu verstricken, dass wir die Realität des gegenwärtigen Augenblicks vergessen. Diese Übung ist der perfekte Weg, nicht nur um zu üben, präsent zu sein, sondern auch, um sich von unnötigen Sorgen zu befreien und sich daran zu erinnern, dass in diesem Moment alles in Ordnung ist.

Indem Sie Ihrem Atem ein Mantra zuordnen, hilft es Ihnen, den Fokus des Geistes aufrechtzuerhalten und sich im Hier und Jetzt zu verankern.

1. Nehmen Sie sich einen Moment Zeit, um sich auf den natürlichen Rhythmus Ihres Atems einzustellen.
2. Sagen Sie beim Einatmen innerlich die beruhigenden Worte: „Ich atme ein."
3. Wenn Sie ausatmen, sagen Sie innerlich: „Ich atme aus."
4. Wiederholen Sie dieses Mantra in aller Ruhe, während Sie die Atemrunden durchlaufen.

Denken Sie daran, dass das Mantra eher zu Ihrer Atemfrequenz passt als umgekehrt. Lassen Sie sich nicht von den Worten den Atem diktieren, stattdessen beobachten und kommentieren sie den gegenwärtigen Moment.

Atmen mit Worten

Zur Veränderung der Stimmung

Wenn Sie sich damit wohl fühlen, ein einfaches Mantra zusammen mit Ihren Ein- und Ausatmungen zu verwenden, können Sie Worte nutzen, um über die Achtsamkeit hinauszugehen und sie zur Veränderung Ihrer Stimmung oder Perspektive einzusetzen. Bei dieser Übung kommt es darauf an, dass Sie offen für ihre Durchführung sind und ihr erlauben, sich wirklich in Ihrem Körper niederzulassen und Ihren Geist zu verändern. Sie kann verwendet werden, wenn Sie sich in einer Stimmung befinden, die Sie sofort loswerden wollen, aber auch für eine längerfristige Veränderung der Perspektive.

1. Schließen Sie die Augen und nehmen Sie sich einige Augenblicke Zeit, um zu beobachten, wie Sie sich emotional und geistig fühlen. Es könnte eine klare, dominante Emotion geben oder es könnte sich wie eine mehrdeutige Mischung anfühlen. Akzeptieren Sie, was immer Ihnen in den Sinn kommt.
2. Wenn Sie eine gute Vorstellung davon haben, wo Sie damit stehen, denken Sie über Ihre Absicht für diese Sitzung nach. Welche Gedanken oder Emotionen sind Ihnen nicht dienlich? Wie würden Sie sich gerne in diesem Moment fühlen?

3. Sobald Sie sich auf Ihre Absicht festgelegt haben, beginnen Sie, auf Ihren Atem zu achten. Wenn Sie es noch nicht getan haben, beginnen Sie damit, lange, beruhigende Ein- und Ausatmungen einzuführen.
4. Wenn Sie sich bereit fühlen, beginnen Sie, Ihren Ein- und Ausatmungen Worte zuzuordnen, die Ihrer Absicht entsprechen. Hier sind einige Beispiele:
    - „Ich atme Frieden ein. Ich atme Angst aus."
    - „Ich atme Stärke ein. Ich atme Angst aus."
    - „Ich atme Positivität ein. Ich atme Negativität aus."
    - „Ich atme Dankbarkeit ein. Ich atme Eifersucht aus."
5. Fahren Sie fort, bis Sie das Gefühl haben, dass Sie Ihre Absicht erreicht haben, und seien Sie offen für die Kraft dieser Übung.

Tipp

Es kann hilfreich sein, eine Visualisierung zu verwenden, z. B. verschiedene Farben, um die eingehenden und ausgehenden Emotionen darzustellen.

4-7-8

Zum Loslassen

Diese Technik nutzt dasselbe Gefühl des Loslassens wie das Ausatmen mit offenem Mund auf den Seiten 76–77, aber indem sie auch das Zählen des Atem-Anhaltens einführt, erhöht sie die Kraft, mit der das Loslassen beim Ausatmen kommt.

Es wird auch ein stimmhafter Klang verwendet, um beim Ausatmen eine Kraft der Luft zu erzeugen. Dies kann eine großartige Methode sein, um Ärger oder Stress loszulassen. Stellen Sie sich vor, dass Sie alle negativen Emotionen ausatmen, während Sie diese kraftvollen Ausatmungen erzeugen.

1. Bereiten Sie sich auf die Übung an einem Ort vor, an dem Sie sich geistig und körperlich wohl fühlen.
2. Wenn Sie bereit sind, atmen Sie ein und zählen bis vier.
3. Halten Sie den Atem bis sieben an.
4. Zählen Sie beim Ausatmen bis acht und erzeugen Sie dabei ein „Whoosh"-Geräusch. Versuchen Sie, dieses Geräusch während des gesamten Ausatmens beizubehalten, indem Sie Ihren Bauch benutzen, um das gesamte lange Ausatmen herauszupressen.
5. Zählen Sie beim Einatmen bis vier.
6. Wiederholen Sie diesen Zyklus so lange wie nötig.

Wenn Sie sich mit den Längen und Ihrer Atemkapazität nicht ganz wohl anfühlen, passen Sie die Übung an und bauen Sie sie langsam auf. Versuchen Sie nur, halb so lang einzuatmen wie auszuatmen, mit einer langen Phase des Luftanhaltens dazwischen.

Löwen-Atmung

Für Selbstvertrauen

Als Erwachsene verlieren wir oft unsere Fähigkeit zu spielen und albern zu sein. Unsicherheiten machen sich breit, während wir durch das Leben navigieren und unseren Platz in der Gesellschaft suchen, und die Angst vor Beurteilungen kann dazu führen, dass wir uns zurückhalten, unser authentisches Selbst zu sein.

Diese Atemtechnik hat nicht nur körperliche Vorteile, wie die Aktivierung der Stimmbänder und das Lösen von Verspannungen in Gesicht und Kiefer, sondern sie baut auch mentale Barrieren ab und ermöglicht es uns, uns selbstbewusster zu fühlen. Es kann sich anfangs überwältigend anfühlen, aus seiner kontrollierten Komfortzone herauszutreten, aber ermutigen Sie sich selbst, den Sprung zu wagen, und genießen Sie das neu gewonnene Gefühl von Selbstvertrauen und Kommunikation.

1. Suchen Sie sich eine bequeme Sitzposition.
2. Lehnen Sie sich leicht nach vorn und stützen Sie Ihre Handflächen mit gespreizten Fingern auf Ihre Knie oder den Boden.
3. Atmen Sie tief durch die Nase ein.
4. Öffnen Sie den Mund weit, strecken Sie die Zunge heraus und führen Sie sie nach unten zum Kinn.
5. Wenn Sie kräftig ausatmen, machen Sie einen „Ha!"-Laut. Setzen Sie Ihre Bauchmuskeln ein, um den Laut zu forcieren.
6. Atmen Sie dann einige Male normal, bevor Sie den nächsten Löwenatem ausführen.

Tipp

Die körperlichen Vorteile dieser Praxis sind ideal für Sänger oder Redner in der Öffentlichkeit. Es wärmt die Stimmbänder, stimuliert das Zwerchfell und löst Verspannungen im Gesicht.

Tagebuch

Wenn Sie Ihren Atem sehen könnten, wie würde er aussehen?

Welche Farbe hätte er? Verändert er sich zwischen Ein- und Ausatmen? Schreiben Sie Ihre Erkenntnisse hier auf.

....

....

....

....

....

....

....

....

Denn Atem ist Leben, wenn du also gut atmest, wirst du lange auf Erden leben.

Sanskrit-Sprichwort

Der Atem des Feuers

Zum Aufwärmen

Hoffentlich spüren Sie, wie sich Ihr Selbstvertrauen und Ihre Kontrolle über Ihre Atmung verbessern. An diesem Punkt können wir weitere körperliche Techniken einführen, um noch größere und unmittelbarere Vorteile zu erfahren.

Die Feueratmung besteht aus einer Mischung aus normalem Einatmen und kraftvollem Ausatmen unter Einsatz der Bauchmuskeln. Das schnelle, körperliche Ausatmen hilft, den Körper schnell zu erwärmen, was gut ist, wenn man eine Belebung oder Motivation braucht, um in Bewegung zu kommen.

1. Suchen Sie sich eine bequeme Sitzposition, halten Sie die Wirbelsäule aufrecht.
2. Legen Sie eine Hand sanft auf Ihren Bauch, sodass Sie das Auf und Ab Ihrer Atmung spüren können.
3. Atmen Sie tief ein und spüren Sie, wie sich Ihr Bauch ausdehnt.

4. Atmen Sie scharf und kräftig durch die Nase aus und spüren Sie, wie sich Ihre Bauchmuskeln zusammenziehen. Ihr Ausatmen sollte laut und kräftig sein.
5. Setzen Sie diesen Zyklus fort – passiv einatmen, kräftig ausatmen – ohne Pausen zwischen den Atemzügen und mit gleich langen Ein- und Ausatmungen. Wiederholen Sie dies einige Male, bis Sie sich mit der Übung vertraut gemacht haben.
6. Wenn Sie sich bereit fühlen, können Sie die Zyklen für kurze Zeit beschleunigen.

Denken Sie daran: Nehmen Sie sich Zeit, um Geschwindigkeit und Dauer dieser Übung aufzubauen. Wenn Sie sich zu irgendeinem Zeitpunkt benommen fühlen, beenden Sie das Atemtraining umgehend und kehren Sie zu Ihrer normalen Atemweise zurück.

Kühlende Atmung

Zur Abkühlung

So wie der Atem kontrolliert werden kann, um unser inneres Feuer zu entfachen, kann er auch zur Abkühlung eingesetzt werden, sowohl mental als auch körperlich. Dies ist die perfekte Technik, wenn Ihnen unangenehm heiß ist oder Sie einen Moment brauchen, um Ihre geistige und körperliche Temperatur zu senken.

1. Suchen Sie sich eine bequeme Position und atmen Sie ein paar Mal tief durch.
2. Rollen Sie Ihre Zunge, indem Sie die Seiten in die Mitte rollen, sodass eine Röhre entsteht. Stecken Sie das Ende der gerollten Zunge zwischen den zusammengepressten Lippen heraus. Wenn Sie Ihre Zunge nicht rollen können, spitzen Sie Ihre Lippen und formen Sie ein kleines "O". Halten Sie die Zunge an die Rückseite der unteren Zähne, damit die kühle Luft über die Oberseite strömen kann.
3. Atmen Sie langsam durch Ihre gerollte Zunge oder Ihre Lippen ein.
4. Schließen Sie den Mund und atmen Sie durch die Nase aus.
5. Atmen Sie in diesen Runden weiter, bis Sie den gewünschten Kühleffekt erreicht haben.

MEIN KÖRPER
BESTEHT
AUS MILLIONEN
VON WUNDERN.

MEIN ATEM IST
EIN MAGISCHER AKT.

Tagebuch

Wie fühlt sich Ihr Atem in diesem Moment an? Wie würden Sie jemandem beschreiben, wie sich das Atmen in Ihrem Körper anfühlt? Achten Sie auf den Rhythmus, die Tiefe und die Stelle, an der Sie ihn am deutlichsten spüren, und schreiben Sie Ihre Gedanken hier auf.

....

....

....

....

....

....

....

....

Tiefes Atmen

Für Aktivität

Wir werden uns unserer Atmung oft bewusst, wenn wir Sport treiben, da sich unsere Atemfrequenz erhöht, um den Anforderungen der Muskeln gerecht zu werden, die mehr Sauerstoff benötigen. Das kann das Gefühl einer brennenden Brust und eines keuchenden Atems hervorrufen. Diese Technik hilft, die Atmung im Körper zu vertiefen, und ist daher ideal für die Anwendung vor dem Training, um den Körper mit Sauerstoff zu versorgen, und auch nach dem Training, um die Erholung der Atemwege zu unterstützen.

1. Legen Sie Ihre Hände sanft hinter Ihren Kopf, mit weit gespreizten Ellbogen.
2. Stellen Sie sich beim Einatmen vor, dass sich Ihre Ellbogen voneinander wegbewegen, um Ihren Brustkorb vollständig aufzublähen. Atmen Sie langsam und gleichmäßig ein.
3. Halten Sie den Atem an, zählen Sie bis zwei und lassen Sie dabei die Ellbogen ausgestreckt.
4. Atmen Sie sanft aus und versuchen Sie, die Luft kontrolliert ausströmen zu lassen, indem Sie die Arme leicht entspannen.
5. Wiederholen Sie diese Zyklen und atmen Sie dabei ganz tief in die Lunge ein.

Atmung von Seite zu Seite
Zur Mobilisierung

Diese Technik kombiniert den Feueratem (Seite 100–101) mit einer Körperlichkeit, die eine tiefere Atmung fördert und die sehr belebend wirkt.

Wie bei der Feueratmung sollten Sie auch bei dieser Technik das Tempo langsam steigern, da es eine Weile dauern kann, bis Sie sich an die drehende Bewegung in Verbindung mit der schnellen Atmung gewöhnt haben. Seien Sie auch vorsichtig, wenn Sie Probleme mit dem Rücken oder der Wirbelsäule haben.

1. Suchen Sie sich eine bequeme Sitzposition mit viel Platz um Sie herum. Setzen Sie sich aufrecht hin.
2. Legen Sie die Fingerspitzen sanft an die Schläfen, die Ellbogen sind weit geöffnet.
3. Drehen Sie sich beim Einatmen sanft zu einer Seite, sodass ein Ellbogen nach vorne und einer nach hinten zeigt.
4. Drehen Sie sich beim Ausatmen auf die andere Seite und atmen Sie dabei scharf und kräftig aus.
5. Wiederholen Sie dies mit zunehmender Geschwindigkeit.
6. Nach ein paar Runden wiederholen Sie die Übung, wobei Sie sich beim Einatmen in die entgegengesetzte Richtung drehen. Dies wird Ihnen helfen, sich ausgeglichen zu fühlen.

Wechselatmung mit den Nasenlöchern

Für Ausgeglichenheit

Manchmal fühlen wir uns unausgeglichen, ohne zu wissen, warum. Diese Technik kann Ihnen helfen, ein Ungleichgewicht in Ihrer Atmung zu erkennen und es zu beheben. Sobald Sie ein körperliches Gleichgewicht erreicht haben, kann dies auch Ihrem Geist helfen, sich ausgeglichener zu fühlen.

Die körperlichen Anforderungen dieser Übung machen sie zu einem sehr effektiven Mittel, um die Konzentration auf die Ausübung aufrechtzuerhalten, da Sie ein sich wiederholendes Muster haben, das Ihre Aufmerksamkeit auf sich zieht. Wenn Sie krank sind oder Ihre Nase verstopft ist, ist die Wechselatmung weit weniger erfolgreich und wird nicht empfohlen.

1. Legen Sie Ihren rechten Daumen auf Ihr rechtes Nasenloch und atmen Sie durch das linke Nasenloch ein.
2. Lassen Sie den Daumen los und legen Sie den rechten Ringfinger auf das linke Nasenloch.
3. Atmen Sie durch das rechte Nasenloch aus.
4. Atmen Sie durch das rechte Nasenloch ein.
5. Entfernen Sie Ihren Ringfinger und legen Sie Ihren rechten Daumen auf Ihr rechtes Nasenloch.
6. Atmen Sie durch das linke Nasenloch aus.
7. Beginnen Sie den Zyklus erneut und fahren Sie fort: links einatmen, rechts ausatmen, rechts einatmen, links ausatmen.

Einige Ausübende empfehlen, den rechten Zeigefinger und Mittelfinger sanft auf das „dritte Auge" (den Raum zwischen den Brauen) zu legen, während Daumen und Ringfinger verwendet werden. Vielleicht möchten Sie auch Ihre Augen schließen und Ihrem inneren Blick bis zum „dritten Auge" folgen.

ICH BIN
DIESER ATEM.

ICH BIN
DIESER MOMENT.

Tagebuch

Wenn Sie jemandem einen Top-Tipp für die Atmung geben könnten, welcher wäre das und warum?

....

....

....

....

....

....

....

....

....

....

Zirkuläre Atmung

Um Giftstoffe freizusetzen

Bei den meisten meditativen Atemübungen atmen wir durch die Nase ein; bei dieser Technik atmen wir jedoch durch den offenen Mund ein, um ein größeres Luftvolumen in den Körper zu bekommen.

Versuchen Sie, einmal tief durch die Nase und einmal tief durch den Mund einzuatmen, und sehen Sie selbst, welche der beiden Atemtechniken die Lungen und den Bauch mehr füllen. Auf diese Weise wird sowohl beim Ausatmen als auch beim Einatmen durch den offenen Mund verbrauchte Luft aus den tiefen Lungen verdrängt und frische Atemluft angesaugt.

1. Setzen oder stellen Sie sich aufrecht hin, sodass viel Platz um Ihren Oberkörper herum ist.
2. Öffnen Sie den Mund weit und atmen Sie ein.
3. Konzentrieren Sie sich beim Einatmen darauf, zuerst den Bauch zu füllen, bis der Atem sich in den Brustkorb und die Brust ausdehnt, so als ob Sie einen Behälter mit Flüssigkeit füllen würden.
4. Ohne eine Pause zu machen, atmen Sie gleichmäßig aus, als ob sich der Behälter von oben nach unten entleeren würde.
5. Wiederholen Sie diese zirkulären Atemzüge und stellen Sie sich dabei ein ständiges Füllen und Entleeren des Behälters im Inneren Ihres Rumpfes vor.

Brummender Bienenatem

Für den geistigen Raum

Viele von uns leben in einer Welt der ständigen Stimulation. Es gibt immer etwas zu sehen, zu hören oder zu lesen. Das kann nicht nur überwältigend sein, sondern es kann sich auch fremd anfühlen, mit unseren Gedanken allein zu sein. Bei vielen meditativen Praktiken ist es zum Beispiel schwirig, den Geist zur Ruhe zu bringen, weil er so oft mit Geschwätz gefüllt ist.

Das Summen des Bienenatems zielt darauf ab, die Außenwelt auszuschließen und unsere Gedanken zur Ruhe zu bringen, indem wir ein alles verzehrendes „weißes Rauschen" in unserem Kopf erzeugen. Es ist eine großartige Übung, um den Geist zu reinigen und unerwünschte oder nicht hilfreiche Gedanken auszublenden, bevor man sich auf ruhigere Atemübungen einlässt.

1. Suchen Sie sich einen Ort, an dem Sie sich nicht unsicher fühlen oder gestört werden.
2. Schließen Sie sanft Ihre Augen und bedecken Sie Ihre Augenlider mit Ihren Zeigefingern.

3. Drücken Sie Ihre Daumen sanft auf den Tragus (den äußeren Knorpel direkt außerhalb des Gehörgangs), sodass sie die Ohrlöcher abdecken und Außengeräusche dämpfen.
4. Atmen Sie tief ein.
5. Drücken Sie dann Ihre Mittelfinger über Ihre Nasenlöcher – nicht ganz zu, da Sie durch die Nase ausatmen werden. Legen Sie die Ringfinger nach unten auf die Oberlippe und die kleinen Finger nach oben auf die Unterlippe und schließen Sie den Mund.
6. Lassen Sie beim Ausatmen ein konstantes Brummen bis zum Ende Ihres Atemzuges erklingen. Sie sollten spüren, wie der Ton in Ihrem Kopf widerhallt und Ihren eigenen Kokon aus Klang und Dunkelheit schafft.
7. Heben Sie sanft die Finger, um vollständig durch die Nase einzuatmen, und wiederholen Sie die Übung.

Wenn sich die Platzierung der Finger sich nicht angenehm anfühlt, können Sie einfach die Augen schließen und nur auf den Ohrknorpel drücken. Sie können auch mit hohen und tiefen Brummgeräuschen spielen, aber es sollte ein konstanter Ton für ein ganzes Ausatmen sein.

Ozean-Atem

Für die Yoga-Praxis

Wie auf den Seiten 36-37 beschrieben, ist die Atemtechnik oder Pranayama ein grundlegender Bestandteil der Yogapraxis, sowohl in der physischen Asanapraxis als auch in den eher meditativen Zweigen. Traditionell sollten Sie während der gesamten Yogapraxis durch die Nase ein- und ausatmen und dabei die sanft-geräuschvolle Ujjayi-Atmung oder den „Ozeanatem" verwenden.

Es gibt viele Gründe, warum die Ujjayi-Atmung im Yoga verwendet wird:

- Wenn Sie Ihren Atem hören, können Sie sich darauf konzentrieren, mehrere Runden von Ein- und Ausatmungen zu vollenden, und Sie bekommen eine klare Vorstellung davon, ob Ihr Körper in einer Haltung angespannt ist.
- Die Körperlichkeit der Ujjayi-Atmung erwärmt den Körper und verbessert Ihre körperliche Praxis.
- Wenn Sie an einem Kurs teilnehmen, in dem der Lehrer Ihre Ausrichtung physisch korrigiert, kann er durch das Geräusch des Atems hören, wann Sie ausatmen, und seine Korrekturen entsprechend zeitlich anpassen.

1. Es ist am einfachsten, die Technik durch Ein- und Ausatmen mit dem Mund zu beginnen.
2. Ziehen Sie beim Ausatmen den hinteren Teil Ihres Rachens leicht zusammen, so als ob Sie ein Glas beschlagen wollten. Dies sollte sich nicht wie eine Anstrengung oder übermäßig angespannt anfühlen (Haaaa). Es sollte ein leiser Hauch ertönen, der sich wie das Meeresrauschen anhört.
3. Sobald Sie sich wohl fühlen, wenden Sie die gleiche sanfte Verengung des Rachens beim Einatmen an.
4. Das gleiche Geräusch sollte beim Ein- und Ausatmen zu hören sein, sodass es wie die Gezeiten klingt, daher der Name „Ozeanatem".
5. Wenn Sie diese Praxis etabliert haben, schließen Sie den Mund und atmen Sie durch die Nase, mit der gleichen Kehlkopfverengung und dem gleichen Meeresgeräusch.
6. Verwenden Sie diese Pranayama-Technik während Ihrer gesamten Praxis, bis Sie am Ende in Shavasana (Tiefenentspannungs-Haltung) kommen. Da der Ujjayi-Atem zur Erwärmung und Belebung verwendet wird, ist er während der Entspannung von Shavasana nicht erforderlich.

Tagebuch

Welche Atemtechnik haben Sie bisher als die effektivste empfunden? Warum hat sie bei Ihnen Anklang gefunden?

....

....

....

....

....

....

....

....

....

....

Atmen mit zusammengepressten Lippen

Bei Kurzatmigkeit

Wenn wir außer Atem sind, reagiert unser Körper, indem er durch den offenen Mund ausatmet. Das hilft uns, uns abzukühlen und den Körper von Kohlendioxid zu befreien. Diese Übung basiert auf dieser natürlichen Reaktion, wobei die Ausatmung durch den Mund dazu beiträgt, die Atemfrequenz zu verlangsamen.

Der Schlüssel zu dieser Technik liegt darin, sich auf die Kontrolle des Ausatmens zu konzentrieren. So schwierig es sich auch anfühlen mag, wenn man kurzatmig ist: Je gleichmäßiger Sie ausatmen, desto tiefer atmen Sie ein und desto schneller kehren Sie zur normalen Atemfrequenz zurück.

1. Spüren Sie beim Einatmen, wie die Luft in den Bauch einströmt, nicht nur in die Brust.
2. Schließen Sie beim Ausatmen die Lippen und atmen Sie langsam aus, und zwar länger als Sie eingeatmet haben.
3. Setzen Sie diesen Zyklus fort, bis Sie spüren, wie sich Ihr Atem in einen regelmäßigen Rhythmus einpendelt.

Tagebuch

Wie hat sich Ihre Beziehung zu Ihrem Atem im Lauf Ihrer Atemübungen verändert?

....

....

....

....

....

....

....

....

....

....

Fazit

Sie sollten nun das Gefühl haben, dass Sie eine umfassende Einführung in die Welt der Atmung erhalten und selbst erfahren haben, wie viele Vorteile sie bietet und welche verschiedenen Zwecke sie erfüllen kann.

Denken Sie daran, dass Atemtechniken, wie alle anderen Übungen, Hingabe und Erforschung erfordern, um Ihre Fähigkeiten zu verbessern und zu entdecken, wie sie Ihnen am besten dienen kann. Kehren Sie immer wieder zu den verschiedenen Techniken zurück und beobachten Sie, wie sich Ihre Beziehung zu ihnen entwickelt, während Sie Ihre Fähigkeit verbessern, Ihren Atem zu kontrollieren und ihn für sich arbeiten zu lassen.

Mit einer soliden Grundlage in diesen Atemtechniken können Sie sie so oft abrufen, wie Sie sie brauchen, um Ihren Körper und Ihren Geist zu beruhigen, zu reinigen oder zu mobilisieren.

Es ist ein herrliches Geschenk, frei zu atmen, also atmen Sie tief ein und gehen Sie in Ihren Tag mit großer Wertschätzung für das Wunder des Ein- und Ausatmens.

Hilfreiche Links

Webseiten

www.wimhofmethod.com

www.nhs.uk/mental-health/self-help/guides-tools-and-activities/breathing-exercises-for-stress

www.lung.org/lung-health-diseases/wellness/breathing-exercises

www.rebirthingbreathwork.com

www.holotropic.com/holotropic-breathwork/about-holotrope-atmung-arbeit

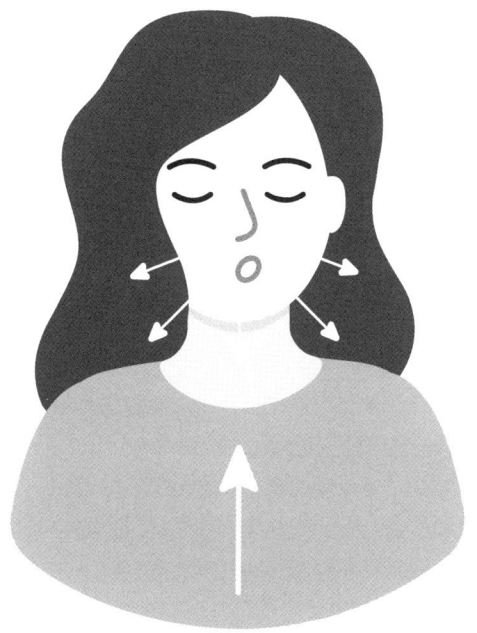

LESEN SIE AUCH:

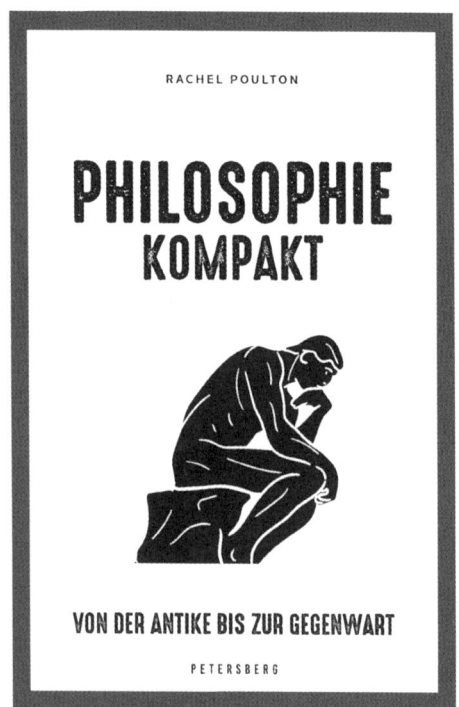

Grundwissen der Philosophie in kompakter Form von den Vorsokratikern über die Big Three (Sokrates, Platon, Aristoteles), die fernöstliche Philosophie und wichtige Fragen des Mittelalters bis zu modernen Themen der politischen Philosophie oder der Ethik. Das Buch erläutert die Begriffe der Metaphysik ebenso wie die der Erkenntnistheorie und erklärt in Grundzügen die wichtigsten Philosophieschulen von der Antike bis heute. Denker, Themen, Theorien alles, was Sie wissen müssen, um zu verstehen, welche Ideen unsere Welt geformt haben und wie wir heute denken.

192 Seiten, 125 x 190 mm, Hardcover
ISBN: 978-3-7553-0008-3
€ (D) 6,95

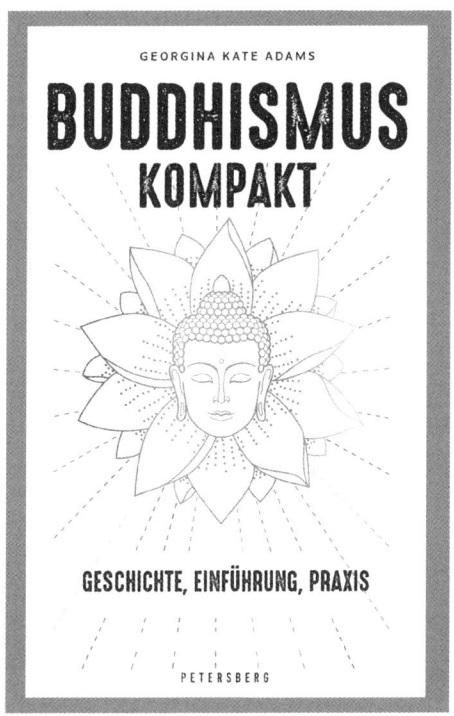

In diesem Kompaktratgeber finden interessierte Leserinnen und Leser Antworten auf zahlreiche Fragen, was Buddhismus bedeutet, wie man Buddhist werden kann, welche philosophischen Eckpfeiler es gibt und wie die fünf Silas in das Leben integriert werden können. Leben Sie glücklich, leben Sie in Frieden und erfahren Sie alles über den Kreislauf von Tod und Wiedergeburt, von Dharma, Sangha und den vier Edlen Wahrheiten.

128 Seiten, mit s/w-Illustrationen, 125 x 190 mm, Hardcover
ISBN: 978-3-7553-0057-1
€ (D) 9,95

Fotos: Cover © triutamis/Shutterstock.com;
© Adobe Stock, Gvais (Windhauch)

Color Vision

COLOR VISION

Perspectives from Different Disciplines

Editors

Werner G. K. Backhaus
Reinhold Kliegl
John S. Werner

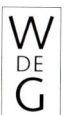

Walter de Gruyter
Berlin · New York 1998

Editors

Werner G. K. Backhaus
Theoretical and Experimental Biology
Department of Biology
Freie Universität Berlin
Thielallee 63
D-14195 Berlin
Germany
e-mail: backhaus@zedat.fu-berlin.de

John S. Werner
Department of Psychology
University of Colorado
Boulder, CO 80309
U.S.A.
e-mail: jwerner@clipr.colorado.edu

Reinhold Kliegl
Department of Psychology
University of Potsdam
P.O. 60 15 33
D-14415 Potsdam
Germany
e-mail: kliegl@rz.uni-potsdam.de

With 237 mostly four-colored figures

⊚ Printed on acid-free paper which falls within the guidelines of the ANSI to ensure permanence and durability

Library of Congress Cataloging-in-Publication Data

Color vision: perspectives from different disciplines/editors
Werner G. K. Backhaus, Reinhold Kliegl, John S. Werner.
Includes bibliographical references and index.
ISBN 3-11-016100-1 (cloth: alk. paper).
ISBN 3-11-015431-5 (pbk.: alk. paper)
1. Color vision. I. Backhaus, Werner. II. Kliegl, Reinhold, 1953– .
III. Werner, John Simon.
QP483.C646 1998
612.8'4--dc21
                                                                97-46863
                                                                CIP

Die Deutsche Bibliothek – Cataloging-in-Publication Data

Color vision: perspectives from different disciplines/
ed. Werner G. K. Backhaus ... – Berlin; New York: de Gruyter, 1998
ISBN 3-11-015431-5 brosch.
ISBN 3-11-016100-1 gb.

© Copyright 1998 by Walter de Gruyter & Co.,
D-10785 Berlin
All rights reserved, including those of translation into foreign languages. No part of this book may be reproduced or transmitted in any form or by any means, electronic or mechanical, including photocopy, recording, or any information storage and retrieval system, without permission in writing from the publisher.
Reproductions and typesetting: City-Repro, Berlin
Printing: Druckhaus Berlin-Mitte GmbH, Berlin
Binding: Heinz Stein, Berlin
Cover design: Hansbernd Lindemann, Berlin
Printed in Germany

Preface

This book, *Color Vision – Perspectives from Different Disciplines*, originated in an interdisciplinary "Symposium on Color Vision" that took place at the Einstein Forum in Potsdam in February 1996, with workshops in Berlin at the Freie Universität Berlin (FUB), the Federal Institute of Material Research and Testing (Bundesanstalt für Materialforschung und -prüfung) and the School of the Arts (Hochschule der Künste). The main goal of the symposium was to review the current state of color vision research, bringing together scientists from such different disciplines as neurobiology, psychology, color metrics, medicine, philosophy and art.

The resulting book is conceptualized in the first place as a text book for introductory courses at the graduate level. It provides an introduction to the exciting field of color vision for students and readers who are new to the field. The second intention of this book is to give established scientists an overview and an update on research activities in related fields. We hope that the material gathered from the diversity of fields will motivate students and experts alike to take a broader perspective with regard to color vision from the different disciplines.

Acknowledgements

The successful completion of this project depended on the commitment of a number of valued colleagues. We want to thank the contributing authors who prepared their chapters according to the aims of this book and who responded constructively to the suggestions for revisions that were made to them. Valuable comments were provided by Hans Irtel, Rainer Mausfeld, Brooke Schefrin, Lothar Spillmann, and Michael Wertheimer. We also thank Gary Smith, director of the Einstein Forum in Potsdam, whose initial encouragement and continued support launched the book project. Sybille De Vito-Egerland (Division for External Affairs, FUB), Mary Gaebel, Johannes Haack (Interdisciplinary Center for Cognitive Studies, University of Potsdam), Matthias Kross (Einstein Forum), Katharina Misch (FUB), Konstanze Pistor (Ministry of Science, Research, and Culture, Brandenburg), and Christiane von Alten (The Permanent Commission for Research and Academic Recruitment, FUB) contributed much time and energy both to the organization of the symposium and the realization of the book. The symposium as well as the color illustrations in the book were made possible by the generous financial support of the Freie Universität Berlin, the Einstein Forum Potsdam, the Interdisciplinary Center for Cognitive Studies at the University of Potsdam, the Brandenburg Ministry for Science, Research and Culture, and the Council on Research and Creative Work of the University of Colorado. Christiane Bowinkelmann and Mario Noyer-Weidner, of Walter de Gruyter Publishers Berlin, brought the book to completion. We are grateful to each of them. J. S. W. is especially grateful to the Alexander von Humboldt Foundation and the University of Potsdam for a guest professorship related to a senior scientist award during the time of the symposium.

Berlin, 31 July 1997

Werner G. K. Backhaus
Reinhold Kliegl
John S. Werner

Contents

Introduction xiii
Werner G. K. Backhaus, Reinhold Kliegl
and John S. Werner

I. Color Vision in Art and Science

1. Aging through the Eyes of Monet
John S. Werner

1.1 Introduction 1
1.2 A Link between Sunlight and Aging . 5
1.3 The Trivariance of Color Mixture:
Maxwell and Helmholtz 9
1.4 Monet's Early Impressionistic Style . 12
1.4.1 Possible Influences of Turner and
Goethe 13
1.4.2 Possible Influences of Chevreul
and Delacroix 17
1.5 Monet's Years in Argenteuil and
Vètheuil 23
1.6 The Opponent Code for Color
Appearance: Hering 23
1.7 Monet's Response to Pointillism and
Divisionism................... 27
1.8 Hay Stack and Cathedral Series..... 30
1.9 Monet Returns to London 33
1.10 Water Lilies and Cataracts......... 33
1.11 Summary 38
References 39

II. Physiology and Neuroethology

2. Physiological and Psychophysical Simulations of Color Vision in Humans and Animals
Werner G. K. Backhaus

2.1 Introduction 45
2.1.1 Phenomenology of Color Vision 45
2.1.2 Disciplines 45
2.1.3 Psychophysical Simulations 46
2.1.4 Physiological Simulations 46
2.2 Color Stimuli 47
2.3 Psychophysics of Color Vision 48
2.3.1 Psychophysical Judgments 50
2.4 Psychophysical Color Spaces 51
2.4.1 The Color Similarity (MDS) Space.. 51
2.4.2 The Elementary Color Space (Color Sensations Space)................ 52
2.4.3 The jnd Scale 54
2.5 Neurophysiology of Color Vision ... 54
2.5.1 Humans and Other Vertebrates 54
2.5.2 Honeybees and Other Invertebrates.. 56
2.6 Physiological Color Spaces........ 57
2.6.1 Physical Description of the Color
Stimulus 57
2.6.2 The Color Stimulus Space......... 57
2.6.3 The Photoreceptor Sensitivity
(Light Absorption) Space
(1st Physiological Color Space)..... 60
2.6.4 The Photoreceptor Excitation Space
(2nd Physiological Color Space) 61
2.6.5 The Color-Opponent Coding Space
(3rd Physiological Color Space) 61
2.6.6 Color Spaces and jnd Scales 62
2.7 Psychophysical and Physiological
Simulations of Color Vision....... 62
2.7.1 The Psychophysical (MDS) Color
Space in Honeybees 62
2.7.2 Neuronal Color-Coding and
Color-Choice Behavior in Honeybees 64
2.7.3 Identification of the Physiological
COC Space and the Psychophysical
MDS Space................... 65
2.8 Conscious vs. Unconscious
Judgments.................... 71

2.8.1	Color Sensations in Animals	71	5.5	Variation in Normal Color Vision ... 115
2.9	Conclusions	74	5.6	What Can Visual Pigment Gene Expression Tell Us about the Architecture of the Retina? 116
	References	75		References 117

3. Receptors, Channels and Color in Primate Retina
Barry B. Lee

3.1	Introduction	79
3.2	Physiology and Anatomy in the Retina	80
3.3	Conclusions	86
	References	87

4. Chromatic Processing in the Lateral Geniculate Nucleus of the Common Marmoset (*Callithrix jacchus*)
Jan Kremers, Eberhart Zrenner, Stefan Weiss and Sabine Meierkord

4.1	Introduction	89
4.2	Spectral Responsivities	91
4.3	Responses of LGN Cells to Various Photoreceptor Contrasts	93
4.4	Selective Photoreceptor Stimulation in Human Observers	95
4.5	Summary	98
	References	98

5. Molecular Genetics and the Biological Basis of Color Vision
Maureen Neitz and Jay Neitz

5.1	Introduction	101
5.2	Background	101
5.2.1	Types of Congenital Color Vision Defects	101
5.2.2	Genome Organization and Inheritance Patterns of Color Vision Defects	102
5.2.3	Genes and Gene Expression	103
5.3	Spectral Tuning of M- and L-Cone Pigments	104
5.4	Color Vision Defects	108
5.4.1	What Distinguishes Normal from Anomalous Pigments?	111
5.4.2	What Distinguishes Photopigments Underlying Dichromacy from Normal Pigments?	113

6. Source Analysis of Color-Evoked Potentials in a Realistic Head Model Confirmed by Functional MRI
Walter Paulus, Renate Kolle, Jürgen Baudewig, Nora Freudenthaler, Mathias Kunkel, Michael Finkenstaedt and Hans-Heino Rustenbeck

6.1	Introduction	121
6.2	Methods	127
6.3	Results	128
6.4	Discussion	129
6.5	Summary	129
	References	129

7. Wavelength Information Processing *versus* Color Perception: Evidence from Blindsight and Color-Blind Sight
Petra Stoerig

7.1	Introduction	131
7.2	Wavelength Information Processing	134
7.2.1	Wavelength Information Processing in Cortical Blindness	134
7.2.2	Wavelength Processing in Cortical Color Blindness	138
7.3	Segregation of Wavelength and Intensity Information and Constancy	141
7.4	Color Perception	143
	References	145

8. Color Vision in Lower Vertebrates
Christa Neumeyer

8.1	Introduction	149
8.2	Wavelength Discrimination in Lower Vertebrates	150
8.2.1	Goldfish	150
8.2.2	Turtles	151
8.2.3	Amphibia	154
8.3	Color Constancy and Color Contrast	155

8.4	Color Vision and Other Visual Functions: Evidence for Parallel Processing of Visual Information ... 157
8.5	Color Perception 159
8.6	Summary 160
	References 161

9. Color Vision: Ecology and Evolution in Making the Best of the Photic Environment
Peter G. Kevan and Werner G. K. Backhaus

9.1	Introduction 163
9.2	Palaeontological Record 164
9.3	Daylight and Color Vision......... 165
9.4	Colorimetry 167
9.5	Color Spaces.................. 168
9.6	Evolution of Floral Colors and Color Vision....................... 171
9.7	Color Patterns in Flowers 175
9.8	Trichromacy and Tetrachromacy 177
9.9	Conclusions 178
	References 178

III. Psychology and Philosophy

10. The Perception of Blackness: An Historical and Contemporary Review
Vicki J. Volbrecht and Reinhold Kliegl

10.1	Introduction 187
10.2	The Phenomenology of Blackness... 187
10.2.1	Helmholtz: Trichromatic Theory of Color Vision 189
10.2.2	Hering: Opponent-Process Theory of Color Vision 189
10.2.3	Criticism and Other Theories 191
10.3	Historical Review 194
10.3.1	Induction Experiments 194
10.3.2	Blackness-Induction Experiments ... 195
10.4	Physiological Mechanisms 201
10.5	Conclusion 202
	References 202

11. Basic Color Terms and Basic Color Categories 207
Clyde L. Hardin

Discussion and Summary 215
References 216

12. Color Perception: From Grassman Codes to a Dual Code for Object and Illumination Colors
Rainer Mausfeld

12.1	Introduction 219
12.2	Elementaristic vs. Ecological Perspectives in Color Research 220
12.3	Attributes of Color 222
12.4	Early Color Coding and the Elementaristic Approach.......... 224
12.4.1	Newton and Helmholtz's Approach to Color Perception............... 224
12.4.2	The Young-Helmholtz Theory and Grassmann's Laws............... 225
12.4.3	Opponent-Color Theory 226
12.4.4	Relating Psychophysical and Neurophysiological Color Codes.... 228
12.4.5	Elementary Color Codes Accounting for Variations in Spatial and Temporal Context....................... 231
12.5	Ecological and Computational Perspectives 236
12.5.1	The Problem of Approximate Color Constancy from a Computational Point of View 238
12.5.2	Qualitative Observations on the Dialectic Relationship of Illumination and Object Color................. 240
12.6	Center-Surround Configurations as Minimal Stimuli for Triggering a Dual Code for 'Object Colors' and 'Illumination Colors' 242
12.6.1	Laminar Segmentation and a Dual Code for 'Object Color' and 'Illumination Color' 243
12.6.2	Segregation of 'Object Color' and 'Illumination Color' in Minimal Seurat-type Configurations........ 245
	References 248

13. Color Contrast Gain Control
Michael D'Zmura

- 13.1 Introduction 251
- 13.1.1 What is Contrast Gain Control? 251
- 13.1.2 Selectivity for Spatial Frequency, Orientation and Color 252
- 13.1.3 Feed-Forward, Matrix-Multiplicative Circuitry 253
- 13.1.4 Spatial Pooling of Contrast 254
- 13.2 Model Components 254
- 13.3 Color Image Processing 256
- 13.3.1 Channel Responses 256
- 13.3.2 Channel Contrasts 257
- 13.3.3 Channel Interaction 261
- 13.3.4 Channel Gains 261
- 13.3.5 Multichannel Contrast Gain Control . 263
- 13.4 Discussion 264
- 13.5 Summary 265
- References 265

14. Binocular Brightness Combination: A Mechanism for Combining Two Sources of Rather Similar Information
Hans Irtel

- 14.1 Intensity Invariance of Binocular Brightness 267
- 14.2 Methods 269
- 14.3 Results 270
- 14.4 Discussion 271
- 14.5 Summary 273
- References 273

15. Inferences about Infant Color Vision
Kenneth Knoblauch, Michelle L. Bieber and John S. Werner

- 15.1 Introduction 275
- 15.2 Inferences from Luminosity 275
- 15.3 Inferences from Silent Substitution . . 277
- 15.4 Inferences about Rod Intrusion 278
- 15.5 Inferences about M- and L-Cones ... 279
- 15.6 Summary 281
- References 281

IV. Color Metrics and Application

16. Dichromacy – The Simplest Type of Color Vision
Horst Scheibner

- 16.1 Introduction: An Initial Overview ... 285
- 16.2 The Trichromatic Instrumental Color Space $^3V_{BGR}$ 286
- 16.3 Measuring the Deuteranopic Missing Color and Reducing Trichromacy to Deuteranopia 287
- 16.4 The Transition from the Instrumental Trichromatic Space to the Instrumental Deuteranopic Space ... 290
- 16.5 The Transformation from the Trichromatic Instrumental Color Space to the Deuteranopic Opponent-Color Space 291
- 16.6 The Role of the Fundamental Color Space 294
- 16.7 Construction of the Fundamental Color Spaces $^3V_{PTD}$ and $^2V_{PT}$ and the Deuteranopic Opponent-Color Channels 295
- 16.8 A Synopsis of Deuteranopia 298
- 16.9 A Synopsis of Dichromacy 299
- 16.10 A Lattice-Theoretical Classification of Dichromacy and Other Color Deficiencies 301
- 16.11 Concluding Remarks 301
- 16.12 Summary 302
- References 302

17. Current CIE Work to Achieve Physiologically-Correct Color Metrics
János Schanda

- 17.1 Introduction 307
- 17.2 Cone Excitation Spectra 308
- 17.2.1 Choice of the Color-Matching Functions 308
- 17.2.2 Deriving L-, M-, S-Cone Excitation Spectra from Color-Matching Data . . 309
- 17.2.3 Intra-Ocular Screening 310
- 17.2.4 Derivation of the Fundamental Response Curves 311

17.3	Further Aspects...............	314
17.3.1	Rod Intrusion	314
17.3.2	Color Appearance.............	315
17.3.3	Color Management Studies.......	315
17.4	Summary	316
	References	316

18. Use of Computer Graphics in PostScript for Color Didactics
Klaus Richter

18.1	Introduction	319
18.2	Multiplicity of Colors...........	321
18.3	Color Solid, Basic Colors and Color Attributes	322
18.4	Spectrum and 3-Dimensional Color Values......................	324
18.5	Color Measurement, Mixture and Contrast	325
18.6	Colors: Equally Spaced and Thresholds	327
18.7	Opponent Achromatic Color Vision..	328
18.8	Sensitivity, Saturation and Chromaticity...................	329
18.9	Summary	332
	References	332

List of Contributors 333

Index 337

Introduction

Werner G. K. Backhaus, Reinhold Kliegl and John S. Werner

The colors of objects appear, at first glance, to be inherent properties of those objects. We say, for example, "this flower is blue," "this apple is red," "the grass is green," and "this painting is colorful." The tendency to treat color as a property of objects is strengthened by mechanisms that maintain a color constant world with changes in the illumination. The flower, the apple and the grass appear to have more or less the same color under the various phases of daylight illumination. It is easy to show, however, that color constancy is not perfect. The hue of an object is strongly affected by certain light sources, as well as by preceding and/or surrounding light, as scientists and artists have observed in many circumstances described in this book. These latter observations suggest that color, as we experience it, is not an inherent property of objects but is associated with the spectral distribution of light reflected from them in the context of preceding and surrounding illumination.

Just as experienced color is not a property of objects, color is also not a property of the light. The perceived color of an object depends on the spectral content of the light that is absorbed by the cone photoreceptors which initiate a cascade of physiological reactions in the retina and the brain. Newton (1704) recognized this when he wrote "For the Rays to speak properly are not coloured" (p. 124). He came to this view by observing that there are numerous combinations of physically different lights that appear identical, called metamers. Maxwell (1860) and Helmholtz (1867) later established an empirical basis for three-dimensional metameric-matching spaces from which they concluded, correctly, that color vision is made possible by three classes of photoreceptors.

The appearance of color is also not explained, however, solely by the activity of three classes of cone photoreceptors, although like the physical properties of the stimulus, trivariance represents an indispensable component in color vision processing. Introspection shows that all experienced colors can be described in terms of six elementary sensations: red, green, blue, yellow, black and white. This is represented in Figure 1. Hues are represented on the circumference, with blue and

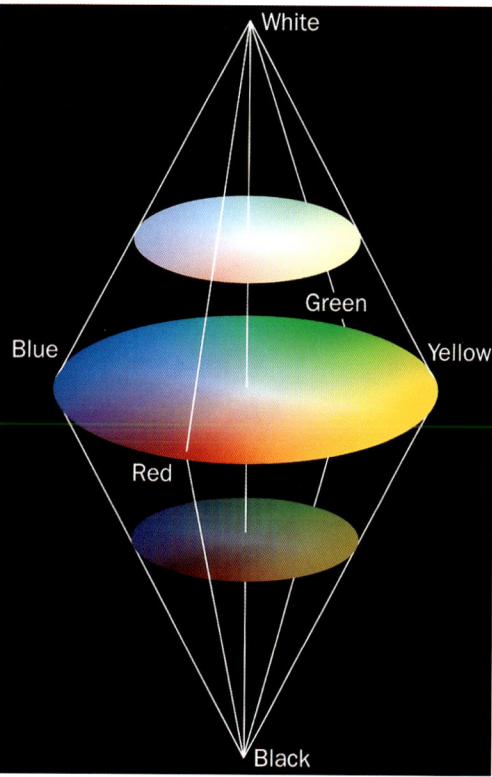

Fig. 1: The color solid: perceptual color space following Hering's (1920) proposal that there are six elementary color sensations.

yellow, and red and green, plotted opposite each other because the pairs red/green and blue/yellow never occur co-spatially and/or co-temporally. They are thus called opponent colors (Hering, 1920). The achromatic colors, black and white, are shown at the apices. The three planes orthogonal to the black-white axis illustrate colors having different levels of lightness and darkness. Hering recognized that constraints on how colors appear imply constraints on how colors are coded by the nervous system. The perceptual bases for Hering's ideas have been verified by psychophysical experiments and their physiological foundations have been proven in general to be correct by neurophysiological measurements.

Perspectives from Different Disciplines

What is left to explain in color science? This depends on one's discipline and perspective within that discipline. This book provides a sampling of perspectives beginning with an historical discussion of research on color vision in art and science. The artist who composes a picture must know about the effects of light on our perception (e.g., color assimilation, contrast and color constancy) to avoid unintended side effects. While artists continue to show provocative effects that beg for physiological and psychological explanation, color scientists sometimes look at the problem the other way around: asking to what degree artistic achievements can be explained by what is currently understood from color science.

Color perception is based on a number of neural processing stages and while each level of processing is essential to understanding color appearance, there is not a one-to-one mapping between physical stimuli, physiological responses and color appearance. The physiological concept of three photoreceptor types and the psychological experience of six elementary colors obviously do not match each other. Von Kries (1882), however, proposed a zone theory in which the activity of the three receptor types is transformed at a stage of opponent-color processing. This view is now well accepted but, as discussed in several chapters in this book, the mathematical transformations used to map the photoreceptor activity to the neural code, and ultimately to perception, are still being investigated.

The links among a number of physiological processing stages are also explored in this book through research from several different disciplines: the relations between photoreceptor signals and various transformations into a color-opponent code carried through processing stages in the retina and higher-levels of the brain; the molecular genetics of the cone photopigments and their influences on color-matching; and, the relations between neural computations and behavior, not only in normal and color deficient primates, but in animals such as the honeybee where the neuronal circuits are simpler and more tractable both electrophysiologically and computationally.

Despite extraordinary leaps in technical methods for investigating color vision (such as electrophysiology, brain imaging, molecular genetics, etc.), the meaning of the information yielded is not always self-evident. Ultimately, we can never be sure that two humans have the same color experience, even if they identify the same stimulus using the same words. Inferences about sensations are even more difficult in the case of different animal species with which we can only communicate via behavioral experiments. For this reason, philosophers remain useful in guiding our thinking about further criteria that, if satisfied, might allow a reasonable person to infer whether two people or two different species experience the world in the same way.

Finally, the transformations from color metrics to displayed colors is a matter of great practical importance. The use of color has become more prevalent in everyday life. Until very recently, books containing as many color illustrations as this one were reserved for those wealthy popes and dukes who could afford illuminated manuscripts. Color television and computer displays are now common place. While engineering moves ahead, principles from other disciplines also come to the fore. Precise color management is in the process of being developed in some cases on the basis of results from basic color science, but the practical issues in color imaging can also raise thorny questions for color theory.

Integrative Views

It seems clear from the chapters in this book that progress in the various disciplines of color science often depends not only on progress within that discipline, but also on conceptual developments in related fields. The successful search for single cells in the visual pathway that respond in a spectrally-opponent manner was motivated by perceptual studies implying that our nervous system must be organized in this manner (although not necessarily at the level of single cells). In this example, as in many others, there was a period during which interdisciplinary interest surged to the benefit of several disciplines interested in color coding. Often, however, the disciplines are widely out of step with one another as witnessed by the long lag between Hering's proposal of perceptual-opponent coding and the much later discovery of its possible cellular basis. Following a period of interdisciplinary progress, some concepts lose their energizing force for one or the other discipline and new cycles ensue. We now see, for example, a search for specific neural mechanisms to explain the more complex aspects of color perception such as color contrast, color constancy or the filling-in of color information beyond the spatial coverage of receptive fields of single neurons. While one approach, usually the perceptual, moves ahead of the other for a period of time, the lag between disciplines today is shorter than in the past.

Nowadays, as in the past, color vision is not so much investigated by interdisciplinary teams but by researchers working in different disciplines. The investigations usually aim to solve specific problems within their specific area, but because of the causal chain structure of color processing, ideas and methods are imported from other disciplines as the problem dictates. Thus, the separation amongst the disciplines varies over time and ultimately vanishes into an integrative view on color vision. At the risk of being called "color vision chauvinists," we submit that there is no other field where our understanding of the physical, physiological and perceptual foundations of a behavior are better understood than in color vision. Thus, the area of color vision stands as a model for investigations of other aspects of brain and behavior where disciplinary barriers must be broken to make further progress.

References

Helmholtz, H. v. (1867) Handbuch der Physiologischen Optik. (Hamburg: Voss). [third edition translated as: Helmholtz's Treatise on Physiological Optics; J. P C. Southall, Ed. Rochester, New York: Optical Society of America, 1924.]

Hering, E. (1920) Outlines of a Theory of the Light Sense. L. M. Hurvich and D. Jameson, trans. (Harvard U. Press, Cambridge, Mass., 1964; originally published by Springer, Berlin).

Kries, J. v. (1882) Die Gesichtsempfindungen und ihre Analyse. (Leipzig: Veith & Co.).

Maxwell, J. C. (1860) On the theory of compound colours and the relations of the colours of the spectrum. Philos. Trans. R. Soc. London *150*, 57–84.

Newton, I. (1704) Opticks: Or, a Treatise of the Reflexions, Refractions, Inflexions and Colours of Light. (London: S. Smith and B. Walford). [based on the fourth edition (Dover, U.S.A.: Dover Publications), 1952].

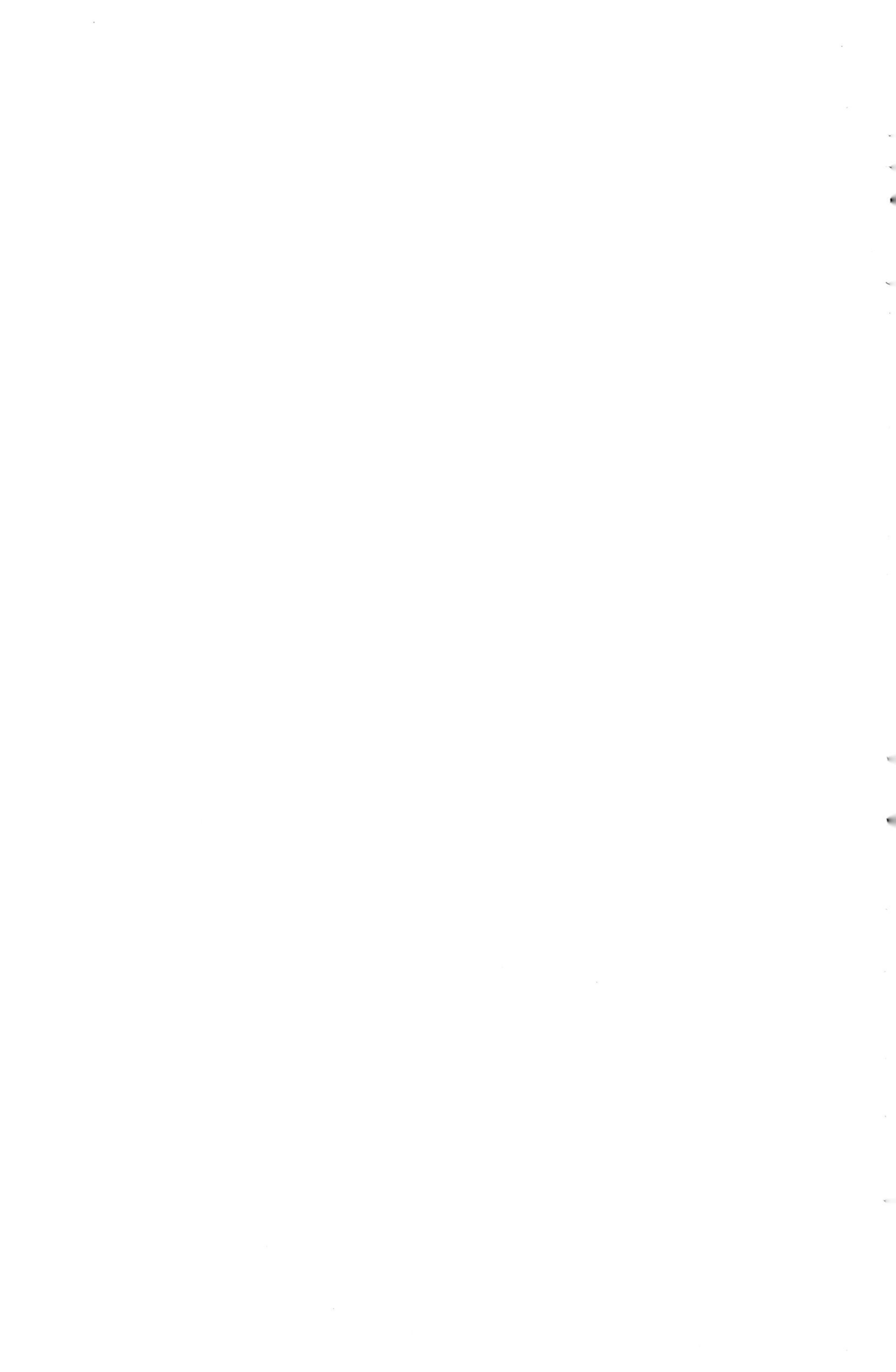

I Color Vision in Art and Science

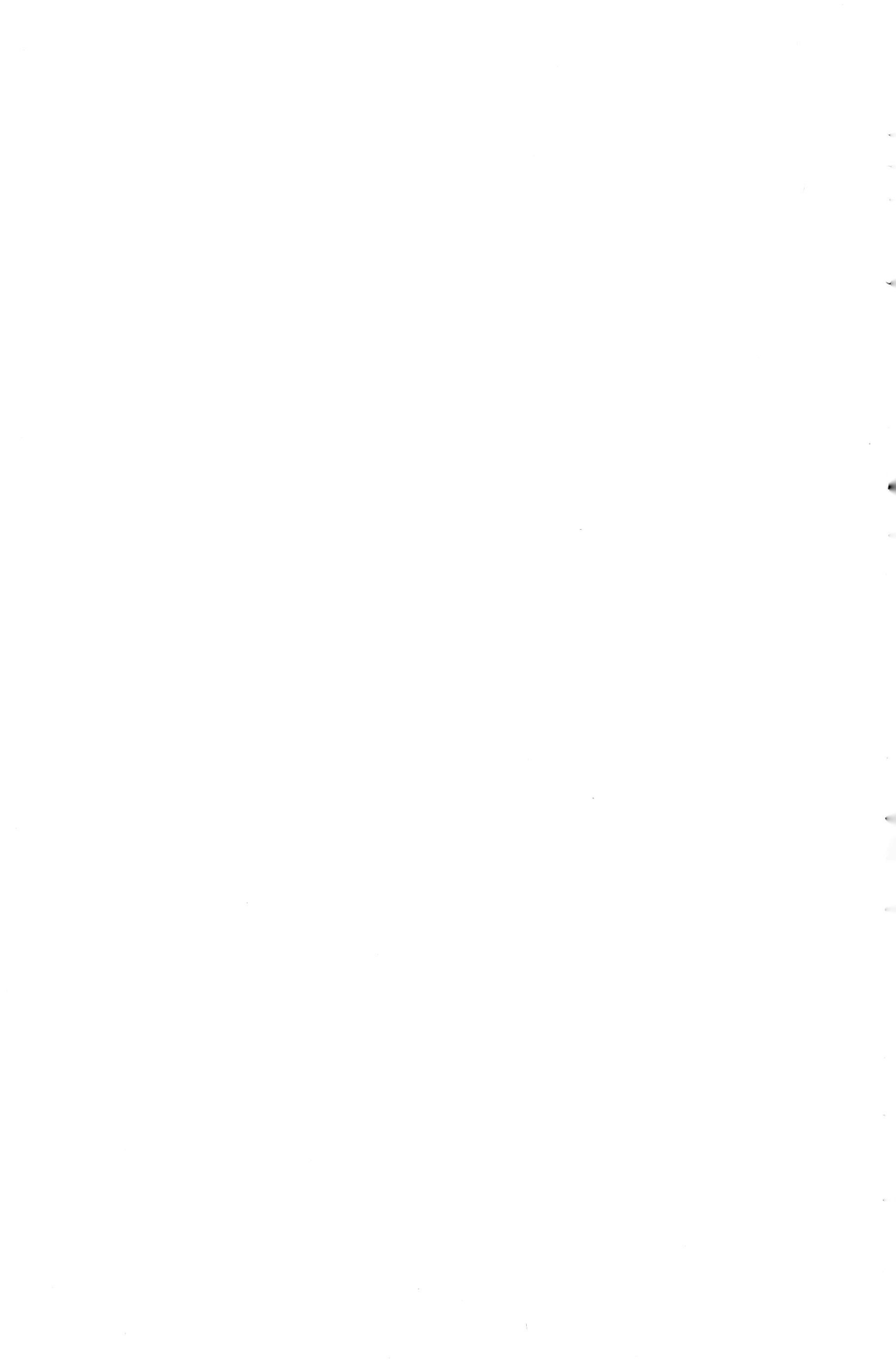

1. Aging through the Eyes of Monet

John S. Werner

1.1 Introduction

One of the most eventful periods for our understanding of color, both in art and in science, occurred between 14 November 1840 and 5 December 1926 – the life span of Oscar Claude Monet. In art, Monet's life encompassed the period between the Romantic pictorial tradition and Abstract Expressionism. In science, the physical principles pertaining to light and color laid down by Newton in the preceding century (Newton, 1704) were used to discover processes of color coding by the eye and brain. In short, the way both artists and scientists think about color today was shaped from 1840 to 1926 to a degree that may be unparalleled by any other period of 86 years.

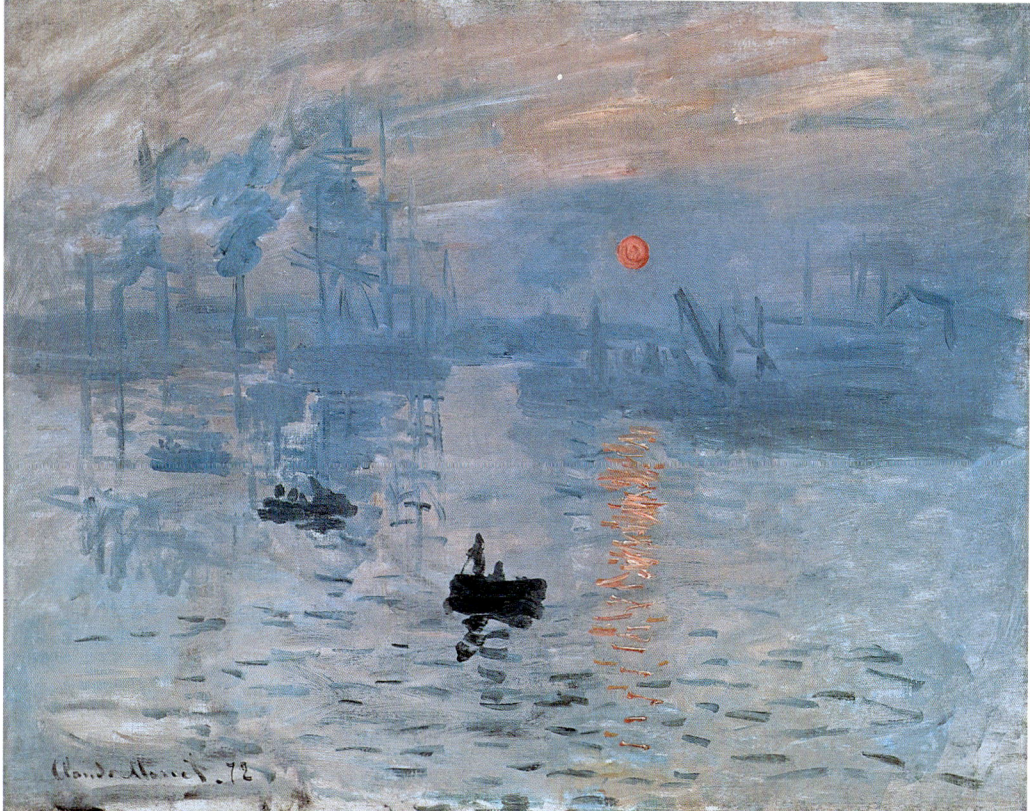

Fig. 1.1: Claude Monet (1872) *Impression: Soleil levant (Le Port du Havre par la brume). [Impression: Sunrise (Port of Le Havre Through the Mist.]* Oil on canvas, 48 × 63 cm. (After restoration.) Musée Marmottan, Paris. (Photo credit: Giraudon/Art Resource, New York.)

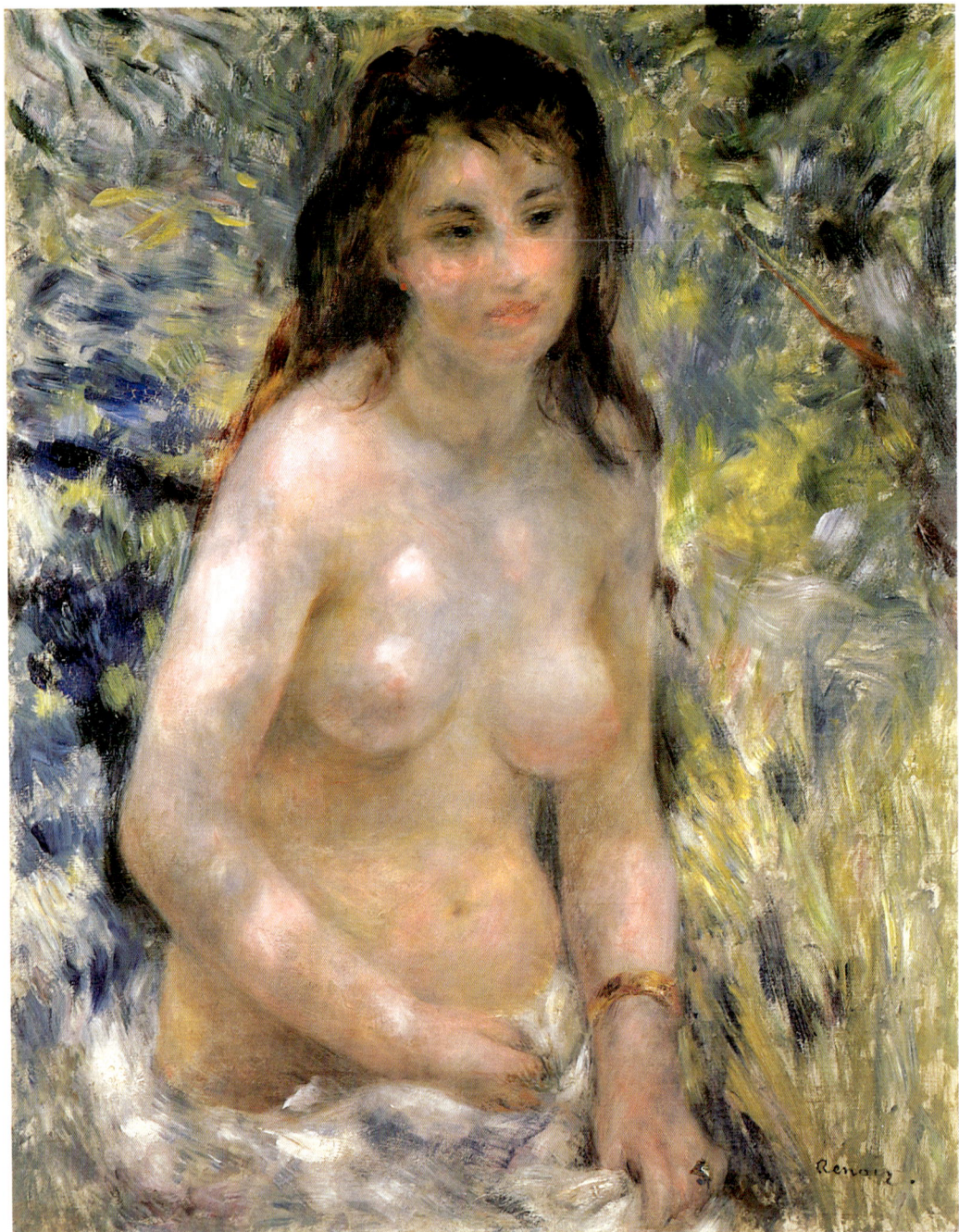

Fig. 1.2: Pierre Auguste Renoir (1875-76) *Torse de femme au soleil. [Torso of a Woman in the Sun.]* Oil on canvas, 81 × 65 cm. Musée d'Orsay, Paris.

Art and science have at least one purpose in common: to enrich the human spirit. Whatever else one might say about Monet, he has certainly enriched our civilization. For when he unveiled the painting shown in Figure 1.1 at the first exhibition of the Société Anonyme des Artistes in 1874, he became the *de facto* leader of a movement that would alter the course of Western art history. This painting was originally called *"The Port of Le Havre"* but is now known by its subtitle *"Impression: Sunrise,"* from which a school of art was given its name, Impressionism. The picture captures what we now expect from an Impressionist painting – light, atmosphere, color and movement, all in the service of rendering the feelings of the moment.

The Impressionists were individualists, with different styles, preferred subject matter, and aspirations. What united them, however, was a rebellious spirit against the Paris Salon and a desire to capture the fleeting effects of light and color. Consider Pierre Auguste Renoir's *Torso of a Woman in the Sun* (Fig. 1.2) presented in the second Impressionists' exhibit in 1876. Although he preferred to paint the human form, he did so in a way that captured the delicate shades and shadows that were previously not recorded on canvas. But it was not just the handling of light and color that made the movement controversial; those pretty pictures of the Impressionists had said "No" to the classical pictorial tradition. Great art no longer had to depict kings, popes and saints: ordinary experience would do.

Someone once asked Renoir how it is that he obtained the delicate flesh tones of his nudes for which he became famous, and he said in effect, I just keep painting and painting until I feel like grabbing (Vollard, 1925). When pushed further about the possible scientific basis of his techniques, Renoir said that if any of his work could be subjected to scientific analysis, he would not consider it art. Such a reaction is not atypical in the history of art, but it is somewhat atypical for the Impressionists. Many of them had a deep and abiding interest in color science. Camille Pissarro, for example, studied scientific literature in order to perfect his use of color.

The eyes of Monet changed over his life span, and so too did the way he portrayed the world. One must admit, of course, that changes in Monet's vision are confounded by changes in his style of painting, notwithstanding that his stated goal was always to portray the subtle modulations of light without interpretation. Monet once said:

When you go out to paint, try to forget what objects you have before you, a tree, a house, a field or whatever. Merely think, here is a little square of blue, here an oblong of pink, here a streak of yellow, and paint it just as it looks to you, the exact color and shape, until it gives your own naive impression of the scene before you. (Perry, 1927, p. 120)

Monet's changing portrayal of nature throughout his life has drawn attention to important processes of visual aging but has also perpetuated myths about the aging visual system. The purpose of this chapter is to offer a personal interpretation of color science and art in Monet's lifetime, with an analysis of his aging eye as it may be derived from his art and as related to current research on senescence of human color vision.

1.2 A Link between Sunlight and Aging

Paul Cézanne once remarked (Barnes, 1990, p. 6) that "Monet is just an eye but my god what an eye!" The human eye is shown schematically in Figure 1.3. Light, if it is to be seen, must first travel through the various ocular media, the cornea, the anterior chamber filled with aqueous, the lens and the vitreous humor. It then passes through the layers of cells comprising the retina, shown in an enlarged view, where it can be absorbed by the rods and cones, the receptor cells that initiate vision.

The clinically normal eye appears rather stable over much of the life span. Barring disease or trauma, senescent deterioration is seldom noticed until mid- to late-life. At first glance, then, aging of the eye is a phenomenon of later life. Unfortunately, first impressions can be quite misleading. A closer look at the visual system shows that it is constantly changing throughout life (Weale, 1982; Werner et al., 1990).

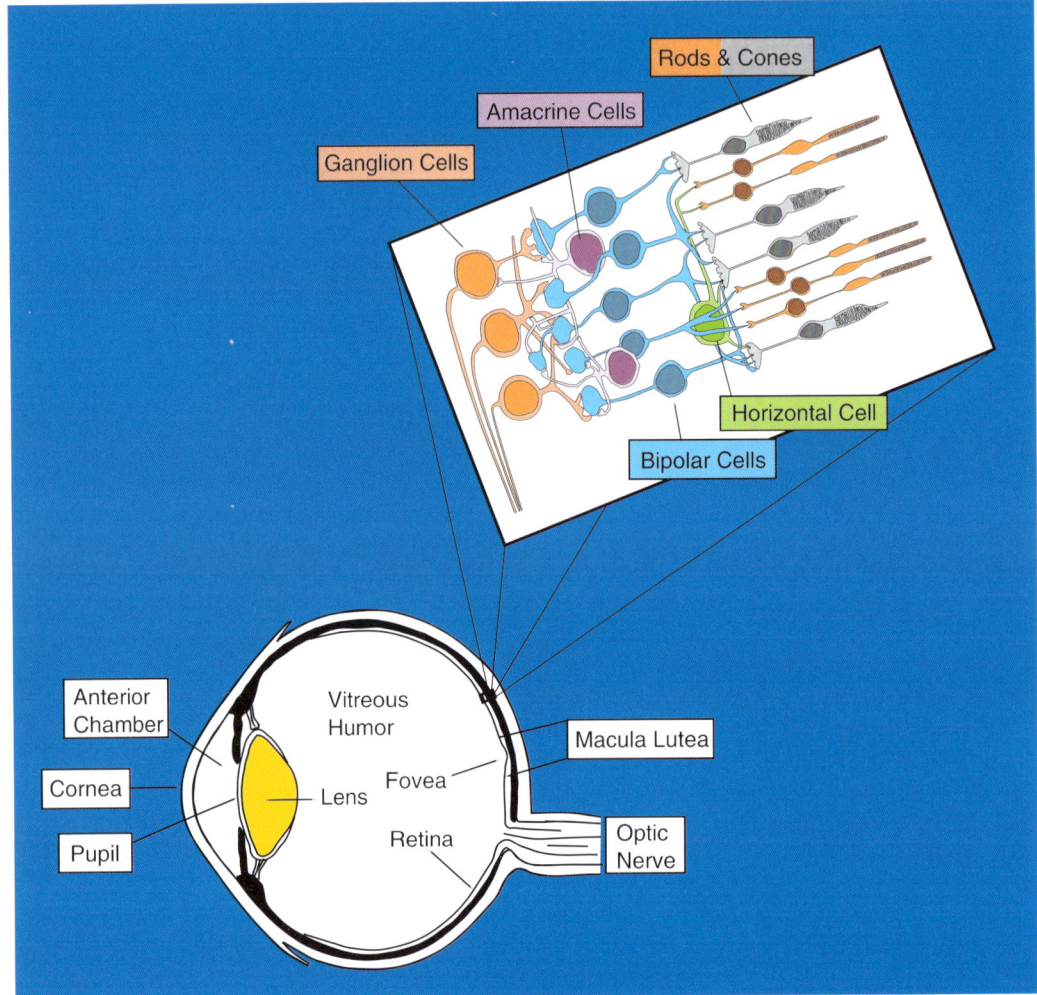

Fig. 1.3: Schematic cross-section of the human eye with the retina shown in an enlarged view. The ocular media include the cornea, aqueous contained in the anterior chamber, lens and vitreous humor. The retina, shown in a magnified view, includes five principal cell types, photoreceptors (rods and cones), horizontal cells, bipolars, amacrines and ganglion cells (the axons of which form the optic nerve).

One factor that is believed to contribute to age-related changes in the eye is exposure to light itself (Werner, 1991). This factor may be especially pertinent to understanding Monet. Although other artists had painted in the open, Monet was perhaps the first to do so on a large scale and seemingly under all weather and seasonal conditions. His careful observations of the varying effects of sunlight and his insistence on painting *en plein air* virtually guaranteed that he would receive more than the usual cumulative exposure to sunlight. Even as early as 1867, at age 27, Monet had trouble with his vision following hours of painting in sunlight, and he received medical advice to abandon his outdoor painting (Stuckey, 1995). Several times thereafter he reported visual disturbances following a day of painting in the sun.

To understand the effects of light on the eye, it is necessary to define the spectrum of optical radiation. The visible spectrum includes wave-

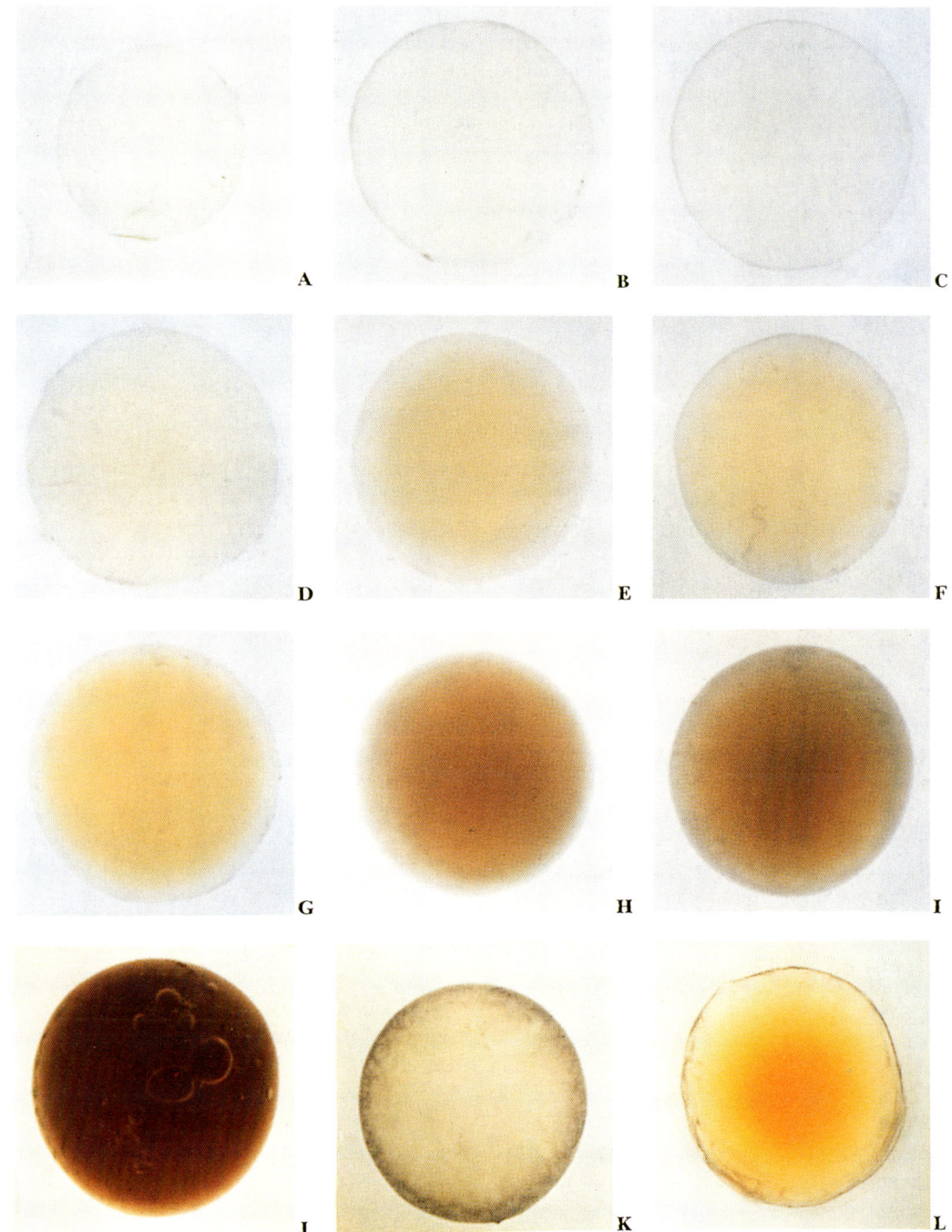

Fig. 1.4: Extracted lenses of humans at various ages: (A) six months, (B) eight years, (C) 12 years, (D) 25 years, (E) 47 years, (F) 60 years, (G) 70 years, (H) 82 years, and (I) 91 years. Also shown are three types of cataractous lenses: (J) nuclear cataract, age 70; (K) cortical cataract, age 68; and (L) mixed nuclear and cortical cataract, age 74 years. (From Lerman, 1980.)

lengths between about 400 and 700 nm. At 400 nm the light normally appears violet in the light-adapted state, and shorter wavelengths are called ultraviolet (or UV) light. Because of absorption in the stratospheric ozone layer, very little light below 300 nm reaches the earth's surface so, for practical purposes, the UV spectrum of sunlight encompasses the range from approximately 300 to 400 nm. At the other end of the visible spectrum at 700 nm, the light normally appears red under light-adapted conditions; longer wavelengths are called infrared.

The energy contained within a single quantum is inversely related to its wavelength; quanta in the UV may contain enough energy to alter molecules in the eye that absorb them, primarily by initiating a cascade of oxidative reactions that are harmful to cells. This type of light damage is usually called photochemical or actinic (Werner and Spillmann, 1989). These photochemical reactions occur as long as we are exposed to high-energy photons and because we are exposed to them from birth, we can be assured that cellular deterioration, or senescence, begins even from the first days of life.

Experiments with non human animals verify that any wavelength of light, in sufficient intensity, may damage the eye, but the shorter the wavelength, the more effective it is. For example, light at 325 nm in the UV is about 1,000-fold more effective in damaging the photoreceptors and retinal pigment epithelium than light at about 580 nm (usually appearing yellow) in the visible region of the spectrum (Ham et al., 1982). This damage is not fundoscopically visible until about 48 hours after exposure, indicating that it is due to photochemical processes and not a burn. A retinal burn seldom occurs with natural light exposure because there is usually insufficient energy to raise the temperature of the retina by $\geq 10\,°C$, the approximate threshold for thermal damage. Exposures that are insufficient to reach the threshold for retinal damage may nevertheless add to the effects of other exposures, accumulating over time to produce cellular changes associated with normal aging (Marshall, 1985; Werner 1991).

Under normal circumstances the eye has several natural defenses to protect it from the photochemical insult associated with sunlight. For example, distributed throughout the eye are various antioxidant molecules (e.g., superoxide dismutase, α-tocopherol, glutathione, melanin, selenium and ascorbic acid) that neutralize phototoxic reactions. Especially important in this respect is the presence of the yellow macular pigment around the fovea (a depression in the retina where the cone photoreceptors are most densely packed and which provides our best spatial resolution; it typically corresponds to the center of gaze) which not only reduces the intensity of short-wave visible light reaching the retina, but which also consists of carotinoid pigments that are excellent at neutralizing some of the phototoxic reactions that occur in the eye (Kirschfeld, 1982). A second line of defense lies in the ability of cells to replace their parts by molecular renewal. Visual cells continuously reconstruct or replace virtually all of their parts except DNA (Young, 1982). As a result, damaged constituents of cells are replaced in a piecemeal fashion. A third defense against the most damaging wavelengths of light results from the tendency of these wavelengths to be absorbed by the ocular media, primarily the lens, before they can reach the retina. Figure 1.4 shows that the lens becomes an even more effective absorber of short wavelength light as an increasing function of age. One can see how clear the lens is in the newborn, and that it becomes distinctly yellow in adulthood and brown in old age. Quantitative studies with larger numbers of individuals reveal that the density (log of the reciprocal of transmission) of the ocular media increases as a function of age from infancy through the end of life (Werner, 1982; Weale, 1988; Pokorny and Smith, 1997).

Figure 1.4 illustrates common types of cataract. Nuclear cataract, which is what Claude Monet ultimately developed, is shown by lens J. Cataract is only an extreme of normal aging; we call the aged lens a cataract when it interferes with functional vision. Considerable experimental and epidemiological evidence has shown that lenticular senescence and cataract are, in part, due to the absorption of high-energy photons of UV (Young, 1991). In other words, exposure to sunlight accelerates aging of the lens and is one of the significant risk factors for cataract.

1.3 The Trivariance of Color Mixture: Maxwell and Helmholtz

Once light reaches the retina, it can be absorbed by three different classes of cones, the photoreceptors of color vision. The foundation for our understanding of these processes was laid by James Clerk Maxwell and Hermann von Helmholtz in the mid 19th Century, although Thomas Young (1802) and others before him (Weale, 1957) had speculated earlier that normal human vision may be trichromatic. Maxwell and Helmholtz understood the difference between additive and subtractive light mixture, a distinction that would be discovered somewhat later by the Impressionists.

Subtractive mixture is familiar to most people through playing with paints in childhood. As illustrated by Figure 1.5, the mixture of blue and yellow paint typically appears green. In this example, the blue pigment absorbs many of the long-wave quanta and the yellow pigment absorbs many of the short-wave quanta. What reaches the eye is primarily middle wavelengths, the band that is reflected by both pigments. This is analogous to passing a white light with all wavelengths through two successive filters, a blue and a yellow. In Figure 1.5 the blue filter transmits quanta primarily of short and middle wavelengths while the yellow filter transmits primarily the middle and long wavelength quanta. Light of specific wavelengths is subtracted out at each stage and all that reaches the eye is that which both filters transmit, the middle wavelengths, which we usually call green. In subtractive color mixture the result is always a loss of light compared to that which would be transmitted (reflected) by either filter (pigment) alone. This can be appreciated by comparing the individual paint reflectances or the filter transmittances in the top row of Figure 1.5, with the resultant subtractive mixture shown on the right of the middle row.

Consider now a case of additive color mixture which can be effected using the same blue and yellow paints or filters shown in Figure 1.5. In the case of paints, a blue spot is placed next to a yellow spot so that light from each is reflected to the eye in parallel. If the spots are small enough, the two reflected lights will not be resolved as individual spots and will, in the words of Pointillist painters, "optically blend." The mixture in this example will appear achromatic (gray or white). The light distribution that reaches the eye in this example is equivalent to that obtained when the same broad-band light is passed in parallel through each filter so that both beams enter the eye and are superposed at the retina. The resultant mixture within the eye appears neither yellow nor blue, but achromatic. Such pairs of lights, that can be mixed to appear white, are called complementary lights. There is a large number of complementary light pairs, but they are most conveniently found using monochromatic lights, essentially single wavelengths of light (e.g., 470 and 570 nm). More generally, three relatively arbitrarily chosen lights are required to match any other light distribution. Physically different lights that appear identical are called metamers. The existence of metamers shows that the appearance of a color is not explicable on the basis of the physics of light alone, but is due to the processes that the light initiates in the eye and brain.

Maxwell's (1860) studies of additive light mixture carefully documented the proportions of three lights required to match an achromatic standard. He described the results by algebraic or color mixture equations, and because only three variables were required, he could illustrate the results in a triangular diagram. He realized that the trivariance of color mixture implies the existence of three kinds of color mechanisms in the eye. In related experiments, Helmholtz showed that any light of the spectrum can be matched by an appropriate combination of three others. From this observation, he too correctly concluded that the retinal receptors of daylight vision, the cones, are trivariant. Helmholtz's estimates of the relative sensitivities of the three cone types presented in his *Handbuch der Physiologischen Optik* (Helmholtz, 1867) are close to more modern estimates (Vos and Walraven, 1971; Smith and Pokorny, 1975) such as those shown in Figure 1.6 for infants and adults.

Although correct about this fundamental point, Helmholtz took another step that went beyond his data. To account for color appearance, he proposed that the response of each class of receptor is di-

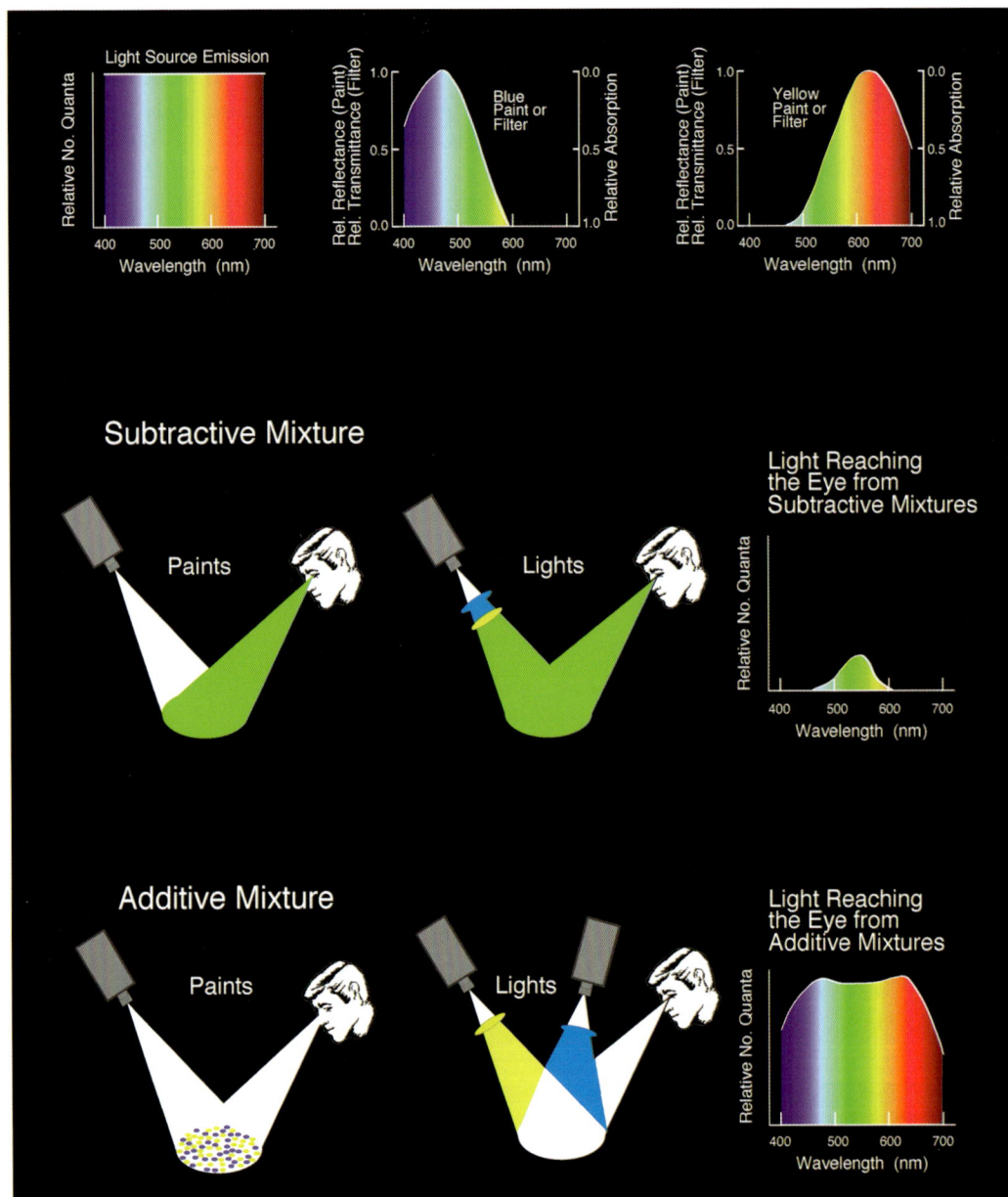

Fig. 1.5: Top row: The number of quanta emitted from a hypothetical light source is plotted as a function of wavelength. Graphs in the middle and right show hypothetical paints and filters; the reflectance axes refer to the proportion of incident quanta (plotted from 0.0 to 1.0) reflected by the individual paints and the transmittance axes refer to the proportion of incident quanta (plotted from 0.0 to 1.0) transmitted by the individual filters. What is not reflected by the paint or transmitted by the filter is shown on the right axes as absorption (plotted from 1.0 to 0.0). A blue paint (filter) contains pigment that reflects (transmits) primarily short and middle wavelength quanta, but absorbs long wavelength quanta. A yellow paint (filter) contains pigment that reflects (transmits) quanta primarily at middle and long wavelengths, but absorbs short wavelength quanta. **Middle row:** Subtractive mixture using the blue and yellow paints (in a uniform mixture) or the blue and yel-

1.3 The Trivariance of Color Mixture: Maxwell and Helmholtz

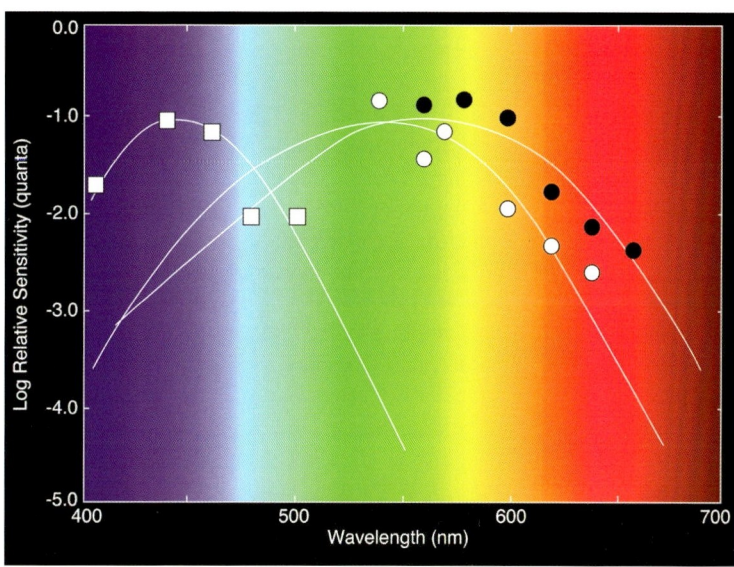

Fig. 1.6: Relative log quantal sensitivity of the three classes of human cone photoreceptor. Smooth functions show the sensitivities of short- (S), middle- (M) and long-wave (L) cones in the adult (Vos, 1978), adjusted in sensitivity according to the less dense ocular media (Werner, 1982) and absence of macular pigment of infants. Squares show sensitivity of S-cones from an infant obtained by Volbrecht and Werner (1987), while white and black circles show sensitivities of an infant's M- and L-cones, respectively, obtained by Bieber et al. (in press).

rectly linked to perception. Therefore, he labeled the three classes of receptors as blue, green and red. For reasons to be described later, this aspect of his theory is not correct and it is more accurate to label the receptors according to their wavelength of maximal sensitivity at either short-, middle- or long-wavelengths.

Using psychophysical methods, Werner and Steele (1988) measured the sensitivity of the different cone pathways for 75 observers between the ages of 10 and 85 years. All three cone types were found to decrease significantly in sensitivity as a function of age. A linear function describes the data well and there is no statistical justification for supposing that the true function is non-linear over this age range. In addition, the rate of change with age appears to be similar for the three cone types; approximately 0.13 log unit (26%) per decade. One can think of these results as showing that the elderly visual system, at least at this stage of pro-

low filters (in series) from the top row are illustrated. While these two figures show the approximate appearance with neutral adaptation, the figure on the right shows the physical light distribution reaching the eye from these mixtures.
Bottom row: Additive mixture occurs when the light is reflected by the two (unmixed) paints applied in small dots that cannot be resolved as discrete dots by the visual system; the appearance is achromatic. Additive mixture also occurs when the light is passed through the two filters in parallel; the appearance is achromatic. As illustrated by the graph on the right, the light reaching the eye is the sum of that reflected (transmitted) by each of the pigments (filters) alone.

cessing, is similar to the young visual system operating at a reduced light level.

Several sites in the visual pathway are responsible for age-related losses in sensitivity, but the largest proportion of the sensitivity loss appears to be at early stages of processing. These include increased absorption of light by the ocular media, a loss in the ability of the photoreceptors to capture quanta (Schefrin et al., 1992), and/or an elevation in neural noise (Schefrin et al., 1995).

One also sees a great deal of individual variation in cone sensitivity within each age. The sources of this variation are no doubt multi-faceted, but an important one is likely to be exposure to sunlight. Psychophysical studies (Werner et al., 1989) and an anatomical study (Marshall, 1978) suggest that retinal aging, as with aging of the lens, is accelerated by exposure to light, especially UV and shortwave visible light.

1.4 Monet's Early Impressionistic Style

While Maxwell and Helmholtz were developing theories about the physiological basis of color mixing, Monet and Renoir were in La Grenouillère experimenting with additive and subtractive mixtures on canvas. Here, many of the fundamentals of Monet's style were developed, including painting *en plein air* and representing complex aspects of reflections and shadow on canvas. More and more, his brushstrokes consisted of a pure, unmixed color, except when dark colors were formed through subtractive color mixtures.

In 1921, the Neo-Impressionist painter Paul Signac (1921) published an historical account that characterized Impressionism as based on these four aspects of technique:

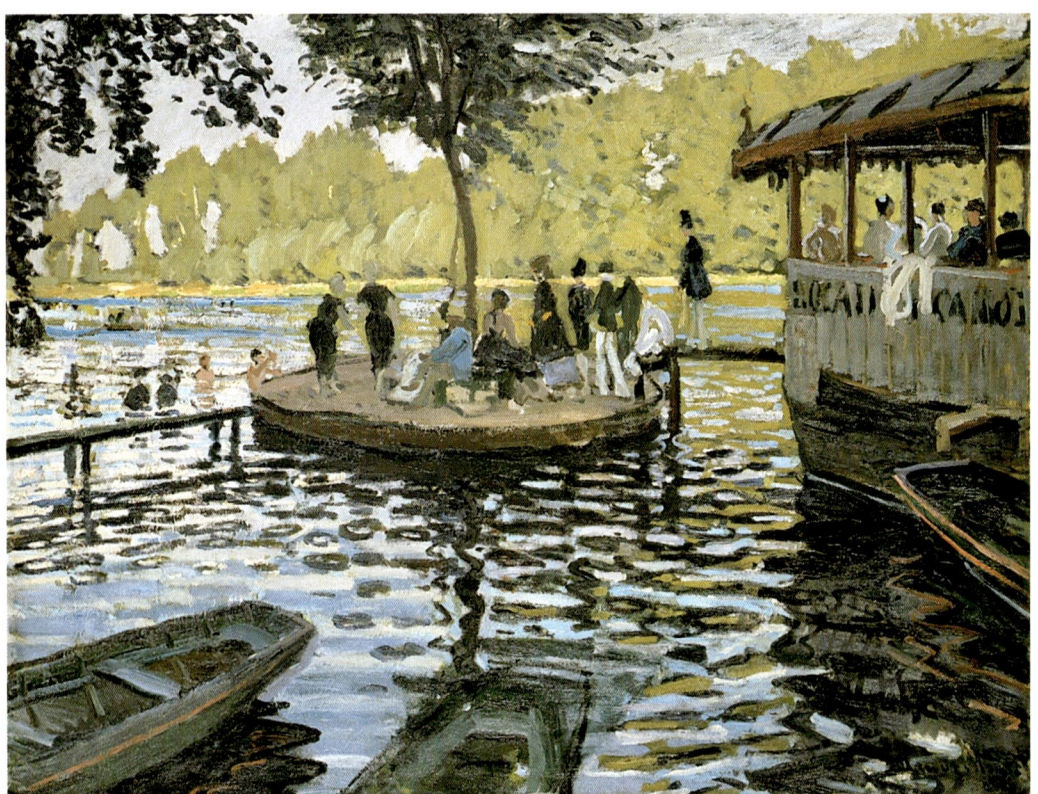

Fig. 1.7: Claude Monet (1869) *La Grenouillère.* Oil on canvas, 74.6 × 99.7 cm. The Metropolitan Museum of Art, Bequest of Mrs. H.O. Havemeyer, 1929. The H.O. Havemeyer Collection.

1. Palette composed solely of pure colors approximating those of the solar spectrum;
2. Mixing on the palette and optical mixture;
3. Comma-shaped or swept-over brushstrokes;
4. Technique of instinct and inspiration. (p. 266)

All of these characteristics can be seen to some degree in Monet's 1869 painting, *La Grenouillère* (Fig. 1.7).

Signac's first point is clear, although the term "pure" is not necessarily used in any perceptual sense. He seems to have meant only that the Impressionists used the most saturated pigments available. The second point, mixing on the palette and optical mixture, refers to the use of subtractive and additive color mixture, respectively. This point is also related to the fourth point, which merely refers to an unwillingness of most Impressionists to follow strict divisionist techniques associated with Pointillism and Neo-Impressionism.

With respect to Signac's third point, Monet's comma-like brushstrokes can certainly be identified in many of his paintings. His brushstrokes, however, were quite varied (Seitz, 1956). He might use dapples of paint to represent the ripple of water, or swirls to depict smoke and steam. Multi-colored periodic patterns that recede in contrast and size are used in *La Grenouillère* to show shadows shimmering on the water. Or, as in some of his water lily paintings, Monet captures shadows reflected on the water with mostly vertical lines, while the lily pads are contrasted with thick horizontal brushstrokes. These and other brushstrokes were combined with a variety of textures (Herbert, 1979) which were also quite complex, but which generally varied from coarse in the foreground to fine in the background, corresponding to the surface variations on the retinal image. At times criticized as unskilled, some of the patterns seen in his 1869 *La Grenouillère* may be considered a prelude to abstract art.

Close inspection of Monet's paintings also shows another interesting feature – the weave of his white canvases can often be seen through the background because they are not completely covered by paint. The choice of a white canvas was not accidental. Canvas was available in a variety of colors in the 19th Century, but Monet always used white (Callen, 1982). Unpainted areas provided contrasting textures, and the high reflectance of a white canvas could be exploited to capture quickly certain highlights in natural scenes by having to apply little or no paint.

Monet described still another reason for his choice of a white canvas; he said it was to establish a scale of (color) values. He studied the light intensely and is said to have attempted to understand the color of the prevailing illumination before attempting to evaluate the colors of the landscape. Our sense of illumination was later discussed by the Gestalt psychologist David Katz (1911), but it is still poorly understood.

In describing this period of his life when he and Renoir, among others, would paint together, Monet said, "It was as if a veil was torn from my eyes and I understood what painting could be" (Barnes, 1990, p. 8). Soon, however, another veil would be torn from Monet's eyes when in 1870 he and his wife, Camille, moved to London. He wanted to escape conscription in the Franco-Prussian war as did Pissarro, whom he met there. In London, Monet and Pissarro saw the works of that lone English genius, J. M.W. Turner, almost certainly one of England's most creative painters.

1.4.1 Possible Influences of Turner and Goethe

Not only Monet and Pissarro, but many of the budding Impressionists went to London to see, for example, Turner's *The Fighting Temeraire* (1838) and his *Rain, Steam and Speed* (1844). Captivated by light and color, Turner attempted to achieve in his paintings a luminosity and brightness that approached those visual experiences where light and color reach their highest levels of complexity for the painter – when light is reflected from water or seen through rain, steam and fog.

How did he do it? First of all, he seemed to grasp the difference between additive and subtractive color mixture. In many of his paintings Turner strategically placed small dots of light color so that the additive mixture provided luster and brilliance. This was about 40 years before the Impressionists would exploit this technique more fully, and some 50 years before the Neo-

Impressionists would carry it to its limit. Turner also experimented extensively with blocks of color placed side-by-side to study the ways colors influenced each other (Clark, 1960).

Despite having very little formal education, Turner painstakingly worked his way through a translation of Johann Wolfgang von Goethe's (1810) *Zur Farbenlehre* (Reynolds, 1969). To appreciate the impact of Goethe on Turner, it is necessary to describe briefly ideas of Goethe that have taken hold.

Goethe wanted to be a painter, but lacked the

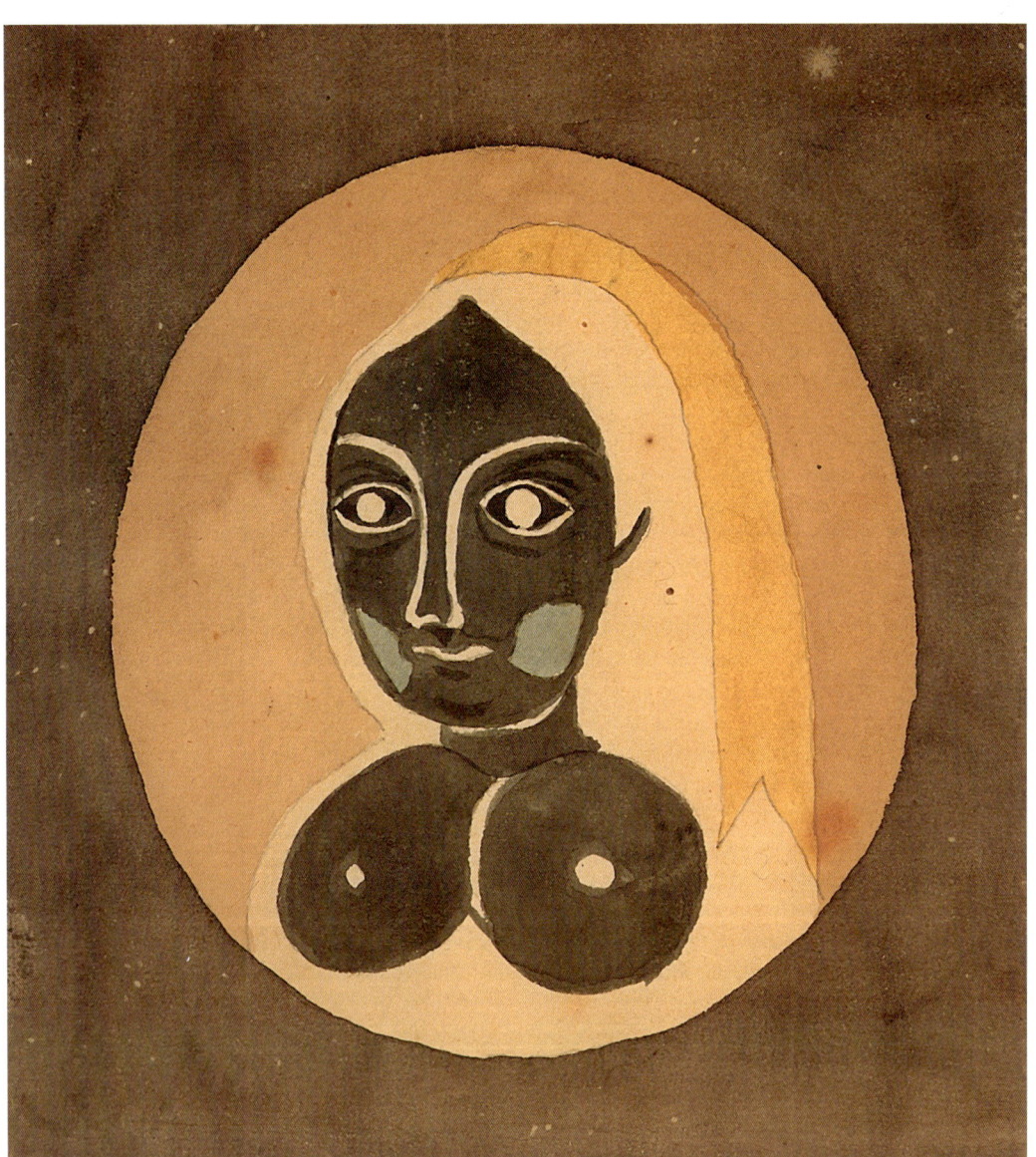

Fig. 1.8: Johann Wolfgang von Goethe (1810). *Bild eines Mädchen in umgekehrten Farben. [Picture of a Girl in Reversed Colors.]* Watercolor with penciled outlines, 15.8 × 14.6 cm. Stiftung Weimarer Klassik Museen, Weimar, Germany.

talent. Many modern scientists dismiss his *Farbenlehre* because of his polemic against Newton; history does not look kindly on attacks against Newton. Nevertheless, there is much in Goethe's book that is worthwhile, beginning with his attempt to analyze sensations independently of the stimuli that produce those sensations. His statement that "the theory of colors in strictness may be investigated quite independently of optics" (Goethe, 1810, p. 163) anticipated an oft-quoted statement by Maxwell (1872) who asserted that "the science of color must ... be regarded as essentially a mental science" (p. 261). Goethe also anticipated Hering's opponent-color theory (described below) when he indicated that there are pairs of primary colors (at least four, perhaps six) and that the paired members interact with each other antagonistically. He came to this view by careful observations of afterimages, successive contrast effects, as he describes in the following example:

> I have entered an inn toward evening, and, as a well-favoured girl, with a brilliantly fair complexion, black hair, and a scarlet bodice, came into the room, I looked attentively at her as she stood before me at some distance in half shadow. As she presently afterward turned away, I saw on the white wall, which was now before me, a black face surrounded with a bright light, while the dress of the perfectly distinct figure appeared a beautiful sea-green. (Goethe, 1810, p. 83)

Goethe painted the negative image shown in Figure 1.8 so that this "well-favoured girl" can be appreciated in all her splendor through an afterimage. To produce the afterimage, carefully fixate a salient point and hold the eyes steady for about 15 seconds; then shift your gaze to a blank field such as a neutral wall. It helps to blink when looking at the blank field. Notice that the colors of the afterimage are complementary, or approximately so, to those of the original image.

Goethe described analogous phenomena in the spatial domain based on colored shadows, a topic that would later engage Helmholtz and Hering (Hering, 1887) in heated debate. According to Goethe's illustration, shown in Figure 1.9, a surface is illuminated by a whitish light from the left and a yellowish light from the right. Each beam will be partially obstructed by the object in the center, re-

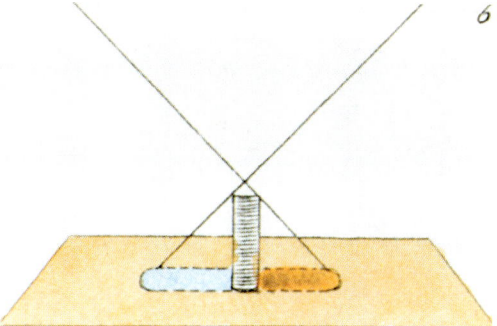

Fig. 1.9: Goethe's (Goethe, 1810) illustration of colored shadows (see text).

sulting in a shadow on either side. The shadow on the right is lacking the whitish light so, having only the yellow illumination, it appears a more saturated yellow than the surround. One might expect that the shadow on the left, lacking the yellowish light and being illuminated only by the whitish light, would appear white, but it does not. Rather, it appears bluish, that is, tinged with the opposite hue to that surrounding it. This is an example of what is more generally known as simultaneous contrast. As Goethe correctly concluded from this phenomenon, blue and yellow oppose each other not just in time, as with afterimages, but also in space.

Goethe described how perceptual principles could be exploited to good effect in painting. Turner accepted this view and used it to his advantage to exaggerate light yellow areas by surrounding them with dark blue areas. In a tribute to Goethe, he painted *Light and Colour (Goethe's Theory) – the Morning after the Deluge* (Fig. 1.10). This painting is predominantly yellow, the color that Goethe considered the first derivative of light. It stands in marked contrast to Turner's (1843) companion painting (*Shade and Darkness – the Evening of the Deluge*) which is dominated by blue, Goethe's first derivative of darkness. At this point, Turner had obviously become extremely abstract, anticipating aspects of Impressionism and Expressionism. This work is without precedent in Western Art and it is safe to say that Monet could not have seen anything remotely similar to it in Europe at the time.

Turner also became quite a profound pessimist

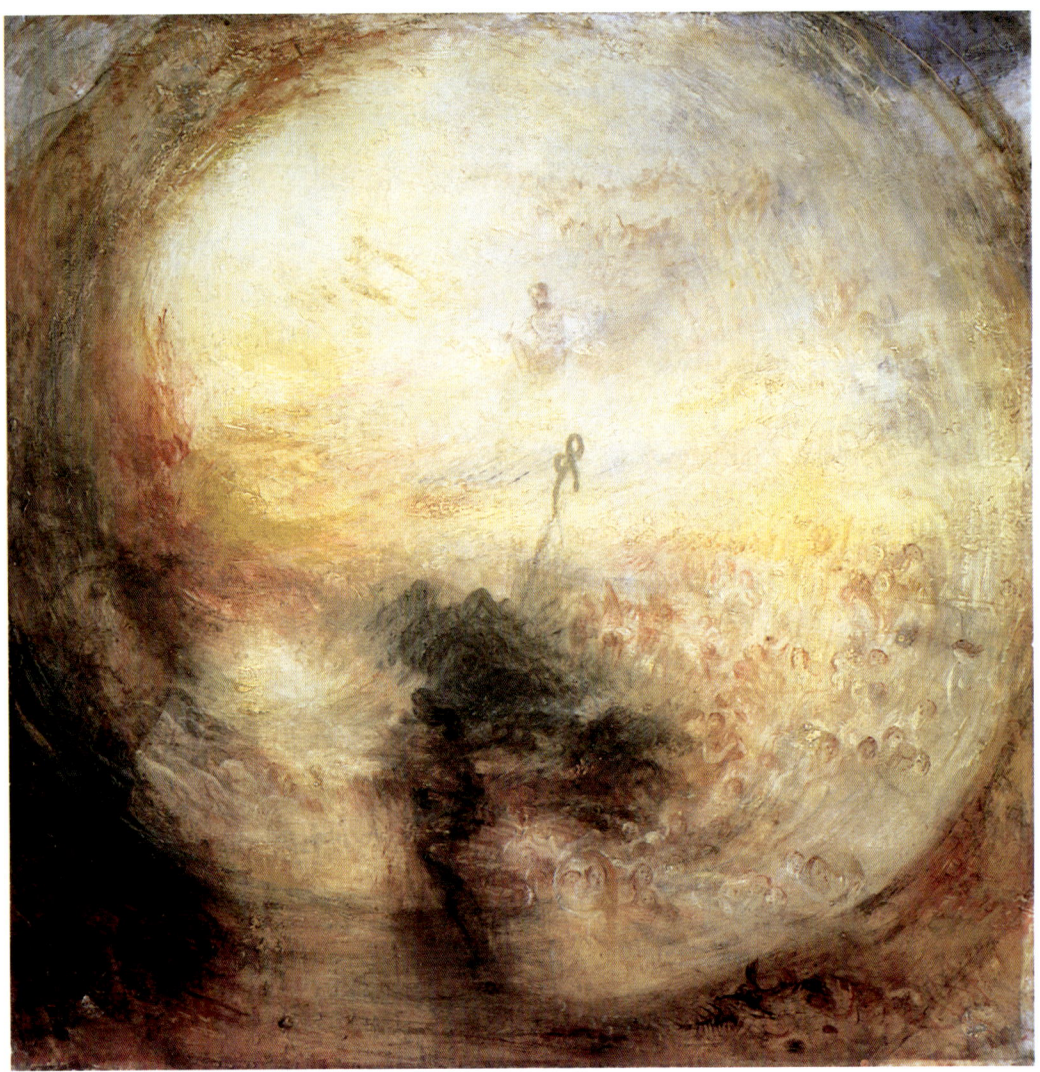

Fig. 1.10: Joseph Mallord William Turner (1843) *Light and Colour (Goethe's Theory) – the morning after the Deluge – Moses writing the Book of Genesis*. Oil on canvas, 78.8 × 78.8 cm. Tate Gallery, London.

as exemplified by the verses attached to the title of this painting taken from his poem, *The Fallacies of Hope.* He wrote: "hope, hope, where is thy market now?" This aspect of Turner would not have appealed to the Impressionists. Renoir said he simply wanted to paint pretty pictures. And Vincent van Gogh, more a Post-Impressionist, said that he hoped that their art could "give comfort, and make life possible, in the way that Christianity once did" (Russell, 1974, p. 22).

Pissarro was enthralled with Turner, and although Monet rarely commented on other paintings, he did make complimentary statements about *Rain, Steam and Speed* (interestingly, an etching of this Turner masterpiece by Félix Bracquemond was shown in the first Impressionist exhibit). Generally, however, Monet denied being much impressed by Turner and was critical of his exuberant romanticism. In truth, Paul Signac noted that the Impressionists studied Turner's work and marveled at effects that he produced that they had not been able to achieve. Signac (1921) writes:

> They were in the first place struck by his snow and ice effects. They were astonished to see how he had succeeded in producing the sensation of whiteness of the snow while they had so far been unable to achieve this with their large patches of ceruse (white lead) spread out flat with broad brushstrokes. They say that this marvelous result was obtained not by a uniform white, but by a number of touches of diverse colors, placed side by side and reconstituting the desired effect at a distance. (pp. 239–240)

Turner and Monet had much in common besides their interest in additive color mixture and color contrast effects. They were both fascinated by the changing effects of light at different times of day. John Ruskin (1843) catalogued some 60 Turner paintings according to the lighting conditions associated with various times of day, as modified by weather, atmosphere and the objects themselves. Later, Monet would illustrate the changing effects of light and atmosphere in more compelling fashion through series of paintings of the same subject. Both artists went to great extremes to observe nature. For example, Turner claimed to have tied himself to the deck of a ship to observe a raging storm at sea and was nearly killed. Monet described a similar experience. But their differences were equally compelling; while Turner depicted nature in her fury, Monet seems to have preferred her more pastoral, but elegant, simplicity.

1.4.2 Possible Influences of Chevreul and Delacroix

If Monet had been inclined to study the work of any scientist, it would probably have been Michel Eugène Chevreul rather than Goethe. Whereas an emotion-laden analysis of color appealed to Turner and Goethe, a less passionate analysis appealed to Chevreul and Monet. Chevreul was the Director of Dyes for the Gobelins tapestry works, and in that capacity he conducted detailed experiments on the interactions between threads placed side by side, either when the colored regions were small enough to mix additively or large enough to create simul- taneous contrast. These experiments are described in his 1839 book (Chevreul, 1839), *De la Loi du Contraste Simultané des Couleurs,* a book that was hailed by the Impressionists and studied by Helmholtz. Chevreul's studies of contrast culminated in a set of descriptive laws. Figure 1.11 shows one of his beautiful illustrations of how a hue induces its complement in surrounding regions, analogously to Goethe's colored shadows.

Many of Chevreul's ideas were tested on the canvas by Eugène Delacroix. Like Turner, Delacroix offended his contemporaries by his bold use of color, although it is doubtful that his paintings ever realized the luminosity of Turner's. Figure 1.12 shows his painting called *The Lion Hunt* (1860–61). The carnage in Delacroix's picture is made vivid enough by his use of saturated pigments, and perhaps it is done so well because it was said that he never missed a feeding at the Paris zoo (Clark, 1960). The Impressionists studied the work of Delacroix and seemed particularly enamored by his thoughts on simultaneous contrast, about which he is said to have remarked: "Give me the mud of the streets and I will turn it into the luscious flesh of a woman" (Signac, 1921, p. 238) [if you will allow me to surround it as I please].

If it is assumed for the moment that the "luscious flesh" that Delacroix had in mind was white, it can be shown by experiment that he was correct. Figure 1.13 presents results from an experiment (Werner and Walraven, 1982) in the CIE x,y chromaticity diagram, which represents all possible additive color mixtures. The perimeter of the diagram represents the loci of monochromatic lights and the light mixtures (between 400 and 700 nm) that enclose the space. The colored areas illustrate the approximate appearance of these light mixtures in the neutral state of adaptation (i.e., when the colors are viewed in an unilluminated surround). The subject's task in the experiment was to vary the ratio of two lights (complementary colors) until the mixture looked white. The central x shows the light mixture that appeared white without any background or surrounding light. The experiment was then repeated in the presence of various larger chromatic adapting backgrounds. The spokes connect the neutral white point and the adapting backgrounds, which were all located on the perimeter of the color dia-

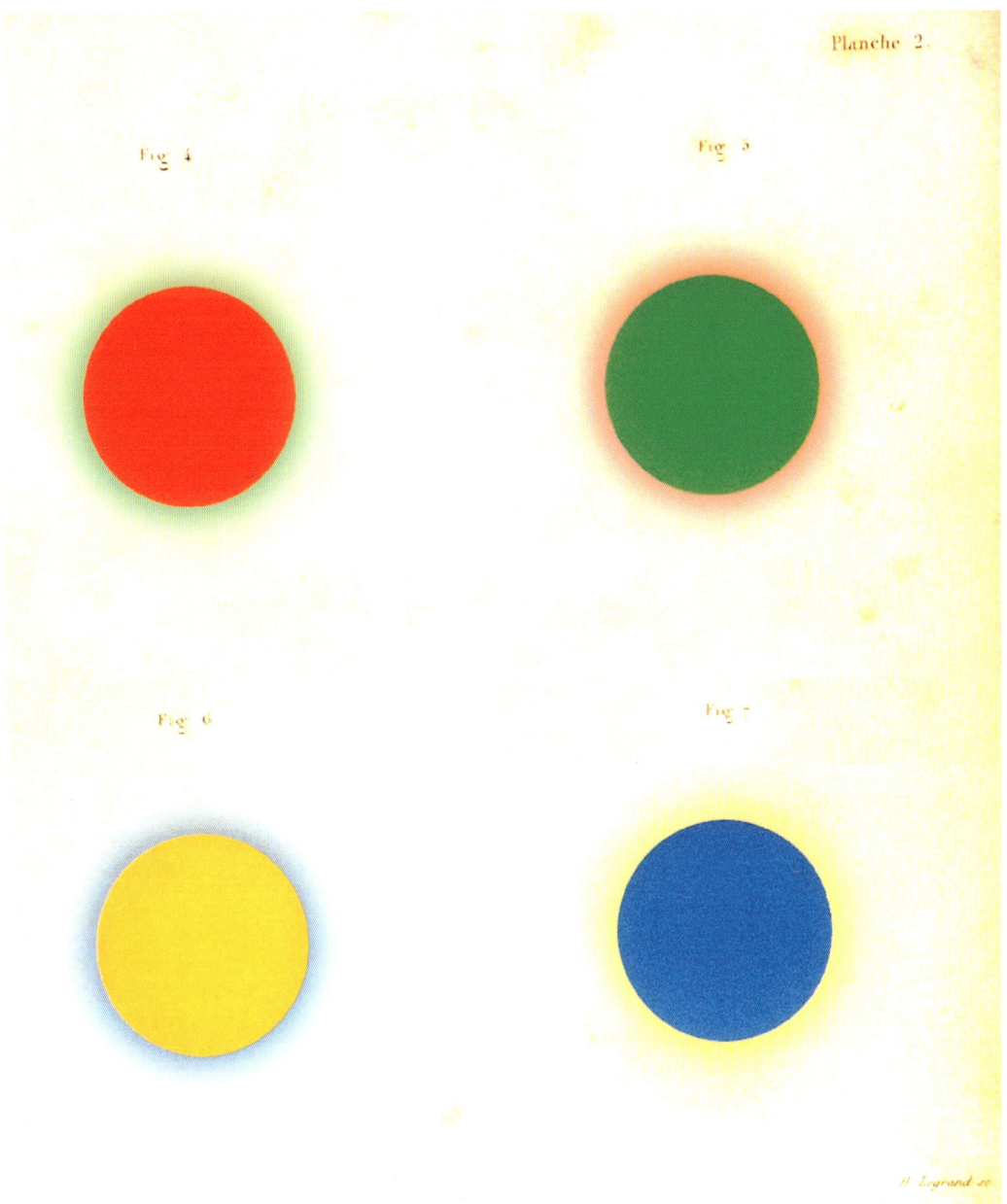

Fig. 1.11: M. E. Chevreul's (Chevreul, 1839) illustration of simultaneous hue contrast. In this figure, the colors that would normally be induced by a colored disk into a neutral surround are exaggerated by painting the surround regions. (Colors are digitally enhanced by the author to compensate for fading of the original plate.)

gram. The data points show the stimulus that looked white after adaptation to various colors and for various contrasts (i.e., intensity ratios of test and background). The dashed contours are model predictions assuming von Kries adaptation and a subtractive process; that is, separate sensitivity adjustments in each class of receptor in proportion to their activation by the background light (Werner

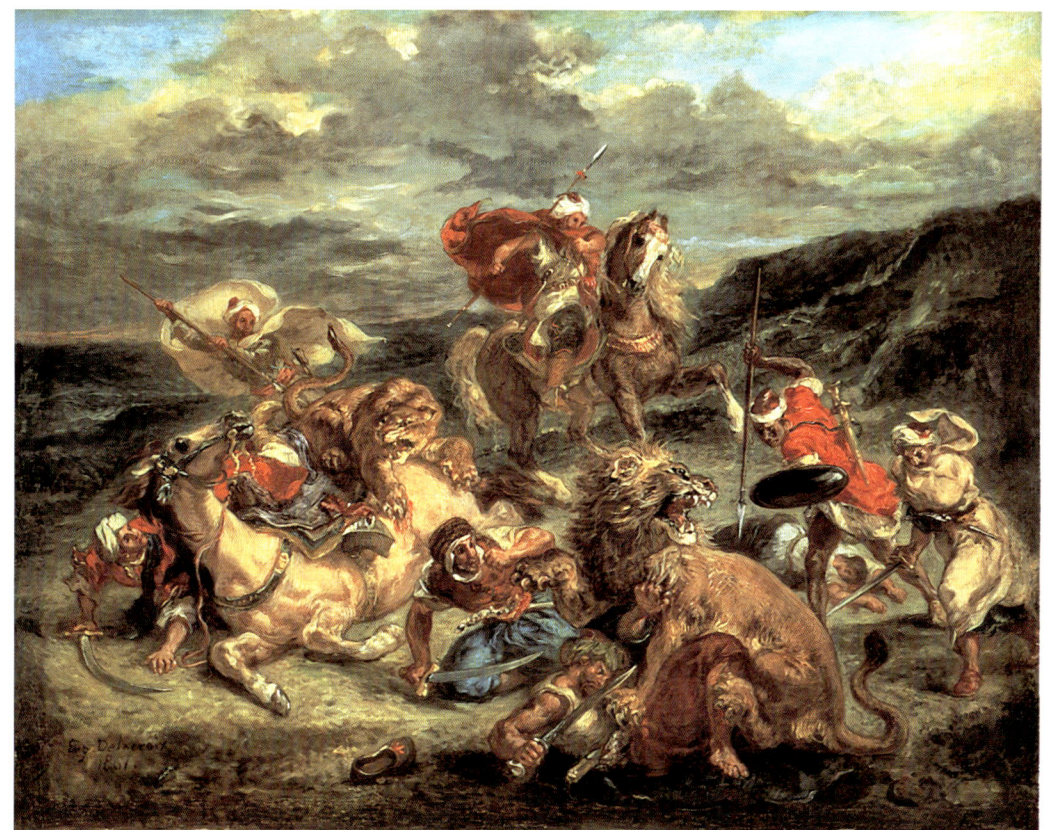

Fig. 1.12: E. Delacroix (1860/61) *La chasse aux lions. [The Lion Hunt.]* Oil on canvas, 76.5 × 98.5 cm. Potter Palmer Collection, Art Institute of Chicago. (Photograph © 1996, The Art Institute of Chicago. All rights reserved.)

and Walraven, 1982; see chapter 12). Without discussing the experimental details, one can readily appreciate that Delacroix was correct: that any light can appear white under the right conditions of contrast and adaptation.

Delacroix also advocated the use of hatchings to influence colors based on a complementary phenomenon to contrast called assimilation or the Bezold Spreading Effect (Bezold, 1874). This occurs when a background and interlaced pattern of different color fail to oppose each other as in simultaneous contrast, but seem to blend together. Figure 1.14 illustrates assimilation with four different hues that have black or white hatching superimposed; although the background hue within each panel is physically uniform, it appears different depending on whether it is interlaced with black or white.

Assimilation is still not well understood, but it is known that it cannot be explained by light scatter from one region of the image to another. When the hatching is fine relative to the diameters of individual receptors, additive light mixture occurs, but in this case the hatching itself will not be visible. If the elements in the hatching are small relative to the postreceptoral elements that sum inputs from a number of cones, assimilation may occur. When the hatching is courser, contrast typically occurs, but depends on a number of factors such as the luminance of the pattern relative to the background (de Weert and Spillmann, 1995). By varying the viewing distance of a suitable pattern, one can observe light mixture, assimilation and contrast. Thus, assimilation, although not due to optical mixture, could be due to a neural blending in some color channels

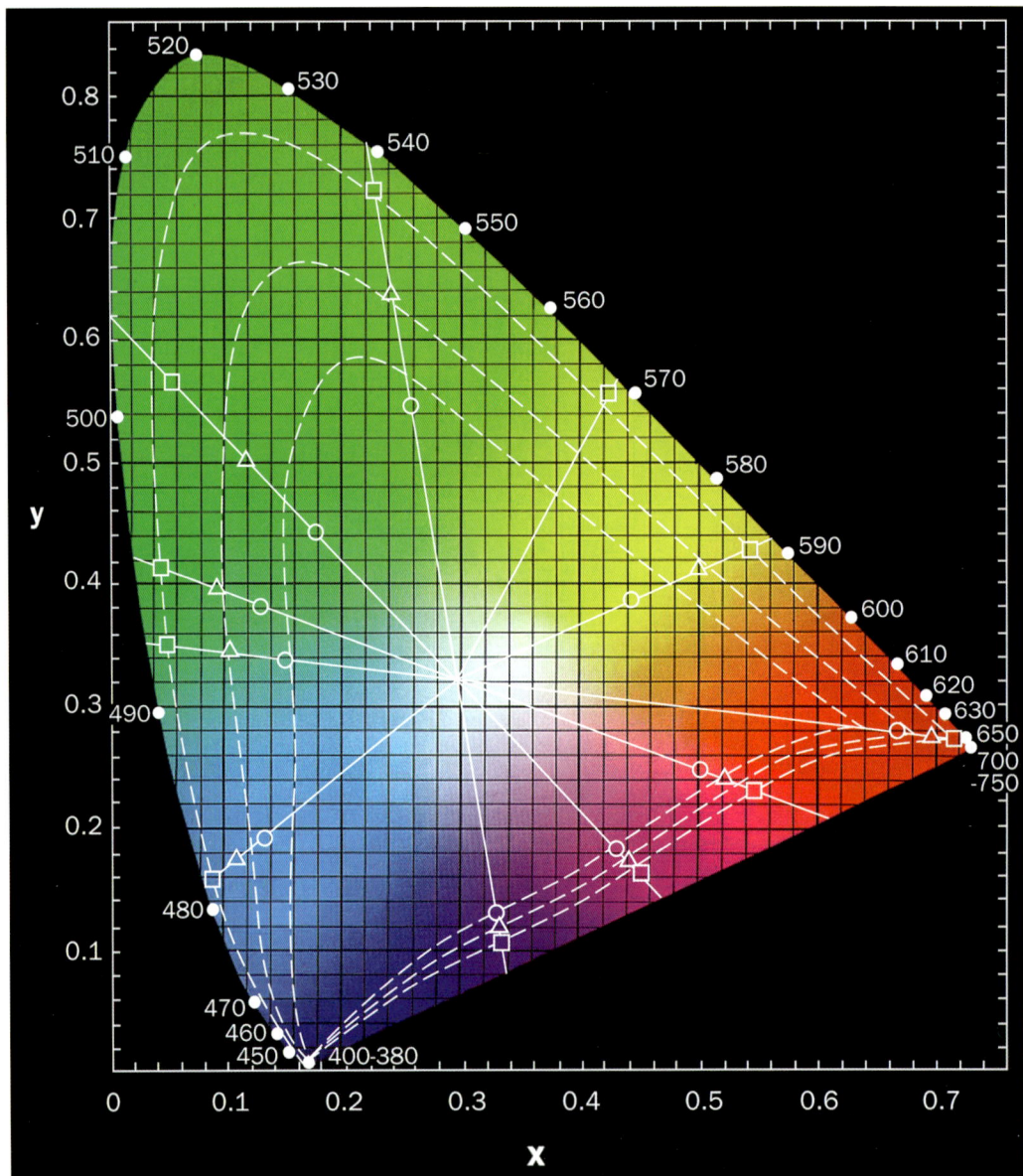

Fig. 1.13: The loci of lights that appear white under various states of adaptation presented in the CIE x,y chromaticity diagram. Colored areas within the diagram represent the approximate appearance of additive color mixtures in a neutral state of adaptation. The central x represents the light mixture that appeared white in a neutral state of adaptation for one observer, while the data points show the chromaticity of the light that appeared white following adaptation to the continuously presented chromatic backgrounds (250 Troland retinal illuminance). The backgrounds tested are all on the perimeter of the diagram and connected to the central x by lines. Squares, triangles and circles represent illuminance contrasts (test/background intensity) of 0.2, 1.0 and 5.0, respectively. (After Werner and Walraven, 1982.)

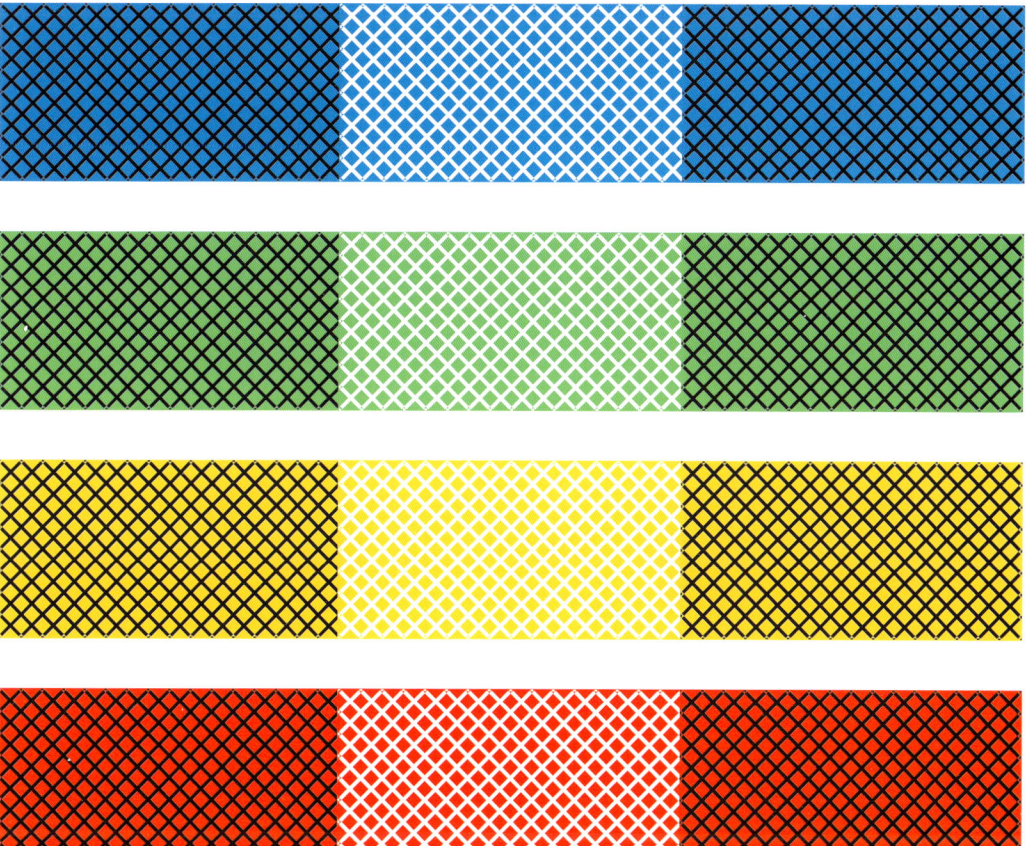

Fig. 1.14: Illustration of assimilation or the Bezold Spreading Effect. The background color is the same within a panel, but it appears darker when interlaced with black hatching compared to when it is interlaced with white hatching.

while other color channels still respond differently to the form and the background (Jameson and Hurvich, 1989). Assimilation probably occurs as much in nature as contrast, but we know much less about its physiological basis (de Weert, 1991).

It may seem from these phenomena of adaptation, assimilation and contrast that the visual system is easily fooled and subject to illusion, but the mechanisms producing these effects are what make normal color vision possible. As Hering (1920) pointed out:

"The most important consequences of reciprocal interactions are not at all those expressed in contrast phenomena, that is, in the alleged false seeing of 'real' colors of objects. On the contrary, it is precisely the so-called correct seeing of these colors that depends in its very essence on such reciprocal interactions" (pp. 123–124).

In full agreement, Monet would later say:

For me, a landscape does not exist in its own right, since its appearance changes at every moment; but its surroundings bring it to life – the air and the light which vary continually ... For me, it is only the surrounding atmosphere which gives objects their true value. (Barnes, 1990, p. 36)

Thus, while some of these phenomena of adaptation, assimilation and contrast do illustrate imperfect color constancy, they seldom lead to confusion about an object's identity based on color. More generally, they support correct identification of object color by accentuating differences between object

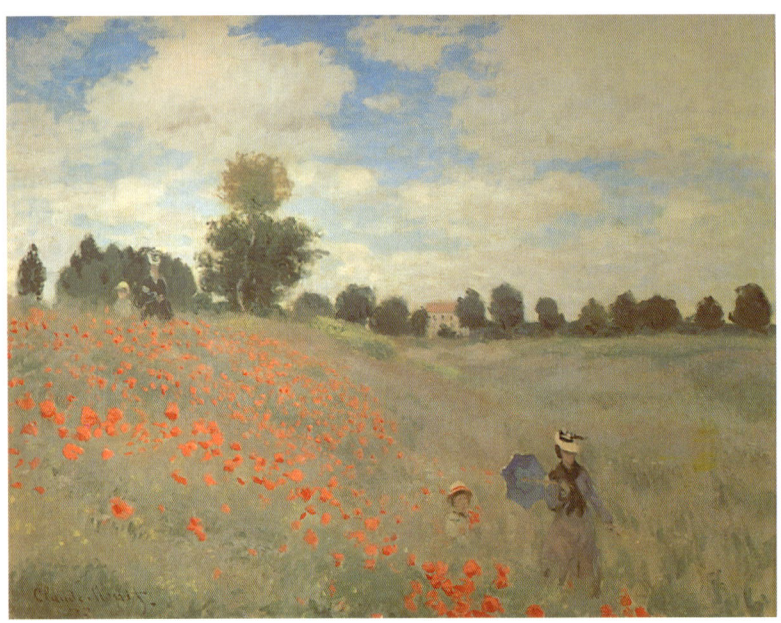

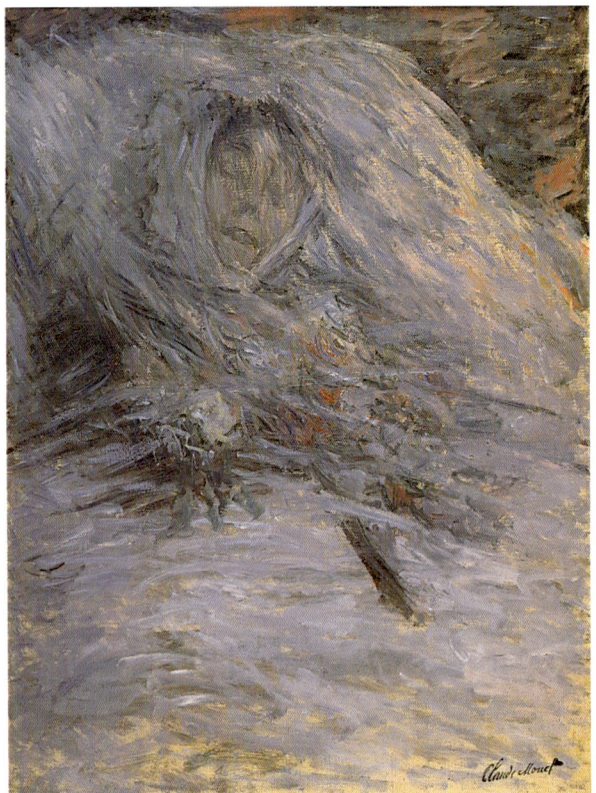

Fig. 1.15: Top: Claude Monet (1873) *Les coquelicots à Argenteuil. [Poppies at Argenteuil.]* Oil on canvas, 50 × 65 cm. Musée d'Orsay, Paris. (Photo credit: Erich Lessing/Art Resource, New York.)
Bottom: Claude Monet (1879) *Camille Monet sur son lit de Mort. [Camille Monet on her death-bed.]* Oil on canvas, 90 × 68 cm. Musée d'Orsay, Paris.

and shadow, with assimilation enhancing the uniformity of a single surface and contrast enhancing differences between figure and ground. These examples provide important probes to visual scientists for identifying properties of the visual system that are normally not apparent at all. The mechanisms mediating these effects are what keep us from being fooled most of the time about the reflectance or color of objects when the color of the illumination changes – they make color constancy possible. This refers to the experience that the colors of most objects appear to be about the same in a wide variety of lighting conditions, even though they may reflect very different spectral distributions to the eye. Color constancy would not be possible if the visual system were not able to adjust its chromatic sensitivity as illumination varies.

1.5 Monet's Years in Argenteuil and Vètheuil

Monet lived in Argenteuil and Vètheuil from 1871 to 1881. During this time he created some of the most beloved masterpieces of the Impressionist movement. Many of these paintings illustrate an idyllic country lifestyle with his wife Camille and young son Jean, such as in his painting, *The Luncheon* (1873) or the *Poppies at Argenteuil* (Fig. 1.15, top). This was a happy time for Monet – until 1879 when his wife Camille died. Out of this tragedy we gain insight into Monet's seemingly irrepressible obsession with the changing effects of color. He went so far as to portray Camille's changing coloration on her death bed (Fig. 1.15, bottom) and described his feelings as follows:

> You cannot know ... the obsession, the joy, the torment of my days. To the point that, one day, when I was at the death-bed of a lady who had been, and still was, very dear to me, I found myself staring at the tragic countenance, automatically trying to identify the sequence, the proportions of light and shade in the colors that death had imposed on the immobile face. Shades of blue, yellow, gray, and I don't know what. That's what I had become (Clemenceau, 1929, p. 350–351).

1.6 The Opponent Code for Color Appearance: Hering

During these years, Germany was developing its own Impressionist school through the wonderful paintings of Adolph Menzel, Max Liebermann, Gotthardt Kuehl and others (Düchting and Sagner-Düchting, 1993), although the most significant events from the point of view of this essay were probably being carried out in the laboratory.

Ewald Hering, Professor of Physiology in Vienna and later in Prague and Leipzig, pointed out that the Helmholtz view nicely accounted for the trivariance of color mixture, but the second part of the Helmholtz theory – that there are three fundamental hue sensations – is inconsistent with our color experience. Hering (1920) proposed that there are four elemental hues, red, green, yellow and blue, and that all hue experience is based on combinations of these elements. (For a complete account of color experience, Hering also proposed that there are two fundamental achromatic colors, black and white; see chapter 10, Shinomori et al., 1997.) He was not the first to make this proposal. It could be pointed out that Leonardo appreciated this centuries before. To which Hering replied that:

> "If one were to designate the nomenclature used ... as a four-color theory, then ... language itself would be its author, for language has long since singled out red, yellow, green and blue as the principle colors of the multiplicity of chromatic colors" (Hering, 1920, p. 48).

Hering further postulated that the hue variables are organized physiologically in antagonistic pairs that involve processes of excitation and inhibition, with the result that the sensations of red and green never occur at the same time and place, nor do the sensations of blue and yellow. He, therefore, referred to these paired colors as opponent. To explain phenomena of successive and simultaneous contrast, Hering also proposed that these physiological processes are organized in an antagonistic or opponent fashion across time and space.

Since Berlin and Kay's (1969) anthropological survey, evidence has supported the view that there are a limited number of hue names needed to describe our color experience and that they are de-

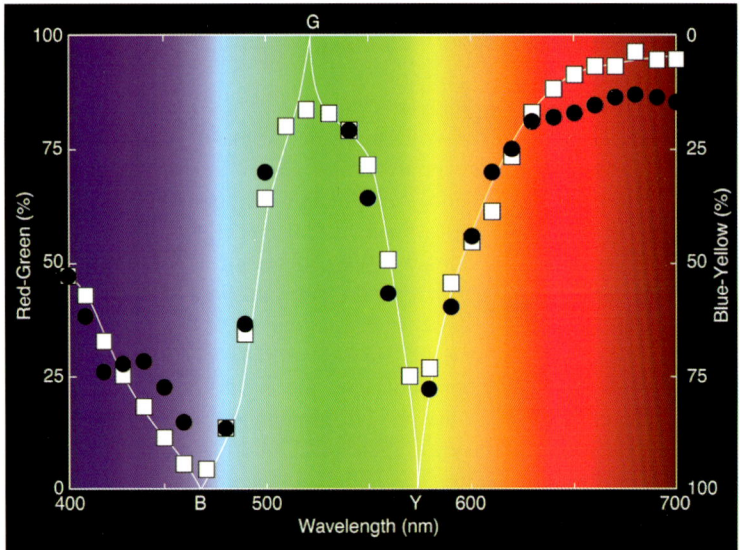

Fig. 1.16: Mean hue-naming data (white squares) and average predicted hue-naming (black circles) based on opponent-cancellation functions (Figure 1.17) for three observers plotted as a function of wavelength. Red-green is plotted from 0 to 100% on the left axis; blue-yellow is plotted from 100 to 0% on the right axis. The letters B, G, and Y denote the average wavelength of the same observers' unique hues. (After Werner and Wooten, 1979.)

pendent on the organization of neurophysiological mechanisms in the eye and brain (Ratliff, 1976). One example is shown in Figure 1.16. Observers were asked to describe lights of different wavelength using the terms red, green, yellow and blue (Werner and Wooten, 1979). Results are shown by the white squares. Red or green is plotted from 0 to 100% on the left axis, and blue or yellow is plotted in the opposite direction, from 100 to 0%, on the right axis. The data could be plotted in this way because, consistent with Hering's theory, the observers almost never used the terms red and green together or the terms blue and yellow together. The letters (B, G, Y) on the horizontal axes designate the wavelengths of the lights that were uniquely blue, green or yellow for the average of the same three persons whose hue-naming data are presented.

Jameson and Hurvich (1955) developed methods to measure psychophysically the opponent processes of Hering using a hue-cancellation task. The strength of each hue (e.g., red) was quantified by the energy of the opponent hue (e.g, green) necessary to produce an equilibrium state (e.g., neither red nor green). Hue cancellation functions presented in Figure 1.17, based on their method, show the response of the red-green and yellow-blue opponent channels as a function of wavelength. Responses of single cells of the macaque monkey at various levels of visual processing look remarkably similar to these functions (see chapter 3; Zrenner et al., 1990), and there is compelling reason to believe that these opponent processes, via cortically-rectified signals (DeValois and DeValois, 1993), are an important part of the neural network responsible for perceived hue. Figure 1.16 (circles) compares hue naming and the mean ratio of red-green to yellow-blue response at each wavelength measured by the cancellation task. The opponent responses measured by cancellation agree quite well with color naming, consistent with the idea that these opponent processes are the neural substrate of color appearance.

While some researchers, even as recently as 20 years ago, seemed to find the Hering view incompatible with the Maxwell-Helmholtz theory,

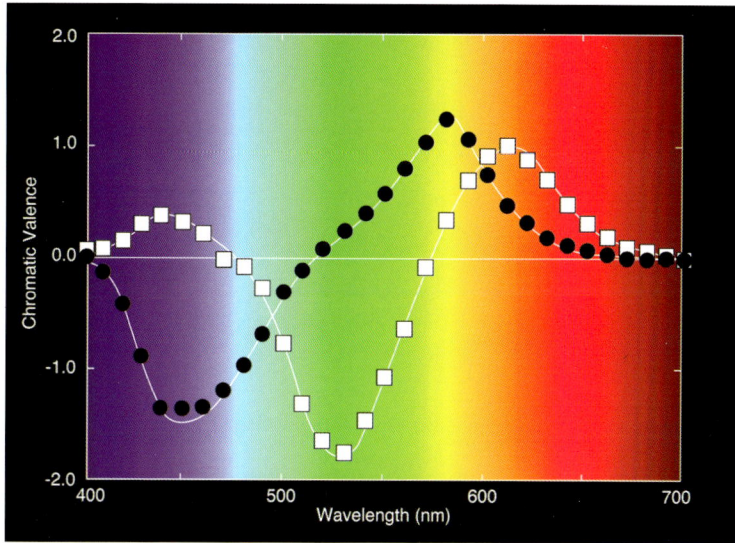

Fig. 1.17: Opponent-hue cancellation functions averaged for three observers plotted as a function of wavelength. Red-green is shown by white squares, with red plotted as positive and green as negative. Blue-yellow is shown by black circles, with blue plotted as negative and yellow as positive. (After Werner and Wooten, 1979.)

Johannes von Kries (1882), Professor of Physiology in Freiburg, put forth a zone theory before the turn of the century in which color vision begins with the activity of three classes of cone photoreceptor which is re-mapped onto the neural-opponent processes of Hering. A more modern version of such a zone model based on equations of Jameson and Hurvich (1968) is presented in Figure 1.18. It utilizes the idea that receptors activate neural processes in either an excitatory or inhibitory fashion, and different combinations of all three receptors produce the two opponent-chromatic processes. The direct connections between receptors and opponent mechanisms shown in Figure 1.18 are a considerable oversimplification to illustrate functional relations. Anatomical and physiological studies have demonstrated numerous interactions between cells at various levels between the photoreceptors and higher-level color mechanisms. It should also be noted that more complex non-linear models are required to describe some aspects of color perception, even though the linear equations used in Figure 1.18 provide an excellent first-order description of cancellation functions.

The data on age-related changes in color vision presented so far have dealt only with the first zone (i.e., photoreceptors), but there might also be age-related changes in the later stages of color processing. Schefrin and Werner (1990) measured the balance points of the opponent mechanisms (that is, the spectral unique hues) in 50 observers ranging in age from 13 to 74 years. Of particular interest are the loci of unique blue and unique yellow, because they can be described under many conditions by a linear model and will, therefore, be unaffected by age-related losses in light intensity associated with lenticular senescence. The results show that there is no significant change in the wavelength of these unique hues over this wide age range. That these results reflect a more general pattern of stability in color perception across the life span was confirmed in a color-naming experiment using more naturalistic, broad-band surfaces, color chips from the Uniform Color Samples of the Optical Society of America (Schefrin and Werner, 1993). Not only did young and old use the same words to describe hues, but they did not differ significantly in the proportions of different

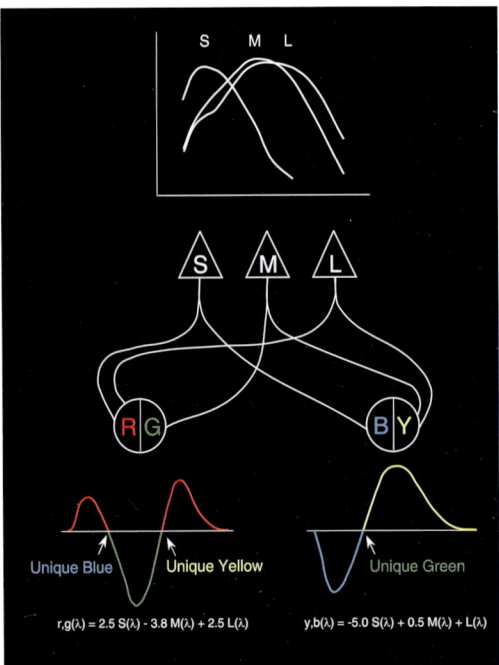

Fig. 1.18: A modern version of von Kries's 1882 zone theory (Kries, 1882), based on the equations of Jameson and Hurvich (1968) linking the activity of the three classes of cone photoreceptors (S, M and L) to red-green (left) and yellow-blue (right) opponent mechanisms as a function of wavelength from 400 to 700 nm. The shapes of the opponent-response functions depend on the sign (+ or -, corresponding to neural excitation or inhibition) of the signals from the cones and their neural weights. The parameters (specified in terms of quanta at the cornea) and equations used to generate the functions are shown at the bottom.

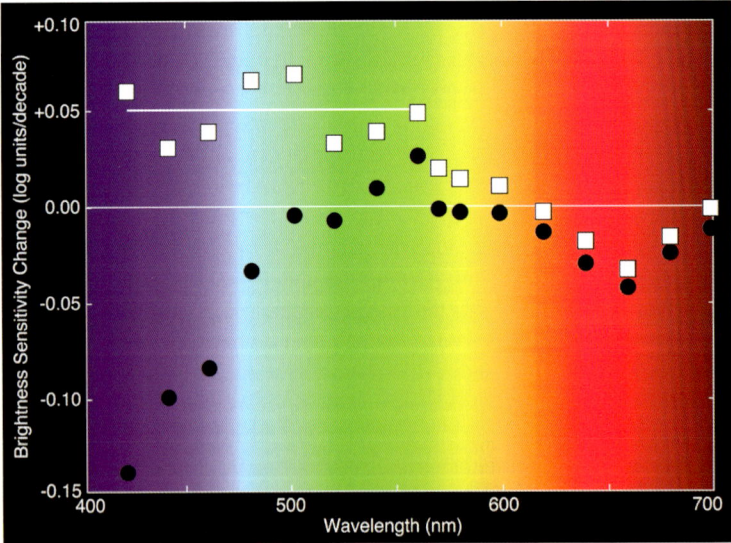

Fig. 1.19: Heterochromatic brightness sensitivity change per decade is plotted as a function of wavelength at the cornea (black circles) and at the retina (white squares). The horizontal line at zero denotes no age-related change. The thicker horizontal line at +0.05 shows the mean increase in brightnesss sensitivity per decade between 420 and 560 nm. (After Kraft and Werner, 1994.)

hues needed to describe the stimuli. Similarly, when asked to describe the percentage of chromatic and achromatic components of spectral lights (Kraft and Werner, 1997), and when asked to find a mixture of unique blue and yellow that appeared white (Werner and Schefrin, 1993), young and old did not differ significantly.

These results demonstrate a surprising degree of stability in color perception across the life span, even though age-related changes in the lens alter the spectral distribution of light reaching the retina. This would seem to be possible only if the visual system compensates for or adapts to those changes in retinal illumination that occur with lenticular senescence. Clear evidence for this compensation was found in a study by Kraft and Werner (1994) of the brightness of monochromatic lights for 50 observers ranging in age from 19 to 85 years. Each monchromatic light (420–700 nm; 16 wavelengths) was matched in brightness to a white standard. In the same individuals, the density of the ocular media was estimated so that brightness sensitivity could be *specified at the retina,* as shown in Figure 1.19 (white squares). On average, brightness sensitivity at middle and long-wavelengths does not change significantly, but at short wavelengths it actually *increases* with age. This increase occurs only at the retina, and under natural conditions it is not enough to eliminate some brightness loss (at the cornea) for violet lights in the elderly. However, across 6 decades it implies a doubling of brightness sensitivity, which goes a long way toward restoring constancy that would otherwise be disrupted by the yellowing of the lens.

1.7 Monet's Response to Pointillism and Divisionism

In the eighth Impressionist exhibit in 1886, Georges Seurat showed how the Neo-Impressionists would take the next step in applying the color science of the time to painting. His (1884) *A Sunday Afternoon on the Island of the Grand Jatte* (Fig. 1.20) is one of the most celebrated examples of the technique of Pointillism. The technique is, in principle, not different from that used by Turner, although in practice it was an extraordinary leap from Turner because the points were applied by Seurat in a much more systematic and consistent manner. Seurat had studied all the color science available to him including work by Chevreul and Helmholtz. His masterpiece includes dots of varying sizes to achieve the Pointillist goal of increasing the luminosity of paintings by placing small dots of pure color side-by-side to produce an optical mixture in the eye or to achieve strong hue contrasts with larger dots.

Pissarro, van Gogh and Matisse tried their hand at Pointillism but were not satisfied and soon abandoned the technique. Their disillusionment was due, in part, to the fact that the appearance of a Pointillist painting depends so critically on the viewing distance. At some distances, the paintings do not have the brilliant hues intended, but just the opposite – the hues appear drab and desaturated. Even Seurat's (1887–88) *Les Poseuses,* with its tiny dots, is a disappointment in this regard (Ratliff, 1992). Interestingly, the mechanism that underlies the success of the Pointillist technique as an art form also underlies its limitations. The problem arises because the signals from cone photoreceptors are integrated in the visual pathways to form receptive fields, areas of the retina that activate a particular cell by excitation or inhibition, depending on where the light falls within the receptive field (Wiesel and Hubel, 1966), as illustrated by Figure 1.21. The three-dimensional profile on the left illustrates the response increase when stimulated by green in the receptive field center and the inhibition by red in its surround. The other cell shown has a blue-yellow, antagonistic center-surround organization. These receptive field profiles are spatial filters for color processing, modeled here as the difference of two Gaussian functions, one representing the distribution of excitation and a second, having lower amplitude but broader area, representing the distribution of inhibition. Many individual cells can be modeled in this way, although their responses often do not follow the perceptual red-green or blue-yellow axes (Lennie and D'Zmura, 1988). Nevertheless, the combined activity of many such cells having overlapping receptive fields appears to result in a network that forms

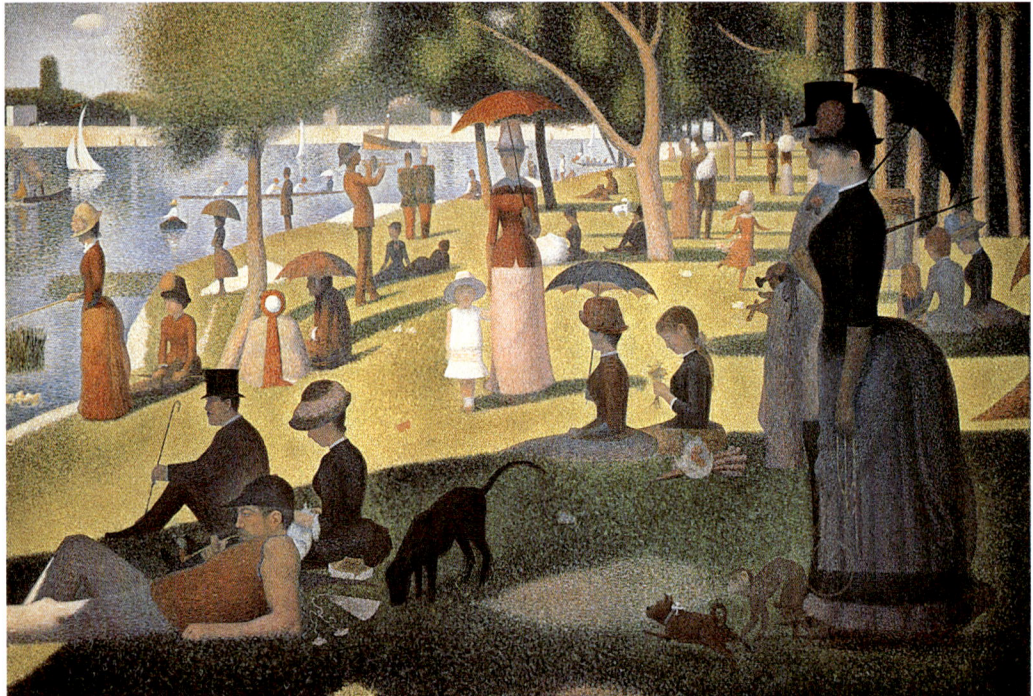

Fig. 1.20: Georges Seurat (1884) *Un Dimanche après-midi à Ile de La Grande-Jatte. [A Sunday Afternoon on the Island of the Grand Jatte.]* Oil on canvas, 207.5 × 308 cm. Helen Birch Bartlett Memorial Collection, Art Institute of Chicago. (Photograph © 1996, The Art Institute of Chicago. All rights reserved.)

a mosaic consistent with Figure 1.21. Such receptive fields provide the kind of mechanism required to explain the spatial-chromatic opponency described by Hering (1920). Of course, each individual receptive field will produce a response only to stimulation by an edge, but if the entire receptive field is uniformly illuminated by a particular color it will not respond. These receptive fields help to explain hue contrast at borders, but not the induction of hue across large areas of the visual field such as observed with Goethe's colored shadows. How an entire area is filled-in perceptually with a uniform hue is not clear, although a number of neurophysiological hypotheses involving propagation across cortical regions beyond the area of the classical receptive field have been described (Spillmann and Werner, 1996).

Consider the consequences of this kind of neural organization for how we perceive a Pointillist painting. Suppose an artist places small dots of paint, say a blue and yellow dot, side-by-side. If the dots, at a particular viewing distance, are small enough to approach the size of individual cone receptors, additive color mixture would be expected and the region would appear achromatic. If the dots were somewhat larger, but small enough so that the yellow and blue fell within the excitatory and inhibitory regions of the receptive field, respectively, they would likely cancel each other's effects, rather than produce contrast. The result would be an achromatic color. Notice that in this case, the effect is similar to additive color mixture, but it is really a neural mixture that depends on the size of the areas over which information is summed in the visual pathways. Whether small dabs of paint produce cancellation, contrast or assimilation depends upon the "fit" between the size of the dots imaged on the retina (and hence the viewing distance) and the size of the receptive fields. Receptive fields are known to increase in size with retinal eccentricity, although there is a range of receptive field sizes representing each re-

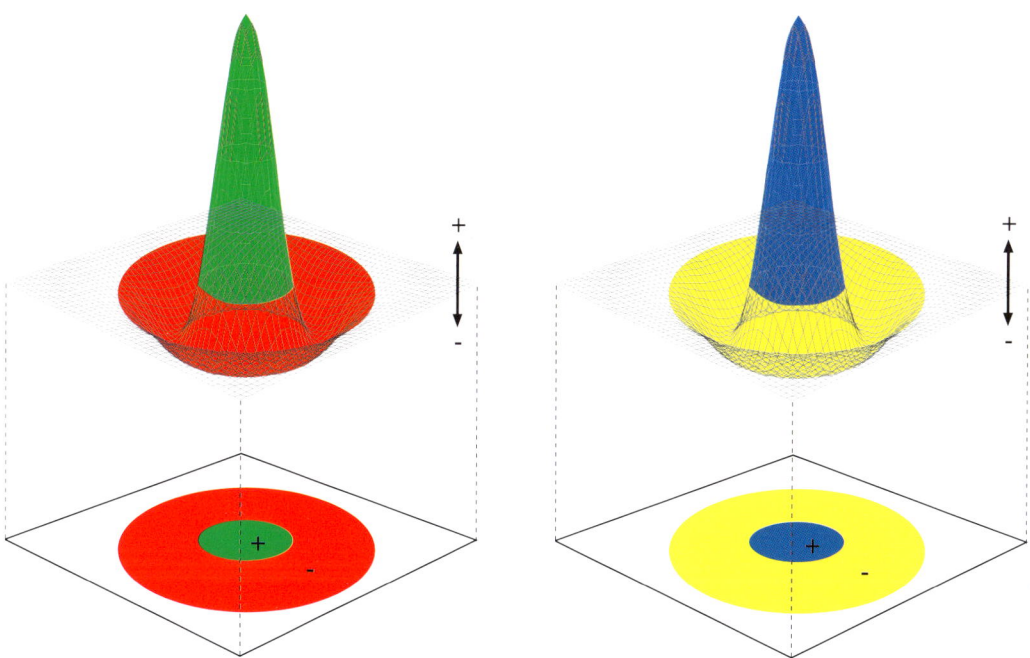

Fig. 1.21: Receptive field profiles for red-green and blue-yellow cells. These cells have an antagonistic center-surround spatial organization such that one color in the center produces excitation and the opponent color in the surround produces inhibition.

gion of the visual field. The Neo-Impressionists did not know about receptive fields, but certainly knew about the perceptual phenomena that they produce. At just the right distance, the receptive fields will be activated to produce the additive mixtures and contrasts intended by the artist. How does one know what that distance is? In noting that the brilliance of Pointillist paintings depended on the viewing distance, Pissarro suggested the general rule that a Pointillist painting be viewed at a distance that is three times the diagonal. Of course, this advice only makes sense if the size of the dots has a fixed relation to the size of the painting as a whole (Weale, 1971) - which was apparently not always the case.

Paul Signac emphasized that the best technique practiced by Neo-Impressionists was "Divisionism" not "Pointillism," by which he meant that the paint should be applied with small distinctive strokes, not tiny points. Signac wrote: "The Neo-Impressionist does not paint with dots, he divides" (1921, p. 207). It is difficult to see how this solves the problem; rather, it only defines a new set of distances at which one has hue cancellation vs. contrast. Perhaps anticipating this rejoinder, Signac referred to Rembrandt:

"A painting is not to be sniffed," said Rembrandt. When listening to a symphony, one does not sit in the midst of the brass, but in the place where the sounds of the different instruments blend into the harmony desired by the composer. Afterwards one can enjoy dissecting the score, note by note, and so study the manner of orchestration. Likewise, when viewing a divided painting, one should first stand far enough away to obtain the impression as a whole, and then come closer in order to study the interplay of the colored elements, supposing that these technical details are of interest. (Signac, 1921, p. 264).

In the meantime, Monet tried other approaches that used elements of Divisionism, but without a rigid application of the technique. One example is shown in Figure 1.22, *Bend in the Epte River near*

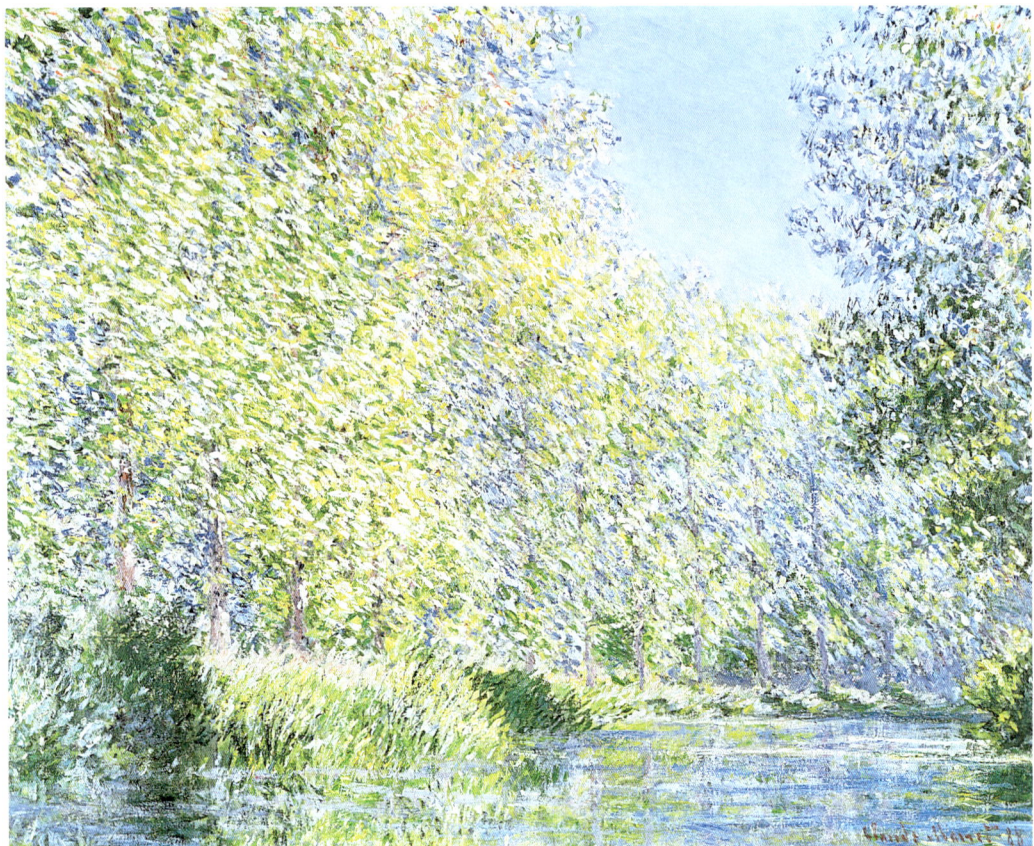

Fig. 1.22: Claude Monet (1888) *Un Tournant de l'Epte. [Bend in the Epte River near Giverny.]* Oil on canvas, 74 × 93 cm. Philadelphia Museum of Art: The William L. Elkins Collection.

Giverny (1888). The foliage of the trees follows very much the style of Seurat, but it is set apart from the water and sky which maintain his comma-like strokes. The result is just as luminous as the Pointillist and Divisionist attempts, but seems altogether more spontaneous and natural.

1.8 Hay Stack and Cathedral Series

By 1890, at the age of 50, Monet had reached a high standing in the art world and had found financial security. He rebuilt an old farmhouse in Giverny and employed six gardeners to indulge his love of horticulture and flowers. It was a magnificent site which he captured in numerous paintings. Glorious though his gardens were, Monet also illustrated the subtle undulations of light and color in more mundane spots such as in the hay stacks behind his house. There he painted a series of canvases capturing different conditions of light, atmosphere and weather. His approach was methodical; rising early in the morning even in the depth of winter, he caught the first glimpse of sunrise at his chosen location, typically rested at midday and then returned to catch the setting sun.

Figure 1.23 shows how splendidly Monet captures the light in the hay stacks. On the top, the morning light falls upon the snow, and the yellow hay stacks are surrounded with the blue colored shadows described by Goethe. On the bottom, Monet shows a greenish shadow induced by the reddish color of the

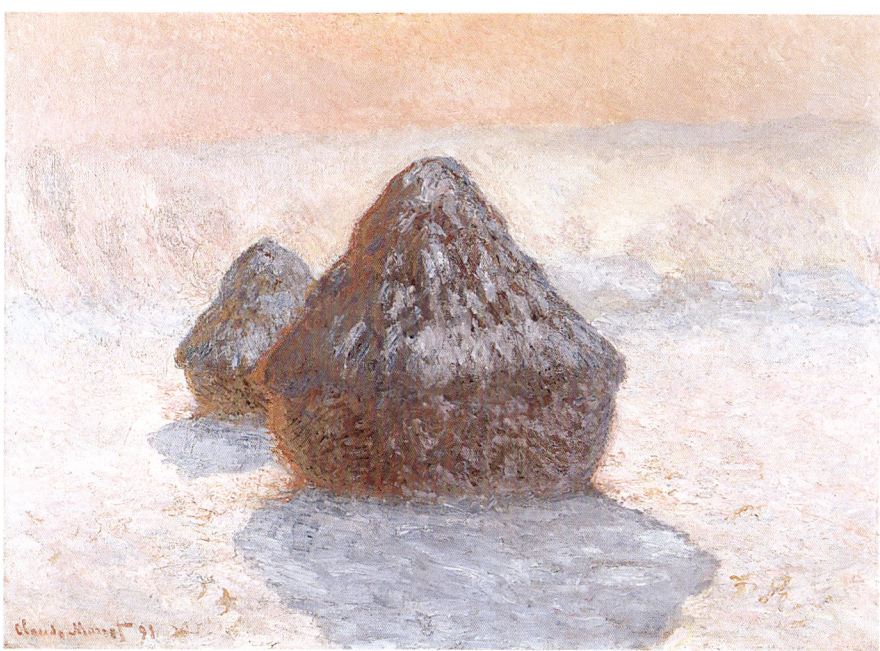

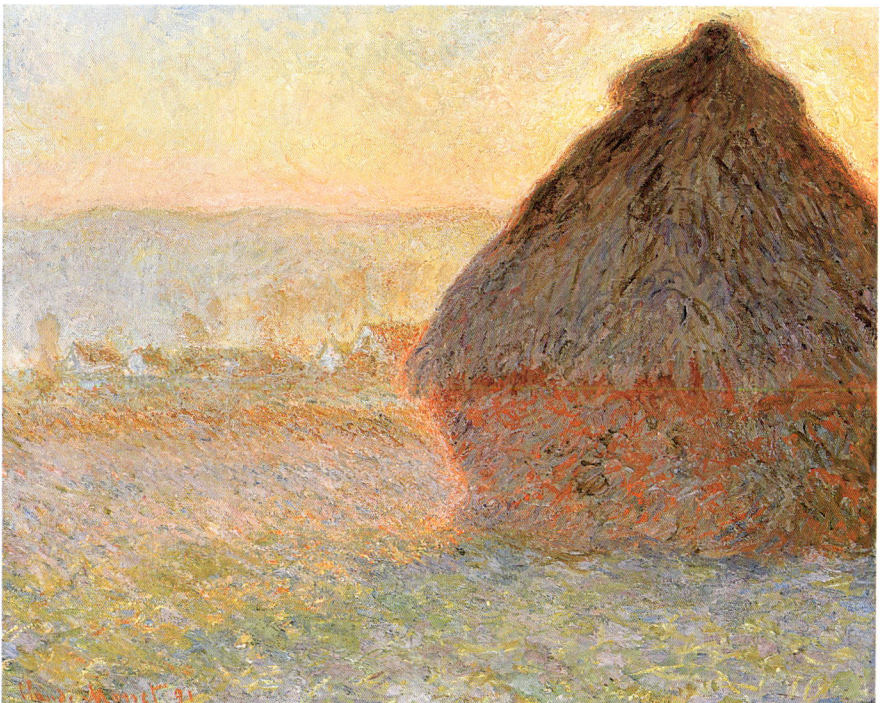

Fig. 1.23: Top: Claude Monet (1891) *Meules, Effet de Gelée Blanche. [Hay Stacks. Snow Effect. Sunshine.]* Oil on canvas 65 × 92 cm. National Gallery of Scotland, Edinburgh.
Bottom: Claude Monet (1890–91) *Meule, Soleil couchant. [Hay Stack. (Sunset).]* Oil on canvas, 73.3 × 92.6 cm. Juliana Cheney Edwards Collection, Museum of Fine Arts, Boston.

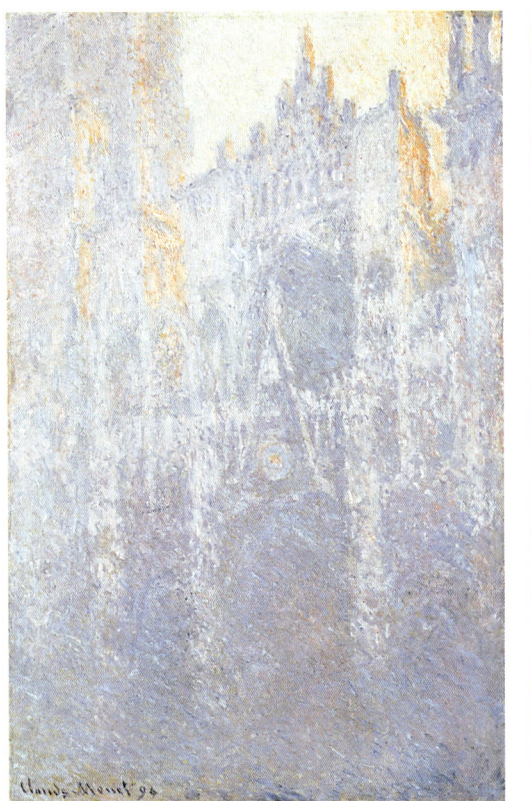 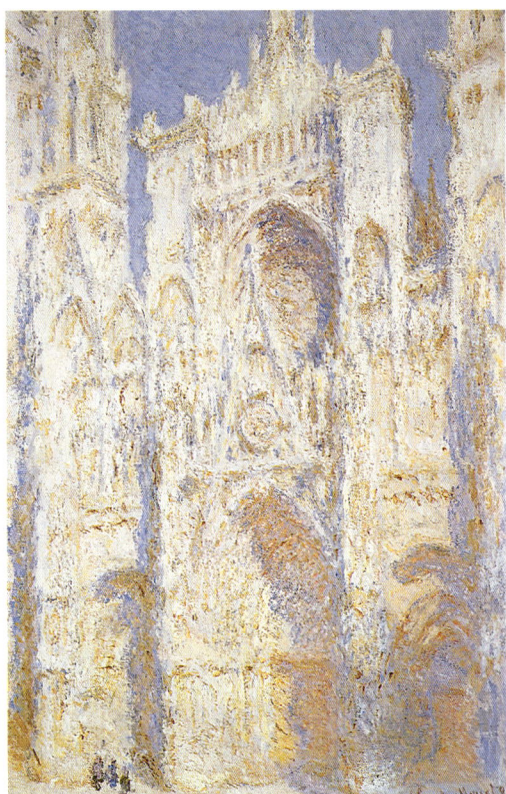

Fig. 1.24: Left: Claude Monet (1894) *Le portail, brouillard matinal. [Rouen Cathedral: The Portal (Early Morning).]* Oil on canvas, 100 × 65 cm. Museum Folkwang, Essen.
Right: Claude Monet (1894) *Le portail (soleil). [Rouen Cathedral: The Portal (Early Afternoon).]* Oil on canvas, 100 × 65 cm. Board of Trustees's, National Gallery of Art, Washington.

hay stack in the late afternoon sun. We now regard this simultaneous contrast effect, exaggerated by Monet on the canvas, as due to the reciprocal neural-opponent responses across the visual field.

Monet's hay stack series includes more than 30 canvases, from different vantage points and distances, and in different lighting. In order to depict fugitive effects, he worked on as many as seven canvases simultaneously, apparently dashing from one to another as the light would change. The canvases would then be taken to the studio and placed side-by-side for retouching. The series was intended to be displayed together. That the subject matter is monotonous and uninspiring to many people is beside the point. Monet said: "I was trying to do the impossible ... to paint light itself" (Myers, 1990, p. 92).

Monet painted several other series, including the Gare St. Lazare, the Seine near Giverny and various scenes from his gardens. In the cold winter of 1892, the 52-year-old Monet rented a large room directly across from the Cathedral of Notre Dame in the nearby city of Rouen. For the first time, he would paint an outdoor scene from indoors. Unlike many cathedrals, there was little space to afford an unobstructed vantage point so we see the cathedral facade cropped (Fig. 1.24), due apparently to the restricted view through the window. Monet was apparently frustrated, not so much from the view, but from what he was trying to accomplish. No other paintings occupied so much of his time.

He left Rouen after the winter and returned again the next year, but still failed to complete his project until he returned home and painted from memory. In all, he managed 30 canvases which he placed side-by-side in his studio to finish. They all are signed 1894, the year of their completion. Once again, the content of the series is not particularly critical to Monet (cf., Pissarro, 1990). Each canvas represents a moment in time associated with different light and atmosphere. In Figure 1.24, the painting on the left represents early morning, and the sun can be seen gently breaking through the mist near the spires while the light is occluded nearer the ground. On the right, it is afternoon, and the entire facade basks in the sunlight. The shadows are created with sculpted mounds of paint, whereas the bright areas include patches where the canvas is not completely covered.

If Monet had wanted to represent the physical situation accurately he would have had to make the afternoon scene reflect several thousand times more light to the eye compared to the canvas depicting the morning scene. He could not have done that, but he didn't need to because our visual system is remarkably insensitive to ambient light level over a large range. How, then, does his painting convey the obvious impression that the afternoon scene is much brighter than the morning scene when there is relatively little difference between the two paintings in their average light reflectance?

Monet seems to have discovered another fundamental characteristic of the visual system. As the overall light level increases, so does the perceived contrast - yellows and blues become more yellow or blue, blacks become blacker and whites become whiter. The loss of sensitivity to absolute light level may result largely from sensitivity adjustments of the cone pathways, but the changes in contrast require an explanation at a neural level in the opponent pathways (Jameson and Hurvich, 1975).

1.9 Monet Returns to London

In the fall of 1899, Monet traveled back to London. From the Savoy Hotel and St. Thomas's Hospital he would paint Waterloo Bridge and the Houses of Parliament. He made several trips over the next five years, during which he completed more than 100 canvases (Tucker, 1995). It is interesting to compare his *Boats on the Thames* in 1871 with his *Houses of Parliament* painted 30 years later (Fig. 1.25). The atmosphere in the latter is richer, as we see the fiery sun barely penetrating the dense clouds. Indeed, the pageant of colors in many canvases from this series anticipated Fauvism. It is almost as though Monet is now challenging Turner on his own turf, as Turner had once done with the great French landscapist, Claude Lorrain. Turner not only copied some of Lorrain's paintings, but insisted in his bequest to the National Gallery that his copies hang next to Lorrain's originals for comparison, a request that is still honored. Some critics pointed out that now Monet's paintings should be hung next to Turner's, calling them both great Impressionists worthy of comparison (Gage, 1972).

1.10 Water Lilies and Cataracts

Monet's final motif, which occupied him for well over 25 years, was based on his garden at Giverny, particularly his water lilies and his Japanese-style bridge. The bridge on the top in Figure 1.26 was painted in 1899 and the one on the bottom about 20 years later. What was the basis for the enormous difference? In the intervening years, Monet's cataracts had matured. One sees not only a shift in colors from blues and greens to yellows and browns, but also less distinct forms on the bottom painting, no doubt due to the scattering of light caused by his cataracts. This is an optical effect that neural processes previously described cannot compensate.

Although the onset of his visual loss was gradual, he seems not to have remarked about it until about 1908, at age 68. Four years later, a Paris doctor confirmed the diagnosis of bilateral cataracts made by Monet's country physician. As his cataracts became worse, he found it impossible to paint in bright light or to depict scenes with bright backgrounds – again, to be sure, due to the scattering of light and the concomitant degradation of the retinal image.

Despite his poor vision, Monet pursued his dream of many years to create vast canvases that

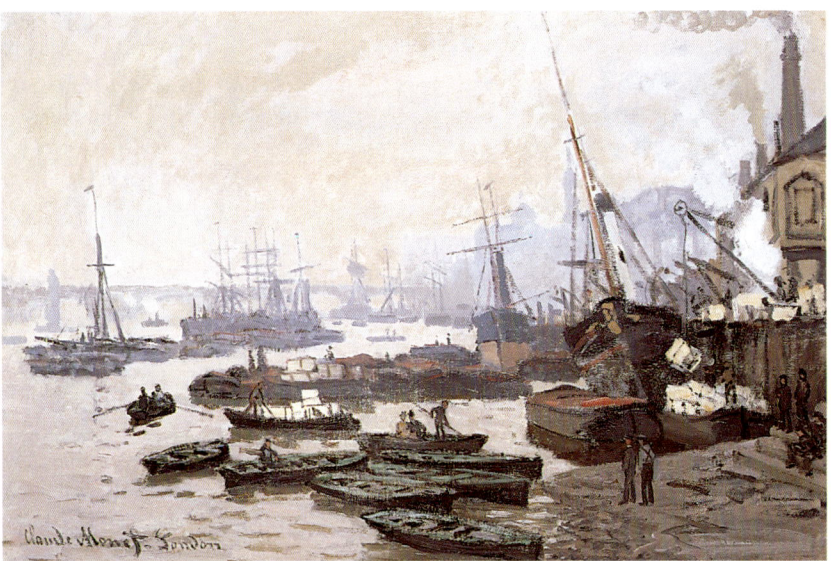

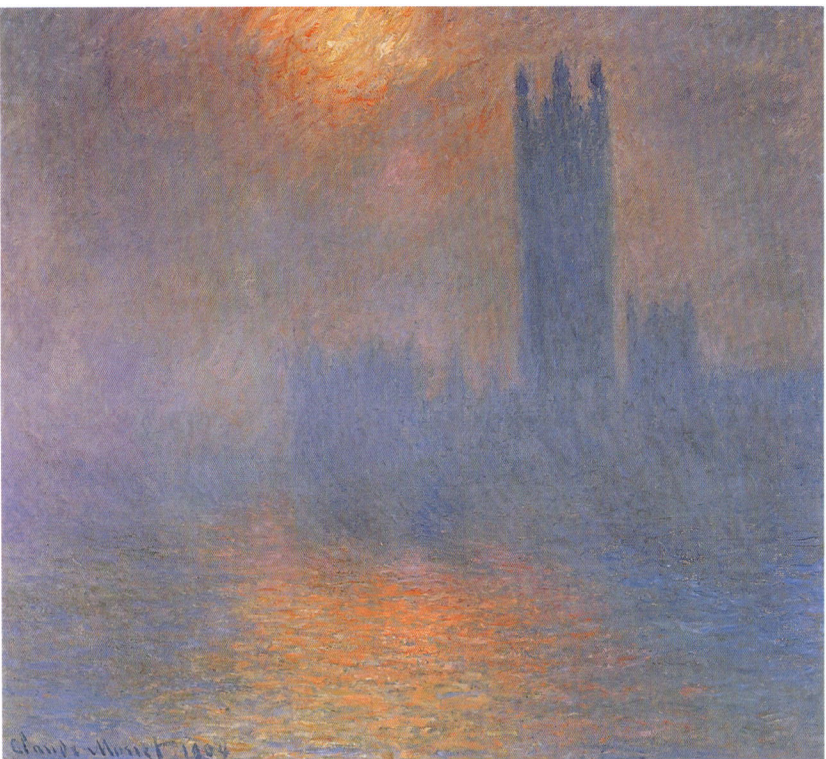

Fig. 1.25: Top: Claude Monet (1871) *Bateaux dans le Bassin de Londres. [Boats on the Thames, London.]* Oil on canvas, 47 × 72 cm. Private Collection, Monte Carlo.
Bottom: Claude Monet (1904) *Londres, le Parlement, Trouée de soleil dans le brouillard. [Houses of Parliament (Rays of Sun in the Fog).]* Oil on canvas, 81 × 92 cm. Musée d'Orsay, Paris.

1.10 Water Lilies and Cataracts 35

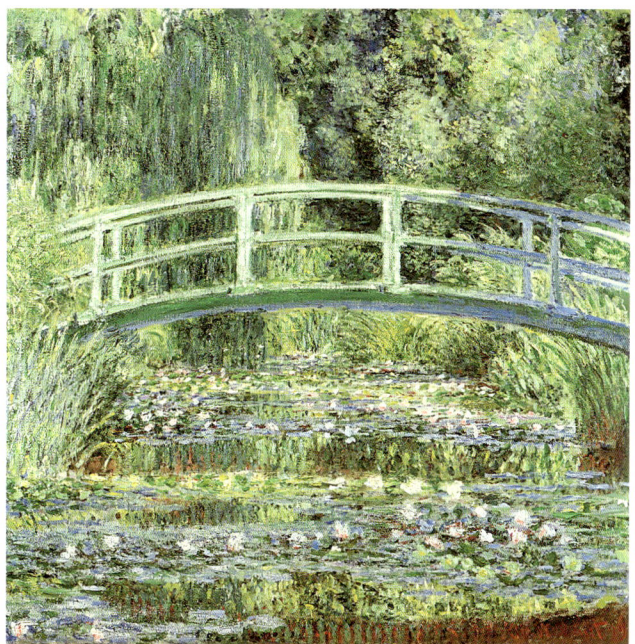

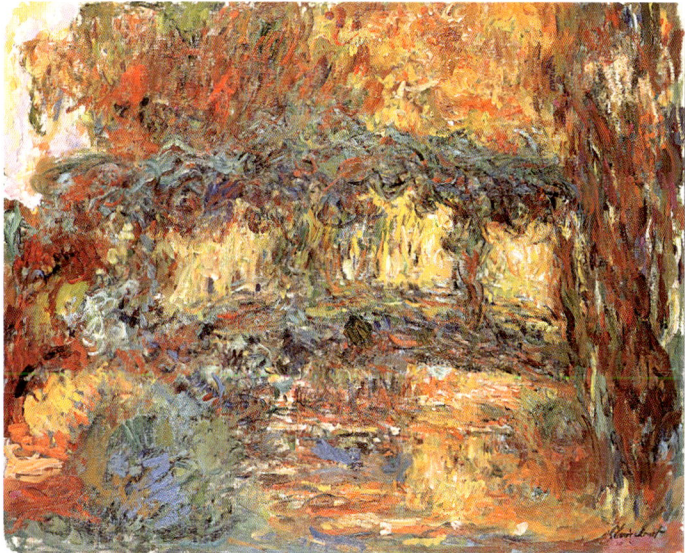

Fig. 1.26: Top: Claude Monet (1899) *Le bassin aux nymphéas. [Water-lillies and Japanese Bridge.]* Oil on canvas, 91 × 90 cm. The Art Museum, Princeton University. From the Collection of William Church Osborn, Trustee of Princeton University (1914–1951), President of the Metropolitan Museum of Art (1941–1947); given by his family. (Photo credit: Clem Fiori.)
Bottom: Claude Monet (1918–22) *Nymphéas: Le pont Japanais. [Japanese Bridge.]* Oil on canvas, 89 × 116 cm. The Minneapolis Institute of Arts.

would surround the entire interior of a room, depicting water and plants in a manner that revealed the elusive brilliance of nature. He pursued the project with vigor and even built a large new studio to accommodate his large-scale canvases. Monet called this project a bit of a folly and referred to the paintings as his "Grandes Décorations." At this point he refused cataract surgery, fearing it would make his vision even worse. Yet he could no longer discriminate between many of his paints, relying instead on reading the labels for selecting his colors and then remembering their precise arrangement on his palette. He realized that many of his pictures were quite dark; and on several occasions, after comparing these canvases with his earlier works, he slashed and destroyed them.

During these years, Monet received frequent visits from his long-time friend, Georges Clemenceau, a remarkable man who had ascended to the rank of Premier of France. By the beginning of 1917, the end of the first World War was in sight, and Monet had agreed to donate two large panels of his "Grandes Décorations" to France to celebrate the armistice. Clemenceau, however, convinced him to donate not two panels but all 12 that Monet had planned, with the stipulation that a building would be constructed to house them in the manner that Monet had envisioned. The number was later increased to 19 panels in order to accommodate the architect's plan to house them in the Orangerie des Tuileries in Paris. There was, of course, some question in Monet's mind about whether he would have the energy and the eyesight needed to complete this enormous undertaking.

Monet had once said that he wished he had been born blind and then suddenly made to see so that he could paint his impressions without the bias of prior experience. Soon, a version of his wish would be granted. By 1922, at the age of 82, he had become essentially blind in the right eye and had only a little useful vision in the left eye, according to his medical records. Determined to continue, he said that "I will paint almost blind as Beethoven composed completely deaf" (Stuckey, 1995, p. 251). To improve his vision for a few hours at a time, he used a prescribed mydriatic to dilate his pupils (Ravin, 1985). Monet used very little blue in his paintings at this time, presumably because his dense cataracts would have transmitted so little short-wave light that blue would have been indistinguishable from black. The compensation processes described above may have reached the physiological limit so that by the summer of 1922 he found it necessary to stop painting. Clemenceau finally convinced Monet to go ahead with cataract surgery in his right eye that year.

Within six months of cataract extraction, Monet developed a secondary cataract, an opacification of the posterior capsule of the operated eye. This is a common complication of cataract surgery; and, although it did not surprise his physician, the opacity was a traumatic development for Monet. In July 1923 the cloudy membrane was extracted in Monet's home in Giverny. Monet was prescribed glasses, but they caused him to experience double vision and optical distortion. He discovered that his vision improved if he covered one eye, usually the left. Now Monet complained that through his left eye, with a remaining cataract, everything was too yellow, while through the eye with the cataract removed (aphakic eye), he experienced everything as too blue. Figure 1.27 shows his paintings of his *House Seen from the Rose Garden* which are believed to be painted with only one eye or the other (Lanthony, 1993). The difference between the views through the different eyes is striking.

One might wonder why the difference in yellow filters in Monet's eyes should so strikingly affect his choice of colors. After all, in the aphakic eye, Monet's retina should receive more short-wavelength light reflected not only from the scene he is trying to depict but equally from the blue paints on his palette. The net effect would therefore seem to require the same match between the scene and the canvas with or without a dense yellow cataract. From this point of view, the yellow filter should have no effect on Monet's paintings because it lies in front of both the original scene and his palette.

This analysis would be correct if our visual system were capable of responding to each wavelength of light separately and if there were enough pigments to match each wavelength. However, neither of these two requirements is met. As Clemenceau put it to Monet, "The steel of your eyesight breaks the crust of appearances, and you

1.10 Water Lilies and Cataracts 37

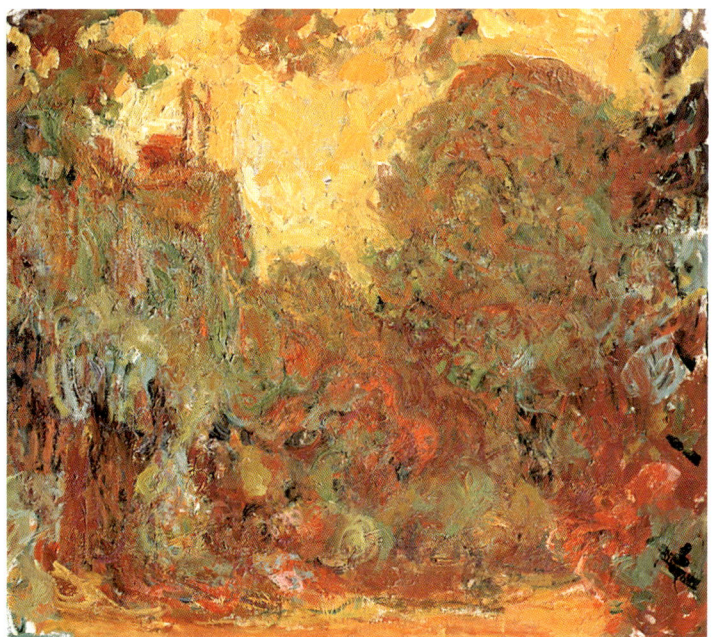

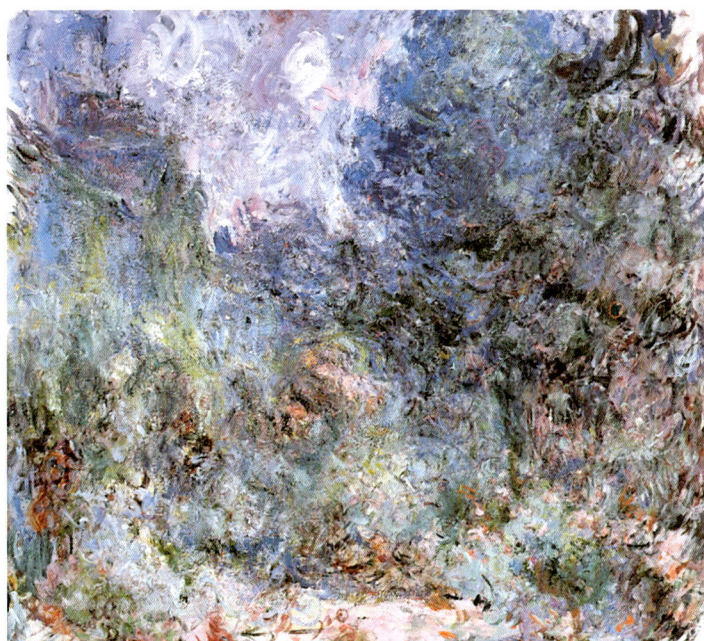

Fig. 1.27: Top: Claude Monet (1925) *La maison vue du jardin aux roses. [House Seen from the Rose Garden.]* Oil on canvas, 81 × 92 cm. Musée Marmottan, Paris.
Bottom: Claude Monet (1925) *La maison vue du jardin aux roses. [House Seen from the Rose Garden.]* Oil on canvas, 89 × 100 cm. Musée Marmottan, Paris.

penetrate the inner substance of things in order to decompose it into projectors of light which you recompose with the brush so that you may reestablish subtly upon our retinas the effect of sensations in their fullest intensity" (Clemenceau, 1930, pp. 18–19). Expressed less poetically, the painter does not make a physical match between the original scene and the canvas but a visual (approximately metameric) match. These matches depend on the shapes of the receptor action spectra (Fig. 1.6), and the latter are modified (as specified at the cornea) by age-related changes in the lens (Wright, 1928–29). In short, the senescent or cataractous lens modifies the receptor sensitivities in two ways: First, it *alters the shapes* of the receptor action spectra (specified at the cornea) by reducing sensitivity more at short wavelengths than at middle and long wavelengths. Second, it *reduces the relative heights* of the action spectra, affecting S-cones more than M- or L-cones. Processes such as color matching which depend on the shapes of the photoreceptor action spectra cannot be compensated neurally because each cone type obeys the principle of univariance (i.e., all *absorbed* quanta produce the same response in a photoreceptor), while relative sensitivities or heights of the curves can be compensated to a large extent. The net effect is that lenticular senescence affects color matches more than color appearance (Werner, 1996).

Following cataract surgery, patients often report a resurgence of blue experienced through the operated eye, as would be expected due to the removal of their dense yellow lens, but they adapt rather quickly over the course of weeks or months. Monet did not adapt so quickly, but some of his difficulty may have been with his impatience, which led his physician frequently to change the prescribed colored lenses that were intended to equate color appearance in the two eyes (Ravin, 1985). This process commenced when a Paris ophthalmologist, Jacques Mawas, prescribed a pair of glasses that were tinted yellowish-green. This eliminated Monet's previous complaint that he sees nothing but blue. Up to that point, he relied on his left eye for painting, but now switched to his right eye. Monet and Dr. Mawas tried glasses with various tints during the next two years. In the end, they settled on a pair of untinted glasses that Monet described as quite satisfactory. No doubt this outcome was due to chromatic adaptation in his visual system over this period.

In July 1925, three years after his original cataract extraction, Monet declared that his color vision was completely restored and his mood was ebullient. Now 85 years old, he resumed his work and completed not the 19 promised canvases for his "Grandes Décorations" but 22.

Monet never saw these canvases displayed in the room that he had envisioned. He died on 5 December 1926. Next to his bed was a book opened to Baudelaire's poem, "The Stranger" (Vidal, 1956). It goes, "Tell me, enigmatical man, whom do you love best, your father, your mother, your sister, or your brother?" To which the man replied, "I love the clouds." It was fitting that Clemenceau was by his side and was the one to close his eyes. Monet once said to Clemenceau, "Put your hand in mine and let us help one another to see things better" (Tucker, 1995, p. 225). Two months after closing Monet's eyes, Clemenceau helped the world to see better through Monet by opening the Orangerie des Tuileries with his "Grandes Décorations."

1.11 Summary

The life span of the Impressionist Claude Monet, 1840 to 1926, encompassed some of the most important developments in how color is now understood in art and science. In his paintings, Monet made the ephemeral effects of light and color his central subject matter. He is likely to have been influenced by J. W. v. Goethe via J. M. W. Turner and M. E. Chevreul via E. Delacroix, who exploited new ideas about additive color mixture and simultaneous contrast. Paintings from this period provide useful illustrations of the discoveries and theories of Monet's contemporaries in science, including J. C. Maxwell, H. v. Helmholtz, E. Hering and J. v. Kries, although he was probably not directly influenced by them. Their scientific theories are cornerstones for current thinking about color vision and provide a useful framework for analyzing age-related changes in color perception.

Monet's vision changed during his life, perhaps due in part to accelerated aging caused by sunlight to which he was often exposed by virtue of his painting *en plein air*. Light, especially UV light, may accelerate the normal age-related changes in the lens and photoreceptors. The cone pathways lose sensitivity on a continuous basis from early adulthood to old age. When expressed in terms of sensitivity at the cornea, S-, M- and L-cones appear to lose sensitivity at approximately the same rate with age. This is somewhat surprising because senescent changes in the lens produce a selective loss in the amount of short wavelength light that can reach the retina, a reduction commonly thought to reduce sensitivity of the visual system to blue hues. Monet's reaction to his own senescent lens, culminating in a cataract, has been taken to support this view. Recent studies, however, show that the visual system adapts to normal lenticular senescence and actively rebalances the sensitivity of color mechanisms to support constancy of color perception across the life span.

Acknowledgements

I am grateful to the Alexander von Humboldt Foundation (Bonn, Germany) for a Senior Scientist Award. Studies conducted in my laboratory were made possible through the support of the National Institute on Aging (grant AG04058). The helpful comments of Michelle L. Bieber, Philippe Lanthony, Jonathan O. Roberts, Brooke E. Schefrin, Elizabeth J. Smith, Vivianne Smith, Lothar Spillmann, Floyd Ratliff and Michael Wertheimer are gratefully acknowledged.

References

Barnes, R. (1990). Monet by Monet. (New York: Alfred A. Knopf).
Berlin, B. and Kay, P. (1969). Basic Color Terms, Their Universality and Evolution. (Berkeley: University of California Press).
Bezold, W. v. (1874) Die Farbenlehre. (Braunschweig: Westermann).
Bieber, M., Knoblauch, K., and Werner, J. S. (in press). M- and L-cones in early infancy: II. Action spectra at 8-weeks of age. Vision Res.
Callen, A. (1982). Techniques of the Impressionists. (London: QED Publishing).
Chevreul, M. E. (1839). De la Loi du Contraste Simultané des Couleurs. Paris: Pitois-Levrault. [trans. by F. Birren (1967) as The Principles of Harmony and Contrast of Colors and their Applications to the Arts.] (New York: Van Nostrand Reinhold Company, Inc.).
Clark, K. (1960). Looking at Pictures. (London: John Murray).
Clemenceau, G. (1929). Claude Monet. Reprinted in: Monet: A Retrospective, C.F. Stuckey, ed. (New York: Spadem, 1985), pp. 350–366.
Clemenceau, G. (1930). Claude Monet: The Water Lilies. (Garden City, New York: Doubleday, Doran & Company)
de Weert, C. M. M. (1991). Assimilation versus contrast. In: From Pigments to Perception, A. Valberg and B. B. Lee, eds. (New York: Plenum), pp. 305–311.
de Weert, C. M. M. and Spillmann, L. (1995). Assimilation: Asymmetry between brightness and darkness? Vision Res. *35*, 1413–1419.
DeValois, R. L. and DeValois, K. K. (1993). A multistage color model. Vision Res. *33*, 1053–1065.
Düchting, H. and Sagner-Düchting, K. (1993). Die Malerei des deutschen Impressionismus. (Köln: DuMont Buchverlag).
Gage, J. (1972). Turner: Rain, Steam and Speed. (London: Allen Lane the Penguin Press).
Goethe, J. W. v. (1810). Zur Farbenlehre. (Tübingen: J.G. Cotta. Diederich, Jena). (Translation arranged and edited by R. Matthaei as: Goethe's Color Theory. New York: Van Nostrand, 1971.)
Ham, W. T., Mueller, H. A., Ruffolo, J. J., Guerry, D., and Guerry, R.K. (1982). Action spectrum for retinal injury from near-ultraviolet radiation in the aphakic monkey. Am. J. Ophthalmol. *93*, 299-306.
Helmholtz, H. v. (1867). Handbuch der Physiologischen Optik. (Hamburg: Voss). [third edition translated as: Helmholtz's Treatise on Physiological Optics; J. P. C. Southall, Ed. Rochester, New York: Optical Society of America, 1924.]
Herbert, R. (1979). Method and meaning in Monet. AIA *67*, 90–108.
Hering, E. (1887). Ueber die Theorie des simultanen Contrastes von Helmholtz. Pf. A. *40*, 172–191.
Hering, E. (1920). Outlines of a Theory of the Light Sense. L.M. Hurvich and D. Jameson, trans. (Harvard U. Press, Cambridge, Mass., 1964; originally published by Springer, Berlin).

Jameson, D. and Hurvich, L. M. (1955). Some quantitative aspects of an opponent-colors theory: I. Chromatic responses and spectral saturation. J. Opt. Soc. Am. *45,* 546–552.

Jameson, D. and Hurvich, L. M. (1968). Opponent-response functions related to measured cone pigments. J. Opt. Soc. Am. *58,* 429–430.

Jameson, D. and Hurvich, L. M. (1975). From contrast to assimilation: In art and in the eye. Leonardo *8,* 125-131.

Jameson, D. and Hurvich, L. M. (1989). Essay concerning color constancy. A. Rev. Psychol. *40,* 1–22.

Katz, D. (1911). The World of Colour. [English translation by R. B. MacLeod and C. W. Fox, published in 1935)], (London: Kegan Paul, Trench, Trubner & Co).

Kirschfeld, K. (1982). Carotenoid pigments. Proc. R. Soc. London B. *216,* 71–85.

Kraft, J. M. and Werner, J. S. (1994). Spectral efficiency across the life span: Flicker photometry and brightness matching. J. Opt. Soc. Am. A. *11,* 1213–1221.

Kraft, J. M. and Werner, J. S. (1997). Age-related changes in saturation of non-spectral lights. In: John Dalton's Color Vision Legacy, C.M. Dickinson, I. J. Murray and D. Carden, eds. (London: Taylor & Francis), pp. 553–560.

Kries, J. v. (1882). Die Gesichtsempfindungen und ihre Analyse. (Leipzig: Veith & Co.).

Lanthony, P. (1993). La cataracte et la peinture de Claude Monet. Points De Vue No. *29,* 12–25.

Lennie, P. and D'Zmura, M. (1988). Mechanisms of color vision. CRC Critical Rev. Neurobiol. *3,* 333–340.

Lerman, S. (1980). Radiant Energy and the Eye. (New York: Macmillan Publishing Co.).

Marshall, J. (1978). Ageing changes in human cones. In: XXIII Concilium Ophthalmologicum, Kyoto, K. Shimizu and J. A. Oosterhuis, eds. (Elsevier North-Holland, Amsterdam), pp. 375–378.

Marshall, J. (1985). Radiation and the aging eye. Ophthalmic Physiol. Opt. *5,* 241–263.

Maxwell, J. C. (1860). On the theory of compound colours and the relations of the colours of the spectrum. Philos. Trans. R. Soc. London *150,* 57–84.

Maxwell, J. C. (1872). On color vision. Proc. R. Inst. G.B. *6,* 260–271.

Myers, B. (1990). Methods of the Masters: Monet. (London: Park Lane).

Newton, I. (1704). Opticks: Or, a Treatise of the Reflexions, Refractions, Inflexions and Colours of Light. (London: S. Smith and B. Walford).

Perry, L. C. (1927). Reminiscences of Claude Monet from 1889 to 1909. Am. Mag. Art *18,* (March, No. 3), 119–126.

Pissarro, J. (1990). Monet's Cathedral: Rouen 1892–1894. (New York: Alfred A. Knopf).

Pokorny, J. and Smith, V. (1997). How much light reaches the retina? In Colour Vision Deficiencies XIII, C. R. Cavonius, ed. (Dordrecht: Kluwer), pp. 491–511.

Ratliff, F. (1976). On the psychophysiological bases of universal color terms. Pro. Am. Phil. Soc. *120,* 311-330.

Ratliff, F. (1992). Paul Signac and Color in Neo-Impressionism. (New York: The Rockefeller University Press).

Ravin, J. G. (1985). Monet's cataracts. J. Am. Med. Ass. *253,* 394–399.

Reynolds, G. (1969). Turner. (London: Thames and Hudson).

Ruskin, J. (1843). Modern Painters. Vol. 1. Of General Principles and of Truth. (London: Smith, Elder & Co.).

Russell, J. (1974). The Meanings of Modern Art. Vol. 1. The Secret Revolution. (New York: The Museum of Modern Art).

Schefrin, B. E. and Werner, J. S. (1990). Loci of spectral unique hues throughout the life span. J. Opt. Soc. Am. A. *7,* 305–311.

Schefrin, B. E. and Werner, J. S. (1993). Age-related changes in the color appearance of broadband surfaces. Color Res. and Appl. *18,* 380–389.

Schefrin, B. E., Shinomori, K., and Werner, J. S. (1995). Contributions of neural pathways to age-related losses in chromatic discrimination. J. Opt. Soc. Am. A. *12,* 1233–1241.

Schefrin, B. E., Werner, J. S., Plach, M., Utlaut, N., and Switkes, E. (1992). Sites of age-related sensitivity loss in a short-wave cone pathway. J. Opt. Soc. Am. A. *9,* 355–363.

Seitz, W. (1956). Monet and abstract painting. Reprinted in: Monet: A Retrospective, C. F. Stuckey, ed. (New York: Spadem, 1985), pp. 367–374.

Shinomori, K., Schefrin, B. E., and Werner, J. S. (1997). Spectral mechanisms of spatially induced blackness: data and quantitative model. J. Opt. Soc. Am. A. *14,* 372–387.

Signac, P. (1921). D'Eugène Delacroix au Néo-Impressionnisme. (Paris: H. Floury). [trans. and ed. by W. Silverman in F. Ratliff (1992) Paul Signac and Color in Neo-Impressionism. New York: The Rockefeller University Press, pp. 193–285]

Smith, V. C. and Pokorny, J. (1975). Spectral sensitivity of the foveal cone photopigments between 400 and 500 nm. Vision Res. *15,* 161–171.

Spillmann, L. and Werner, J. S. (1996). Long-range interactions in visual perception. TINS *19,* 428–434.

Stuckey, C. F. (1995). Claude Monet: 1840–1926. (Chicago: The Art Institute of Chicago).

Tucker, P. H. (1995). Claude Monet: Life and Art. (New Haven: Yale University Press).

Vidal, H. (1956). Remembering Claude Monet. Reprinted in: Monet: A Retrospective, C. F. Stuckey, ed. (New York: Spadem, 1985), pp. 349–350.

Volbrecht, V. J. and Werner, J. S. (1987). Isolation of short-wavelength-sensitive cone photoreceptors in 4-6-week-old human infants. Vision Res. *27,* 469–478.

Vollard, A. (1925). Renoir, an intimate record. Reprinted in: Renoir: A Retrospective, N. Wadley, ed. (New York: Hugh Lauter Levin Associates, 1987), pp. 304–308.

Vos, J. J. (1978). Colorimetric and photometric properties of a 2° fundamental observer. Color Res. and Appl. *3,* 125–128.

Vos, J. J. and Walraven, P. L. (1971). On the derivation of the foveal receptor primaries. Vision Res. *11,* 799–818.

Weale, R. A. (1957). Trichromatic ideas in the seventeenth and eighteenth centuries. Nature *179,* 648–651.

Weale, R. A. (1971). The death of Pointillism. The Listener (4 March), 273–275.

Weale, R. A. (1982). A Biography of the Eye. (London: H.K. Lewis & Co. Ltd.).

Weale, R. A. (1988). Age and transmittance of the human crystalline lens. J. Physiol., Lond. *395,* 577–87.

Werner, J. S. (1982). Development of scotopic sensitivity and the absorption spectrum of the human ocular media. J. Opt. Soc. Am. *72,* 247–258.

Werner, J. S. (1991). The damaging effects of light on the eye and implications for understanding changes in vision across the life span. In: The Changing Visual System: Maturation and Aging in the Central Nervous System, P. Bagnoli and W. Hodos, eds. (New York: Plenum), pp. 295–309.

Werner, J. S. (1996). Visual problems of the retina during ageing. In: Prog. Retinal Res., N. N. Osborne and J. Chader, eds. (Oxford: Pergamon Press), pp. 621–645.

Werner, J. S. and Schefrin, B. E. (1993). Loci of achromatic points across the life span. J. Opt. Soc. Am. A. *10,* 1509–1516.

Werner, J. S. and Spillmann, L. (1989). UV-absorbing intraocular lenses: Safety, efficacy, and consequences for the cataract patient. Graefe's Arch. Clin. Exp. Ophthalmol. *227,* 248–256.

Werner, J. S. and Steele, V. G. (1988). Sensitivity of human foveal color mechanisms throughout the life span. J. Opt. Soc. Am. A. *5,* 2122–2130.

Werner, J. S. and Walraven, J. (1982). The effects of chromatic adaptation on the achromatic locus: Role of luminance, contrast, and background color. Vision Res. *22,* 929–943.

Werner, J. S. and Wooten, B. R. (1979). Opponent-chromatic mechanisms: Relation to photopigments and hue naming. J. Opt. Soc. Am. *69,* 422–434.

Werner, J. S., Peterzell, D. H., and Scheetz, A. J. (1990). Light, vision, and aging. Optom. Vision Sci. *67,* 214–229.

Werner, J. S., Steele, V. G., and Pfoff, D. S. (1989). Loss of human photoreceptor sensitivity associated with chronic exposure to ultraviolet radiation. Ophthalmology *96,* 1552–1558.

Wiesel, T. N. and Hubel, D. H. (1966). Spatial and chromatic interactions in the lateral geniculate body of the rhesus monkey. J. Physiol., Lond. *29,* 1116–1156.

Wright, W. D. (1928–29). A re-determination of the trichromatic coefficients of the spectral colors. Trans. Opt. Soc. *30,* 141–164.

Young, R. W. (1982). The Bowman lecture, 1982. Biological renewal. Applications to the eye. T. Ophth. Soc. *102,* 42–75.

Young, R. W. (1991). Age-Related Cataract. (New York: Oxford University Press).

Young, T. (1802). On the theory of light and colors. Philos. Trans. R. Soc. London *92,* 12–48.

Zrenner, E., Abramov, I., Akita, M., Cowey, A., Livingstone, M., and Valberg, A. (1990). Color perception: Retinal, geniculate, and cortical mechanisms. In: Visual Perception: The Neurophysiological Foundations, L. Spillmann and J. S. Werner, eds. (San Diego: Academic Press), pp. 163–203.

II Physiology and Neuroethology

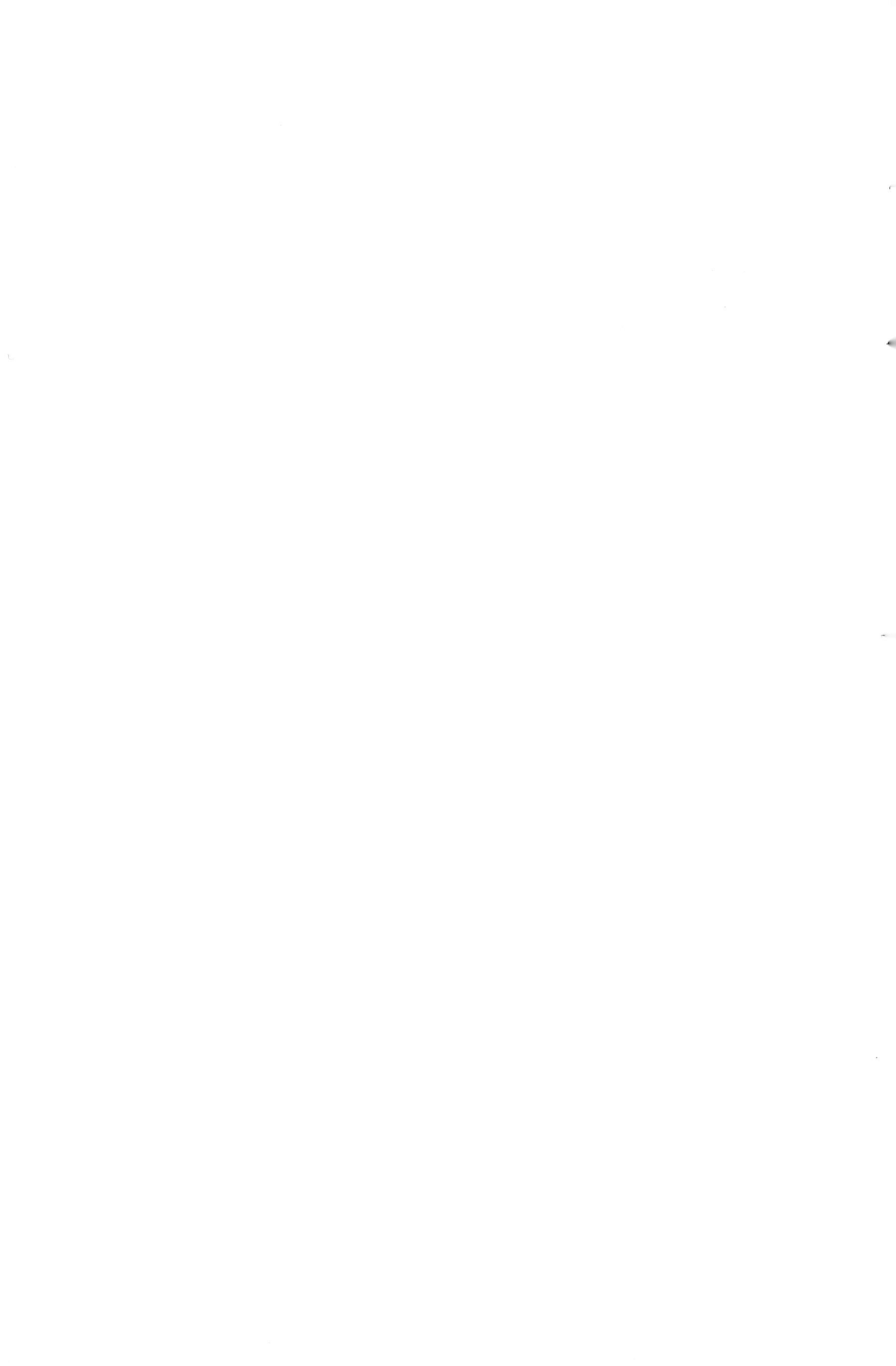

2 Physiological and Psychophysical Simulations of Color Vision in Humans and Animals

Werner G. K. Backhaus

2.1 Introduction

2.1.1 Phenomenology of Color Vision

When light enters our eyes, we experience color sensations. Under constant viewing conditions, identical lights cause comparable color sensations. This holds to a good approximation in different subjects with normal color vision and allows us to perform systematic investigations of the subjective phenomena of color vision in psychophysical experiments. Depending on the wavelength intensity distribution of the light, we are able to experience about a million different colors. A closer inspection shows that all color sensations are composed of only six elementary color sensations (German: Urfarben, English: unique-colors, elementary colors) red, green, blue, yellow, black and white, of different amounts (Hering, 1874; 1920). Black is indeed an elementary color sensation and not "no sensation at all" which just occurs when no light is present (see chapter 10). This can easily be demonstrated in color contrast experiments with "black" cardboards which do not reflect any light at all and "white" cardboards which reflect almost all light. Simultaneous illumination of both cards, for example, by daylight shows that in a small region to both sides of the contrast border "black" looks darker and "white" looks brighter compared to an independent presentation. This phenomenon is called the Mach band, first quantitatively described and explained by the physicist and philosopher, Ernst Mach (1886) in physiological simulations.

2.1.2 Disciplines

Light entering our eyes is absorbed by the photoreceptors in the retina. The neuronal color-coding system processes the information from the

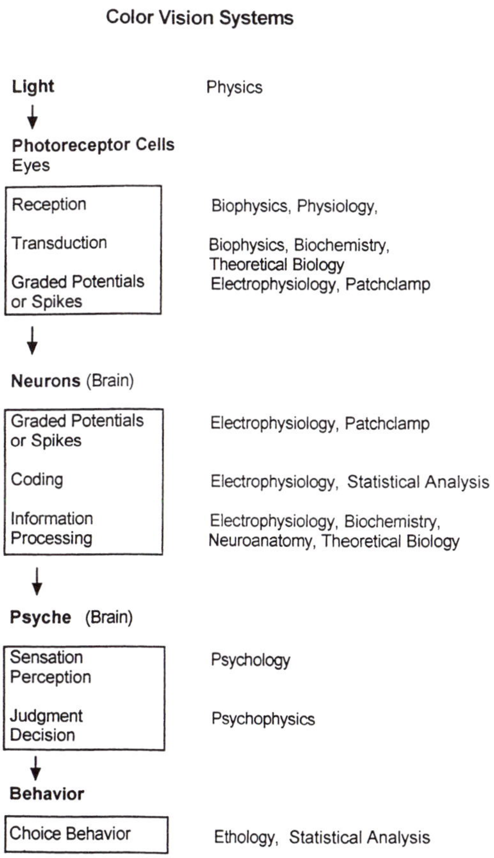

Color Vision Systems

Light	Physics
↓	
Photoreceptor Cells Eyes	
Reception	Biophysics, Physiology,
Transduction	Biophysics, Biochemistry, Theoretical Biology
Graded Potentials or Spikes	Electrophysiology, Patchclamp
↓	
Neurons (Brain)	
Graded Potentials or Spikes	Electrophysiology, Patchclamp
Coding	Electrophysiology, Statistical Analysis
Information Processing	Electrophysiology, Biochemistry, Neuroanatomy, Theoretical Biology
↓	
Psyche (Brain)	
Sensation Perception	Psychology
Judgment Decision	Psychophysics
↓	
Behavior	
Choice Behavior	Ethology, Statistical Analysis

Fig. 2.1: Integrative view of the color vision process and related research disciplines. Color vision systems possess a causal chain structure (left side).

photoreceptors further and finally provides the information for the color sensations. Humans can verbally report about their color sensations. Color vision in non-human animals, can be tested only in behavioral experiments. The specific color-choice behavior of the species is most relevant, in addition in these cases. Figure 2.1 gives an integrative view to the major components of color vision systems and the different disciplines working on the respective parts. Since processing of color information is a causal chain, from the photoreceptors via the neuronal color-coding system to the color sensations produced in the brain, excitations at different stages of this chain may be used as an unequivocal description of the respective color produced at the end of this chain. Research on color vision is obviously only possible by integrative research of different disciplines.

2.1.3 Psychophysical Simulations

Since under constant viewing conditions identical lights cause identical color sensations, the simplest way to denote color sensations is in terms of characteristics of the light stimuli (e.g., by the respective spectral intensity distributions that produce a criterion response). It is furthermore possible to denote a color by a dot in linear coordinate systems (i.e., color spaces). A basis for these color spaces may also be provided by different parts of the neuronal color-coding chain. The different color spaces thus have different properties and are thus used for different purposes. As a basis for these color spaces one may use:

1) the light intensities of three lights (primaries) of constant relative spectral intensity distributions (e.g., colored lamps, phosphors of monitors), which are used for light mixture (tristimulus space);

2) the photon fluxes (photons per second) absorbed in the different spectral types of photoreceptors (light absorption space);

3) the membrane potentials of the spectral types of photoreceptor cells (photoreceptor space);

4) the numbers on three abstract scales derived, for example, by multidimensional scaling (MDS) analysis from the results of color discrimination and color similarity experiments (color similarity space, e.g., MDS color space);

5) the excitation values of the color-opponent coding (COC) neurons (COC space);

6) the amounts of elementary colors (EC) which constitute the color sensation (EC space);

7) the choice proportions measured in the color-choice behavior in terms of just noticeable difference (jnd) scales.

2.1.4 Physiological Simulations

Mach (1886) derived a quantitative model which explains black and white contrast effects in terms of a mathematical description of a neuronal net-

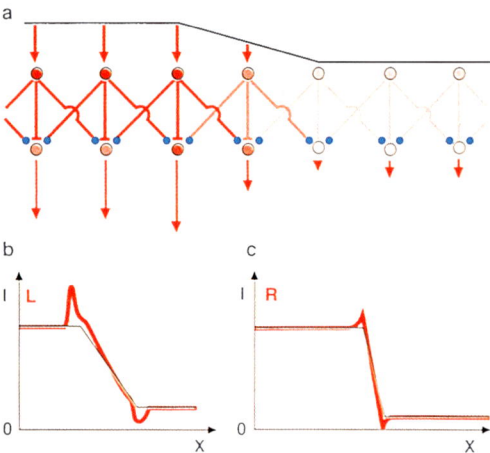

Fig. 2.2: **a:** Model of the retina describing photoreceptors (upper circles) and neurons (lower circles) as interconnected via inhibitory (blue dots) and excitatory (red bars) synapses (see eq. 1, lateral inhibition, Mach, 1886). The contrast boarder of brighter (longer arrows) and dimmer (shorter arrows) light is increased (lower red arrows) at the neuronal level (x: retina position).
b: subjective brightness L (red line) of Mach's intensity profile I (black line).
c: Brightness R (red line) of the intensity profile I (black line) calculated from the retina model. A comparison of the graphs in (b) and (c) shows that the black and white color contrast effect, as measured in psychophysical experiments, is well explained by the model (see text). (After Ratliff, 1965; Backhaus, 1996.)

work. The physiological model takes lateral inhibition between neurons of the human retina into account:

$$R_p = I_p(I_p K / \sum_{j=1}^{n} I_j k_{pj}) \tag{1}$$

The light intensity (I) reaches the photoreceptor cells (p) in the retina. Each of p photoreceptors is connected to a fixed number (n) of p neurons with excitations R, via an excitatory synapse of weighting K and inhibitory synapses with weightings k_{pj}. Figure 2.2 shows a comparison of experimental (psychophysical) data with the predictions of respective simulations with the model (Ratliff, 1965). These results imply two further properties of the neuronal color-coding system which appear to be most helpful for further physiological simulations of color vision systems: 1) Mach's results clearly demonstrate that it is not always necessary for explaining color vision phenomena to take the entire neuronal color-coding system into account. It is rather sufficient to describe the essential parts which determine the respective phenomena. 2) The model describes only the nonlinear interactions of the peripheral part (retina) of the neuronal color-coding system. From this it follows that the further parts of the neuronal color-coding network perform almost linear coding.

In the following sections, the determination of the properties and applications of the color spaces will be described. First physiological interpretations of the abstract psychophysical scales of the subjective color spaces will be presented and the implications for conscious and unconscious color vision in man and animals will be discussed.

2.2 Color Stimuli

The color vision system analyzes the light stimulus at first by absorbing photons in the different types of photoreceptors according to their spectral sensitivities. The photons are absorbed in the photoreceptors of the eye with a probability depending exclusively on the spectral sensitivity of the respective photoreceptor, not on the energy of the photons. Thus, photoreceptors perform measurements of the photon fluxes rather than of the light energy. So the spectral intensity distribution contains the entire information about the light relevant to color vision.

From the intensity values of the photoreceptors the neuronal network derives the color information which is finally represented by our color sensations. The visible wavelength range for our own color vision is about 400 nm–700 nm (Fig. 2.3), whereas the visible ranges of insects (Menzel and Backhaus, 1991; see below) and several lower vertebrates (see chapter 8) appear to be shifted to shorter wavelengths (UV range: <400 nm). In these cases, the long wavelength photoreceptor appears either to be replaced by a UV-receptor (trichromats) or the visible wavelength range is extended to the UV range (300 nm–700 nm) (tetra- and higher polychromats). The UV-component of daylight is, therefore, most relevant for the color vision systems of many animals but is irrelevant for color vision of higher vertebrates including our own. This has to be accounted for in experiments with animals because light that is white for us may not be white for many animals.

Since light is the stimulus for color sensations it is necessary to measure light in terms of spectral intensity functions over time. Nowadays this can be performed by simultaneous spectral photometers via a stationary grid and an array of photocells. Simultaneous spectral photometers allow us to measure spectral intensity distributions, even at lower light intensities, e.g. each 4 ms, with high accuracy (e.g., in the range of 250 nm–800 nm in 1 nm steps). This allows one to determine the physical properties of even rapidly changing light stimuli. For further processing of the measured light spectra in physiological simulations of color vision, it is thus convenient to express the light intensities as photon fluxes (unit: trolands) over wavelength. Otherwise wavelength dependent conversion factors have to be taken into account before comparing light intensity spectra and spectral sensitivities measured in different units.

In color vision experiments, it is most suitable to mix a light from a daylight simulating source (comparable to illuminant D65) with monochromatic light with independently adjustable intensities at different mixing ratios. Changing the mix-

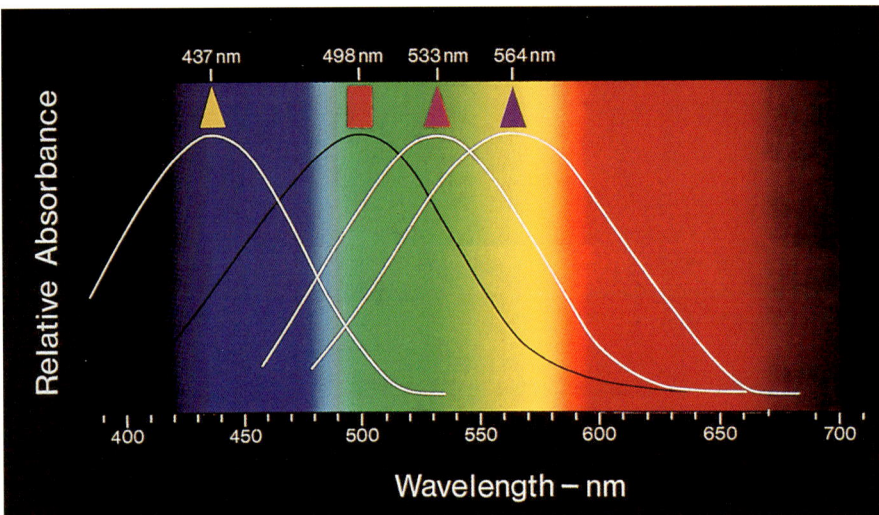

Fig. 2.3: Relative absorbance of the three cone types and rods in the human retina plotted as a function of wavelength. Although the relations between color appearance are slightly distorted by photographic reproduction, one can still appreciate that the purest hues (elementary hues) are not visible near the wavelengths of maximal sensitivity of the photoreceptors. Rather, the information from the photoreceptors is further processed by the retina and the brain (see text). (After Dowling, 1987.)

ing ratio from pure monochromatic light over diluted monochromatic light to pure daylight causes sensations reaching from most saturated colors via whitish, grayish or blackish colors to the achromatic colors white, gray or black.

We are nowadays able to produce millions of different color stimuli on color monitors. Nevertheless, lamps of higher intensities and classical optical equipment did not become old-fashioned. UV light can only be produced by lamps and modified by optics of quartz glass up to now. Also for light in our visible wavelength range, color monitors can only partially replace the optical equipment.

Color monitors possess three types of phosphors; the spectral intensity distribution of the emitted light is broad (i.e., not at all monochromatic) and of rather low intensity compared to bright daylight. Consequently, the range of lights which can be produced by light mixture is very much restricted and thus allows us to only produce unsaturated colors. Furthermore, prediction of the outcome of light mixtures is much more difficult (e.g., crosstalk between the phosphors) than it is for the additive light mixtures which can be produced by classical optical devices. Nevertheless, if the system – computer and monitor – is calibrated, color patterns can be easily produced, which are indeed most helpful in many psychophysical investigations. In total, in modern color vision labs classical optical equipment and color monitors, both of course computer controlled, compliment each other. The technical devices became more and more sophisticated, so that it became necessary to perform color vision experiments also at optical and other more technical institutes (see chapters 17 and 18).

2.3 Psychophysics of Color Vison

Psychophysics of color vision originally developed as a special discipline of experimental psychology. Experimental psychology measures perceptual processes (effects) in order to scale the internal representations of sensory stimuli in the brain (psyche). The stimuli have to be well defined so that they can be repeatedly presented with high accuracy (e.g., photographs of faces, handwritten texts, paintings). Usually the stimuli cannot be described in simple physical terms. Nevertheless the stimuli can be labeled by numbers and subjective scales can be determined, for example, the similarity of faces, the wellness of handwritings, the beauty of paintings, on which each of the stimuli is represented by a certain number (see chapter 1). If the stimuli are more simple and thus can be described in physical terms, we speak of psychophysics as part of experimental psychology. Most of the experiments performed on color vision are of the latter type, with light as the physical stimulus. The first systematic psychophysical experiments were performed by Weber (1834) and Fechner (1860).

Color vision experiments on animals are performed traditionally at neurobiology and behavioral biology institutes. At present, physiological models of color vision are ongoing developed, which allow simulation of the subjective judgments of animals and humans in order to 1) obtain neurobiological and psychological explanation models for color vision in animals and in man which will finally allow us 2) derivation of color difference formulas for human color vision for specific purposes, also providing the basis for more precise technical color management.

In a first approach, psychophysics relates the measured subjective scales of the internal representation of stimuli to the intensities of the sensations. In the cases of more simple modalities, as the sense for heaviness which Weber investigated in his earlier experiments, the internal representation can be described mathematically by one subjective scale only. This is because the subjective internal representation of the sensational intensity (e.g., color brightness X which is related to light intensity S) has only one degree of freedom. In the cases of one-dimensional representations, a psychometric function X(S) can be derived which allows one to predict the sensational intensity (X) from the intensity of the physical stimulus (S). Weber measured the threshold ΔS at which a stimulus S appears in 50% of the cases to be different from a second stimulus $S + \Delta S$. It turned out that ΔS is proportional to the stimulus intensity S which can be written in terms of Weber's law (1st psychophysical law) with the Weber constant c:

$$\Delta S / S = c \qquad (2)$$

Fechner interpreted the constant c as the intensity of the sensational representation X of the stimulus, with the assumption that equally large X's are detected equally often by the subject. Thus eq. 2 became:

$$\Delta S / S = c = c' \, \Delta X. \qquad (3)$$

Integration of eq. 3 for infinitesimally small thresholds gives Fechner's psychometric function (2nd psychophysical law):

$$X = 1/c' \, \ln(S/S_0) = k \log(S/S_0). \qquad (4)$$

This equation can also be read as a definition of the sensational intensity X with respect to stimulus intensity S and absolute threshold intensity S_0.

Thurstone described the psychophysical process by the statistical model shown in Figure 2.4. The stimuli S are mapped by the neuronal processes to certain but fluctuating sensational intensities X. The decision process is described as due to the

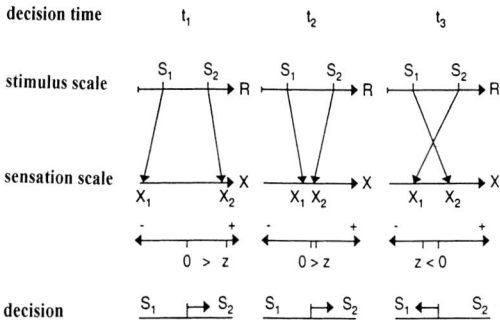

Fig. 2.4: Psychophysical model of the decision-making process in color vision experiments based on Thurstone's law of comparative judgment (see text). The color stimuli S are mapped onto the scale of color sensations X according to the respective fluctuations of the neuronal network which performs this process. The fluctuations of the stimuli usually are negligible. The decision-making process is described as instantaneous (i.e., the decision is performed by comparison of the actual values on the color sensation scale at decision time). Since no memory is involved in this process, the precision of the decisions does not depend on the time between two decisions.

actual difference $\Delta X = X_1 - X_2$ at time t. So, the same results of Weber's threshold experiments were interpreted by Thurstone (1927) using exclusively subjective terms (law of comparative judgment, 3rd psychophysical law):

$$X_1 - X_2 = z_{12}\sqrt{\sigma_1^2 + \sigma_2^2 - 2 r_{12}\, \sigma_1\, \sigma_2} \qquad (5)$$

σ is the standard deviation of the fluctuations of the sensational intensities X caused by the stimuli S, r is the correlation coefficient between the fluctuations of the sensational intensities X, z's are the probability transformed choice percentages of correct choices of the reference stimulus (e.g., S_1).

Thurstone's formulation is more general than the formulation of Fechner. The assumption of Fechner (1860) that equally large $\Delta X = X_1 - X_2$ are equally often detected by a subject, is only realized if the square-root expression is a constant, which is, for example, the case if the standard deviations σ are identical, constant and uncorrelated (r = 0). This important case is known in psychophysics as Thurstone's case V. The results of psychophysical experiments on color vision and other modalities are well described by this case. In the special case of complete correlation (r =1) and $\sigma \sim S^n$, the psychometric function derived from eq. 5 deviates from Fechner's logarithmic psychometric function and takes the form of a power function $X = k' S^n$, with a constant exponent n (Plateau, 1872; Stevens, 1975). The different cases are obviously related to the noise properties of the neuronal color-coding systems. Thus, the question of the appropriateness of different psychometrical functions will best be investigated in more detailed physiological and psychophysical simulations based on respective measurements.

Since eq. 5 does not contain any physical quantities, the law of comparative judgment cannot only be used for scaling choice percentages measured in psychophysical experiments but is also used for the wider class of data measured in experimental psychology. Weber's and Fechner's formulation of the psychophysical law describes one-dimensional cases only. Thurstone's law allows a generalization to multidimensional modalities and thus provides a most helpful tool for describing color vision, which in the case of humans is indeed three-dimensional.

2.3.1 Psychophysical Judgments

2.3.1.1 Color difference judgments

Subjects may be asked to discriminate a color stimulus from a dark surround or to discriminate two color stimuli from each other by answering "yes" when a difference is seen and "no" when no difference is seen. The repeated judgments of the subject can be accumulated to choice percentages which represent the detection probability of a difference between a light and the surround or between two lights (Fig. 2.5). This experimental method is called "indirect scaling". The first experiments of this type were performed by Weber (1834). The sensations that were caused had only one quality (dimension) of which only the sensational intensity X can vary. Repeated measurements of absolute thresholds (with respect to no stimulus) or incremental thresholds (with respect to another stimulus of certain intensity) were performed, e.g., by adjusting the stimulus until it is just detected or judged as different from the reference stimulus in 50% of the cases (i.e., 75% correct choices of the reference stimulus). The differ-

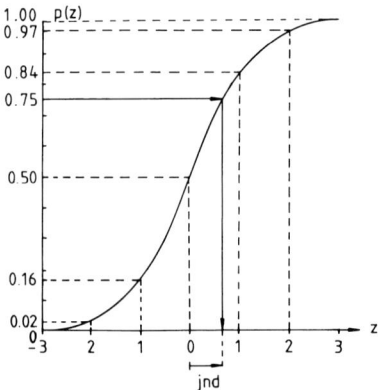

Fig. 2.5: The psychophysical measurement process. According to the statistical model described in Figure 2.4, a difference of two colors on the linear color sensation scale z is one jnd if the choice percentages for the reference color is 75% (identical colors: 50%). The assumption of Fechner that one jnd on the sensation scale is detected equally often does not hold in general, but does for the most important case of the law of comparative judgment (i.e., Thurstone's case V).

ences between two stimuli at 50% (resp. 75%) threshold (ΔS) is said to be a just noticeable difference (jnd).

2.3.1.2 Color similarity judgments

In the case of color vision, the subjects may be asked to judge which of two color stimuli is more similar to (or different from) a reference stimulus (method of triads, Torgerson, 1958). The results of color similarity experiments of this type showed: 1) two identical sensations have to be represented at one locus in a perceptual color space, and the difference between the two sensations is, therefore, represented by a distance of zero (identity axiom). 2) Differences of two sensations A and B are symmetrical (i.e., Δ(A, B) = Δ(B, A)). 3) If sensation A is different from sensation B and B is different from C, then the difference between A and C cannot be greater than the difference between the sum of the differences Δ between A and B, and A and C: Δ(A, C) ≤ Δ(A, B) + Δ(B,C) (triangle inequality). For one-dimensional sensations the inequality sign reduces to the equal sign.

The method of complete triads measures the similarities of all color stimuli against a reference stimulus and every color stimulus in the experiment is taken once as the reference stimulus. Multidimensional scaling (MDS) analysis allows the determination of the subjective color space which allows us to specify the number of dimensions, the scale values of the color stimuli on these dimensions and the composition rule (Minkowski metric, see below) which fulfills the axioms above and allows us a derivation of the total differences of each two colors from the differences on the individual dimensions.

2.3.1.3 Content analytical judgments

In content analytical experiments on color vision, the subjects are asked to judge the proportions of elementary color sensations (elementary colors) of which the total color sensations (colors) consist (see above). The members of the pairs red/green and blue/yellow do not occur simultaneously in a color sensation, they appear to exclude each other and so are called opponent colors. All other combinations of elementary colors may indeed occur simultaneously, for example, blue and green (blue-green), green and yellow (yellowish green), yellow-red (orange), red and blue (purple), black and white (gray). This means that only four percentages (red or green, blue or yellow, black and white) have to be judged for any color. Since the percentages sum up to 100%, only three of the percentages are sufficient for unequivocally denoting the color sensations (see below).

2.4 Psychophysical Color Spaces

2.4.1 The Color Similarity (MDS) Space

The subjective color space of humans and animals can be determined, for example, by multidimensional scaling (MDS) analysis of choice percentages obtained in color difference and color similarity experiments (see above). The MDS analysis assumes that every (color) sensation is represented as a locus in a linear multidimensional vector space. Color discrimination (reference stimulus and one alternative stimulus) and color similarity judgments (reference stimulus and two alternative stimuli) are described as simply related by a probability transformation (% → z-values, see Fig. 2.5) to the distances between each two color loci in the subjective color space. The color distance D between two colors (1, 2) is derived from the differences of the respective scale values x_i on the d coordinates (dimensions) according to a general calculation rule, the Minkowski-Metric with the exponent n:

$$D_{12} = (\sum_{i=1}^{d} |x_{i1} - x_{i2}|^n)^{1/n}. \quad (6)$$

The Minkowski metric is the simplest metric which fulfills the axiomatic conditions discussed in the previous section (see e.g., Kolmogorof and Fomin, 1957; Ahrens, 1974). The Minkowski metric contains three different cases: 1) n = 2: the Euclidean metric (square-root of the sum of the squared coordinate differences, see Fig. 2.6),

2. Physiological and Psychophysical Simulations of Color Vision in Humans and Animals

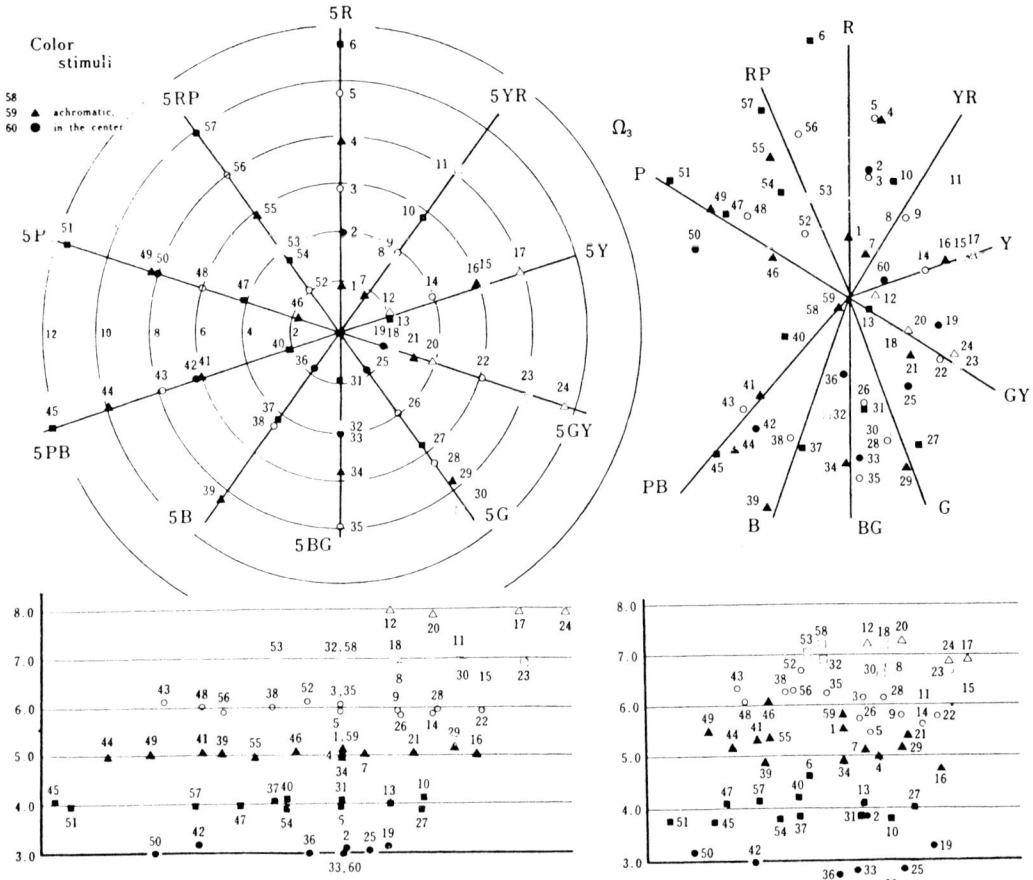

Fig. 2.6: Comparison of the relative loci of 60 colored chips in the Munsell system (left side) and in the MDS color space (right side) obtained by multidimensional scaling of a color similarity experiment with these chips. Because of the Euclidean metric of the human color space, the MDS scales are usually not drawn, but the relative positions of the color loci are compared instead (see text). (After Indow and Ohsumi, 1972.)

2) $n = 1$: city-block metric (sum of the absolute coordinate differences, see Fig. 2.7) and
3) $n \to \infty$: the dominance metric (largest coordinate difference).

Several color-choice experiments of this kind were performed with humans and the obtained choice percentages were investigated by metric (Euclidean space) and non-metric (Minkowski space) MDS analysis. The results showed, at least to a good approximation, that the human color space is three-dimensional with a Euclidean metric. This result agrees with other subjective color-order systems, such as the Munsell atlas (see Fig. 2.6), obtained when subjects are asked to sort all kinds of different color chips according to their similarity (e.g., Indow and Ohsumi, 1972).

2.4.2 The Elementary Color Space (Color Sensations Space)

The three-dimensional color space spanned by the elementary colors (see above) is based on content analytical judgments and thus is quite different from the three-dimensional light mixture space and also from the physiological color spaces, which are based on color discrimination and color similarity judgments (see above). The six proportions can be

2.4 Psychophysical Color Spaces

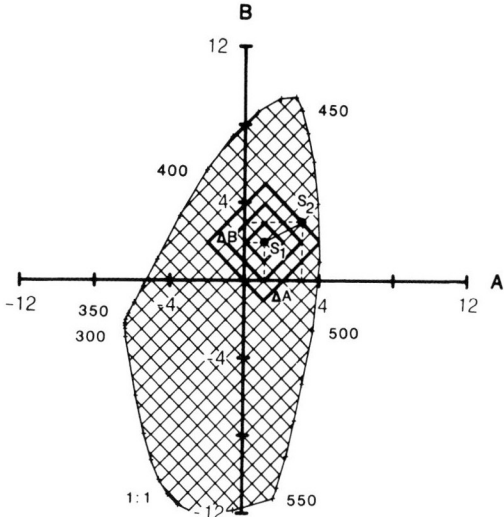

Fig. 2.7: Geometry of the subjective COC space of the honeybee. Because of the city-block metric of the COC diagram, the loci of most similar colors lie on a square around the reference color locus. The color difference between two colors or between the respective color stimuli, S1 and S2, can be calculated according to the city-block metric (see text) or graphically from the COC diagram by counting the concentric squares crossed (jnd's) when moving on a straight line from S1 to S2. Because of the city-block metric, the same number of jnd's is obtained when moving on axis A and then perpendicular on axis B from S1 to S2 (see text).

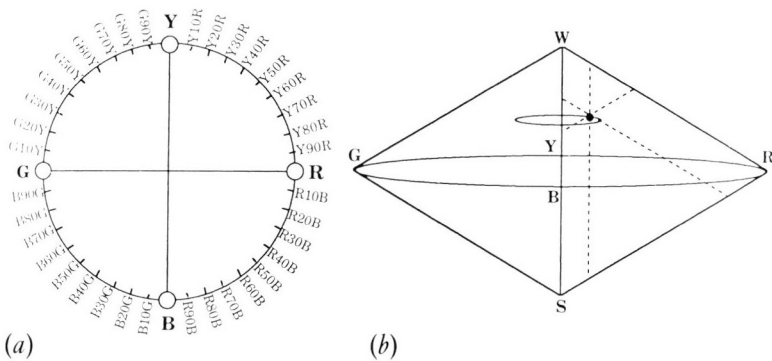

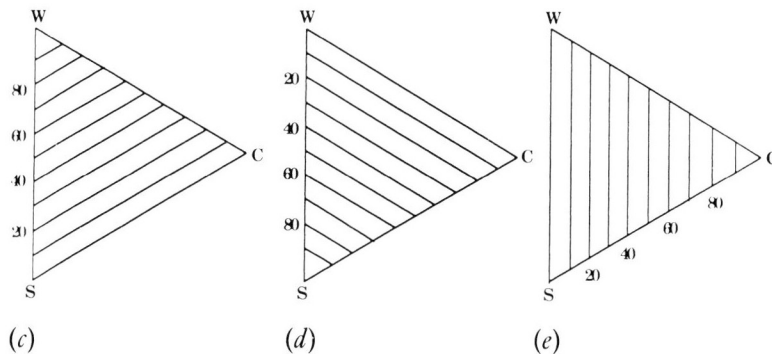

Fig. 2.8: Geometry of the natural color system NCS (see text).

represented in a three-dimensional elementary color space. Two coordinates represent the amounts of the opponent-color pairs, elementary red or green and elementary blue or yellow. The third dimension represents the amounts of elementary black and white. This color space is called the Natural Color System (NCS, Hering, 1874; 1920; see Introduction). Figure 2.8 shows a graphical representation of the Swedish Standard (1979) notation of the Natural Color System based on the respective color order systems of Hering and Ostwald (see Derefeldt, 1991).

From the amounts of elementary colors, three values of blackness, chromaticness (here: saturation), and hue are derived according to the formula as in the following examples: chromaticness = greenness (G) = 30 + 40 = 70 / yellowness (Y); hue = G x Y, with x = yellowness / (yellowness + greenness) * 100 = 30/70 * 100 = 43 (G43Y). Because of the judgment type this space is based on (see above), the elementary color space does not possess a metric for deriving color differences.

2.4.3 The jnd Scale

Two color stimuli possess a just noticeable difference (jnd) to each other, if a difference is observed in 50% of the cases presented (see above). If the two color stimuli are more different than one jnd from each other, the smallest possible number of jnd's between the two color stimuli can be taken as a measure of color difference or color similarity. This allows for an experimental determination of subjective color differences by successive threshold experiments, especially with animals for which the subjective color space is not known.

2.5 Neurophysiology of Color Vision

2.5.1 Humans and Other Vertebrates

Color vision systems consist of the following components: light entering the eye is absorbed in the photoreceptor cells according to their respective spectral sensitivities. The absorbed photons excite the photopigments in the photoreceptor membranes. The chromophore of the photopigments in the human eye and that of most of the other vertebrates is retinal, so the photopigments are rhodopsins (fishes and amphibians can have porphyropsins instead). The excited rhodopsin (metarhodopsin) molecules trigger a biochemical phototransduction cascade. This finally closes cation channels, which steer the flux of cations (mainly sodium) through the membrane, causing variations of the membrane potential. The total ion flux is affected in addition by the activity of ion-pumps. The light intensity absorbed in the photoreceptors is thus coded as hyperpolarization (more negative values) of the membrane potential. Paradoxically, the cation flux is highest at night when no light is present, whereas during daytime, the flux of cations is reduced.

Our eye possesses four different spectral types of photoreceptors: 1) one type of rod with maximum spectral sensitivity at about 498 nm (Dowling, 1987; Fig. 2.3), and 2) three different cone types: 433 nm, 532 nm, and 564 nm (Tab. 2.1, Fig. 2.3). The central region of highest spatial resolution in our eye, the fovea, has a visual angle of 2° and contains exclusively cones. Extrafoveally, the rods dominate more and more from the center to the periphery. The rods are more sensitive than the cones. Under dim light conditions vision relies exclusively on the rods (scotopic vision), whereas under daylight conditions (photopic vision) vision is dominated by the cones (normal color vision).

The information from the photoreceptors is further processed by the neuronal color-coding system, which is finally represented as the six elementary colors in our color sensations. This processing starts in the neuronal network of bipolar cells, horizontal cells, amacrine cells, and ganglion cells in our retina. The axons of the ganglion cells form the optic nerve which projects via the optic chiasm and the lateral geniculate nucleus (LGN) to the prestriate and striate cortex. The signals from the cones are further processed in an antagonistic fashion (i.e., neurons in the LGN and cortex receive inhibitory and excitatory inputs from the photoreceptors via the neuronal network

Table 2.1: Maxima of cone spectral sensitivity determined with different methods.

S-cone	M-cone	L-cone	method	author
444 nm	533 nm	571 nm	psychophysics	Estévez, 1979
419 nm	531 nm	558 nm	microspectrophotometry	Dartnall et al., 1985
437 nm	533nm	564 nm	microspectrophotometry	Dowling, 1987
433 nm	**532 nm**	**564 nm**	(average)	

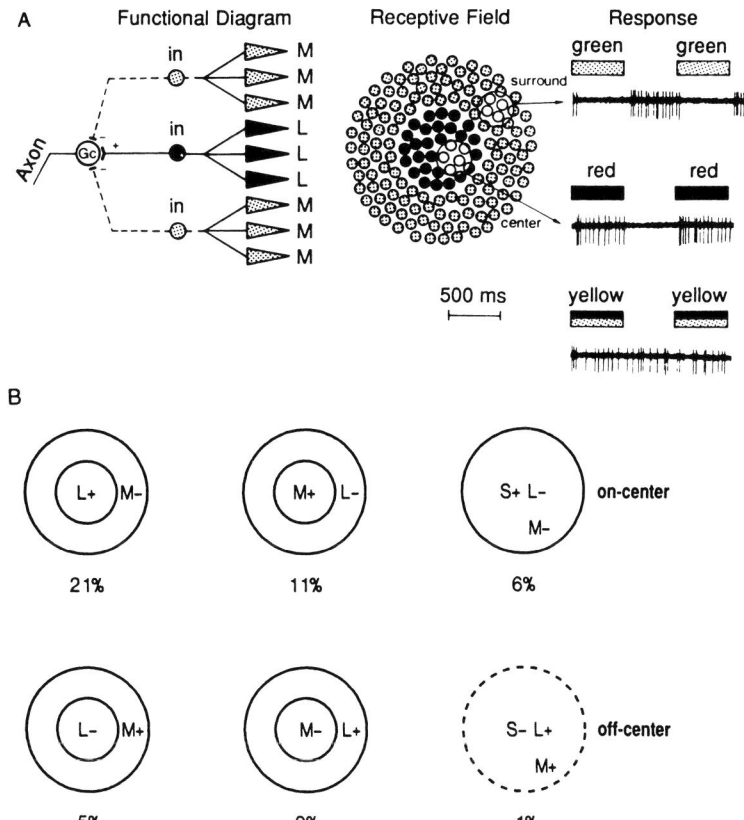

Fig. 2.9: Functional diagram, receptive fields and responses of photoreceptors and color opponent-coding ganglion cells in the macaque retina (see also chapters 3 and 4). **A:** In this example the L cones in the center of the receptive field of the ganglion cell are surrounded by M cones. Increasing the intensity of "red" light illuminating the center, excites the cell. Cells of this type are called ON-center cells (OFF-center cell when inhibition occurs when the center is illuminated by "red" light). Increasing the intensity of "green" illumination of the surround inhibits the cell. A "yellow" light which excites both the L and M cones has no effect because excitation and inhibition cancel each other (see spike responses, right column). **B:** Spatial structure of the receptive fields of the six most common types of color-opponent ganglion cells and frequency of incidence. (After Zrenner et al., 1990.)

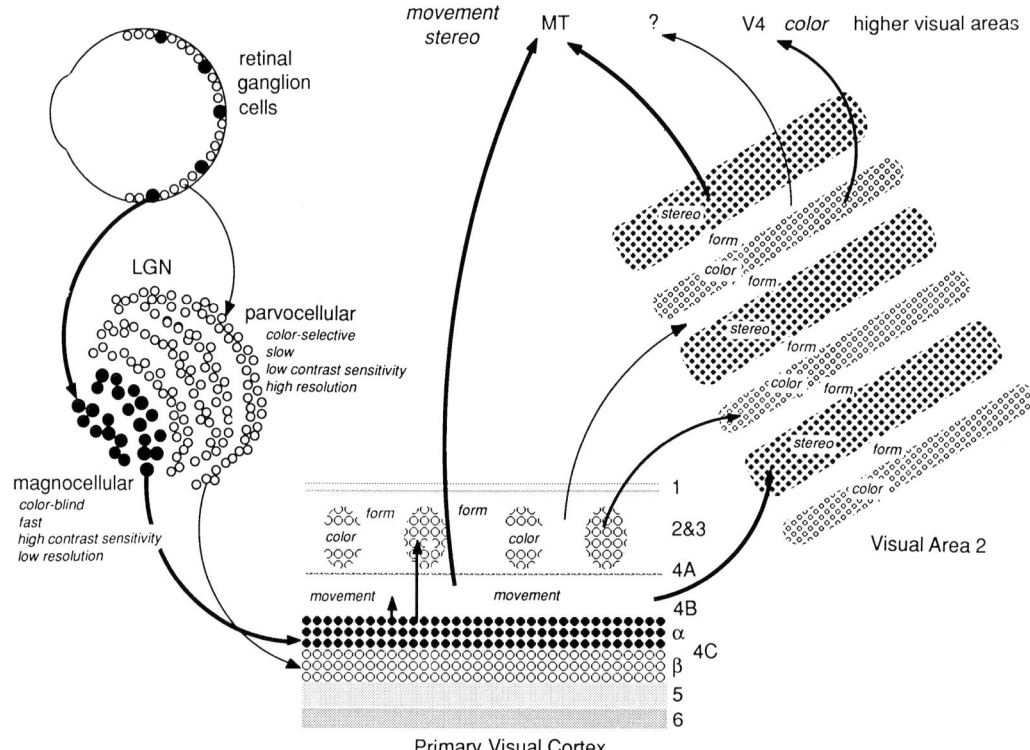

Fig. 2.10: Anatomical interconnection scheme of the neurons of the human color-coding system. The retinal ganglion cells project into the parvocellular lateral geniculate nucleus (LGN) and via the β-band of the primary visual cortex and visual area 2 (V2) to visual area V4. (After Livingstone and Hubel, 1988.)

in the retina). Human color perception appears to rely on the excitations of two color-opponent coding neuron types having antagonistic inputs from the S, M, and L cones: a) L_+ center – M_- surround (L_- center – M_+ surround, M_- center – L_+ surround, and M_+ center – L_- surround) coding for red/green with spectrally/spatially antagonistically organized receptive fields, and $S_+L_-M_-$ ($S_-L_+M_+$) with simple receptive fields, coding for blue/yellow. A non-opponent coding system b) $S_+L_+M_+$ ($S_-M_-L_-$) codes for black and white (Zrenner et al. 1990; Gouras, 1991a,b). Figure 2.9 shows the receptive fields of the respective LGN neurons which project via area V1 to area V4 (see Fig. 2.10).

2.5.2 Honeybees and Other Invertebrates

The compound eye of the honeybee contains about 5,000 facets (ommatidia). Each ommatidium consists of nine photoreceptor cells (3 UV, spectral sensitivity: $\lambda_{max} = 344$ nm, 2 "blue" (B), $\lambda_{max} = 436$ nm, and 4 "green" (G), $\lambda_{max} = 544$–556 nm, Fig. 2.11) which build a fused rhabdom of their rhabdomers (microvilli). Light entering an ommatidium via the cornea lens is absorbed successively in the light-guiding rhabdom by the rhodopsin molecules in the microvilli membranes. As in the eyes of other invertebrates, an absorbed photon converts the rhodopsin molecule into metarhodopsin which triggers a biochemical phototransduction cascade, finally opening cation channels. The resulting ion currents depolarize (more positive values) the

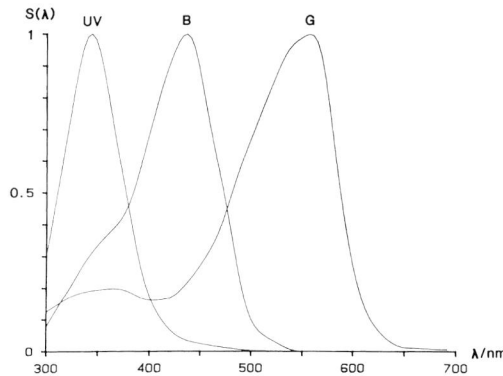

Fig. 2.11: Best-estimate functions based on intracellular recordings of the spectral sensitivities of the photoreceptors of the honeybee compound eye (from Backhaus, 1991).

membrane of the photoreceptor (i.e., the absorbed photon fluxes are coded in the graded membrane potentials). In the honeybee and other insects neuronal coding for color vision is realized by further processing of the membrane potentials of the photoreceptor cells of the retina by the monopolar cells of the lamina (1st optical neuropile) and the medulla (2nd optic neuropile). In the bee, the monopolar cells mainly sum the potentials of several photoreceptor cells of exclusively one spectral class of ca. 19 neighboring ommatidia. The graded potentials of the monopolar cells are further processed by two types of spiking color-opponent coding (COC) neurons of the lobula (3rd optic neuropile), which mainly sum the membrane potentials of all three spectral classes of monopolar cells weighted by the inhibitory and excitatory synapses (type A: $UV_- B_+ G_+$, type B: $UV_- B_+ G_-$).

2.6 Physiological Color Spaces

2.6.1 Physical Description of the Color Stimulus

The color stimuli presented in psychophysical experiments are sufficiently physically described in terms of spectral light intensity distributions (see above). The spectral intensity distributions of several lights can be superimposed (summed) to the total intensity distribution of the mixture, over wavelength. The physical properties of light mixtures can be determined from such a diagram, but nothing can be said about the physiological weightings of the lights by the photoreceptors or the neuronal color-coding system or about color appearance. Since under constant viewing conditions identical lights cause identical color sensations, the purely physical description of light may be used as an objective "color" notation. These diagrams allow to predict mixtures of completely different lights which are nevertheless physically identical and thus produce identical color sensations (metameric light mixtures, see below).

2.6.2 The Color Stimulus Space

The physicist Newton (1643–1727) spread daylight by a prism into a continuum of monochromatic lights of different wavelengths. He explained the phenomenon in quantitatively exact fashion by his theory of light waves. Besides the physical aspects of light he was also interested in the color sensations (colors) caused by the light entering our eyes. He remixed parts of the spectrum and found lights (metameric lights) which are physically different (i.e., different spectral intensity distributions) but nevertheless look identical (i.e., produce the same color). A white sensation occurs, for example, by mixing selected pairs of monochromatic lights (complementary lights) with accordingly adjusted intensities. The physical properties of light (intensity and wavelength) therefore have to be carefully distinguished from the color sensations caused by the light. He wrote in his Opticks:

> "The homogeneal Light and Rays which appear red or rather make Objects appear so, I call Rubrifick or Red-making; those which make Objects appear yellow, green, blue, and violet, I call Yellow-making, Green-making, Blue-making, and Violet-making, and so of the rest. ... For the Rays to speak properly are not coloured. In them there is nothing else than a certain Power and Disposition to stir up a Sensation of this or that Colour." Newton (1704, 1952)

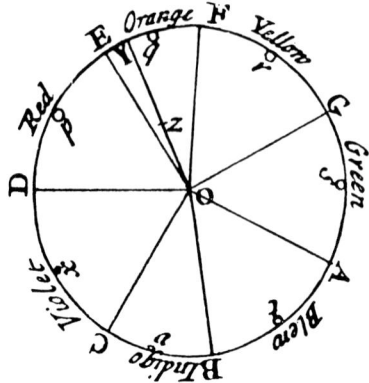

Fig. 2.12: Newton's color plate. The lights are ordered according to the subjective similarity of the color sensations they cause in a human observer. White-making light rays are located in the center. Chromatic lights which cause the purely chromatic color sensations are located at the round boundary of the plate, equidistant from the white-point. Newton could not determine the proper form of the boundary curve on which the monochromatic lights are located (spectral curve, compare Figs. 2.7, 2.8, 2.14, 2.15 and 2.22) because of optical limitations of the instruments available at his times (see also chapters 17 and 18). (After Newton, 1704, 1952.)

On the basis of the results of his light mixture experiments, he developed an idealized model for the prediction of the colors caused by different light mixtures (color table, Fig. 2.12) within the range of accuracy at which optical experiments could be performed at his time. Daylight which looks white to us (white light) is located at the center of the round "weightless" table. Equidistant from the center (i.e., at the periphery of the table) the monochromatic lights are located. The amounts (intensities) of the mixed lights were represented by "masses" at the loci of the lights used for mixture. The locus of the light mixtures of each of the two lights is simply found as the center-of-gravity which lies on the straight line through the two light (color) loci. The locus and amount of the mixture is found when the distance between the two loci is divided in the inverse proportions of the two masses (center-of-gravity method). Although Newton had not derived a vector space, his model is nevertheless three-dimensional. The color plate is two-dimensional; the third dimension of light intensity corresponds to the masses which represent the amounts of the mixed lights. In this sense Newton was first to demonstrate that human color vision is three-dimensional.

Based on the center-of-gravity method for color mixture and emphasizing the three-dimensionality of human color vision, the physicist and physiologist v. Helmholtz (1852; 1867) and the mathematician Grassmann (1853) suggested a color triangle as a mathematical representation of metameric light mixtures. The corners of the triangle represent three primary lights (primaries) used for light mixture. The color triangle can be interpreted as a plane section (chromaticity plane) through the three-dimensional color space (vector space) spanned by the primary values R, G, B:

$$R = \int I(\lambda)\, r'(\lambda)\, d\lambda, \quad G = \int I(\lambda)\, g'(\lambda)\, d\lambda,$$
$$B = \int I(\lambda)\, b'(\lambda)\, d\lambda, \tag{7}$$

with the spectral intensity distributions $I(\lambda)$ weighted by the spectral weighting functions $r'(\lambda)$, $g'(\lambda)$, $b'(\lambda)$. The chromaticity coordinates r, g, b of the color triangle (chromaticity plane) are the proportions of the primary values (Fig. 2.13 a, b):

$$r = R / (R+G+B), \quad g = G / (R+G+B),$$
$$b = B / (R+G+B), \text{ thus } r + g + b = 1. \tag{8}$$

The spectral weighting functions describe the effectiveness of monochromatic light intensity in the eye of the observer. For a specific set of primaries, these functions can always be obtained in color-matching experiments in which an observer is asked to adjust the intensities of the three primary lights R, G, B so that the resulting light mixture looks identical to a given monochromatic light of wavelength λ (judgment: color of I_λ is identical to color of $r'(\lambda)\, R_{max} + g'(\lambda)\, G_{max} + b'(\lambda)\, B_{max}$; see chapter 12). In the cases in which these matches can be obtained, the corresponding chromaticity coordinates are positive and the color loci lie within the chromaticity triangle spanned by the primaries. If such a direct match cannot be achieved, one or two of the primaries have to be mixed with the monochromatic light and the resulting mixture has to be adjusted to match the color of the mixture of the

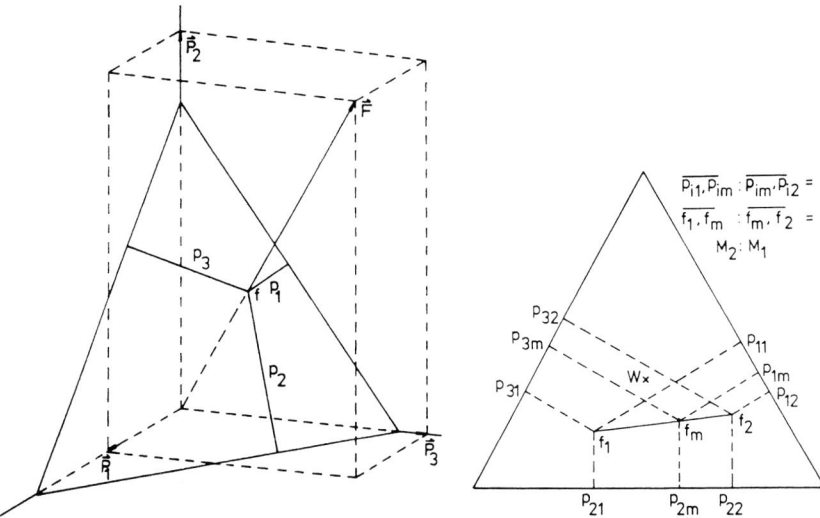

Fig. 2.13a: Photoreceptor sensitivity (light absorption) color space and respective chromaticity diagram. The color space is spanned by three vectors P which represent the photon fluxes absorbed in the three types of photoreceptors. A color is represented by the tip of the resultant vector F. Color brightness can be approximately derived as the sum of the coordinate values P. The length of the color vector F has no special meaning. The chromaticity diagram can be derived as a plane section through the color space. The chromaticity coordinates p represent colors of equal totally absorbed photon flux (ΣP_i = const., eqs. 9–10). The color loci in the chromaticity diagram can be determined as the intersection points of the color vectors F through the color plane.
b: Determination of the locus of a light mixture f_m from the loci of two color stimuli f_1 and f_2 mixed. According to the Graßmannian (1853) mixture rules based on Newton's (1704) center-of-gravity method the straight line through the two loci has simply to be divided into the inverse proportions of the amounts of light (M = $P_1+P_2+P_3$) used for mixture (the procedure is the same in the color space). It has to be pointed out that the chromaticity coordinates are only a rough denotation of chromaticness (the two-dimensional aspect of color, different from brightness). The chromaticness of a color depends on the light intensity (i.e., the Bezold-Brücke effect) which is not at all described by the chromaticity diagram because the chromaticity coordinates are independent of variations in light intensity (see eq. 10). Thus, color differences between the color loci cannot be derived in a simple way (e.g., as the geometrical distance between two color loci) from chromaticity diagrams (see text). (After Backhaus and Menzel, 1987.)

remaining primaries (indirect color matching). The respective chromaticity coordinates become negative and the loci of the monochromatic lights lie outside of the color triangle in this case (see e.g., Richter, 1981).

The light spectrum was first gauged by Maxwell (1855, 1860) who determined the weighting functions r'(λ), g'(λ) and b'(λ) in precise color mixture experiments with rotating disks consisting of light reflecting sectors (color top). The loci of the monochromatic lights proved to lie on a slightly distorted circle around the white point. Mixtures of the ends of the visible spectrum, which look purple (blue/red), lie at the respective centers-of-gravity on the straight mixture line between the loci of the visible ends of the spectrum (see e.g., Fig. 2.14). For special applications in human color vision (color metrics), linear transformations of the RGB color stimulus space and color plane are in use (e.g., CIE diagram, see chapter 17).

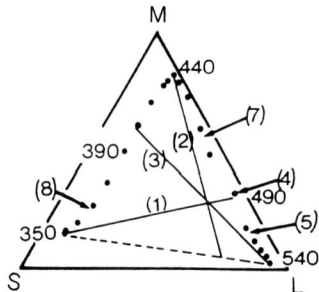

(1) 350 ⟶ 490 (= 65% 590 + 35% 440)
(2) 440 ⟶ 80% 590 + 20% 360
(3) 590 ⟶ 66% 440 + 34% 360

(4) 490 = 65% 590 + 35% 440
(5) 530 = 60% 616 + 40% 490
(6) 588 = (20-80)% 616 + (80-20)% 530
(7) 474 = (40-60)% 440 + (60-40)% 490
(8) 375 = 20% 440 + 80% 360

Fig. 2.14: Daumer's 1956 color-choice percentages measured in light mixture experiments with honeybees, redrawn in the photon absorption color triangle for the honeybee. (After Menzel and Backhaus, 1991.)

The concept of the RGB color stimulus space can also be applied to other animal species when the respective loci of the monochromatic lights (spectral curve) have been determined in color choice experiments. The RGB space is especially useful if the physiology of the color-coding system of an animal species is only incompletely known (honeybees: Daumer, 1956, see Fig. 2.14; bumblebees: Mazokhin-Porshnyakow, 1962; for other animals see Jacobs, 1981). The form of the spectral curve allows for an examination of the dimensionality of the respective color vision system, for predicting light mixtures and their discriminability in terms of metameric color stimuli (see above).

In the case of dichromatic (two photoreceptors) color vision (see chapter 16), there exists for any light mixture a monochromatic light of certain intensity which is metameric to the mixture. Color vision is at least three-dimensional if there exist light mixtures which are not metameric to any monochromatic light (e.g., white light, mixture of monochromatic lights of the extreme ends of the visible spectrum or "purple"-line, see Fig. 2.14). Spectral curves are thus most useful for a quantitative comparison of the color vision systems of different species.

It has to be pointed out that in all the color stimulus spaces only the light (color) loci have a meaning. Subjective color differences (see above) may not be read from these diagrams directly as the geometric distance between the color loci.

2.6.3 The Photoreceptor Sensitivity (Light Absorption) Space (1st Physiological Color Space)

Palmer (1777) and Young (1802) already hypothesized about the physiological basis of human color vision on the basis of psychophysical measurements, to be based on three spectral types of resonators for light of different wavelengths. These resonators were much later identified in electrophysiological investigations to be the three spectral types of photoreceptors (cones) in the retina. If the spectral sensitivity functions are electrophysiologically measured for a specific color vision system, the absorbed photon fluxes may be used as the basis vectors of a physiological color space and a respective color triangle (Cornsweet, 1970; Rushton, 1972; Rodieck, 1973). The linear light mixture rules (Graßmann, 1853) hold in both the color spaces. This is because the absorbed photon fluxes are calculated as the integral over the spectral intensity distribution weighted by the spectral sensitivity of the photoreceptors (see Fig. 2.13a, b), which are, mathematically speaking, linear functionals of the light intensity, which do not affect the linearity of the mixture rules (Krantz, 1975):

$$P_i = R_i \int_{i=1}^{m} I(\lambda) \, s_i(\lambda) \, d\lambda, \qquad (9)$$

where $I(\lambda)$ is the spectral light intensity distribution, $s(\lambda)$ the spectral sensitivity function of the (m) types of photoreceptors ($i = 1 - m$) and the range sensitivity R which accounts for the reduction of the sensitivity during light adaptation (Laughlin, 1981). The color space is spanned by the relative photon fluxes P_i absorbed in the photoreceptors. The chromaticity plane again is calculated according to eq. 7–8 which holds for an arbitrary number (m) of photoreceptors (honeybees: v. Helversen, 1972b; insects: Menzel and Backhaus, 1991):

$$p_i = P_i / \sum_{i=1}^{m} P_i \quad (10)$$

The chromaticity diagram, spanned by the (m) chromaticity coordinates p_i, represents light stimuli which cause constant total absorbed photon fluxes. Polychromatic color spaces and polychromatic chromaticty planes allow us a description of color vision systems for species with more than three types of photoreceptors (tetrachromatic systems: e.g., the wasp *Tentredo* and the solitary bee *Callonychium petuniae*, vertebrates: e.g., goldfish (see chapter 8) and pentachromatic systems: e.g., butterfly *Papilio xuthus* (see Menzel and Backhaus, 1991). All color stimuli with constant totally absorbed photon flux lie in the general polychromatic case within a (m−1)-dimensional subspace ($\Sigma p_i = 1$) of the m-dimensional color space. In the case of two-dimensional color vision, this subspace is a straight line (see chapter 16), in the case of three-dimensional color vision, a flat triangle (see above) and in tetrachromatic color vision, a tetrahedron (see Neumeyer, 1988). These chromaticity subspaces allow a three-dimensional representation (for coordinates and respective transformations of three-dimensional representations of tetrachromatic color vision, see Menzel and Backhaus, 1991).

The light absorption color space takes spectral sensitivity as a major property of the photoreceptors into account and thus contains more information for comparison of color vision in different species. Again in this case, the geometrical distances between the color loci may not be directly interpreted as the subjective color differences. The color stimulus space as well as the light absorption space both belong to the lower color metric (Schrödinger, 1920 a, b).

2.6.4 The Photoreceptor Excitation Space (2nd Physiological Color Space)

The photoreceptors absorb photons with a probability determined by their spectral sensitivity and so exclusively code for the relative absorbed photon flux. The photoreceptors therefore do not analyze the wavelengths of the absorbed photons but just measure absorbed photon fluxes (univariance principle). The membrane potential V is nonlinearly related to the relative absorbed photon flux P according to the general phototransduction function (Naka and Rushton, 1966, 1967; Lipetz, 1971):

$$E = V/V\max = P^n / (P^n + 1), \quad (11)$$

with a species-specific parameter n. The photoreceptor space is spanned by the relative electrical excitations E. The sum of the excitations can be interpreted as the excitation of a neuron which codes for brightness. The plane, $\Sigma E_i = $ const., thus represents the colors of approximately constant brightness. Paradoxically, this color space is less useful than the color stimulus space and the light absorption space. This is because the linear Grassmannian rules for predicting light mixtures neither hold in this space nor can the subjective color difference be read directly in terms of the geometrical distance between the color loci. For the design of psychophysical experiments with animals, thus, the photon absorption space is usually prefered over the photoreceptor excitation space (see chapter 9), also because the color plane ($\Sigma p_i = 1$) appears to be a rather good approximation for equally-bright ($\Sigma E_i = $ const.) colors (see Backhaus, 1992).

2.6.5 The Color-Opponent Coding Space (3rd Physiological Color Space)

Following the physiological approach (see Fig. 2.1) further, we obtained the color-opponent coding (COC) space. The relative membrane potentials of the three types of photoreceptors caused by light are described by eq. 11, taking into account adaptation to bright light as described by eq. 9. The photoreceptor potentials are processed further via several other neurons (honeybees: monopolar cells, humans: neurons in the retina, LGN, and V1) to two (honeybees) or three (humans) types of color-opponent coding neurons (see above). The coding of the neurons via their synapses are assumed to be linear. In the case of the honeybee, the color-opponent coding (COC) space was shown to be identical to the psychophysical MDS color space (Backhaus, 1991). It is expected that a comparable relationship exists between the MDS space and a respective COC space in humans (see below).

2.6.6   Color Spaces and jnd Scales

The minimum number of jnd's is identical to the color difference between two colors (see example, Fig. 2.7). In the case of the city-block metric, the color difference between each two colors is therefore more easily obtained by successive jnd measurements than in the case of the Euclidean metric. In the first case, any line in a wider area has only to be measured, whereas in the second case, a specific mixture line has to be found. As already pointed out above, the geometry of the chromaticity diagram is not equispaced with respect to subjective color differences. The line of the smallest number of jnd's (i.e., the line of most similar colors) is thus curved in the color stimulus space, the light absorption space and in the photoreceptor excitation space as well as in the respective color planes (i.e., chromaticity diagrams).

The psychophysical MDS space and the physiological color opponent-coding (COC) space (see below) both appear to be equispaced with respect to subjective color differences. In the Euclidean space (e.g., human color vision), the difference between each two colors is simply determined as the straight (geometrical) distance between each two color loci. The loci of colors, one jnd different from a certain color, lie on circles (Fig. 2.6). In a color space with a city-block metric (e.g., honeybee color space), the loci of colors one jnd apart from a specific color lie on squares around this color. Figure 2.7 shows the city-block geometry of the COC space which allows for a simple geometrical method for determining the color differences between each two colors by simply counting the lines crossed when moving from one color locus to the other on a straight line (see example). If the subjective color space possesses a Euclidean metric, there exists only one line of the smallest number of jnd's between two colors. If the metric is the city-block metric, there always exists an area within the boundaries of which all lines, between one color stimulus and another, possess the minimum number. This geometrical property allows to determine the number of jnd steps in behavioral experiments much easier when the subjective color space possesses a city-block metric compared to a Euclidean metric.

2.7   Psychophysical and Physiological Simulations of Color Vision

Since the first systematic psychophysical measurements performed by Weber (1834) and Fechner (1860), there have been continuous attempts to interpret and understand the psychophysical results in the field of color vision in progressively detailed neurophysiological and neuroanatomical terms. Nowadays, it is possible to simulate neuronal color-coding systems in detail on the computer. These simulations allow for predictions which motivate more specific electrophysiological measurements. How far this iterative process has come will be illustrated by means of the theory of color vision and color-choice behavior of the honeybee.

2.7.1   The Psychophysical (MDS) Color Space in Honeybees

In order to determine the subjective color space of the honeybee, multiple color-choice experiments were performed with twelve color stimuli, especially for multidimensional scaling analysis (Backhaus, Menzel and Kreißl, 1987). Individual bees were trained on one of twelve color stimuli and the choice percentages towards the alternatives were measured (color similarity experiments). Special care was taken to check whether

2.7 Psychophysical and Physiological Simulations of Color Vision 63

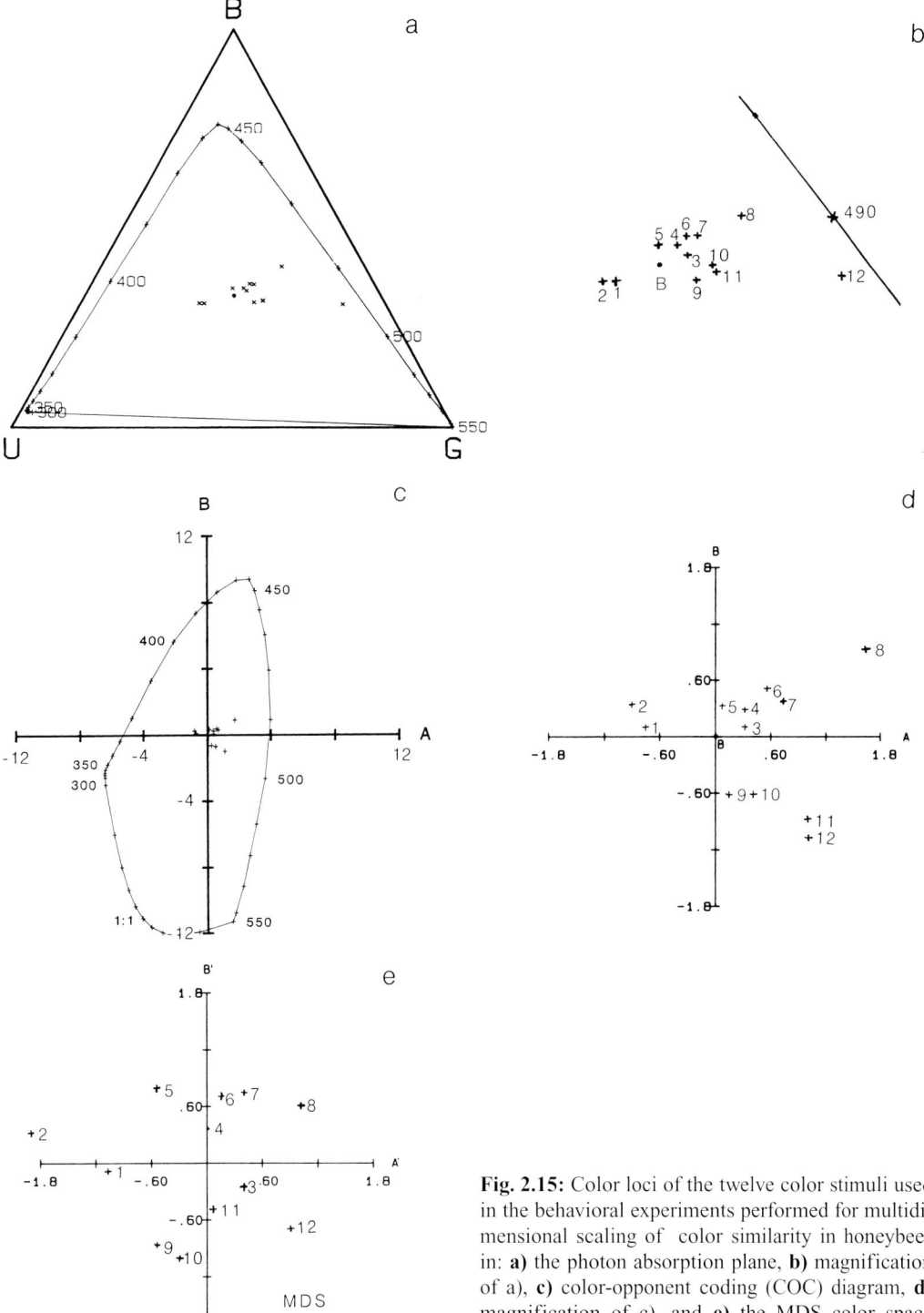

Fig. 2.15: Color loci of the twelve color stimuli used in the behavioral experiments performed for multidimensional scaling of color similarity in honeybees in: **a)** the photon absorption plane, **b)** magnification of a), **c)** color-opponent coding (COC) diagram, **d)** magnification of c), and **e)** the MDS color space (from Backhaus 1991).

the MDS model of color perception in humans is appropriate also for color vision of the honeybee. The choice percentages of bees turned out to be even more reliable (smaller fluctuations) than those of humans. The choice percentages were thus analyzed by metric (Euclidean metric) and non-metric multidimensional (Minkowski metric) scaling (MDS) analysis. According to special goodness-of-fit-measures, the dimension, the metric and the scale values (dimensions, coordinates) of the twelve color stimuli used were determined. The following results were obtained: 1) the internal representation of color information in the bee has the structure of a vector space, comparable to human color vision. 2) The color space is only two-dimensional, compared to the human color space which is three-dimensional. 3) It is without a brightness dimension and 4) with a city-block-metric, which again is different from the human color space which has a Euclidean metric. 5) The scale values for the twelve color stimuli allow for a reliable reconstruction of the measured choice percentages according to the psychophysical (MDS) model of color vision. The geometry of this color space is shown in Figure 2.15c–e. Subjective color differences can be calculated via the city-block metric (eq. 6) or geometrically from the MDS diagram (see example, Fig. 2.7).

2.7.2 Neuronal Color-Coding and Color-Choice Behavior in Honeybees

Color spaces have been derived for humans but also for color vision in animals with the intention of getting an impression of how the lights are weighted and represented in the respective species, in terms of color discrimination and color similarity relations and in terms of elementary colors. For many insect and vertebrate species, color vision is well investigated in terms of color discrimination and color similarity experiments as well as by electrophysiological measurements of the spectral sensitivity of the photoreceptors. Thus, in many cases, color vision in animals can be well described in terms of color stimulus spaces and photon absorption spaces (see above; chapters 8 and 9).

Honeybees have been the most intensively investigated in behavioral as well as physiological respects since the first experiments of v. Frisch (1914), who showed that bees are able to discriminate a "blue" plate from a series of "gray" plates. A bee reaches an acquisition level of color learning which is better than 95% when rewarded several times on a color stimulus with droplets of sucrose solution. In color discrimination experiments, alternative color stimuli are tested for confusion with the training stimulus in unrewarded tests. The experimental bee provides the sucrose solution to other bees in the hive for further processing, and then immediately returns to the experimental setup. An individual bee can be tested up to 14 days. Thus, honeybees are ideal animals for color training experiments. The color-choice percentages that are obtained can be treated like results of psychophysical experiments with humans. Because of the detailed electrophysiological and neuroanatomical knowledge of the neuronal color-coding system, all of the color spaces described above can be used to describe their color vision. Thus, the problem of color vision in animals will be further discussed using the color vision system of the honeybee as a model.

Daumer (1956) showed in light mixture experiments that color vision of the bee is trichromatic. He presented the amounts of the light stimuli used for mixtures that are indistinguishable for the bee from a reference stimulus (metameric colors) in a chromaticity diagram, spanned by the normalized light intensities of the basic lights (primaries) used for the mixture see also chapter 9. It turned out that the color stimulus space needed for describing the results is three-dimensional.

Since the first electrophysiological recordings of Autrum and v. Zwehl (1964), the spectral sensitivity functions of the three types of photoreceptors were determined with increasing accuracy (for a comparison of methods and results, see Menzel, et al., 1986; best estimate functions: Menzel and Backhaus, 1991; Fig. 2.11).

Knowledge of the spectral sensitivity functions of the photoreceptors allows us to construct the photon absorption space for the bee (v. Helversen, 1972a; Backhaus and Menzel, 1987). Daumer showed in his light mixing experiments that honeybee color vision is indeed trichromatic in the sense that three types of photoreceptors are involved. The photon absorption space stands in a linear relationship to the color stimulus space. The linear mixture rules hold and thus Daumer's mixture ratios hold in both the spaces. Daumer's results are redrawn in the photon absorption diagram which makes this conclusion obvious (see Fig. 2.14).

According to eq. 9–11, the photoreceptor space for the honeybee was derived. This space *per se* has no further interesting properties except to represent the membrane potentials of the photoreceptors, i.e., neither the linear light mixture rules hold nor can the color difference between two color loci be derived directly from the diagram (see above). The photoreceptor space was therefore combined with the jnd concept for determination of color differences from this diagram (Backhaus and Menzel, 1987; Backhaus, 1992b). As mentioned above, the jnd concept is most useful as long as the subjective color space is unknown. Indeed the photoreceptor model was developed before the subjective color space of the bee was determined by MDS analysis (see above) and so it was a precursor for the COC model of the honeybee. The photoreceptor model of color vision is still attractive because it allows a generalization to color vision of other animal species if only the spectral sensitivities of the photoreceptors are known (see chapter 9). The photoreceptor model allows in addition a straightforward extension to polychromatic color vision (insects: Menzel and Backhaus, 1991).

In the next step, the neuronal color-coding system was described by steady-state models (Backhaus, 1991) of the three types of photoreceptors with the respective monopolar cells and the two types of color-opponent coding (COC) neurons which were exclusively found in the honeybee brain by intracellular recording techniques (Kien and Menzel, 1977). The photoreceptor model included in this description is identical with that used for the photoreceptor space of the bee (i.e., the best estimate functions based on the measured spectral sensitivities (see above), the phototransduction process and the light adaptation mechanism were taken into account). In the case of adaptation to darkness, the relative membrane potential is zero, and half of the maximum response in the case of adaptation to daylight. Since electrophysiological data must always be suspected to be distorted by artifacts, the spectral sensitivity curves of the COC neurons were only qualitatively used, motivating the physiological model of color-opponent coding. Thus, an additional, independent way for determining the physiological parameters of the model was looked for and found.

2.7.3 Identification of the Physiological COC Space and the Psychophysical MDS Space

The abstract MDS scales and the excitation values of the two types of color-opponent coding neurons might well be identical to each other. This would indeed allow a determination of the physiological parameters of the color-opponent coding (COC) model (see eqs. in Fig. 2.16). Most helpful for this approach was that the city block metric fixes the coordinates (dimensions) of the MDS color space (i.e., the coordinates may not be continuously rotated as is indeed the case for the human color space because of its Euclidean metric). The gain parameters could then be calculated as the unique least-square solution for minimal differences (identification) between the twelve MDS scale values, A' and B' of the color stimuli used in the color similarity experiments and the twelve respective excitation values, A and B of the model COC neurons calculated from the spectral intensity functions of these twelve color stimuli (see Fig. 2.15).

After the scales which span the subjective color space were identified by physiological simulations to be identical to the excitation values of the two color-opponent coding neurons, the physiological model and the psychophysical model could be combined (Fig. 2.16). The physiological model yields the excitation values of the two color-opponent coding neurons A and B. From the two excitation values A and B color distances d were derived via the city-block metric of the subjective color space. The city-block metric can also be realized physiologically by simple neurons. The simplest neuronal network consists of pairs of neurons which show no spontaneous activity (i.e., the rest-

The Theory of Color Vision and Color Choice Behavior of the Bee

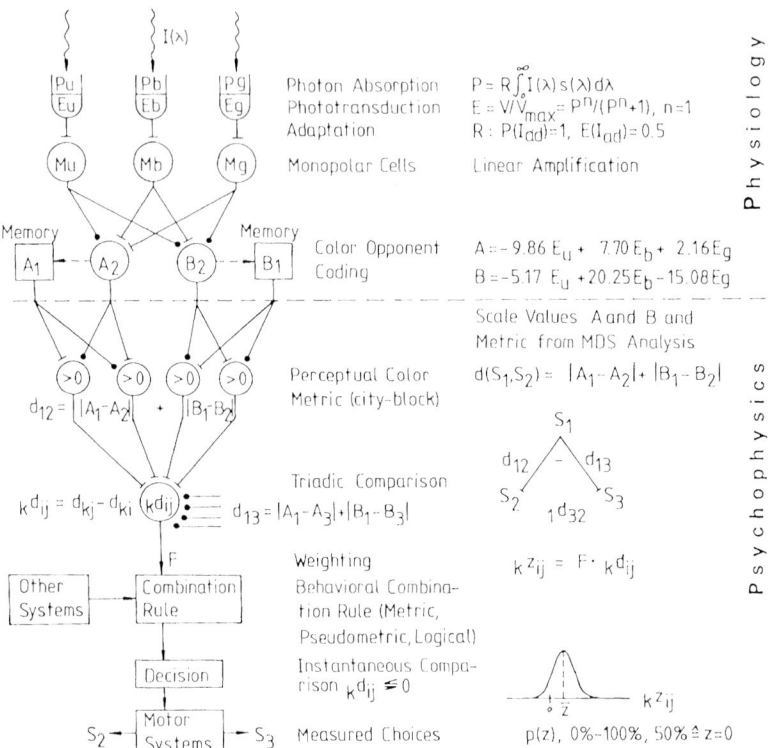

Fig. 2.16: The theory of color vision and color-choice behavior of the bee.
Upper part (above dashed line): physiological model of neuronal color-coding.
Lower part (below dashed line): psychophysical model of color difference (MDS color space) and the model of color-choice behavior.
Left: neuronal interconnection scheme.
Right: mathematical description (from Backhaus, 1993; see text).

ing spike frequency is zero), and receive inputs opposite in sign from the color memory and from the two color-opponent coding neurons A and B, respectively. Cells of this type have additionally been found in the honeybee brain (Kien and Menzel, 1977).

As a check for the appropriateness of this identification, the spectral sensitivity curves of the COC neurons were determined by simulations of the electrophysiological measurements. The form of the wavelength/intensity curves (Fig. 2.17) changes dramatically when the wavelength of the test light is varied. This means that the univariance principle (see above) does not apply in this case.

Certain wavelengths depolarize (higher spike frequency) or hyperpolarize (lower spike frequency) the COC neurons. The intensity to response curves may even be biphasic. Nevertheless, the form of the spectral sensitivity functions do not depend much on the choice of the threshold criterion. This is because the minimum threshold can only be chosen in a range of 1%–6.3% of the maximum response. The reason for this is that the noise amplitude is minimally about 1% of the maximum response in electrophysiological recordings and if the threshold is set to higher values than 6.3%, the criterion is not reached by the test light at all wavelengths of the visual range.

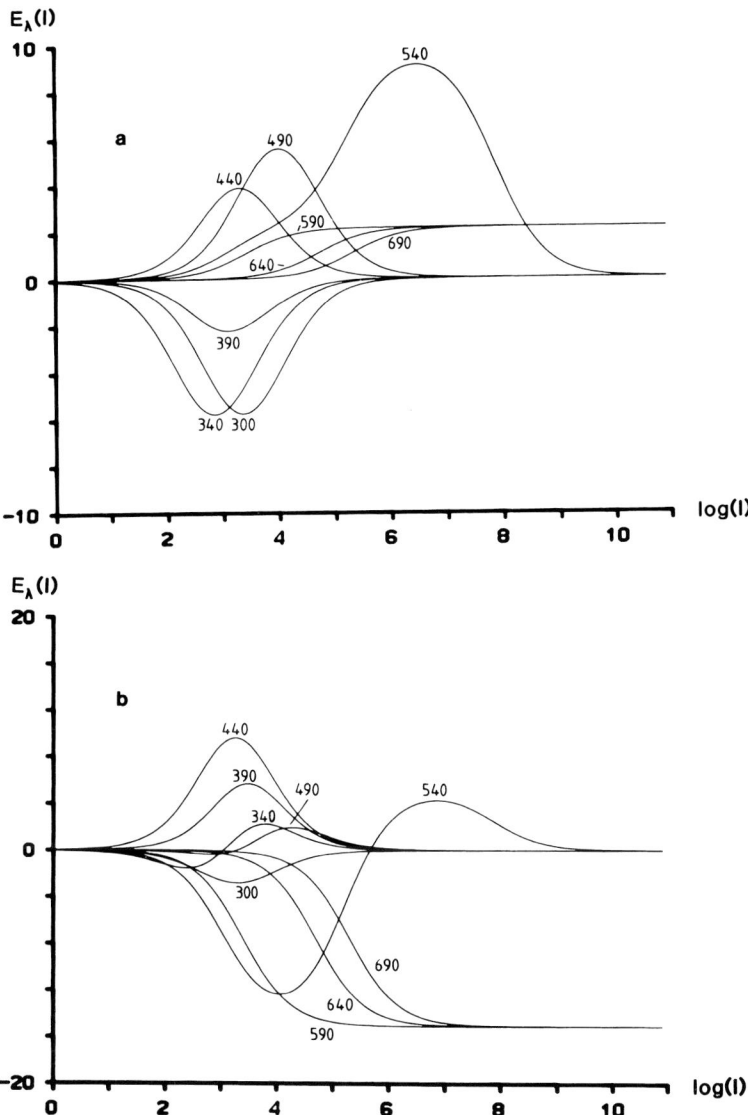

Fig. 2.17: Excitation/intensity curves $E_\lambda(I)$ obtained by simulations of electrophysiological measurements on the two model color-opponent coding neurons A **(a)** and B **(b)** of Fig. 2.16 with dark adapted photoreceptors. The numbers indicate the wavelengths of the monochromatic lights in nm, varied from dark to bright light intensities. Both neurons sum the inhibitory and excitatory inputs from the photoreceptors via the monopolar cells and the respective synapses. At lower as well as at brighter intensities both the neurons show the same relative resting spike frequency (0). The univariance principle (see text) obviously holds only for the photoreceptors. The excitation/intensity of the color-opponent coding neurons decrease or increase with increasing light intensity due to the dominance of the inhibitory or the excitatory inputs from the photoreceptors, and are even biphasic in neuron B (b).

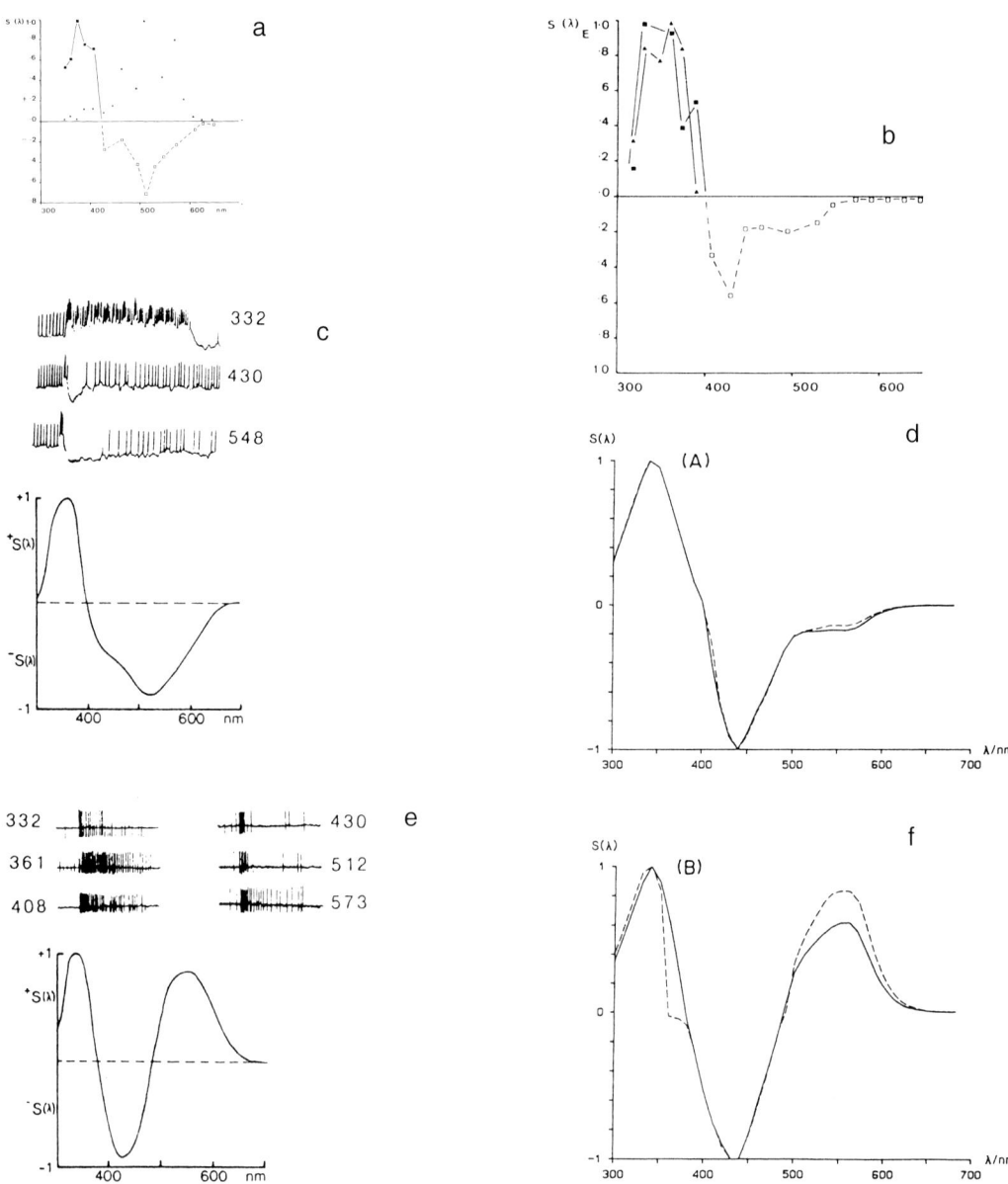

Fig. 2.18: Comparison of the spectral sensitivities derived from the intensity excitation curves in Fig. 2.16 with the spectral sensitivity functions measured by Kien and Menzel (1977). **a)** and **b)** examples of spectral sensitivity functions of which the spectral sensitivity function for neuron type A in **c)** was derived. **d)** spectral sensitivity of model neuron A. **e)** measured spectral sensitivity function of neuron type B. **f)** spectral sensitivity function of model neuron B. The spike trains in c) and e) show typical responses of neuron types A and B with respect to an intensity step of different monochromatic lights. The numbers indicate the wavelengths in nm.
Solid line: minimal criterion of excitation for determining spectral sensitivity: 1% of maximal excitation.
Dashed line: maximal criterion: 6% of maximum response.
The measured and predicted curves from the physiological simulations are in a very good agreement. Only the inhibitory part (minimum) of the measured function in c) could not be obtained. Closer inspection of the indi-

2.7 Psychophysical and Physiological Simulations of Color Vision

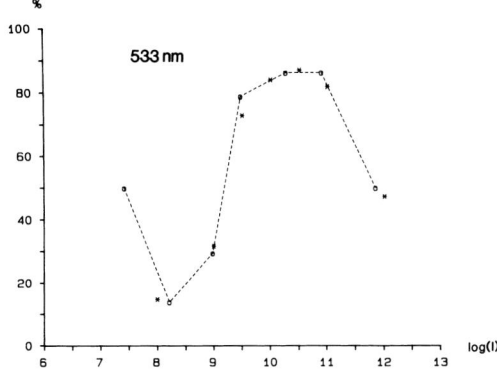
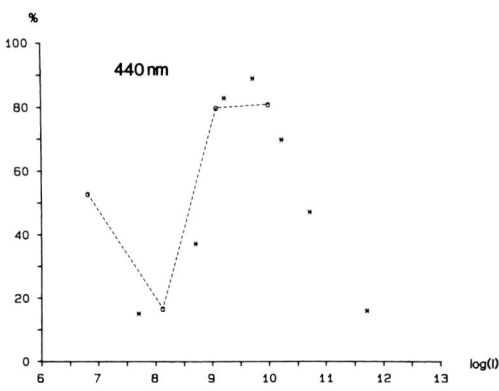
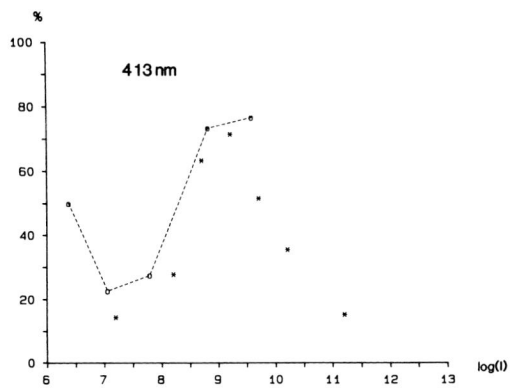

The measured spectral sensitivity functions are in very good agreement with the spectral sensitivity functions predicted from the simulations of these measurements with the COC model (Fig. 2.18). The general form as well as the maxima, minima and zero crossings of the measured and the predicted functions are almost identical. A greater deviation appears to exist only in the inhibitory part of neuron A. The measured minimum is broader than in the respective simulation. Closer inspection of the spectral sensitivity of the individual recordings shows that the form and the halfwidth of the minima agree with that of the simulation. The broadening of the minimum is obviously due to a shift of the minima of the individual functions, which might well be due to artifacts in the recordings. This shows that it was indeed necessary to derive the parameters of the physiological COC model on the basis of behavioral data first, instead of fittting the parameters directly to the electrophysiologically-measured functions.

Fig. 2.19: Comparison of the choice percentages measured (circles, dashed lines) in behavioral color discrimination experiments (Menzel, 1981) and the results of respective physiological simulations (stars) as a function of the intensity I of the monochromatic lights used. In the experiments, dark adapted individual bees were trained to turn to one side (e.g., right) in a T-maze when white light was presented at the decision point and to turn to the other side (e.g., left) when a monochromatic light of an intensity for best discrimination was shown. The intensity of the monochromatic light was varied in the tests and the choice percentages towards the monochromatic light were measured: a) 533 nm, b) 440 nm, and c) 413 nm. The striking agreement between measured and simulated data shows 1) that in color training experiments the color vision system of the bee is at work also at lowest light intenties, and that 2) intensity-dependent color shifts (Bezold-Brücke effect) also exist in the bee (from Backhaus, 1992; see text).

vidual recordings a) and b) from which the curve in c) was derived, look very close to the predicted curve in d). Since the model curves were theoretically derived exclusively from behavioral data, this comparison clearly demonstrates that the color-opponent coding neurons recorded by Kien and Menzel (1977) are essentially involved in color vision of the honeybee (from Backhaus, 1991; see text).

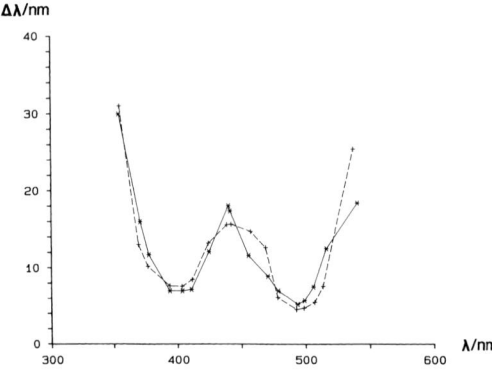

Fig. 2.20: Comparison of the wavelength discrimination curve of the honeybee measured (+, dashed line) in behavioral experiments (v. Helversen, 1972) and the results of the respective physiological simulations (*, solid line) using the COC model and the model of the decision process. Abscissa: wavelengths of the reference monochromatic light. **Ordinate:** wavelength difference necessary for 70% correct choices of the reference light. (From Backhaus, 1991, see text.)

In addition to this physiological test, the steady-state model of color vision and color-choice behavior of the honeybee has also passed all critical tests by behavioral experiments. 1) Menzel (1981) performed a color training experiment in which the bee had to learn to turn to one side in a T-maze when a bright white light was seen at the decision point and to turn to the other side when a monochromatic light of specific wavelength was presented. In the unrewarded tests, the monochromatic light was shown at different intensities. In Figure 2.19, the results of the three experiments performed at 533 nm, 440 nm and 413 nm are compared to the results of the respective simulations with the COC model. The agreement is striking. The results clearly demonstrate that the chromaticness (two-dimensional aspect of a color, different from brightness) depends on the light intensity, i.e., the Bezold-Brücke effect, well known from human color vision, also exists in honeybees (Backhaus, 1992a). It was shown, in addition, that there is indeed no brightness dimension involved in honey-

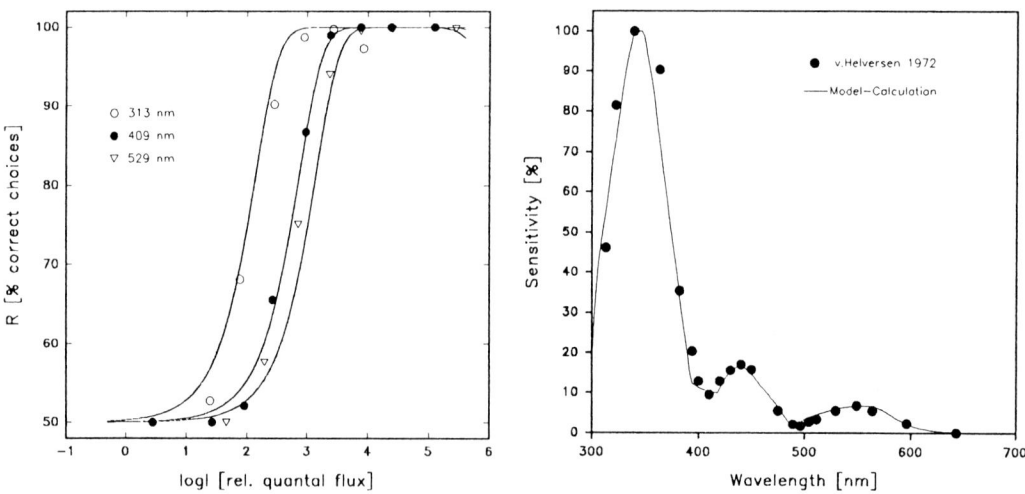

Fig. 2.21: Comparison of a pre-experiment (v. Helversen, 1972) to the behavioral wavelength discrimination experiment of Fig. 2.20 and the respective physiological simulations. After training to a dark color stimulus, the bee was tested against monochromatic stimuli of different intensities. **a)** three typical curves which were measured (symbols) for three different wavelengths and the respective physiological simulations (solid lines). **b)** behavioral spectral sensitivity curve derived from a) with a criterion of 70% correct choices (dots) and the respective physiological simulations with the COC model (Fig. 2.16). (After Brandt, et al., 1993.) The behavioral data are shown to be due again to intensity dependent color shifts (Bezold-Brücke effect) and not to color discrimination on the basis of a color brightness system.

bee color vision even at the highest light intensities. 2) v. Helversen (1972a) measured the wavelength discrimination function of the bee. A comparison of the measured data with the curve obtained in a simulation of the behavioral experiments is shown in figure 2.20. The agreement is again excellent. 3) In a behavioral pre-experiment, v. Helversen (1972a) determined the absolute spectral sensitivity function of the bee with respect to an almost dark color stimulus. This is a standard experiment in human color vision as well as in the color vision of animals. Since only the intensity of monochromatic lights is varied in these experiments, it is usually assumed that the choice behavior would rely on the neuronal color brightness system. The simulation of this experiment with the COC model of the bee (Brandt et al., 1993), which does not possess a brightness dimension, again accurately fits straightforward the measured data (Fig. 2.21). The bee discriminates the intensity differences on the basis of intensity dependent color (chromaticness) shifts (Bezold-Brücke effect), and not on the basis of a brightness system. It must be concluded from this result that care has to be taken when assuming anything about the components of a neuronal color-coding system. The neuronal system in question has rather to be electrophysiologically measured, modeled and tested in detailed physiological simulations.

2.8 Conscious vs. Unconscious Judgments

Because of the causal chain structure of our color vision which we know from introspection, it is not at all obvious which types of judgments rely on our conscious color sensations and which rely on the excitation values of the neurons of the information coding system or on both. Color discrimination and color similarity experiments are also the common experiments performed with animals for investigating their color vision. It is suspected that from this type of experiment nothing may be concluded about color sensations or conscious color vision. Discrimination of a colored light from a series of white lights of different intensities (see above) allows us only the conclusion that the animal possesses a neuronal color-coding system which might code for color sensations as well.

2.8.1 Color Sensations in Animals

The simplest case of conscious color vision is when we experience simple (unstructured, homogeneous) color sensations. The amounts of the six elementary colors constituting a color sensation

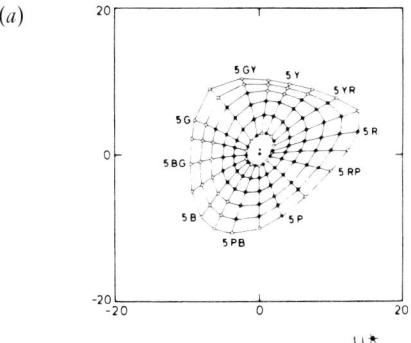

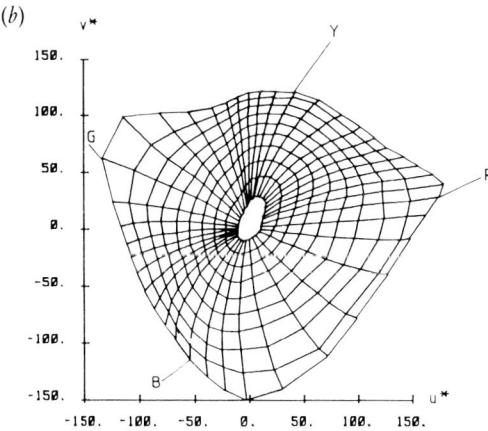

Fig. 2.22: Comparison of **a)** the Munsell color space with lines of constant hue (radial) and constant chroma (concentric) at brightness level value 5 and **b)** the NCS elementary color space with constant-hue lines (radial) and constant-chromaticness (saturation) lines plotted in the CIE 1976 (u*v*) diagram. Both spaces appear to be isomorphic and linearly related to each other (from Derefeldt, G., 1991, Fig. 13.23; after Billmeyer, 1988; and Derefeldt et al., 1987).

are represented in a three-dimensional linear elementary color (EC) space. This color space appears to be isomorphic to the MDS color space as well as to other color order systems, as e.g., the Munsell system (Figs. 2.6, 2.22). Both color spaces represent colors as certain loci. Nevertheless, the EC and the MDS color spaces represent the results of two distinct types of psychophysical judgments. The EC space represents the amounts of the elementary color sensations as measured in color content analytical experiments (see above). The MDS space represents total color differences as distances between each two color loci. The total color distance z is equal to the probability transformed choice percentages p (color distance = $z(p)$) measured in color discrimination and color similarity experiments (see above). This type of experiments, as usually performed also with animals, measures only the similarity relations (differences) between colors and hence does not tell us anything about elementary colors and color sensations *per se*.

Our investigations with honeybees have shown that the coordinates of the respective MDS color space are identical with the excitation values of the respective color-opponent coding neurons (Backhaus, 1993). This allows us predictions of the color-choice percentages from the spectral intensity distributions and the electrical excitations of the neuronal color-coding system alone. There was no need to assume anything about conscious color sensations in animals to explain the results of color discrimination and color similarity experiments so far. Thus, nothing can be concluded about the existence of color sensations in animals from this type of experiment.

This conclusion is supported by the finding that color discrimination experiments can also be performed with cortically color blind patients, who lack conscious color sensations but have the neuronal color-coding system otherwise intact. Although these patients do not see any colors, not even gray shades, they are able to adjust the lights in color discrimination experiments for just-noticeable differences. The wavelength discrimination functions that are obtained possess the same form as those of subjects with normal color vision. Only the absolute discrimination ability is reduced (Stoerig and Cowey, 1989; see chapter 7). Discrimination of color stimuli can obviously be performed on the basis of the (unconscious) electrical excitations of the neuronal color-coding system alone. The elementary colors cannot be identical with the electrical excitations of neurons because we experience our elementary color sensations as six different qualities but the electrical potential is only one physical quality, even if superimposed from several neurons (ontological argument).

In the content analytical experiments mentioned above, the subjects are instructed to inspect the content of the color sensations and to judge the percentages of the elementary colors in a color sensation. Electrophysiologically, no evidence has been found for the existence of neurons which would code for the amounts of elementary colors in simple color sensations (e.g., Gouras, 1991). Cortically color blind patients who lack conscious color sensations thus most likely do not have the information available to perform this task. It therefore appears to be a strong suggestion that there exist color sensations in animals, if an animal could be successfully trained to relate the choice behavior to the amounts of individual elementary colors, and if it could be shown in addition that neuron types which tonically code for the amounts of individual elementary colors are lacking. This indeed seems to be the case in honeybees.

In humans, the MDS space is isomorphic to the space of elementary colors (see above). The color-opponent coding COC system of the bee was shown to be isomorphic to the MDS space of the bee. This motivated the extension of the COC system to a color space spanned by the amounts of elementary colors (EC space, Fig. 2.23). The parameters of the EC space are almost fixed with respect to the COC space because of its picewise linearity and isomorphy to the COC space. This allows us to predict the percentages of elementary colors for all color stimuli of which the spectral intensity distributions are known.

Honeybees show flower constancy (i.e., tend to revisit the flowers of the same plant species), as Aristotle (1951–61) had already reported. Thus, honeybees were alternatingly trained in double color training experiments to two different color

2.8 Conscious vs. Unconscious Judgments

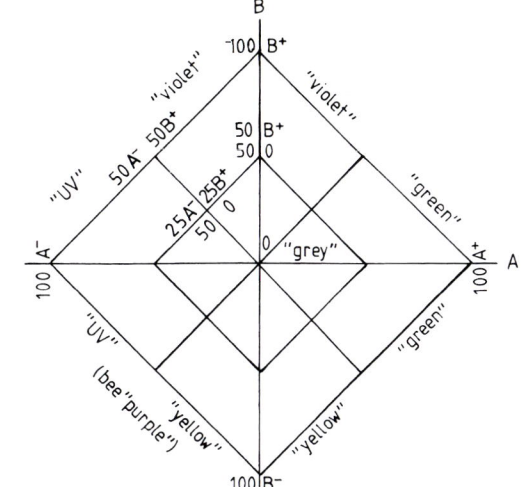

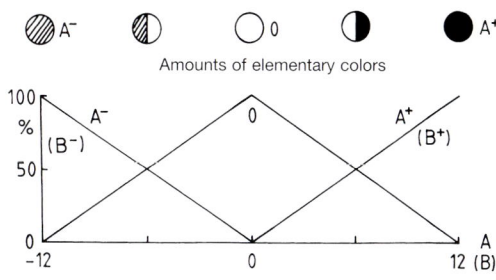

Fig. 2.23: The model of color sensations in honeybees. This diagram is an extension of the COC model in Fig. 2.16. Piecewise linearity is assumed between the COC space and the space of elementary colors which uniquely relates both spaces to each other. The amounts of elementary colors can be read off the diagram as coordinate values of the respective color loci (see examples). (From Backhaus, 1991.)

Fig. 2.24: Linear relationship (solid lines) between the excitation values (abscissa) of the COC neuron type A, resp. (B) and the predicted amounts in % (ordinate) of unique (elementary) colors A–, 0, and A+, resp. (B–, 0, B+). The extreme excitation values (–12 and 12) of the COC neurons are reasonably assumed to cause color sensations which consist of elementary colors A– (B–) and A+ (B+). Dark light as well as very bright daylight does not excite these neurons (0) causing a pure achromatic color sensation of elementary (unique) color 0. Excitations in between these values give rise to mixtures of the respective elementary colors with amounts proportional to the respective excitation values. **Upper graph:** Examples for mixtures of elementary-colors in the color sensations. (From Backhaus, 1995.)

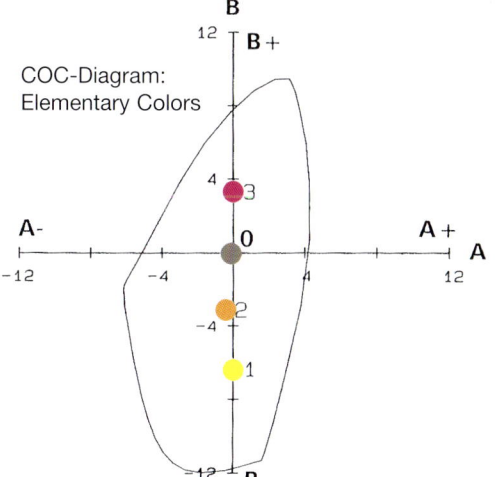

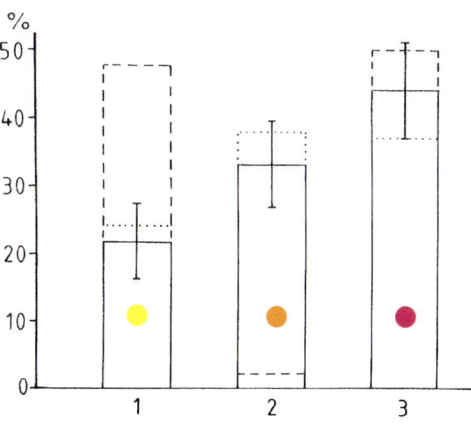

Fig. 2.25a: COC diagram with the color stimuli used in the double-color training experiments below (see text). **b:** Color-choice percentages for the three color stimuli in the tests. **Solid:** measured. Dotted: prediction of the COC model extended by the model of elementary colors (EC space). **Dashed:** prediction according exclusively to the COC model. The behavioral results obviously support the hypothesis of elementary colors and thus color sensations in honeybees. (From Backhaus, 1995.)

stimuli. This was with the idea that they would prefer to learn one color as a food signal instead of two and thus would learn the elementary color which the two rewarded colors have in common. In the unrewarded tests, the bee would then choose the alternatives according to the amounts of the learned elementary color present in the respective colors (Fig. 2.24). Instead, most of the bees learned both colors as two independent color loci in the color space, as in ordinary color discrimination experiments, and ignored an additional alternative in the unrewarded tests, which was clearly discriminable (>95%) from the learned colors and from the "gray" background (Fig. 2.25). But one of the bees showed indeed quite a different choice behavior in these experiments. Although equally often rewarded on both training stimuli, the bee chose one of the rewarded stimuli only about half as often compared to the other rewarded color stimulus. Furthermore, the bee preferred the third stimulus over this training stimulus in the tests, which the other bees had ignored because of the great dissimilarity to both the training stimuli (Fig. 2.25). The bee appears to have indeed learned an elementary color as a food signal and to have chosen the alternatives according to the amounts of the elementary color present in the respective colors. The results obtained agree quantitatively with the predictions of the COC model, extended to the elementary color (EC) model of the bee, and thus support the hypothesis about the existence of elementary colors and thus color sensations in bees (Backhaus, 1995).

2.9 Conclusions

It has been shown that color vision in humans as well as in non-human animals can be described by different color spaces with different properties for different purposes. In the case of the honeybee, the abstract scales of the color space were shown to be identical with the excitations of the two types of color-opponent coding neurons exclusively found in the honeybee brain. A similar relationship is expected for human color vision although this is more difficult to show because the human color space possesses a Euclidean metric which allows a continuous rotation of the axes (scales, dimensions) of the color space.

Because of this identification, the system of six physiological, psychophysical and behavioral models: 1) the photoreceptor model, 2) the model of monopolar cells, 3) the model of COC neurons, 4) the MDS model of color differences, 5) the model of decision making (judgments), and 6) the model of color-choice behavior, allows us to predict the choice behavior of the honeybee exclusively from the spectral light intensity distributions of the color stimuli. In physiological simulations of the color-coding system of the honeybee it could be shown that the color-opponent coding neurons recorded by Kien and Menzel (1977) are indeed essential for color-choice behavior, which could not be demonstrated by intracellular recordings of the neurons alone.

The color vision experiments mostly performed with animals, color discrimination and color similarity experiments, do not need any assumptions about color sensations for explaining the results. The color-choice behavior in this type of experiment appears to be completely described in terms of the electrical excitations of the neuronal color-coding system. Thus, nothing can be concluded about the existence of color sensations from the results of this type of experiment. In order to answer this question, the following further conditions have to be fulfilled:

1) The color sensations must be organized similarly to ours (i.e., must consist of elementary colors of different amounts, adding up to 100%).

2) It must be shown that no neurons exist with excitations strongly correlated with the amounts of elementary colors.

3) The neuronal color-coding system must be modeled physiologically so completely that the color-choice behavior of the respective animal is most accurately described.

4) It must be shown that the neuronal color-coding system does not explain the results of content analytical experiments.

5) On the other hand, the results must be in agreement with the neuronal color-coding (e.g., COC) model extended by the elementary colors (EC) model.

If 1–5 are fulfilled, it can be concluded that the animal indeed relates the color-choice behavior to elementary colors and not directly to the excitations of the neurons. This structural argument would support the hypothesis that the animal possesses color sensations comparable to ours. In one honeybee it has so far been shown that the choice behavior in double-color training experiments cannot at all be described on the basis of the neuronal color-coding systems alone, but is in agreement with the theory of neuronal color-coding and color-choice behavior of the honeybee extended by the elementary colors hypothesis.

Whether color sensations in animals are more or less identical to ours must be further investigated by analyzing the material correlates which might be identical to the color sensations. In this further analysis, the results of color analytical experiments, again, will be most helpful. If these materials (matter) could be identified, the problem of color sensations in animals would be reduced to a standard problem of natural sciences of showing that specific substances are present in the brain.

References

Aristotle, Gohlke, P., (1951–61), ed. Die Lehrschriften. 8.1 Tierkunde. (Paderborn: Schoeningh).
Autrum, H. and Zwehl, V. v. (1964). Die spektrale Empfindlichkeit einzelner Sehzellen im Bienenauge. Z. vergl. Physiol. *48*, 357–384.
Ahrens, H. J. (1974). Multidimensionale Skalierung. Methodik, Theorie und empirische Gültigkeit mit Anwendungen aus der differentiellen Psychologie und Sozialpsychologie (Weinheim: Beltz).
Backhaus, W. (1991). Color-opponent coding in the visual system of the honeybee. Vis. Res. *31*, 1381–1397.
Backhaus, W. (1992). The Bezold-Brücke effect in the color vision system of the honeybee. Vis. Res. *32*, 1425–1431.
Backhaus, W. (1992). Color vision in honeybees. Neuroscience and Biobehavioral Reviews *16*, 1–12.
Backhaus, W. (1993). Color vision and color-choice behavior of the honey bee. In: Recent Progress in Neurobiology of the Honey Bee. Special issue, Apidologie *24*, 309–331.
Backhaus, W. (1995). Unique colors in honeybees? In: Color Vision Deficiencies XII. (ed. B. Drum) (Dordrecht: Kluver), pp. 243–250.
Backhaus, W. (1996). Allgemeine Sinnesphysiologie. In: Neurowissenschaft, J. Dudel, R. Menzel, and R. F. Schmidt, eds. (Berlin: Springer), pp. 278–295.
Backhaus, W. and Menzel, R. (1987). Color distance derived from a receptor model for color vision in the honeybee. Biol. Cybern. *55*, 321–331.
Backhaus, W., Menzel, R., and Kreißl, S. (1987). Multidimensional scaling of color similarity in bees. Biol. Cybern. *56*, 293–304.
Billmeyer, F. W. Jr. (1988). Quantifying colour appearance visually and instrumentally. Color Res. and Appl. *13*, 140–145.
Brandt, R., Backhaus, W., Dittrich, M., and Menzel, R. (1993). Simulation of threshold spectral sensitivity according to the color theory for the honeybee. In: Genes, Brain and Behavior. Proceedings of the 21st Göttingen Neurobiology Conference, N. Elsner and D. W. Richter, eds. (Stuttgart: Thieme), pp. 374.
Cornsweet, T. N. (1970). Visual Perception (New York: Academic Press).
Dartnall, H. J. A., Bowmaker, J. K., and Mollon, J. D. (1983). Microspectrophotometry of human photoreceptors. In: Colour Vision: Physiology and Psychophysics, J. D. Mollon and L. T. Sharpe, eds. (New York: Academic Press), pp. 69–80.
Daumer, K. (1956). Reizmetrische Untersuchung des Farbensehens der Bienen. Z. vergl. Physiol. *38*, 413–478.
Derefeldt, G. (1991). Colour appearance systems. In: Vision and Visual Dysfunction (ed. J. R. Cronly-Dillon), Vol. 6, The Perception of Colour (ed. P. Gouras) (Macmillan, London), pp. 218 to 261.
Derefeldt, G., Hedin, C. E., and Sahlin, C. (1987). Transformation of NCS data into CIELUV colour space. Disp. Techn. Appl. *8*, 183–193.
Dowling, J. E. (1987). The Retina: An Approachable Part of the Brain (Cambridge: Harvard University Press).
Estévez, O. (1979). On the Fundamental Data-Base of Normal and Dichromatic Color Vision. Ph.D. (University of Amsterdam).
Fechner, G. T. (1860). Elemente der Psychophysik (Leipzig: Breitkopf & Härtel).
Frisch, K. v. (1914). Der Farbensinn und der Formensinn der Bienen. Zool. Jb. Physiol. *37*, 1–238.
Gouras, P. (1991a). Precortical physiology of colour vision. In: Vision and Visual Dysfunction (ed. J. R. Cronly-Dillon) Vol. 6, The Perception of

Colour, P. Gouras, ed. (London: Macmillan), pp. 163–178.

Gouras, P. (1991b). Cortical mechanisms of colour vision. In: Vision and Visual Dysfunction (ed. J. R. Cronly-Dillon) Vol. 6, The Perception of Colour, (ed. P. Gouras), (London: Macmillan), pp. 179–197.

Grassmann, H. (1853). Zur Theorie der Farbenmischung. Ann. Phys. Chem. *89*, 69-84. [On the theory of compound colours. Phil. Mag. *7*, 254–264, 1854].

Helmholtz, H. v. (1852). Zur Theorie der Farbenmischung. Poggendorff's Ann. *87*, 45–66. [On the theory of compound colours. Phil. Mag. *4*, 519–534, 1852].

Helmholtz, H.v. (1867). Handbuch der physiologischen Optik (Leipzig: Voss).

Helversen, O.v. (1972). Zur spektralen Unterschiedsempfindlichkeit der Honigbiene. J. Comp. Physiol. *80*, 439–472.

Helversen, O. v. (1972). The relationship between differences in stimuli and choice frequency in training experiments with the honeybee. In: Information Processing in the Visual System of Arthropods (ed. R. Wehner) (Berlin-Heidelberg-New York: Springer), pp. 323–334.

Hering, E. (1874). Zur Lehre vom Lichtsinn. VI. Grundzüge einer Theorie des Farbensinnes. Ber. k. u. k. Akad. Wiss., Wien *70*, 169ff.

Hering, E. (1920). Grundzüge der Lehre vom Lichtsinn (Gerold und Söhne). [translated by L. M. Hurvich and D. Jameson. Outlines of a theory of the light sense (Cambridge, Mass: Harvard University Press), 1964].

Indow, T. and Ohsumi, K. (1972). Multidimensional mapping of sixty Munsell colors by nonmetric procedure. In: Color Metrics (eds. J. J. Vos, et al.) (Holland: AIC), pp. 124–133.

Jacobs, G. H. (1981). Comparative Color Vision (New York: Academic Press).

Kien, J. and Menzel, R. (1977). Chromatic properties of neurons in the optic lobes of the bee. II. Narrow band and colour opponent neurons. J. Comp. Physiol. *113*, 35–53.

Kolmogorof, A. N. and Fomin, S. N. (1957). Elements of the theory of function and functional analysis, Vol. I, Metric and normed spaces (New York: Graylock).

Krantz, D. H. (1975). Color measurement and color theory: I. Representation theorem for Grassmann structures. J. Math. Psychol. *12*, 283–303.

Laughlin, S. B. (1981). Neural principles in the peripheral visual systems of invertebrates. In: Handbook of Sensory Physiology, Vol. VII/6B, (ed. H. Autrum) (Springer: Berlin), pp. 133–280.

Lipetz, L. E. (1971). The relation of physiological and psychological aspects of sensory intensity. In: Handbook of Sensory Physiology, Vol. I (ed. W. R. Loewenstein) (Berlin: Springer), pp. 191–225.

Livingstone, M. and Hubel, D. H. (1988). Segregation of form, color, movement and depth: anatomy, physiology and perception. Science *240*, 740–750.

Mach, E. (1886). Die Analyse der Empfindungen und das Verhältnis des Physischen zum Psychischen (Jena: Fischer).

Maxwell, J. C. (1855). Experiments on colour as perceived by the eye, with remarks on colour blindness. Phil. Roy. Soc. London *21*, 275–297.

Maxwell, J. C. (1860). On the theory of compound colours, and the relations of the colours of the spectrum. Proc. Roy. Soc. *10*, 404–409, 484–486. [Phil. Trans. Roy. Soc. London *150*, 57–84].

Mazokhin-Porshnyakow, G. A. (1962). Colorimetric index of trichromatic bees. Biofisica *7*, 211–217.

Menzel, R. (1981). Achromatic vision in the honeybee at low light intensities. J. Comp. Physiol. A, *141*, 389–393.

Menzel, R. and Backhaus, W. (1991). Colour vision in insects. In: Vision and Visual Dysfunction (ed. J. R. Cronly-Dillon) Vol. 6, The Perception of Colour (ed. P. Gouras) (London: Macmillan), pp. 262–293.

Menzel, R., Ventura, D. F., Hertel, H., Souza, J. M. de, and Greggers, U. (1986). Spectral sensitivity of photoreceptors in insect compound eyes: comparison of species and methods. J. Comp. Physiol. A *158*, 165–177.

Naka, K. I. and Rushton, W. A. H. (1966). S-potentials from colour units in the retina of fish (*Cyprinidae*). J. Comp. Physiol. *185*, 536–555.

Naka, K. I. and Rushton, W. A. H. (1967). The generation and spread of S-potentials in fish (*Cyprinidae*). J. Physiol. *192*, 437–461.

Neumeyer, C. (1988). Das Farbensehen des Goldfisches. Eine verhaltensanalytische Analyse (Stuttgart-New York: Thieme).

Newton, I. (1704). Opticks. Or a Treatise on the Reflections, Refractions, Inflections and Colours of Light. [based on the fourth edition (Dover, U.S.A.: Dover Publications), 1952].

Palmer, G. (1777). Theory of Colours and Vision (London: Leacreft).

Plateau, J. A. F. (1872). Sur la mesure des sensations physiques et sur la loi qui lie l'intensité de ces sensations à intensité de la excitante. Bull. Acad. roy.

Belg., *33,* 376–388. [Poggendorfs Annalen der Physik (1873) *150,* 465–477].

Ratliff, F. (1965). Mach Bands: Quantitative Studies on Neuronal Networks in the Retina (San Fancisco: Holden-Day).

Richter, M. (1981). Einführung in die Farbmetrik, 2. Aufl. (Berlin-New York: de Gruyter).

Rodieck, R.W. (1973). The Vertebrate Retina (San Francisco: Freeman).

Rushton, W. A. H. (1972). Pigments and signals in color vision. J. Physiol. *220,* 1–31.

Schrödinger, E. (1920a). Grundlinien einer Theorie der Farbmetrik im Tagessehen. Ann. Physik *63,* 397–426, 427–456.

Schrödinger, E. (1920b). Grundlinien einer Theorie der Farbmetrik im Tagessehen: Der Farbenmetrik II. Teil: Höhere Farbenmetrik (eigentliche Metrik der Farbe), Ann. Physik *63,* 481–520.

Stevens, S. S. (1975). Psychophysics (New York: Wiley).

Stoerig, P. and Cowey, A. (1989). Wavelength sensitivity in blindsight. Nature *342,* 916–917.

Swedish Standard (1979). Swedish Standard SS 01 91 00 colour notation system (Sweden: Swedish Standards Institution (SIS)).

Torgerson, W. S. (1958). Theory and methods of scaling (New York: Wiley).

Thurstone, L. L. (1927). A law of comparative judgment. Psychol. Rev. *34,* 273–286.

Weber, E. H. (1834). De pulsu, resorptione, auditu et tactu. Annotationes anatomicae et physiologicae (Lipsiae: Koehler).

Young, T. (1802). On the Theory of light and colours. Phil. Trans. R. Soc. *92,* 12–48.

Zrenner, E., Abramov, I., Akita, M., Cowey, A., Livingstone, M., and Valberg, A. (1990). Color perception: retina to cortex. In: Visual Perception: The Physiological Foundations (eds. L. Spillmann and J. S. Werner) (San Diego: Academic Press), pp. 163–204.

3 Receptors, Channels and Color in Primate Retina

Barry B. Lee

3.1 Introduction

The retina transforms the spectral distribution of light falling upon it into a neural signal in two stages. Light is first differentially absorbed by the three types of cone receptor. Then the output of the cones is subtracted or added to generate neural signals which leave the retina to be processed by the cortex or other parts of the brain. Over the past decade, we have learned many of the physiological and anatomical bases of these transformations, and how retinal signals relate to perception of color and form.

The idea of there being three classes of cone in the retina with different spectral sensitivities is usually ascribed to Thomas Young (1802). Young's trichromatic hypothesis is but briefly stated in his Bakerian lecture, almost as an aside. This becomes understandable if we look more closely at the development of ideas about light and color in the 18th century. Many physicists then accepted that the spectrum is a continuous distribution from violet through to red. However, there were two views as to the nature of light. The Newtonian view of light as particles or corpuscles was countered by that of Huygens and Euler (1787), who favored a wave theory. Indeed, Young (1800) was dismissive of Euler until embracing the wave theory in the Bakerian lecture two years later. Contrary to both these views was the empirical fact that spectral colors could be matched by mixing three primaries. Although well known to artists and printers, this finding was first put on a formal basis in a public lecture by Tobias Mayer (1758), an astronomer at Göttingen University, who constructed a three-dimensional color mixture space based on red, yellow and blue as primaries. Mayer was well aware that this was in contradiction to both corpuscular and wave theories, but supposed that there were only three ray types in the spectrum and other spectral colors were a mixture of these. Due to Mayer's early death in 1762, his work was only published in abstract form (in the Göttinger Anzeige) until it was expanded and published with other posthumous papers by G. C. Lichtenberg in 1775, who had just become professor of physics in Göttingen. Figure 3.1 shows

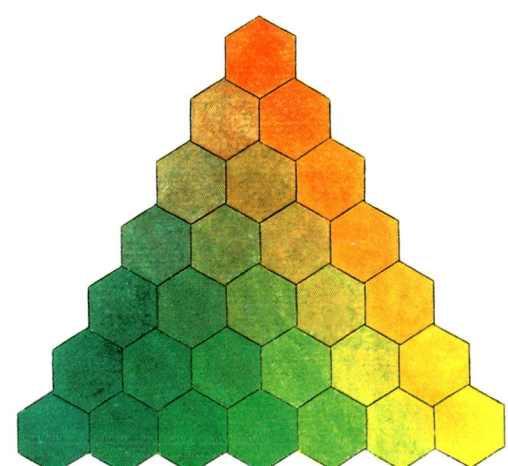

Fig. 3.1: The color triangle of Tobias Mayer. Note that red, yellow and blue are used as primaries. Thomas Young at first used these three colors as well, but later changed his primaries to red, green and blue. In preparing this triangle, Mayer did not in fact follow his prescribed color mixture formula; he cheated to get the correct colors. The distinction between additive and subtractive color mixture was not recognized at that time; Mayer's color mixture solid was based on an additive formula, and printing of course involves subtractive color mixture. Both Mayer and Lichtenberg clearly realised that some problem was present, but it was Helmholtz who was the first to diagnose its origin.

Mayer's color triangle as published in this volume. In Mayer's formal exposition each side of the triangle was divided into thirteen steps, but to simplify printing, each side was reduced to seven for publication. This section through Mayer's color mixture space contained 91 colors. Extension to three dimensions, down to black and up to white, led to a three-dimensional color mixture solid.

Around this time, in 1777, an English glass maker, George Palmer, suggested that there were three types of photoreceptor in the retina (see 3.5), while accepting the Mayer viewpoint of three ray types in physical light. The Palmer theory was reviewed in Lichtenberg's Magazine, published by G. C. Lichtenberg's brother, L. C. Lichtenberg (1781). Thomas Young was a medical student in Göttingen in 1795–96 and wrote his thesis there. He was acquainted with G. C. Lichtenberg, who had maintained a vigorous interest in color vision and physiological optics, and Lichtenberg noted Young's visits in his diary. Unfortunately, he did not note the subjects of their discussions. We can thus see Young's hypothesis as a natural development of ideas current at the time. His great achievement was to see that a continuous distribution of light in the spectrum was compatible with trichromatic matching, if there are only three receptor types in the retina.

Soon after the trichromatic theory became established (Maxwell, 1855; Helmholtz, 1866), Hering put forward an opponent theory of color (1878) based on the perceptual opponency between red and green, and between blue and yellow. These two alternative viewpoints gave rise to controversy, but we can now see that opponent processes reflect in some way post-receptoral mechanisms. DeValois (1966; 1971) was the first to describe cells in the visual pathway of the primate which were, for example, inhibited by red and excited by green light. The rest of this article concerns the transformation of receptor to opponent signals in the retina, and its relation to perceptual opponency.

The presence of three different cone types has now been well established, from spectral absorption measurements on individual cones (Bowmaker, 1991) and through measurements of their physiological responses (Baylor et al., 1987).

Most recently, slight differences in a given cone type between individuals with normal color vision have been found to exist (see chapter 5). Cones with absorption maxima in short (ca. 430 nm), middle (535 nm) and long (565 nm) wavelength regions are designated S-, M- and L-cones. After the receptors, different cell systems carry visual information to the brain. A class of large ganglion cells, termed parasol cells, send axons through the magnocellular (MC) layers of the lateral geniculate nucleus to the visual cortex. These cells appear to sum activity of M- and L-cones. Other classes of small ganglion cells send axons through the parvocellular (PC) layers of the geniculate to the cortex. Most if not all of these cells are cone-opponent; for example, they may be excited by the M-cone and inhibited by the L-cone (+M-L cells). I shall now look at these pathways in more detail.

3.2 Physiology and Anatomy in the Retina

It is possible to directly record from ganglion cells in the intact eye (Gouras, 1968). Combining *in vivo* recordings with visual stimuli carefully matched to those used in standard psychophysical paradigms has yielded much information as to the roles of different cell types in visual performance (see Lee, 1996 for review). However, the anatomical circuitry underlying responses had to be inferred from other studies. Recently it has become possible to maintain the primate retina *in vitro* (Dacey and Lee, 1994a; 1994b). This allows one to record from ganglion cells and other retinal cell types and then inject neurobiotin to fill the cell so that it can be anatomically identified. We can thus learn much more about how the retinal signals are generated.

Figure 3.2 shows responses of a parasol ganglion cell of the MC-pathway to modulation in different directions in an opponent space (Derrington et al., 1984). These directions have been indicated as a black-white axis, which represents luminance modulation, a red-green axis, which represents modulation at equal luminance along a constant S-cone axis (counterphase modulation of the M- and

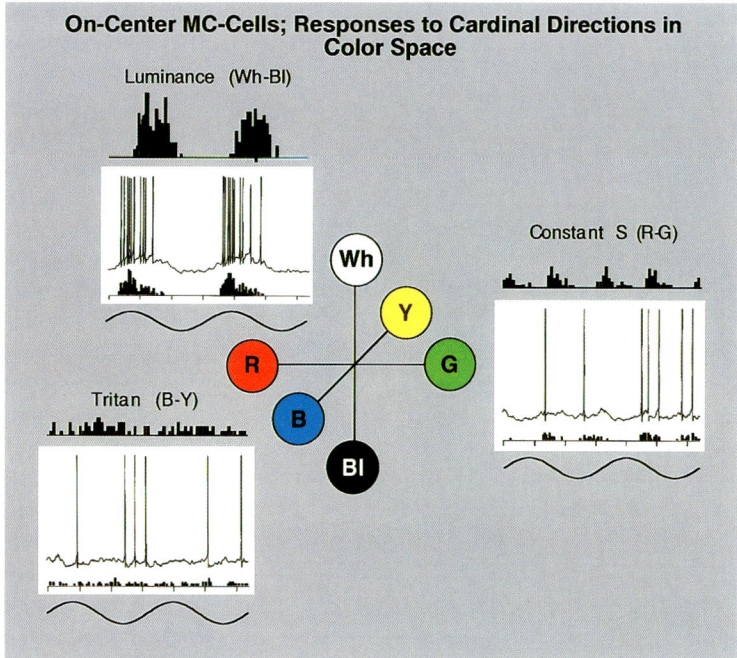

Fig. 3.2: Responses of on-center cells of the parasol, MC system to modulation in cardinal directions in color space. These have been designated as black-white, red-green and blue-yellow as described in the text. Data obtained with luminance, constant S-cone, and pure S-cone modulation are associated with each of the axes. In each, the upper panel shows an impulse histogram from a parafoveal ganglion cell *in vivo* (2 cycles, 10 Hz, 50% contrast, 4.7 deg field, 2000 td; peak response ca. 160 imp/sec). The middle and lower panels show *in vitro* data from a cell from peripheral retina obtained under similar stimulus conditions. The middle panel shows a single response trace. Membrane potential was ca. –60 mV and spike amplitude 65 mV. The lowest histogram shows the averaged spike response from the intracellular recording.

L-cones alone), and a blue yellow axis, representing S-cone modulation along a tritan line. It is important to note that these axes do not exactly correspond to perceptually opponent axes of Hering. The differences are discussed in a later section.

In the panel associated with each of the axes, the top histogram shows the response of a ganglion cell recorded *in vivo* to two cycles of modulation. The middle trace shows the intracellular response of a cell recorded *in vitro* to the same stimuli. The modulation of the membrane potential can be seen, with impulses on top. The lower histogram shows the averaged spike response from the intracellular recording. Both *in vivo* and *in vitro* there is a strong response to luminance modulation, and no response to modulation along the blue-yellow, tritan axis. There is a small response to red-green modulation at twice the stimulus frequency. This appears to be due to a non-linearity of M- and L-cone summation (Lee et al., 1989a); their out-of-phase signals do not perfectly cancel but leave a residual response.

The properties of parasol cells of the MC-pathway closely correspond to those required of a substrate for a psychophysical luminance channel. Those shown in Figure 3.2 correspond to those needed for heterochromatic flicker photometry. In this task, two lights are alternated at, say, 10–20 Hz, and an observer is required to adjust

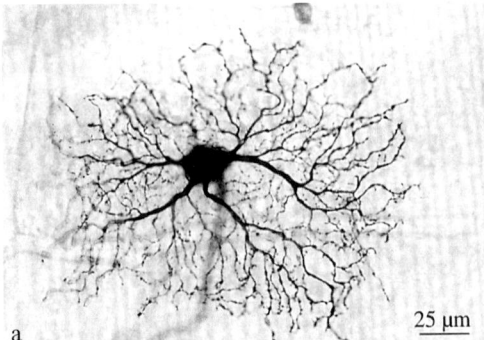

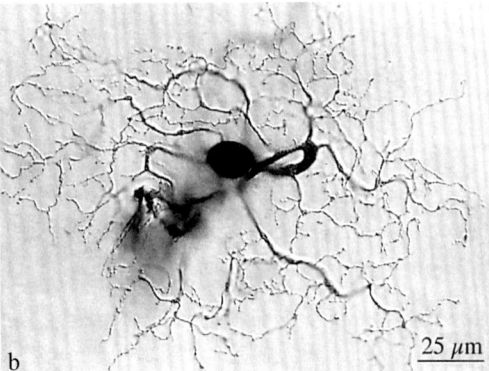

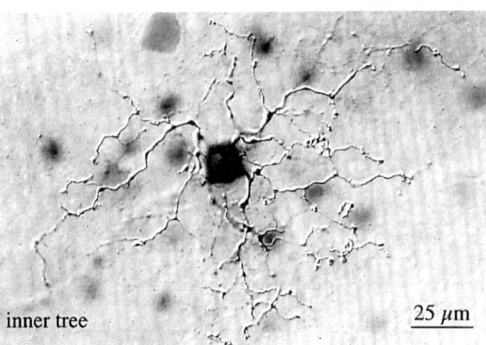

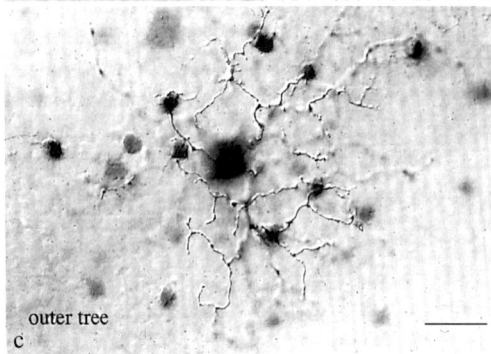

their relative intensity until the sensation of flicker is minimized or abolished. This task provided most of the data used to define the photopic luminosity function, and in a series of experiments we have been able to show that the properties of MC-cells match the psychophysical data in considerable detail (Lee et al., 1988; Smith et al., 1992). Detection of luminance flicker seems likewise to be the responsibility of this pathway (Lee et al., 1989b; 1990).

After intracellular injection of neurobiotin, typical parasol cell morphology is revealed (Fig. 3.3A). MC-cells may have an on- or off-center receptive field structure, and these correspond to two distinct parasol cell types. These are sketched on the left hand of Figure 3.4, which represents a schematic cross-section of primate retina. As in other species (Famiglietti and Kolb, 1976), on and off-center cells have dendritic trees which ramify in the inner, vitreal and outer, scleral sub-layers of the inner plexiform layer (IPL) respectively. At the top of the figure are sketched the array of cones; rod inputs, and their circuitry, have not been included. Parasol ganglion cells probably receive input from only M- and L-cones. Certain diffuse bipolar cell types gather input from about 4–6 cones, and invaginating and flat varieties provide input to on and off-center parasol cells respectively (Boycott and Wässle, 1991). We thus have a specific pathway which carries a luminance signal from the receptors up the brain.

Figure 3.5 shows responses of cone-opponent midget ganglion cells. This is the most numerous type, making up about 60% of ganglion cells, as compared to the MC-cells' 10%. In central retina, from which the *in vivo* recordings were obtained, cells of this type are M,L-cone opponent, with

Fig. 3.3: Morphology of different cell types. **A.** The dendritic tree and cell body of an inner parasol cell, which projects through the MC-layers of the geniculate to cortex. **B.** Morphology of inner midget ganglion cell from peripheral retina. These ganglion cells project through the PC-layers to cortex. **C.** The two dendritic trees of a small bistratified cell. These cells project through the geniculate to cortex, but may strictly speaking belong neither to the MC- or PC-pathways.

3.2 Physiology and Anatomy in the Retina

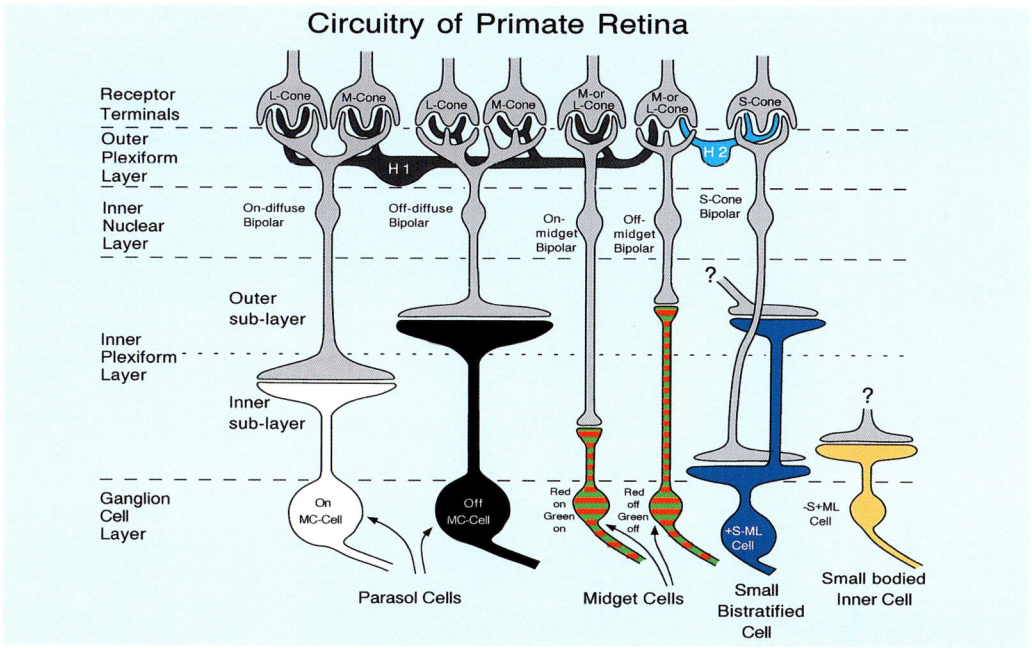

Fig. 3.4: A sketch of hypothetical circuitry in primate retina. On- and off-center cell types (which each form separate mosaics) are connected to the cones through specific bipolar cells. Red and green on-center cells share the same mosaic, as do red and green off-center cells, and they are shown in red and green stripes. The identification of the -S, +ML, yellow on, blue off cell is still tentative. Latest results identifying horizontal cell types are also included.

excitation from one and inhibition from the other cone. The cell shown was of the +M-L type, and gives vigorous excitation to greenward and inhibition to redward modulation. There is a weak on response to luminance modulation and no response to modulation along the tritan line. The *in vitro* recordings were from the same cell type but indicate one of the few differences we have encountered in the *in vivo* and *in vitro* recordings. The *in vitro* cell shows a stronger luminance response than the *in vivo* cell, i.e., less cone opponency. This may be because *in vitro* cells are recorded from peripheral retina, where the larger cell bodies make it easier to record. In central retina, the anatomy suggests midget cells only receive input from a single cone. In peripheral retina, midget ganglion cell dendritic trees are larger and some mixing of cone inputs may take place.

Psychophysical evidence suggests that detection of chromatic and luminance changes are mediated by discrete detection mechanisms. A convenient way of displaying this is shown in Figure 3.6. Based on knowledge of the cone fundamentals, it is possible to calculate M-, L- or S-cone contrast at threshold. In the example shown, M- and L-cone contrast axes are used. Luminance modulation corresponds to in-phase modulation of the M- and L-cones, i.e., a +45 degree vector. Red-green chromatic modulation corresponds to counter-phase modulation of the M- and L-cones, i.e., the vector drawn at −45 degrees. When psychophysical thresholds are measured under carefully controlled conditions and plotted in this space, they can be described by combinations of straight-line segments, as seen in the data replotted in Figure 3.6A (Stromeyer et al., 1985; 1987; Cole et al., 1993). If cell 'thresholds' are plotted in the same space, one finds that different cell types can contribute the different segments, as shown in Figure 3.6B (Lee et al., 1993), where a parasol, MC-cell is seen to have the lowest threshold in the luminance quadrant, and a red-green opponent midget

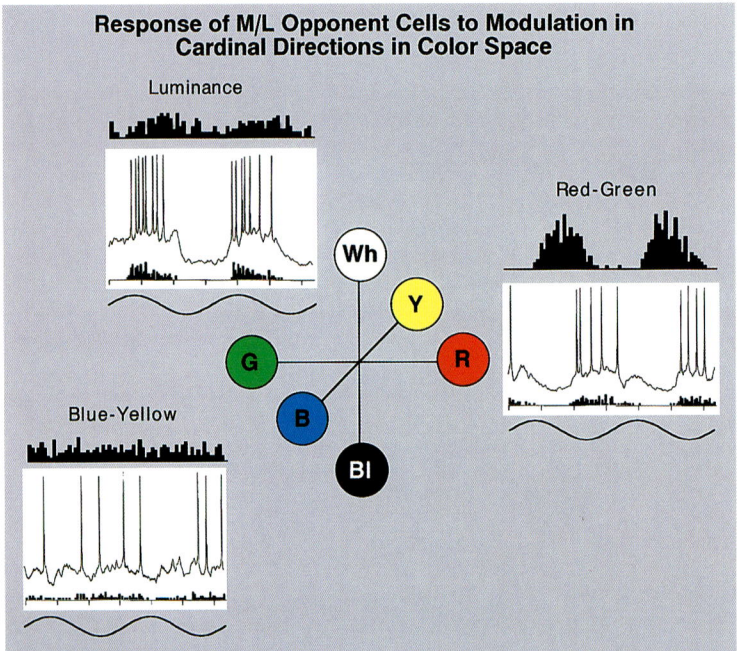

Fig. 3.5: Responses of cells of the midget, PC-pathway as in Fig. 3.2. The *in vivo* recording was obtained from a red-on, +L-M cell, and the *in vitro* recording from a +M-L green on cell. Both give an excitatory response to the luminance modulation, but the response to the red-green modulation is approximately phase inverted. There is a more vigorous response to luminance modulation in the *in vitro* cell.

PC-cell in the chromatic quadrant. Under threshold conditions, peripheral opponent and non-opponent cell systems thus appear to underlie luminance and chromatic detection channels.

The morphology of a peripheral midget cell is shown in Figure 3.3B. It is distinct from the parasol cell in Figure 3.3A, and at a more extreme eccentricity; at the same eccentricity, midget cell dendritic trees are smaller than their parasol counterparts. In the center of Figure 3.4 the circuitry of these cell types has been sketched. There appear to be green, +M-L and red +L-M on-center cells which are currently anatomically indistinguishable. The same holds true for off-center cells. Both have been drawn in red and green stripes. These cell types ramify in the inner and outer sublayers of the IPL, and again specific, midget bipolar cells are associated with them to provide a distinct and separate circuitry for the red-green opponent signal.

Responses of a blue-on cell are shown in Figure 3.7. Cells of this type receive excitatory input from the S-cone and opponent, inhibitory input from the M- and L-cones. The *in vivo* response is vigorous to blue-yellow modulation along the tritan line, weak to luminance modulation and there is no response to red-green modulation. A similar pattern can be seen in the *in vitro* recording.

In psychophysical experiments, it is possible to plot thresholds in an S-, M- and L-cone space, expanding on the representation in Figure 3.6, and then threshold contours indicate the presence of separable blue-yellow, S-cone and red-green chromatic detection mechanisms (Cole et al., 1993). When cellular thresholds are plotted in the space, data are consistent with different cell systems underlying these separable mechanisms.

The blue-on cell has a unique morphology (Dacey and Lee, 1994a). It is the small bistratified cell, with one layer of dendrites in the inner sublayer of the IPL, close to the ganglion cell bodies

3.2 Physiology and Anatomy in the Retina

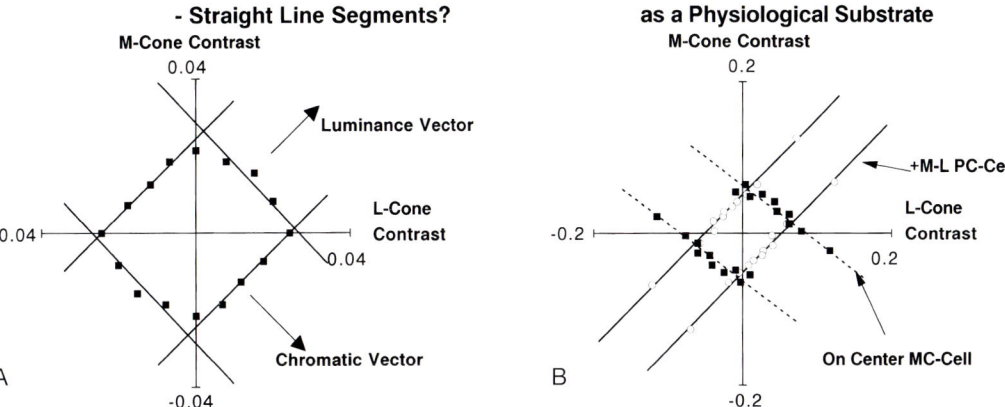

Fig. 3.6: A. Psychophysical thresholds plotted in an M/L-cone contrast space. It appears that the threshold contour can be described by a combination of straight-line segments. Stimuli were 15 Hz modulation of a 3800 td field metameric to 577 nm. Replotted from (Stromeyer et al., 1987). **B.** Thresholds (contrast required to generate a 10 imp/sec first harmonic response) of +M-L opponent cell and parasol MC-cell. Stimuli were 2 Hz modulation of a 2000 td 570 nm field. Each cell's thresholds follow a linear course plotted in this space, and can support the linear segments seen in the psychophysics. Replotted from (Lee et al., 1993).

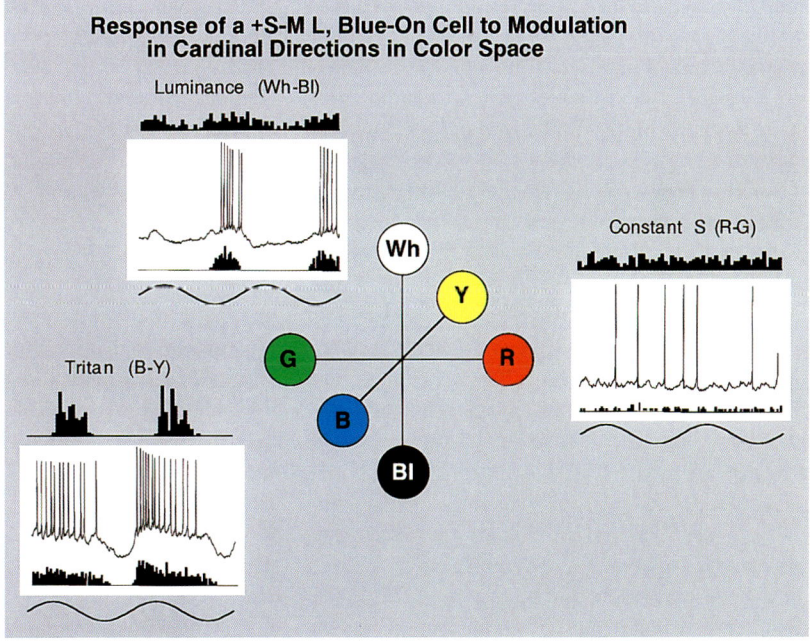

Fig. 3.7: Response of a +S-ML cell to the same stimuli as employed as in Figure 3.2. The cells give a vigorous response to the S-cone stimulus, and no response to the constant S, R-G stimulus.

and another in the outer sublayer. The two layers of dendritic tree of the same cell are separately displayed in Figure 3.3C and they are sketched in Figure 3.4. The inner layer of dendrites matches up with the axonal arborization of a specific bipolar cell associated with the S-cone (Mariani, 1984). The bipolar input to the outer layer is unknown, but these dual inputs seem likely to be involved in the generation of cone opponency. Lastly, there is a physiologically distinctive ganglion cell class with inhibitory S-cone input (Valberg et al., 1986). This has been tentatively identified as a small-bodied ganglion cell with a dendritic tree ramifying in the inner sub-layer of the IPL.

Each of the ganglion cell types drawn in Figure 3.4 represent a mosaic of cells spread across the retina. It may be more useful to think about the retinal signals in terms of their mosaics of origin, rather than in terms of MC- and PC-pathways. The cells of Figure 3.4 constitute the vast majority of cells which project to the visual cortex through the thalamus, and probably make up about 90% of the total ganglion cell population. There are a number of ganglion cell types which project to the brainstem and must fulfill vegetative functions such as pupillary control. They have not yet been fully characterized, but up to now no ganglion cell type has been detected which shows cone opponency apart from the midget and S-cone types drawn in Figure 3.4.

Finally, the *in vitro* technique shows great promise in finding out more about how ganglion cell signals are generated. We have recently recorded from horizontal cells, which are interneurons in the outer plexiform layer. The number of horizontal cell types and their connectivity has been controversial (Boycott et al., 1987; Kolb et al., 1994) but direct recording and anatomical identification has now shown that only two types are present. The H1 type only contacts M- and L-cones while the H2 type contacts preferentially S-cones and M- and L-cones to a lesser degree (Dacey et al., 1996), and these cells have also been drawn into Figure 3.4. It is often assumed that horizontal cells contribute to receptive field surround and/or to visual adaptation, and we now have the means to directly test these hypotheses.

3.3 Conclusions

The picture of the primate retina which has emerged in recent years is one of a simple and elegant structure. After the receptors, very specific circuitry exists with which receptor signals are transformed to neural output signals from ganglion cells. There has recently been some discussion as to how far a degree of randomness may be present in retinal wiring (e.g., Lennie et al., 1991), but so far specificity of connectivity has been a striking feature. Parasol cells of the MC-pathway provide a physiological substrate for the luminance channel of psychophysics, midget ganglion cells for a red-green opponent channel and the small bistratified cell and another cell type for a blue-yellow channel. Thus these psychophysical channels now have a firm physiological and anatomical basis.

A complication lies in the relation of cone-opponent mechanisms to perceptually opponent colors. Although psychophysical threshold experiments seem to match up well with physiological mechanisms at the retinal level (Fig. 3.6), the correspondence fails with suprathreshold color naming. For example, unique green (a green which is neither bluish or yellowish) is located at about 570 nm, whereas unique blue is located at about 470 nm. However, the red-green cone opponent channel is very strongly activated by a change in color from, say, white to 470 nm. Some transformation of cone to perceptual opponency must occur centrally (Guth, 1991; DeValois and DeValois, 1993). Whether it would be sensible to seek for perceptually opponent cells in cortex, or whether this transformation occurs in some kind of neural network remains to be determined; in any event, the locus lies beyond the retina.

The perceptual roles of ganglion cells is most easy to define in detection experiments, under threshold conditions. Under suprathreshold conditions, defining functional roles becomes more difficult. This is especially the case in spatial vision, where high resolution and precision seems to be mediated by an achromatic or luminance channel. The MC-pathway probably supports this channel to a significant degree (Kaiser et al., 1990; Lee et al., 1992; 1995), but midget cells may also be able to contribute due to their high numerosity (e.g., Lennie and D'Zmura, 1988). Perceptual performance may often be flexible enough to make use of neural signals whichever afferent pathway they have traveled, and resolving these pathway's differential contributions remains a challenge.

Acknowledgements

I would like to thank Dennis Dacey for permission to cite unpublished data, and Jan Kremers, Paul Martin and Iris Yeh for their experimental support.

References

Baylor, D. A., Nunn, B. J., and Schnapf, J. L. (1987). Spectral sensitivity of cones of the monkey *Macaca Fascicularis*. J. Physiol. (Lond.) *390*, 145–160.

Bowmaker, J. K. (1991). Visual pigments and color vision in primates. In: From Pigments to Perception, A. Valberg and B. B. Lee eds. (New York and London: Plenum), pp. 1–10.

Boycott, B. B. and Wässle, H. (1991). Morphological classification of bipolar cells of the primate retina. Eur. J. Neurosci. *3*, 1069–1088.

Boycott, B. B., Hopkins, J. M., and Sperling, H. G. (1987). Cone connections of the horizontal cells of the rhesus monkey's retina. Proc. Roy. Soc. Lond. B. *229*, 345–379.

Cole, G. R., Hine, T., and McIlhagga, W. (1993). Detection mechanisms in L-, M- and S-cone contrast space. J. Opt. Soc. Am. A. *10*, 38–51.

Dacey, D. M. and Lee, B. B. (1994a). The blue-ON opponent pathway in primate retina originates from a distinct bistratified ganglion cell type. Nature *367*, 731–735.

Dacey, D. M. and Lee, B. B. (1994b). Physiology of identified ganglion cell types in an in vitro preparation of macaque retina. Invest. Opthalmol. Vis. Sci. *35*, 2001.

Dacey, D. M., Lee, B. B., Stafford, D. M., Smith, V. C., and Pokorny, J. (1996). Horizontal cells of the primate retina: Cone specificity without cone opponency. Science *271*, 656–658.

Derrington, A. M., Krauskopf, J., and Lennie, P. (1984). Chromatic mechanisms in lateral geniculate nucleus of macaque. J. Physiol. *357*, 241–265.

DeValois, R. L. (1971). Physiological basis of color vision. Die Farbe *20*, 151–169.

DeValois, R. L. and DeValois, K. K. (1993). A multistage color model. Vision Res. *33*, 1053–1065.

DeValois, R. L., Abramov, I., and Jacobs, G. H. (1966). Analysis of response patterns of LGN cells. J. Opt. Soc. Am. *56*, 966–977.

Euler, M. (1787). Lettres a une Princesse d'Allemagne sur differentes Questions de Physique et de Philosophie. (Paris, Royez).

Famiglietti, E. V. and Kolb, H. (1976). Structural basis for ON- and OFF-center responses in retinal ganglion cells. Science *194*, 193–195.

Gouras, P. (1968). Identification of cone mechanisms in monkey ganglion cells. J. Physiol. *199*, 533–547.

Guth, S. L. (1991). Model for color vision and light adaptation. J. Opt. Soc. Am. A. *8*, 976–993.

Helmholtz, H. v. (1866). Treatise on Physiological Optics. (New York, Dover).

Hering, E. (1878). Zur Lehre vom Lichtsinne. (Wien, Carl Gerold's Sohn).

Kaiser, P. K., Lee, B. B., Martin, P. R., and Valberg, A. (1990). The physiological basis of the minimally distinct border demonstrated in the ganglion cells of the macaque retina. J. Physiol. (Lond.) *422*, 153–183.

Kolb, H., Fernandez, E., Schouten, J., Ahnelt, P., Linberg, K. A., and Fisher, S. K. (1994). Are there three types of horizontal cell in the human retina? J. Comp. Neurol. *343*, 370–386.

Lee, B. B. (1996). Receptive fields in primate retina. Vision Res. *36*, 631–644.

Lee, B. B., Martin, P. R., and Valberg, A. (1988). The physiological basis of heterochromatic flicker photometry demonstrated in the ganglion cells of the macaque retina. J. Physiol. (Lond.) *404*, 323–347.

Lee, B. B., Martin, P. R., and Valberg, A. (1989a). Nonlinear summation of M- and L-cone inputs to phasic retinal ganglion cells of the macaque. J. Neurosci. *9*, 1433–1442.

Lee, B. B., Martin, P. R., and Valberg, A. (1989b). Sensitivity of macaque retinal ganglion cells to chromatic and luminance flicker. J. Physiol. (Lond.) *414*, 223–243.

Lee, B. B., Martin, P. R., Valberg, A., and Kremers, J. (1993). Physiological mechanisms underlying psychophysical sensitivity to combined luminance and chromatic modulation. J. Opt. Soc. Am. A. *10*, 1403–1412.

Lee, B. B., Pokorny, J., Smith, V. C., Martin, P. R., and Valberg, A. (1990). Luminance and chromatic modulation sensitivity of macaque ganglion cells and human observers. J. Opt. Soc. Am. A. *7*, 2223–2236.

Lee, B. B., Wehrhahn, C., Westheimer, G., and

Kremers, J. (1992). Macaque ganglion cell responses to a stimulus that elicits hyperacuity in man. Invest. Ophthalmol. Vis. Sci. Suppl. *33,* 1343.

Lee, B. B., Wehrhahn, C., Westheimer, G., and Kremers, J. (1995). The spatial precision of macaque ganglion cell responses in relation to Vernier acuity of human observers. Vision Res. *35,* 2743–2758.

Lennie, P. and D'Zmura, M. D. (1988). Mechanisms of color vision. CRC Critical Reviews in Neurobiology *3,* 333–400.

Lennie, P., Haake, P. W., and Williams, D. R. (1991). The design of chromatically opponent receptive fields. In: Computational models of neurobiology, M. S. Landy and J. A. Movshon eds. (Cambridge, MA, USA: MIT Press), pp. 71–82.

Lichtenberg, L. C. and Voigt, J. H. (1781). Des Herrn Giros von Gentilly Muthmassungen uber die Gesichtsfehler bei Untersuchung der Farben. Magazin fur das Neuste aus der Physik und Naturgeschichte *1,* 57–61.

Mariani, A. P. (1984). Bipolar cells in monkey retina selective for the cone likely to be blue-sensitive. Nature *308,* 184–186.

Maxwell, J. C. (1855). Experiments on colour, as perceived by the eye, with remarks on colour-blindness. Transactions of the Royal Society, Edinburgh, *21,* 275–298.

Mayer, T. (1758). De affinitate Colorum. Lecto in Conventu Publico, Göttingen.

Smith, V. C., Lee, B. B., Pokorny, J., Martin, P. R., and Valberg, A. (1992). Responses of macaque ganglion cells to the relative phase of heterochromatically modulated lights. J. Physiol. (Lond.) *458,* 191–221.

Stromeyer, C. F., Cole, G. R., and Kronauer, R. E. (1987). Chromatic suppression of cone inputs to the luminance flicker mechanism. Vision Res. *27,* 1113–1137.

Stromeyer, C. F., III, Cole, G. R., and Kronauer, R. E. (1985). Second-site adaptation in the red-green chromatic pathways. Vision Res. *25,* 219–237.

Valberg, A., Lee, B. B., and Tigwell, D. A. (1986). Neurons with strong inhibitory S-cone inputs in the macaque lateral geniculate nucleus. Vision Res. *26,* 1061–1064.

Walls, G. L. (1956). The G. Palmer story. Journal of the History of Medicine and Allied Sciences *11,* 66–96.

Young, T. (1800). Outline of experiments and inquiries respecting sound and light. Philosophical Transactions (London) *90,* 106–150.

Young, T. (1802). On the theory of light and colours. Philosophical Transactions (London) *92,* 12–48.

4. Chromatic Processing in the Lateral Geniculate Nucleus of the Common Marmoset (*Callithrix jacchus*)

Jan Kremers, Eberhart Zrenner, Stefan Weiss and Sabine Meierkord

4.1 Introduction

Evolution has developed color vision to enable organisms to differentiate between objects of equal brightness by a kind of spectral analysis of the object reflectance. At a given luminance level most visual systems can discern only approximately 20 shades of grey while the analysis of the wavelength of reflected quanta by means of trichromatic color vision allows one to discern millions of different colors with different levels of brightness hue and luminance. Additionally, the usually very subtle differences between the broad spectral reflectance curves of biological objects are enhanced quite admirably by color-opponent ganglion cells so that the small differences between spectral reflectances are transformed to produce the strongest possible neurobiological signal, an electrical sign reversal in the color-opponent ganglion cells (Zrenner, 1983).

On the other hand, mother nature has provided a number of different solutions to this problem of enhancing chromatic differences between objects; photoreceptors of a large variety of spectral sensitivity have developed; animals use two, three or more photoreceptors of different spectral sensitivity to analyze objects. Additionally, it is possible that the interaction between rods and a single class of cones provides a remnant dichromatic type of color vision, e.g. in blue cone monochromats (Reitner et al., 1991). Consequently, the particular influence of the rod system on chromatic differentiation has to be taken into account. Therefore it seems very revealing to compare trichromatic primates and to study the differences between cone spectral sensitivity, rod and cone interaction in trichromatic as well as in dichromatic systems. A well-suited animal in this respect is the common marmoset.

The common marmoset (*Callithrix jacchus*) is a New World primate (suborder: *Anthropoidea* or *Simii*; infraorder: *Platyrrhini*; family: *Callithrichidae*). The New World primates separated from the Old World primates (suborder: *Anthropoidea*; infraorder: *Catarrhini*) about 40 million years ago. The common ancestor probably was a simian (Hershkovitz, 1997). Until recently there was little known of the physiological properties of the platyrrhine visual system. From early observations, it was known that the chromatic processing in platyrrhines might differ from the trichromatic system normal in catarrhines (Grether, 1939; Malmo and Grether, 1947; Miles, 1958; Jacobs, 1963). Subsequent studies mainly from Jacobs, Bowmaker and Mollon and their co-workers confirmed that many platyrrhines were actually dichromats, and that they displayed a sex-linked polymorphism with respect to chromatic processing. In the beginning of the eighties, the idea developed that this polymorphism has a genetic basis. It was hypothesised that there is a single gene on the X-chromosome defining the pigment for the long- and middle-wavelength range. However, there are presumably three different alleles for this gene, each coding for a different type of cone photopigment. Since these three pigments absorb maximally in the long- and middle-wavelength range, they will be summarized as L/M-cone photopigments. As a result, there are three dichromatic and three trichromatic phenotypes. The dichromats are all males and the homozygotic females, whereas the heterozygotic females are trichromats. Confirmation of this hypothesis came from microspectrophotometric measurements and from psychophysical studies (Tovee et al., 1992; Tovee, 1994; Travis et al., 1988; Jacobs et al., 1987; 1993; Mollon et al., 1984).

Apart from these photopigment differences between Old and New World primates there are other differences involving the photoreceptors: the cone density is higher and the rod density is lower in marmoset than in macaques and humans (Troilo et al., 1993; Goodchild et al., 1996). Recent results indicate a lower S-cone density in marmosets (Martin and Grünert, 1996).

In another recent study it was shown that it was possible to determine the phenotype electrophysiologically from measurements in the lateral geniculate nucleus (LGN) of the common marmoset (Yeh et al., 1995). In this study, two lights (from a green and a red LED respectively) were modulated with different relative phases. The response phase of the LGN cells revealed from which cone types the cells received their input. Yeh et al. (1995) also concluded that the retinal processing of the cone information is probably very similar for Old and New World primates. They also found that marmoset retinal ganglion cells had temporal characteristics very similar to those of macaques.

The LGNs of all primates (thus not only all anthropoids or monkeys, but also the prosimians and the tarsiers) are layered. The most important layers are the magnocellular (M-) and the parvocellular (P-) layers. The cells in these layers have different anatomical and physiological properties. They receive their input from morphologically distinct classes of retinal ganglion cells: the midget ganglion cells project to the parvocellular layers whereas the parasol ganglion cells project to the magnocellular layers. Retinal ganglion cells have similar physiological properties as LGN cells and are therefore also distinguished in P- and M-cells. Most probably, the midget ganglion cells are the morphological substrate for the P-cells and the parasol cells of the M-cells. The results of recent intracellular measurements (Dacey and Lee, 1994) seem to confirm this assumption.

P-cells of Old-World monkeys have color-opponent inputs. They receive excitatory signals from either the long- (L-) or the middle- (M-) wavelength sensitive cones and inhibitory signals from the other cone. As a result, P-cells are excited by some colors and inhibited by others, and therefore are probably very important for color vision. In M-cells, both cone types are either excitatory or inhibitory. Therefore they are more sensitive to luminance changes and are not color selective. In dichromatic New World primates, both cell types receive input from only one cone type (the L/M-cone). None of the cells are color selective. The chromatic signals are only carried by a small number of cells, the so-called 'blue-on' cells, which additionally receive input from S-cones.

P- and M-cells also have different temporal and spatial properties. Studies performed in our lab, showed that marmoset LGN cells have temporal properties which are qualitatively the same as in macaque retinal ganglion cells: cells belonging to the magnocellular (M-) layers were more responsive to luminance modulation than parvocellular (P-) cells. Moreover M-cells were temporally more nonlinear than P-cells, and the same types of nonlinearities as in macaques (such as saturation and contrast gain control) were observed in marmoset LGN cells. We, however, found evidence for substantial temporal filtering in the LGN cells (Kremers et al., 1997a). We further found that the spatial processing in the retina is identical for marmosets and macaques. The receptive fields of marmoset LGN cells were larger than those of macaques exactly as would be expected on the basis of the smaller eye of the marmoset. Further, as in macaques, M-cells were spatially more non-linear with similar nonlinearity indices (Kremers and Weiss, 1997).

From these results it can be concluded that retinal processing is probably very similar in platyrrhines and catarrhines. The main differences involve the photoreceptors. In the present paper we want to present the results of some studies on the chromatic processing in the dichromatic marmoset LGN, with emphasis on the interaction between rod and cone signals. Yeh et al. (1995) found some indications for strong rod inputs in some LGN cells. The objective of the present studies was to further pursue this observation. We measured the spectral sensitivities of P- and M-LGN cells to chromatic flashes upon a white background of various intensities. Further, we determined the 'silent substitution' location of a counterphase red-green modulation on a monitor. The concept of silent substitution was first introduced by Estévez and Spekreijse (1974). This idea makes use of the 'principal of univariance' (Mitchell and Rushton, 1971): the hyperpolarization in a photoreceptor is determined by the number of photons absorbed and not by the wavelength of these photons. Thus if two light-sources with different wavelength contents are exchanged without a change in the quantal catches in a certain photoreceptor, this substitution will be 'silent' for this photoreceptor: there will be no change in hyperpolarization. The 'silent substitution' point is characteristic for the present photoreceptor pigment.

The response amplitudes and phases of the cells at various mean luminances allowed some conclusions about the interaction between rods and cones. We further used the results of the electrophysiological studies as a basis for the study of rod-cone interactions in dichromatic human observers.

4.2 Spectral Responsivities

We measured the responses of marmoset LGN cells to chromatic flashes upon a white background (Kremers et al., 1997b) produced by a Xenon arc light source, the output of which was mainly in the visible part of the spectrum (color temperature: 4471° K; measured with a Spectrascan® spectroradiometer). The background intensity was either 1, 10 or 40 cd/m², which resulted in retinal illuminances equivalent to 31, 153 and 615 human trolands respectively (we used an artificial pupil of 2 mm diameter in all marmoset experiments; because of the smaller marmoset eye we calculated that the retinal illumination is 4.9 times larger than in the human eye). The chromaticity of the flashes was determined by interference filters and the same xenon arc source. The responses to various flash intensities were measured. Response amplitude at each condition was determined by the maximal discharge rate in a 50 msec time window after the excitatory stimulus (flash-on for on-center cells and *vice versa*). Response amplitude was plotted as function of the Michelson radiance contrast $\left(=\dfrac{R_{flash}}{2 \times R_{bckgr} + R_{flash}}\right)$ of the stimulus rather than Weber fraction since with Michelson contrast, a good description of only the lower flash intensities could be obtained where the adaptive state of the cells was mainly determined by the background and not by the stimulus. Radiance terms were used instead of quantal terms because of the broad-band spectrum of the background and because the photoreceptor sensitivities were calculated using the whole spectral output rather than the peak output wavelength. Photoreceptor absorptances were therefore divided by the wavelength to get the absorptances in energy units, and were corrected for absorption in the eye media (data kindly provided by Prof. J. Bowmaker). We fitted Naka-Rushton functions through the response vs. contrast plots and responsivity was defined as the initial slope of this function (which is the cell's contrast gain).

Figure 4.1 shows the mean spectral responsivities of LGN cells in one animal. The peak sensitivity for both P- and M-cell at a 1 cd/m² background is at 500 nm, indicating that the response is mainly determined by rod input. The peak sensitivity of P-cells at 10 cd/m² background has shifted to 518 nm and the curve has become broader. We interpret these data as showing that the cells have substantial cone input at this background intensity.

The blood of all animals used in our studies was examined genetically to determine the genotype (Williams et al., 1992; Hunt et al., 1993). In this particular animal the gene for the photopigment which maximally absorbs at 543 nm was present. In a later section we describe that it was actually possible to establish the link between genotype and phenotype, so that we are relatively confident that this animal indeed had the 543 nm photopigment. Through the data we fitted an addition of the sensitivities of rods and the 543 nm cone pigments to the various stimulus conditions. These fits are also shown in Figure 4.1. The spectral responsivities were too broad to determine the present photopigment directly, since the absorption spectra of all three L/M cones gave satisfactory fits. But, the fits with absorption spectra of the genetically determined photopigments were the best in the majority of the cases.

From the strength of the rod and cone input we calculated the ratio of rod to cone input strength to

4. Chromatic Processing in the Lateral Geniculate Nucleus of the Common Marmoset

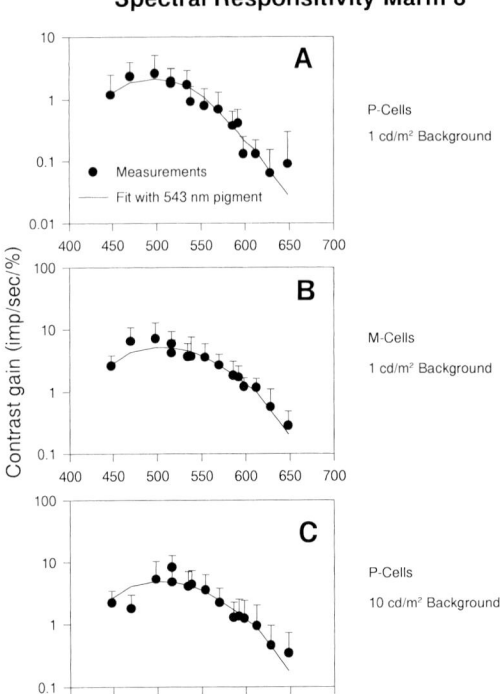

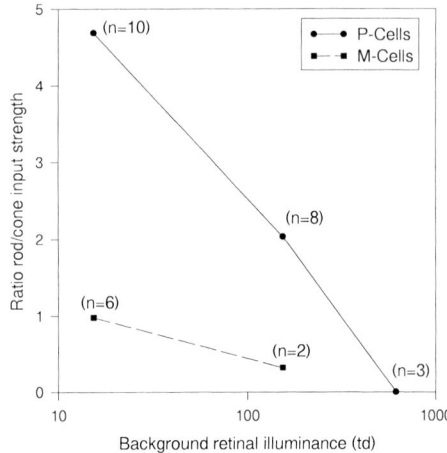

Fig. 4.2: Ratio of rod to cone input to P- and M-cells for different background retinal illuminances. The ratio decreases with increasing illuminance, indicating less strong rod signals. Further, P-cells seem to receive stronger rod signals than M-cells, the cause of which may lie in our way of defining response as discussed in the text.

Fig. 4.1: Mean spectral responsivities of 6 parvocellular (A) and 3 magnocellular (B) cells at a 1 cd/m² background giving a retinal illuminance of 15 equivalent human td. The cells respond maximally at 500 nm. The curve for the M-cells is somewhat broader, indicating stronger cone input. The mean spectral responsivity of 7 P-cells at 10 cd/m² (153 td) background are displayed in panel C. The maximal responsivity has shifted towards longer wavelengths, which is an indication of relatively stronger cone input. Spectral absorptances of the photoreceptors are fitted through the data. These absorptances were calculated using the nomograms of Knowles and Dartnall (1977). The quantal absorptances were divided by the wavelength to obtain the absorption in radiant terms.

the two cell types at various background levels. The ratios are given in Figure 4.2. These data show that there is a negative correlation between rod to cone ratio and background illuminance. Further, P-cells seem to receive stronger rod signals than M-cells.

These data show that LGN cells in the dichromatic marmoset have substantial rod input up to relatively high illuminance levels. But the method of determining spectral responsivities to chromatic flashes has some inherent disadvantages which make it difficult to further study how rods and cones interact. These disadvantages are: Flash stimuli contain many temporal frequencies. When cells have different temporal characteristics then it is difficult to quantify the interaction between both cell types. That seems to be the case with rods and cones. Furthermore, P- and M-cells have different temporal characteristics. The difference between both cell types as found in Figure 4.2 might be the result of these differences rather than real differences in rod or cone input. Since the response was defined as the maximal response within a 50 msec time window, a bias is introduced to get the response in a transient phase after the excitatory response. This transient phase might be more pronounced in M-cells. On the other hand the rod component in the response is possibly too slow to become expressed in this transient phase. A second disadvantage of the flash paradigm is that the state of adaptation changes continuously during the measurements, since the cells also adapt to the stimulus. Finally, the measurements were very time consuming (getting a complete spectral responsivity plot for one cell took about 1.5 hours). Therefore we have only limited numbers of useful response data.

To overcome these disadvantages we developed a stimulus using a monitor. The next section describes this stimulus type and the results of the measurements.

4.3 Responses of LGN Cells to Various Photoreceptor Contrasts

We developed a stimulus on a BARCO monitor that was controlled by a VSG 2/2 graphics card (Cambridge Research Systems). The stimulus consisted of counterphase modulation of the red and green guns of the monitor at a temporal frequency of 4 Hz, which was about the optimal frequency for most P- and M-cells (Kremers et al., 1997a). The spatial configuration of the stimulus was a circular center with a counterphase modulating surround. The center size was chosen to fit the receptive field center optimally. The reason for choosing this spatial configuration was to maximize the signal-to-noise ratio, through reinforcement of the receptive field's center by the surround. The contrast of the red gun was kept constant at 43% (expressed as Michelson contrast). The contrast of the green gun was varied between 5% and 80%, in steps of 5%. From the spectral output of the guns and spectral absorptances of the photopigments (corrected for absorption in the eye media and recalculated into energy terms) we calculated the photoreceptor contrast at each green contrast condition. The photoreceptor contrast of course depends on the absorption spectrum of the photopigments. A photoreceptor contrast of 0% is the 'silent substitution' condition for the pigment. Figure 4.3 shows the calculated photoreceptor contrast as a function of the green contrast for the various photoreceptors. Phase of photoreceptor responses is determined by red

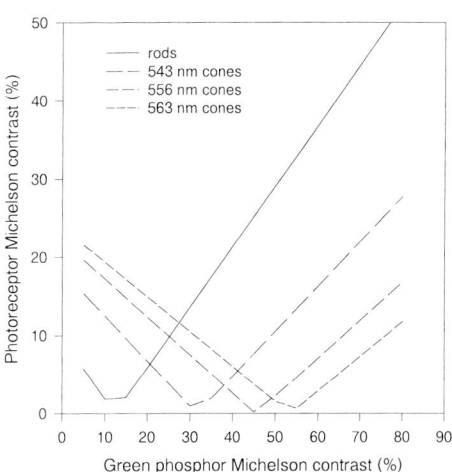

Fig. 4.3: Calculated photoreceptor contrasts for the different stimulus conditions. Red contrast was 43%.

modulation when green contrast is small and by the green modulation (and therefore 180° shifted) when the green contrast is large.

The measurements were repeated at different luminance levels. The responses of an on-center M-cell are displayed in Figure 4.4 as function of green contrast at different luminance levels. At high retinal illuminance the point of minimal response of this cell corresponds best with the 'silent substitution' point of a 563 nm photopigment. The response phase shifts by 180° at this point. Our conclusion that this animal has a 563 nm cone was confirmed by the genetic analysis. At lower retinal illuminances the condition of minimal cell response had shifted towards the 'silent substitution' point of the rods, without reaching it. From this we concluded that under these conditions the cell receives input from rods and the L/M cones. The response phase changes only gradually around the minimum, which indicates that the rod and the cone inputs have different dynamic properties.

We modeled the cell responses by a vector addition of rod and cone inputs. To fit the model to the data, the data were transformed into vectors in polar coordinates where the vector's angle with the abscissa is determined by response phase and the vector length by response amplitude. The rod and

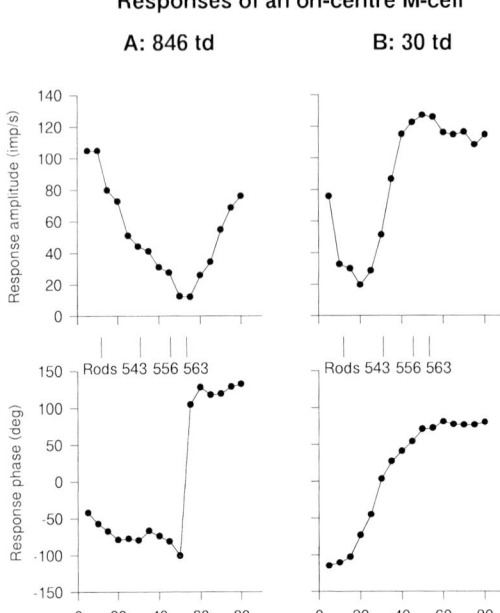

Fig. 4.4: Response amplitude (upper plots) and response phase (lower plots) of an on-center M-cell at two different luminance levels (2 and 40+15 cd/m^2 resulting in 30 and 615+231 equivalent human trolands respectively). The response is minimal close to the 'silent substitution' point of the 563 nm cone at high retinal illuminances. The response phase changes abruptly over 180° at this minimum. At 2 cd/m^2, the minimal response is between the 'silent substitution' points of cones and rods. The response phase changes more gradually.

cone signal vectors were added in such a manner to describe the data best. Figure 4.5 shows the results of the same cell as Figure 4.4 together with the model fits.

From the fits, phases and amplitudes of rod and cone inputs were obtained. For each luminance condition we calculated the ratio of rod to cone input strengths. In Figure 4.6 the mean ratio for P- and M-cells is given as function of retinal illuminance. Even at an illuminance level of 615 human trolands there is some rod input to the cells. For higher retinal illuminances we gave additional unmodulated light of the blue phosphors to selectively adapt the rods. It is only when about 150 td of the blue light is added, that the rod input is negligible, since the ratio does not increase any further.

We further found that the ratio of rod to cone input strength is correlated with retinal eccentricity (Fig. 4.7). This seems to be trivial when taking the rod and cone distribution into account, but to our knowledge this has not been found before on the basis physiological data. The finding is also indicative of the fact that our method is sensitive enough to study rod-cone interactions.

These measurements were repeated in some cells for several different temporal frequencies at an intermediate retinal illuminance level for which we found both substantial rod and cone input at 4 Hz. The data were again consistent with the vector addition model. The phase differences between rods and cones at the different frequencies indicat-

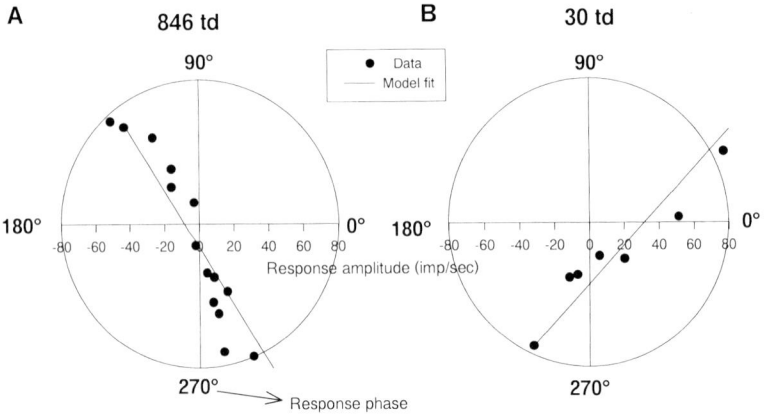

Fig. 4.5: The same data as in Figure 4.4 presented in a polar plot. Data are presented as vector end-points. The response amplitude is depicted by the distance to the origin. The angle of the vector with the abscissa gives the response phase. The lines are best fits with the model of vector addition of rod and cone signals.

ed that the rod signals were delayed relative to cone signals by about 45 msecs. Yeh et al. (1995) found for one cell a latency of 33 msec. These values were relatively close to values found in physiological measurements in macaques (Gouras and Link, 1966; Lee et al., 1997) which gave latencies of about 20–50 msec, and somewhat lower than psychophysically determined latencies (MacLead, 1972; van den Berg and Spekreijse, 1977) of 70–75 msec.

From these measurements we were able to conclude that:
- With this stimulus type it is possible to determine the present L/M photopigment.
- A model which assumes vector addition of rod and cone inputs describes the data well.
- We found that the cells can receive strong rod input up to relatively high retinal illuminances. That is in agreement with the spectral responsivity data and with the observations of Yeh et al.
- The rod input strength increases with increasing retinal eccentricities.

The advantages of this stimulus above the spectral responsivity measurement is that the measurements at all retinal illuminances were performed within about 10 min, in contrast to the 1.5 hours necessary to measure the spectral responsivity at one retinal illuminance level. Further, with the monitor stimulus the time-average retinal illuminance does not change with stimulus condition. Thirdly, the measurements with the monitor stimuli were much more informative about the type of interaction between rods and cones. Moreover by measuring the interaction at several temporal frequencies it is possible to draw some conclusions about the temporal properties of rod and cone signals.

Since the marmoset visual system was found to be relatively similar to those of Old World primates, with the exception of the differences in the photoreceptor density and absorption spectra (Goodchild et al., 1996; Yeh et al., 1995; Kremers and Weiss, 1997), we wondered whether a similar strong rod input can also be found in human dichromats.

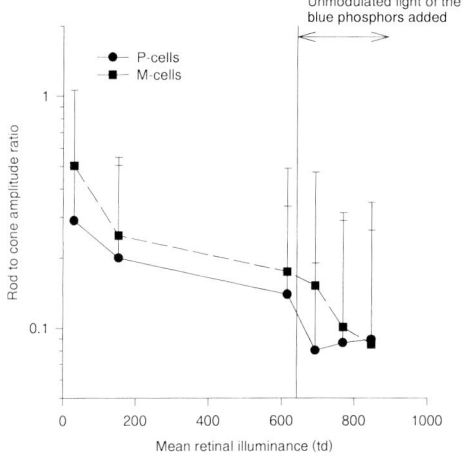

Fig. 4.6: Ratio of rod to cone input strengths as a function of retinal illuminance (expressed as human trolands). The ratio decreases monotonically, indicating decreasing strength of the rod signal. Even at about 600 td significant rod input was measurable. In contrast to the flash data, we did not find differences between P- and M-cells with this paradigm.

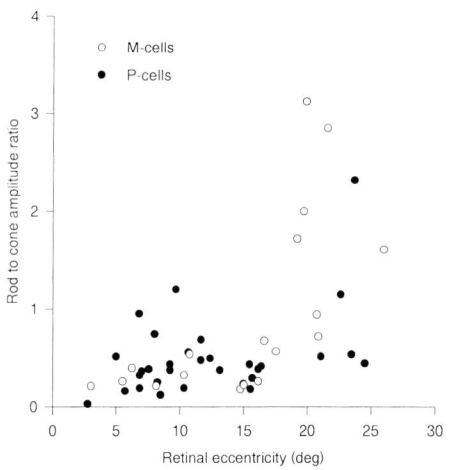

Fig. 4.7: Ratio of rod to cone input strength as a function of retinal eccentricity showing that rod signals are more important in eccentric cells.

4.4 Selective Photoreceptor Stimulation in Human Observers

In this section some preliminary results are presented from psychophysical measurements on human observers for which a similar stimulus as in the physiological experiments was used. All three monitor phosphors were modulated with predefined contrasts at 2 Hz and 10 Hz. The phosphors could modulate either in phase or in counterphase relative to each other. By taking into account the emission spectra of the phosphors and the cone fundamentals (DeMarco et al., 1992), the cone contrast in each of the three cone classes could be calculated. In all the measurements the S-cone contrast was 0% (S-cone silent substitution). Because of the broad emission spectra of the monitor phosphors it was not possible to obtain high cone contrasts, but in most measurements thresholds could be obtained. Thresholds can be presented in a two-dimensional plot displaying the L- and M-cone contrasts. A line through the origin in this plot connects points with the same ratio of L- to M- cone contrast. We measured the thresholds of trichromatic and dichromatic observers along eight directions in this plot. These measurements were performed at a time-averaged retinal illuminance of 470 td, for which the rod signal is probably small. The results are displayed in Figure 4.8 for a trichromat, a deuteranope and a protanope. The dichromatic observers had the largest thresholds along the cone axis which the observer lacks. This is a control that our calculations indeed resulted in the desired cone contrasts. The thresholds in the trichromatic observer were totally different and were more determined by postreceptoral systems. At low temporal frequencies, the thresholds are probably determined by the parvocellular system (Smith et al., 1992; Kremers et al., 1992). Since the parvocellular system is at this frequency least sensitive for luminance modulation and very sensitive for chromatic modulation (Lee et al., 1993), the thresholds are highest for the conditions where the luminance information is maximal and the chromatic information is minimal. That is the case when the L- and M-cones modulate in phase and with equal contrast, thus for conditions along the 45° line. There is however also a chromatic component in this stimulus since in this condition the centers of the blue-on cells are not excited (because these stimuli are all silent substitutions for the S-cone) but the surrounds are excited by the L- and M-cone modulations. At higher frequencies the magnocellular system probably determines the thresholds. Therefore the thresholds now result in a totally different outline in the

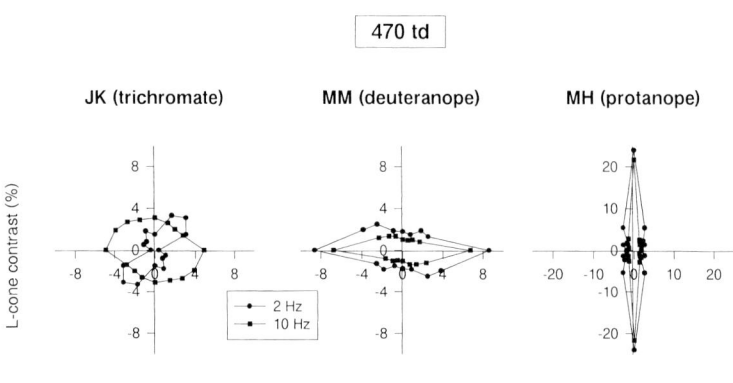

Fig. 4.8: Modulation thresholds for a trichromatic and two dichromatic human observers for different ratios of L- to M-cone modulation. Two different frequencies were used (2 and 10 Hz). Retinal illuminance was 470 td, and retinal eccentricity was 2°. S-cone contrast was 0% for all conditions. The thresholds of the trichromatic observer are determined by the luminance and chromatic contents of the stimulus, whereas the thresholds of the dichromats are determined by the pigment present.

plot, with maximal thresholds along the equiluminance axis, i.e., along the direction when L- and M-cones are modulated in counterphase with the M-contrast twice the L-cone contrast (luminance contrast was calculated along each direction by calculating the multiplication of the phosphor modulations with V_λ).

The monitor stimulus is thus suitable to study rod-cone interactions in dichromats because with the three phosphors we can span the three-dimensional space of the rods and the two cone types. Trichromats have four active photoreceptors, and therefore it is impossible to get each combination of photoreceptor contrast. Analogous to the L/M-cone space described above we created a rod/L-cone space for deuteranopes and a rod/M-cone space for protanopes. S-cone contrast again was 0% in all conditions. Figure 4.9 shows the thresholds of a deuteranopic observer. The stimuli were presented at 2° and 7.5° retinal eccentricity.

At 2° eccentricity and 470 and 47 td, the thresholds along the pure rod modulation axis are larger than along the pure cone modulation axis, indicating that the rod signal indeed was small. With decreasing retinal illuminance the thresholds at 10 Hz increase indicating an overall loss of sensitivity. Only at 4.7 td did the orientation of the threshold ellipse rotate away from the rod axis, indicating substantial rod signals in this condition. From these data it can be concluded that at least at retinal illuminances down to 47 td, rod signals are negligible. That is seemingly in contrast with the electrophysiological data on marmoset LGN cells. But the marmoset data also show that at low retinal eccentricities most LGN cells do not receive strong rod input. Although no electrophysiological data were obtained at 2° it is likely that this is also the case at this eccentricity.

The lower panels of Figure 4.9 show psychophysical thresholds at higher retinal eccentricities. The threshold ellipses indicate that the retinal illuminance at which rod signals are involved

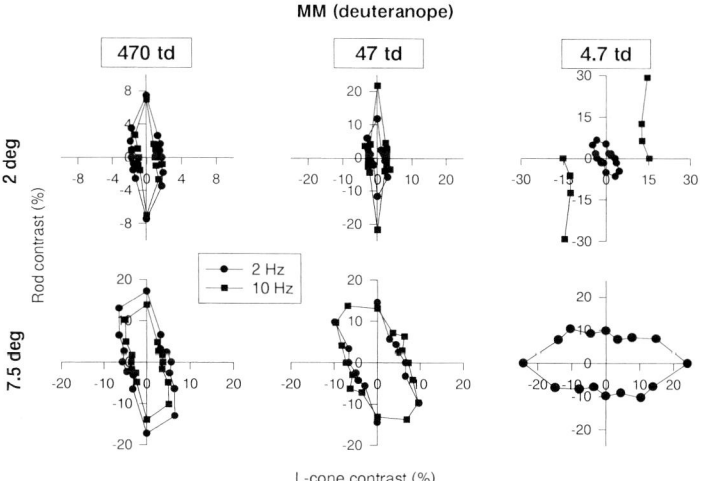

Fig. 4.9: Thresholds of a deuteranopic observer in a rod/L-cone space. Retinal eccentricity for the thresholds shown in the upper panels was 2°. At 470 and 47 td the thresholds are largest along the pure rod modulation axis, indicating only minor rod input at these retinal illuminances. At 4.7 td the threshold ellipse has rotated for the 2 Hz thresholds indicating significant rod signals. The thresholds increase dramatically for the 10 Hz modulation, in agreement with the overall observed loss of sensitivity to high temporal frequencies with decreasing retinal illuminance. The lower panels show thresholds measured at a retinal eccentricity of 7.5°. The threshold ellipses indicate that rods are involved already at 47 td. Thus, the strength of the rod signals increases with increasing retinal eccentricity.

indeed increase when the thresholds are measured at higher retinal eccentricity. It thus seems that, as in the physiological measurements, the retinal eccentricity plays an important role in the strength of the rod signals. The question, however, remains, whether the absolute levels of rod signals differ between humans and marmosets. Further, there might be differences between dichromats and trichromats. This issue is unresolved yet.

4.5 Summary

We measured responses of lateral geniculate cells in dichromatic common marmosets to chromatic flashes and to counterphase modulation of the red and green phosphors of a monitor. Both measurements gave indications of substantial rod input to both magno- (M-) and parvo- (P-) cells up to relatively high retinal illuminances (equivalent to 600 td in the human eye). We found that M-cells and the majority of P-cells had only input from the cone absorbing maximally in the middle- and long-wavelength range. Rod and cone signals to these cells were non-opponent. The response of the cells could be modeled by a vector sum of rod and cone signals. The strength of the rod signal decreased with increasing retinal illuminance and with decreasing retinal eccentricity. In psychophysical threshold measurements in dichromatic human observers at 2° eccentricity, the thresholds were not influenced by rods for retinal illuminances down to 47 td.

Acknowledgements

The authors wish to thank Dr. Tomoaki Usui for help during the experiments and Eva Burkhardt for technical support. We would like to thank Johannes Maurer and Bernd Wissinger for the genetic analysis, and Prof. Jim Bowmaker for providing the microspectrophotometric and absorption data. The project was supported by DFG Grant Zr 1/9-2 and Fortüne programm F.1222120.

References

Dacey, D. M. and Lee, B. B. (1994). Nature *367*, 731–735.

DeMarco, P. J., Pokorny, J., and Smith, V. C. (1992). Journal of the Optical Society of America A *9*, 1465–1476.

Estevez, O. and Spekreijse, H. (1974). Vision Research *14*, 823–830.

Goodchild, A. K., Ghosh, K. K., and Martin, P. R. (1996). Journal of Comparative Neurology *366*, 55–75.

Gouras, P. and Link, K. (1966). Journal of Physiology *184*, 499–510.

Grether, W. F. (1939). Mongr. Comp. Psychol. *15*, 1–38.

Hershkovitz, P. (1977). Living new world primates (Platyrrhini) (Chicago, London, The University of Chicago Press).

Hunt, D. M., Williams, A. J., Bowmaker, J. K., and Mollon, J. D. (1993). Vision Research *33*, 147–154.

Jacobs, G. H. (1963). Journal of Comparative and Physiological Psychology *56*, 616–621.

Jacobs, G. H., Neitz, J., and Crognale, M. (1987). Vision Research *27*, 2089–2100.

Jacobs, G. H., Neitz, J., and Neitz, M. (1993). Vision Research *33*, 269–274.

Knowles, A. and Dartnall, H. J. A. (1977). The characterization of visual pigments by adsorption spectroscopy. In: The Eye. Davson, H. ed. (New York London San Francisco, Academic Press), pp. 53–101.

Kremers, J. and Weiss, S. (1997). Vision Research *37*, 2171–2181

Kremers, J., Lee, B. B., and Kaiser, P. K. (1992). Journal of the Optical Society of America A *9*, 1477–1485.

Kremers, J., Weiss, S., and Zrenner, E. (1997a) Vision Research *37*, 2649–2660.

Kremers, J., Weiss, S., Zrenner, E., and Maurer, J. (1997b). Spectral responsivity of lateral geniculate cells in the dichromatic common marmoset (Callithrix jacchus). In: Colour vision deficiencies XIII. Drum, B. ed. (Dordrecht, Boston, London, Kluwer Academic Publishers), pp. 87–97.

Lee, B. B., Martin, P. R., Valberg, A., and Kremers, J. (1993). Journal of the Optical Society of America A *10*, 1403–1412.

Lee, B. B., Smith, V. C., Pokorny, J., and Kremers, J. (1997). Vision Research *37*, 2813–2828.

MacLeod, D. I. A. (1972). Nature *235*, 173–174.

Malmo, R. B. and Grether, W. F. (1947). Journal of

Comparative and Physiological Psychology *40*, 143–147.

Martin, P. R. and Grünert, U. (1996). Investigative Ophthalmology and Visual Science (SUPPL) 631 (Abstract).

Miles, R. C. (1958). Journal of Comparative and Physiological Psychology *51*, 328–331.

Mitchell, D. E. and Rushton, W. A. H. (1971). Vision Research *11*, 1045–1056.

Mollon, J. D., Bowmaker, J. K., and Jacobs, G. H. (1984). Procedings of the Royal Society B *222*, 373–399.

Reitner, A., Sharpe, L. T., and Zrenner, E. (1991). Nature 352, 798–800.

Smith, V. C., Lee, B. B., Pokorny, J., Martin, P. R., and Valberg, A. (1992). Journal of Physiology *458*, 191–221.

Tovee, M. J. (1994). Trends in Neuroscience *17*, 30–37.

Tovee, M. J., Bowmaker, J. K., and Mollon, J. D. (1992). Vision Research *32*, 867–878.

Travis, D. S., Bowmaker, J. K., and Mollon, J. D. (1988). Vision Research *28*, 481–490.

Troilo, D., Howland, H. C., and Judge, S. J. (1993). Vision Research *33*, 1301–1310.

van den Berg, T. J. T. P. and Spekreijse, H. (1977). Journal of the Optical Society of America *65*, 1210–1217.

Williams, A. J., Hunt, D. M., Bowmaker, J. K., and Mollon, J. D. (1992). EMBO Journal *6*, 2039–2045.

Yeh, T., Lee, B. B., Kremers, J., Cowing, J. A., Hunt, D. M., Martin, P. R., and Troy, J. B. (1995). Journal of Neuroscience *15*, 7892–7904.

Zrenner, E. (1983). Neurophysiological aspects of color vision in primates (Berlin, Heidelberg, New York, Springer-Verlag).

5. Molecular Genetics and the Biological Basis of Color Vision

Maureen Neitz and Jay Neitz

5.1 Introduction

Molecular biology and molecular genetics are beginning to help to answer questions of long-standing interest to color vision scientists. For example, shifts in spectral sensitivity of the middle-(M) and long-(L) wavelength sensitive photopigments have long been known to underlie congenital red-green color vision anomalies, but there have been unanswered questions. What are the spectral sensitivities of the photopigments that underlie the different forms of color blindness? In anomalous trichromacy the X-encoded pigments are less separated in spectral peak than normal, but how large a spectral difference between pigments is required to support color vision? How small can the spectral difference be before color vision is degraded? In the commonly observed congenital color vision defects, how much color vision loss can be explained purely by a decrease in the spectral difference between the underlying pigments, and how much must be attributed to deficiencies in post-receptoral processing? A closely related, but more global question that concerns the relationship between the cone photopigments and color vision is: why, for most humans, is color vision trichromatic, as opposed to tetrachromatic or even pentachromatic? Is trichromacy imposed because the number of spectrally distinct photopigments in the eye is limited to three or is the limitation at a higher level in the nervous system that has the capacity to carry only three color "channels"?

5.2 Background

5.2.1 Types of Congenital Color Vision Defects

To have normal color vision a person needs at least three spectrally different cone photopigments derived from each of three well-separated spectral classes: short-, middle-, and long-wavelength sensitive. These can be abbreviated S, M, and L. Alteration or loss of cone pigments cause color vision defects. The mildest disturbances in color vision are the *anomalous trichromacies* in which two of the cone pigments are less separated in spectral sensitivity than normal. Such mild color vision defects are extremely common, affecting 6% of males in Caucasian populations. The next most severe category of color vision defect are the dichromacies. *Dichromats* have lost one class of pigment and they base their color vision on just two pigments. There are three classes of dichromats categorized by missing either the L, M or S pigments and named respectively *protanopes, deuteranopes, and tritanopes*. Loss of the S pigment (tritanopia) is a rare condition. Protanopia and deuteranopia are much more common. They each occur at a rate of about 1% in Caucasian males. In the final category are the extremely rare *monochromacies* in which individuals are completely color blind. In this group there are two classes. *Rod monochromats* have loss of function of all three classes of cones. *Blue cone monochromats* have functional rods and S cones but have lost function of L and M cones.

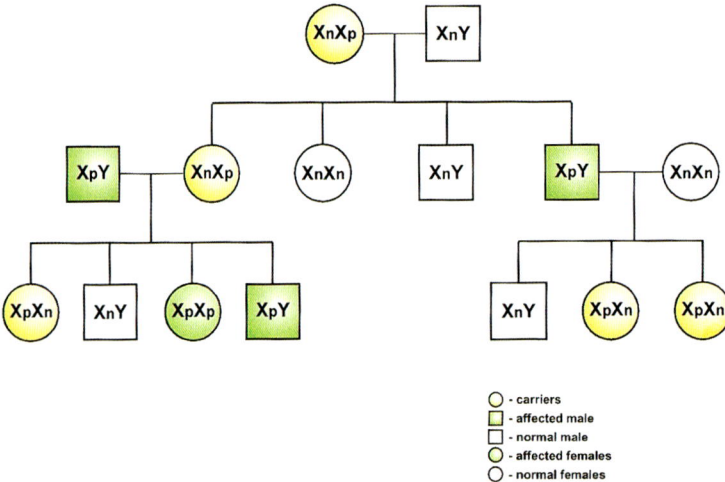

Fig. 5.1: Pedigree showing X-linked segregation of a color vision defect
The circles indicate females, squares indicate males. Females have two X-chromosomes, males have one X- and one Y-chromosome. X-chromosomes conferring normal color vision are denoted X_n, those conferring protanopic color vision are denoted X_p. In the pedigree drawn, the parents of the pedigree (top circle and square) had four children, two males and two females. One daughter ($X_n X_p$) married a protanopic male, and they had four children, two males and two females. One son of the parents of the pedigree married a homozygous normal woman ($X_n X_n$) and they had three children, one male and two females.

5.2.2 Genome Organization and Inheritance Patterns of Color Vision Defects

The human genome is organized into 23 pairs of chromosomes – 1 pair of sex chromosomes, and 22 pairs of autosomes (non-sex chromosomes). The sex chromosomes determine gender. Males have one X-chromosome and one Y-chromosome, females have two X-chromosomes. The majority of the X and Y chromosomes contain different genes, thus males are *hemizygous* for genes on the X-chromosome. Females can either be *homozygous* or *heterozygous* for genes on the X-chromosome depending on whether the genes on the two Xs are the same or different, respectively.

In somatic cells, genes from both members of each pair of autosomes are expressed, however genes from only one X-chromosome are expressed. In females, this is accomplished by a random, functional inactivation (X-inactivation) of one copy of the X-chromosome in each cell.

Red-green color vision defects, including protan and deutan defects, and blue cone monochromacy, are inherited as X-linked traits because the genes encoding the L and M cone opsins are both carried on the X-chromosome. An example of a pedigree segregating the color vision defect, protanopia, is shown in Figure 5.1. A male inherits the X-chromosome from his mother, and the Y chromosome from his father; a female inherits one X-chromosome from her mother and the other from her father. Thus, if a woman is heterozygous for protanopia ($X_n X_p$ in Fig. 5.1) and the father of her children has normal color vision ($X_n Y$), then her sons have a 50% chance of inheriting her X-chromosome carrying protanopia, and thus of being protanopes ($X_p Y$). Her daughters also have a 50% chance of inheriting her protan X-chromosome, but the daughters will inherit a normal X-chromosome from the father.

The daughters, thus, have a 50% chance of being heterozygous carriers of protanopia. A female carrier will have normal color vision because, due to X-inactivation, one-half of her photoreceptor cells will express the genes from the X-chromosome that confers normal color vision, and this rescues her from the color vision defect. In order to have protanopia, a female must inherit an X-chromosome that confers protanopia from both her mother and father. A color deficient man will not pass his genes for protanopia to his sons because his sons inherit his Y chromosome. However, a protanopic father will pass his genes for protanopia to his daughters, and the daughters are said to be obligate carriers. Daughters of carrier females and protanopic fathers have a 50 % chance of being protanopic. The other X-linked color vision disorders follow the same pattern of inheritance as protanopia. One additional consequence of X-inactivation is that females who inherit one X-chromosome that would confer deuteranopia and the other that would confer protanopia have normal color vision. The gene on one chromosome produces M pigment and a gene on the other chromosome produces L pigment. X-inactivation segregates these into two populations of photoreceptors and the nervous system is plastic enough to derive red-green color vision.

The very first studies of the molecular genetics of color vision were done by Nathans and his colleagues (Nathans et al., 1986a; 1986b). They isolated and characterized human L, M and S pigment genes. Their results indicated that the L and M pigment genes are on the X-chromosome and that they are 98% identical to each other. Perhaps the most surprising finding was that most people have more than two cone pigment genes on the X-chromosome. The M and L pigment genes are arranged in a head-to-tail tandemly repeated array. The present evidence indicates that individuals with normal color vision can vary widely in the number of cone pigment genes in the array (Neitz and Neitz, 1995). Two pigment genes – one M and one L – is the minimum requirement for normal vision and three genes is probably the most frequent number, but the range is up to perhaps as many as ten pigment genes. The X-chromosome can have multiple M- or multiple L-pigment genes, but it is more common to have extra M-pigment genes.

The gene encoding the S-cone opsin is located on autosome 7 (Nathans et al., 1986a). The color defect, tritanomaly, is caused by deleterious mutations in the S-pigment gene that render the pigment nonfunctional (Weitz et al., 1992a; 1992b). Tritanomaly is inherited in an autosomal dominant fashion, meaning that heterozygotes who have one mutant and one normal copy of the S-cone opsin gene exhibit the tritanomalous phenotype. The defective gene predominates over the normal one presumably because both are expressed in the same S-cone photoreceptor, and the defective gene product adversely affects the viability of the cell. Curiously, it appears that some people have the defective S-cone opsin gene but do not manifest tritanomaly, and this phenomenon is known as *incomplete penetrance*.

Rod monochromacy is inherited as an autosomal recessive trait. The gene underlying this congenital color vision defect has not been identified, however it appears that it is an autosomal gene, and that two mutant copies (homozygous recessive) are required to produce the disease phenotype. The focus of the remainder of this chapter will be on normal color vision, the common congenital red-green color vision defects and the underlying L- and M-pigment genes.

5.2.3 Genes and Gene Expression

The L-, M-, and S-cone opsin genes are believed to be expressed exclusively in the cone photoreceptor cells of the retina. The steps in the process of gene expression are illustrated in Figure 5.2. The L- and M-cone opsin genes each contain six *exons*, or coding regions, separated by five intervening regions, or *introns*. When a gene is expressed, the genomic copy of the gene is used by the cellular machinery as a template to make an RNA copy. The introns and exons are initially transcribed into heterogeneous nuclear RNA. This initial transcript is processed to remove the introns, and the exons are linked together to form messenger RNA (*mRNA*). The mRNA is used as a template to direct the synthesis of the protein product in the process of translation.

DNA and RNA are chemically very similar.

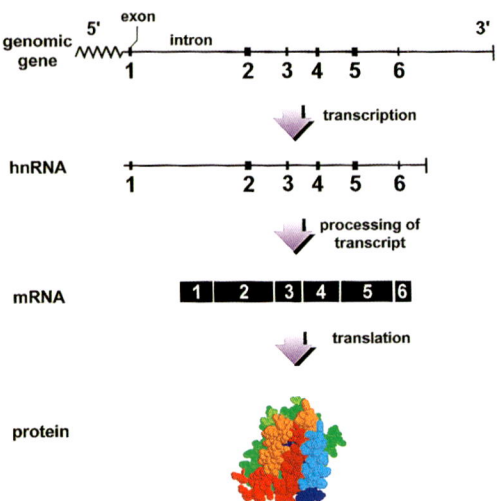

Fig. 5.2: Genes and gene expression. DNA is double stranded with antiparallel strands. The "head" and "tail" of each strand is conventionally designated 5' and 3' respectively. The convention for diagramming DNA is that the 5' end of the top strand is to the left, and the 3' end of the top strand is to the right. The bottom strand has the exact opposite orientation, with the 5' end to the right and the 3' end to the left. Genes are composed of exons connected by introns, indicated here by tiny boxes (exons) connected by lines (introns). Genes are transcribed into heterogeneous nuclear RNA which is then processed by "splicing" out the introns to form messenger RNA (mRNA). The mRNA is translated into a protein.

They both contain linear sequences of four nucleotide building blocks. For DNA the nucleotide building blocks are referred to with the letters G, A, C and T for the bases guanine, adenine, cytosine and thymine. For RNA the nucleotide building blocks are referred to by the letters G, A, C and U for the bases guanine, adenine, cytosine and uracil. The genetic code for the amino acid sequence of a protein is contained within the coding sequence of a gene and its corresponding mRNA. Within the mRNA there is a signal for where the translation machinery should begin translating the mRNA into protein, and the genetic code is read three nucleotides at a time with each series of three nucleotides specifiying the next amino acid to be incorporated into the polypeptide chain, or gene product. Also, included in the genetic code is a signal for where translation is to be terminated. Each set of three nucleotides that specifies an amino acid or specifies termination of translation is termed a *codon*.

When molecular biologists wish to study a gene expressed in a specific tissue, one general approach that is used is to isolate mRNA from the tissue of interest, and make a DNA copy of the mRNA. This DNA copy is termed *cDNA*.

5.3 Spectral Tuning of M- and L-Cone Pigments

A major contribution from molecular biology is an understanding of the role of specific amino acid differences in tuning the absorption spectra of the L and M pigments. This in turn has allowed the use of molecular genetics to deduce the spectral sensitivities of the pigments specified by the genes in individuals. Comparisons of color vision behavior with the deduced spectra of the pigments has provided insight into the photopigment basis of both normal and defective red-green color vision.

Work from a large number of laboratories using a variety of molecular genetic approaches has contributed to our understanding of spectral tuning of the X-chromosome encoded cone pigments (Asenjo et al., 1994; Chan et al., 1992; Ibbotson et al., 1992; Kosower, 1988; Merbs and Nathans, 1992; 1993; Neitz, et al., 1989; 1991; Williams et al., 1992). The genes for the L- and M-pigments each contain six exons. The first and sixth exons are identical between and among L- and M-pigment genes, and thus they do not participate in spectral tuning. Each of the other exons, 2-5, specify amino acid substitutions that produce spectral shifts.

The first identification of which of the differences among the M- and L-pigments contribute most to spectral differences came from a comparison of spectral sensitivities with the deduced amino acid sequences of the X-encoded visual pigments (Neitz et al., 1991). In that study, comparison of two human dichromats and six males from two species of South American primate revealed that most of the spectral difference

5.3 Spectral Tuning of M- and L-Cone Pigments

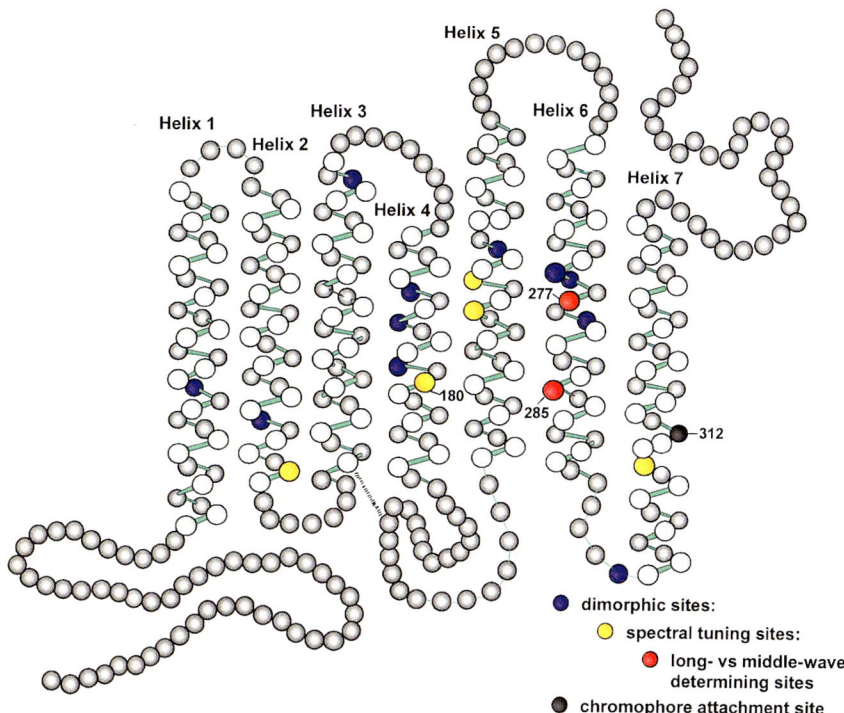

Fig. 5.3: A schematic diagram of an L/M cone opsin molecule.
Amino acids are illustrated as spherical "beads" along the protein strand. There are 18 amino acid dimorphisms that occur among the X-encoded opsins. Two differences, at positions 277, 285, shown in red, located in helix 6, together are responsible for the difference between the two major classes of X-encoded opsin, L and M. Changing these two produces a shift in peak absorption of 16–24 nanometers. Dimorphic changes at five other amino acid positions (shown in yellow) produce relatively smaller spectral differences. The dimorphism at position 180 plays a central role in producing individual differences in normal color vision and also plays a role in modulating the severity of color vision defects. The other spectrally active positions can modulate the severity of color vision defects and probably also play a role in normal color vision variations. It appears that the active changes produce a smaller spectral effect when introduced in an M pigment than when introduced in an L pigment (i.e., when M vs. L are defined by the identity of the amino acids at 277 and 285). An example is that substitution at position 116 produces a spectral change in L but not in M pigments. The 11 amino acid residues shown in blue are dimorphic among the human X-encoded opsins but they are not known to play a role in spectral tuning of M or L pigments. The protein component of the cone visual pigment (opsin) is a chain of amino acids imbedded in the cell membrane lipid bilayer. The seven transmembrane protein segments form alpha helices as they cross the lipid bilayer. In the photoreceptor cell, the helices from a bundle surrounding and completely encasing the light absorbing chromophore, 11-cis retinal. In this diagram, the molecule is opened out to display the inside surface. The chromophore attachment site, Lysine 312 in helix 7, is shown in black. Adapted from Donnelly et al. (1994).

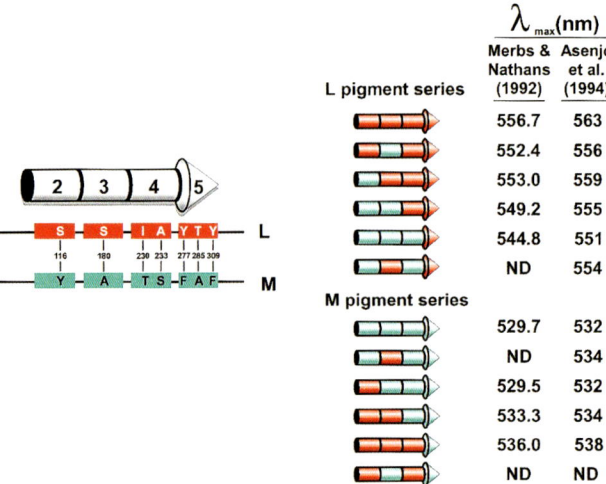

Fig. 5.4: Amino acid substitutions involved in spectral tuning. On the left is a diagram showing the L- and M-pigment gene structure, indicating the seven spectrally active amino acid substitutions encoded by exons 2-5 of the genes. The single letter amino acid code is given and S = serine; I = isoleucine; A = alanine; Y = tyrosine; T = threonine; F = phenylalanine. Red indicates that the encoded amino acids at the spectrally active positions shift the spectrum long, green indicates that the encoded amino acids shift the spectrum short. To the right are the L- and M-pigment genes constructed by Merbs and Nathans (1993) and Asenjo et al. (1994) and the measured spectral peaks (λ_{max}) for each of the encoded pigments are given. The two studies gave different values for the λ_{max} of each pigment but this is not surprising because the two groups used different biochemical methods. ND = not done.

between L and M pigments is produced by two amino acid substitutions encoded by exon 5 of the genes. These substitutions are tyrosine for phenylalanine at position 277 (Y277F) and threonine for alanine at position 285 (T285A), and together they produce a spectral shift of 16–24 nm (Fig. 5.3). These two substitutions, alone, can be thought of as determining whether a pigment is classified as M or L. The results of that study also indicated that substitution of serine for alanine at position 180 (S180A) produces a spectral shift of 4–7 nm. This site was of particular interest, in retrospect, because in the pioneering study of Nathans et al. (1986b) position 180 was not a variant position found to characterize the difference *between* M and L pigments. Instead it was one of four sites that differed *among* three L pigments (two were expressed sequences derived from human donor eyes, the third was a genomic gene)[1]. The discovery that the substitution S180A produces a spectral shift was a direct clue that more than one spectral variant of the L pigment might occur in the color normal population. Earlier microspectrophotometric data had also provided evidence that there

---

[1] It was later discovered that two of the codons which were reported as variant among L-pigments were in error. J. Nathans has generously distributed one of the cDNA clones (hs7). The use of that clone has been invaluable in work on cone pigment genes worldwide. However, several groups, including our own, have determined the sequence of that clone. The originally reported sequence was in error at two sites, in codons 111 and 116.

might be more than one spectral variant of L and M pigments in color normals (Dartnall et al., 1983). Together, these clues suggested a photopigment basis for variation in normal color vision (Neitz and Jacobs, 1986; 1989; 1990).

In vitro and *in vivo* studies confirmed that the substitutions S180A, Y277F and T285A are the three that produce the largest spectral shifts (Asenjo et al., 1994; Chan et al., 1992; Ibbotson et al., 1992; Merbs and Nathans, 1993; Williams et al., 1992). In addition, several other amino acid substitutions encoded by exons 2, 4 and 5 were identified as producing relatively small spectral shifts. Asenjo et al. (1994) demonstrated that seven amino acid substitutions are required to shift the spectral peak (λ_{max}) from that of the shortest M pigment to that of the longest L pigment, a shift of about 27–30 nm. The seven amino acid sites are shown in the protein structure (Fig. 5.3) and on the gene structure (Fig. 5.4).

Merbs and Nathans (1992) and Asenjo et al. (1994) made various gene constructs which encode chimeric pigments designed to investigate the effects of amino acid substitutions on λ_{max}. In Figure 5.4, the gene constructs are diagrammed on the right as arrows showing exons 2, 3, 4 and 5. The color of each exon indicates which amino acids are specified at the spectrally active loci encoded by that exon, and the color is keyed to the red and green genes at the left in Figure 5.4. There is good agreement about the relative influence of the amino acid substitutions on spectral peak.

Merbs and Nathans (1992) and Asenjo et al. (1994) both observed that the magnitude of the spectral shift provided by any given amino acid substitution is influenced by whether the substitution is made in an L-pigment (Y277, T285) or an M-pigment (F277, A285). In general, the shifts are readily apparent in L-pigments, but are either smaller or not detected in the M-pigments, as is evident from the λ_{max} values shown in Figure 5.4. This suggests that spectral subtypes of the L-pigment can be produced by making substitutions at any one of the five spectrally active positions besides 277 and 285. Similarly, subtypes of M-pigments can be produced, but there are perhaps fewer spectral variants of the M-pigment that can be generated by substitutions at these five positions.

To summarize, human pigments can be separated into two main classes by substitution at two amino acid positions encoded by exon 5 of the gene. Other dimorphic sites in the pigments cause smaller spectral shifts that can produce subtypes of L- and M pigments. Subtypes occur as polymorphic variants in normal color vision and they occur in color vision defects. Figure 5.5 summarizes the current thinking about the variety of pigments which may commonly occur in humans.

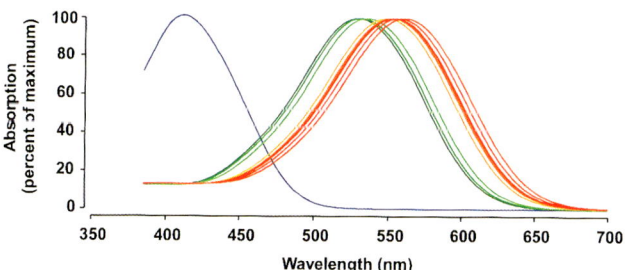

Fig. 5.5: Absorption spectra of the variety of cone photopigments thought to occur in humans. The blue curve is the absorption spectrum of the short-wavelength sensitive pigment. The cluster of green curves that peak near 530 nm are the absorption spectra of the M pigments encoded by the genes shown in Figure 5.4. The cluster of yellow, orange and red curves that peak above 550 nm are the absorption spectra of the L pigments encoded by the genes shown in Figure 5.4. This figure was generated using the λ_{max} values from Asenjo et al. (1994).

The range and variety of M-pigments is proposed to be smaller than L-pigments because some of the substitutions that change the spectral peak of an L-pigment have no effect in an M-pigment, and, in general, the spectrally active substitutions have a greater effect in L pigments than in M-pigments. The L-pigments appear to form a class discrete from the M-pigment class; a span of about 10 nm separates the longest M- from the shortest L-pigment (see Fig. 5.5). The story may not be complete still. Some of the changes made *in vitro* have been confirmed to produce similar effects *in vivo* but others have not. In addition, there are two commonly occurring amino acid dimorphisms, at positions 174 and 178 (Neitz et al., 1995a; Winderickx et al., 1993), that did not occur in the genes that Nathans et al. (1986b) originally studied. The *in vitro* studies summarized in Figure 5.4 were designed to study Nathans' genes, so whether or not these two additional dimorphisms are spectrally active has not been determined. Neither is expected to produce a large spectral change, either alone or in combination with the other dimorphisms that have been tested, but the only way to find out is by experiment.

Understanding the relationship between visual pigment gene sequences and the spectral sensitivities of the encoded pigments provides us with important information with which to test some long standing ideas about the mechanism underlying variation in the severity of color vision defects and in normal color vision.

5.4 Color Vision Defects

In people with normal color vision, the ability to distinguish between colors in the red-to-green region of the spectrum is based on the difference between the L- and M-cone pigments. In contrast, anomalous trichromats are missing one of the nor-

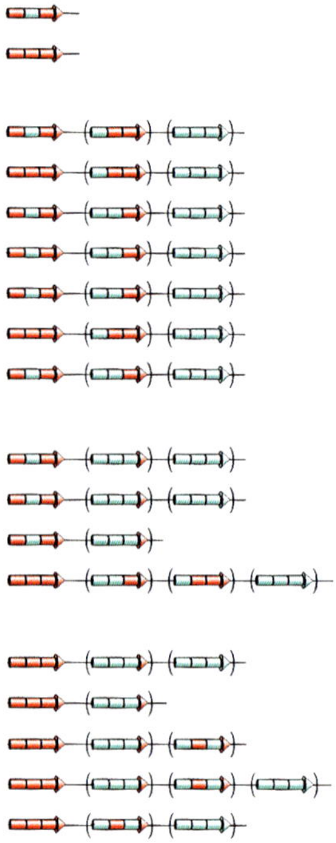

	Subjects	Gene Arrangement	Predicted Spectral Separation Merbs & Nathans (1992)	Asenjo et al. (1994)	D of Most Difficult Plate Read
DICHROMAT	d2		0.0	0	>0.081
	d1		0.0	0	>0.081
SEVERE	189		-0.6	3	>0.081
	187		3.7	4	0.081
	021		3.6	1	0.081
	012		3.6	1	0.072
	022		3.6	1	0.072
	188		3.7	4	0.072
	176		3.6	1	0.072
MILD	191		7.6	5	0.032
	185		7.6	5	0.032
	027		7.6	5	0.032
	028		7.9	8	0.032
VERY MILD	009		11.9	12	0.022
	186		11.9	12	0.022
	017		11.9	12	0.022
	190		11.9	12	0.022
	182		nd	9	0.022

Fig. 5.6: Test of the spectral proximity hypothesis in deuteranomaly. The D value was obtained by measuring the colors in the designs in the AO-HRR plates as specified by their coordinates in units of the Commission International de l'Eclairage (CIE) *u'v'* diagram (following Regan et al., 1994). For normal color vision this represents a two-dimensional color diagram in which equal distances in different locations correspond to equal perceptual differences. The maximal spectral separation between the L pigments encoded by the genes in each subject was calculated using the λ_{max} values from Asenjo et al. (1994) and Merbs and Nathans (1993), given in Figure 5.4. The identity of the first gene in each array is known from experimental data, the relative order of the downstream genes is not known and the orders are arbitrarily drawn here. The parentheses indicate that there may be more than one copy of a gene with that structure.

mal cone pigments, and it has been said that they have an "anomalous pigment". Within a given class of anomalous trichromacy, there is tremendous variability in the degree of color vision loss. One hypothesis that has been proposed to explain this is that individuals differ in the magnitude of the spectral separation between the underlying X-encoded pigments (DeMarco et al., 1992; Neitz and Neitz, 1994; Piantanida, 1976; Pokorny and Smith, 1977; 1982). A modern version of this idea has been termed the spectral proximity hypothesis (Regan et al., 1994). The idea is that if an individual had X-encoded pigments that were quite similar in spectral sensitivity, the individual would have severely impaired red-green color vision. In contrast, an individual whose X-encoded pigments were widely separated in spectral sensitivity would suffer a mild color vision loss.

The amount of information about spectral tuning that is presently available has made a molecular genetic test of the spectral proximity hypothesis possible. This was recently done for deuteranomaly which affects about 5% of men, and is thus the most common form of red-green color vision deficiency (Neitz et al., 1996a). The results of that study are summarized in Figure 5.6. Eighteen men with a deutan color vision defect were identified by Rayleigh matching. Two were dichromats, and sixteen were deuteranomalous trichromats. Among the deuteranomalous men there was a wide range in severity of the color vision defect. This is illustrated quite nicely by their performance on the American Optical Hardy Rand and Rittler (AO-HRR) pseudoisochromatic plate test. This test includes a series of stimuli that are designed to determine the severity of deutan color vision defects. The test relies on the principle that there are saturated colors that a deuteranope cannot distinguish from gray. One of the colors is a very particular blue-green and the other is its complement, a magenta-like color. Most deuteranomalous observers can discriminate from gray the saturated versions of these special colors but fail to see the color in more desaturated (pastel) versions of the same hues. The subject is shown a series of progressively more saturated symbols each printed on a background of gray dots. Severely affected deutan observers can read none or only the most saturated symbols; less severely affected participants are able to read correctly more desaturated symbols. This set of experiments was restricted to the use of the magenta series of symbols in the AO-HRR plates. The extent of each subject's color vision defect was expressed numerically as the distance (D) in color space that must differentiate the symbol on the plate from its gray background before the person could correctly identify the symbol. The D value for the most difficult plate read by each subject is given in Figure 5.6. These ranged from 0.022 indicating a relatively mild defect to 0.081 indicating a relatively severe defect. Three subjects (the two dichromats, d1 and d2, and an anomalous trichromat, subject 189) were unable to correctly identify any of the symbols in the AO-HRR plates meant to diagnose deutan color vision defects. These subjects were assigned D values of >0.081.

For each of the 18 deutan men, molecular genetic analysis was performed to identify the amino acids specified at each of the spectrally active positions. The analysis was done in a way that allowed the first gene in the array, an L-pigment gene, to be characterized independently of the downstream L-pigment genes. The deduced L-pigment gene structures are shown in Figure 5.6. As in Figure 5.4, the arrows in Figure 5.6 show exons 2, 3, 4 and 5 and are color coded according to whether the specified amino acids pull the spectrum long (red) or short (green). We used the λ_{max} values given in Figure 5.4 to determine the maximum spectral separation between the L pigments encoded by the genes in each subject. The genetic analysis suggested that the two dichromats each had a single X-linked pigment gene (Fig. 5.6). Among the deuteranomalous men, there is a nearly perfect correlation between color vision behavior, as indicated by performance on the AO-HRR plates, and the magnitude of the spectral separation between L pigments predicted from the genetic analysis. Together, the molecular genetic and behavioral data define four general categories of deutan defect ranging from the most severe form, dichromacy, to a very mild deficiency.

Alternatives to the spectral proximity hypothesis have frequently been proposed. For example, it has been suggested that differences in the severity of color vision defects derive from the amount of pigment produced (Nagy, 1982; Pokorny and Smith, 1987) or in the stability, quantum efficiency, or signaling of the pigment molecule, or in post-receptoral processing (Jameson and Hurvich, 1956). Proposal of these alternatives seemed necessary because the original version of the spectral proximity hypothesis failed to predict color vision behavior. This failure stemmed from the long held assumption that there was a fixed L-pigment shared by all normal and deuteranomalous people alike.[2] It had seemed natural to assume that everyone with normal color vision had the same L-pigment. Furthermore, the standard idea was that in deuteranomaly only the M-pigment was different from normal, having been replaced with one of a variety of pigments whose spectral peak was in-between the stereotyped normal L and normal M. Known as the "single-shift" hypothesis, this arrangement predicted that the spectral proximity of the X-linked pigments and, thus, color discrimination should decrease with increases in the λ_{max} of the "deuteranomalous pigment". The single-shift hypothesis predicted that deuteranomals would have a systematic pattern of behaviors in a standard color test, the Rayleigh color match.

In the Rayleigh match (after Lord Rayleigh, 1881) a person is shown two primary lights, a red and a green, and is asked to mix them together in a proportion that will exactly match the appearance of a monochromatic orange comparison light. For a trichromat, when the mixture and comparison light appear identical it is because the M and L pigments absorb photons at the same rate when stimulated by the red-green mixture as they do when presented with the monochromatic orange. The S cones are very insensitive to the middle-to-long wavelength lights used in this test so they do not participate in the match. Deuteranomals choose a range of red-green mixtures as matching the comparison light that are much different than normal. The green/red mixture ratios are typically more than four times high-

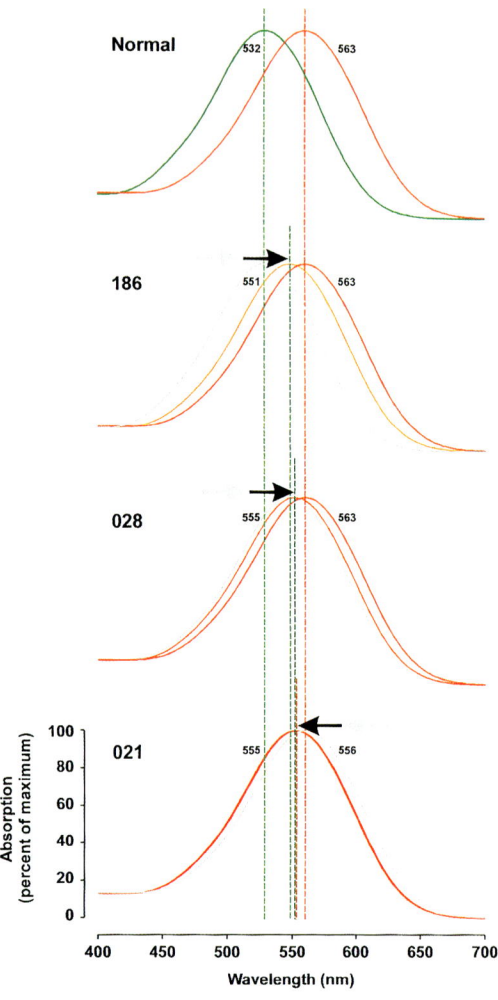

Fig. 5.7: The spectral proximity hypothesis accurately predicts color vision behavior because there are relative spectral shifts in the underlying photopigments.

At the top are the absorption spectra for the furthest separated M (green curve) and L (red curve) pigments underlying normal color vision. Also shown are the L pigments underlying deuteranomalous color vision in three male subjects from Figure 5.6. The λ_{max} values given are those predicted by Asenjo et al. (1994) in Figure 5.4. The vertical dashed green and red lines indicate the position of the λ_{max} for each pigment shown. Arrows indicate the shifts in λ_{max} of pigments underlying deuteranomaly relative to the pigments underlying normal color vision.

---

[2] An exception is a model, progressive for its time, forwarded by Alpern and Moeller (Alpern and Pugh, 1977) who proposed variation in normal L-pigments.

er than normal. This is because with an intermediate pigment replacing the normal M there is a relative decrease in sensitivity to green light and an increase in sensitivity to red. To compensate, the deuteranomals require more green light and less red in the mixture to match the monochromatic standard. People with the more extreme anomalies, because of their poor discrimination ability, will accept a wider range than normal of red/green ratios as indistinguishable from the orange standard.

The single shift hypothesis predicted that as the anomalous pigment's λ_{max} approaches that of the L pigment, there should be a decrease in the red/green mixture ratios chosen as matching the standard and there should be a simultaneous loss of color discrimination ability. The loss of color discrimination would be manifest as a progressively larger range of mixtures chosen as acceptable matches to the monochromatic standard. However, among deuteranomals, Rayleigh matching ranges and the match midpoints are not well correlated as was predicted. This observation is what led to the proposal that there must be defects in post-receptoral processing mechanisms to explain the color vision losses that are not accompanied by progressively more shifted mixture ratios.

Through molecular biology and molecular genetics, we have come to realize that *relative* shifts among the pigments are what account for the differences in behavior, and they also account for why some individuals with very poor color discrimination have a Rayleigh match midpoint that is closer to normal than others who have better color discrimination. This is illustrated in Figure 5.7. Deuteranomalous subjects 189, 028 and 021 are subjects who participated in the study summarized in Figure 5.6, and who were classified as deuteranomalous based on Rayleigh-matching data. Subject 186 only had a mild deuteranomaly, while subject 021 was very severely deuteranomalous, and subject 028 was intermediate between these two. All three subjects have reduced sensitivity to green light compared to normal because all are missing M-pigment function. Subject 186 has increased sensitivity to red light relative to normal, because he has the same 563 nm L-pigment as the normal person, but he also has an L-pigment that peaks at about 551 nm. Subject 028 has the same 563 nm L-pigment as the normal person and subject 186, and he has another L-pigment that peaks at 555 nm, so he is expected to have even greater sensitivity to red light than subject 186. Thus, we would predict that compared to subject 186, subject 028 would have a wider Rayleigh match range and a match midpoint that is further from normal. Subject 021 has an L pigment with a λ_{max} of 556 nm and one with a λ_{max} of 555 nm, and thus would have a greater Rayleigh matching range than either subject 186 or 028. Subject 021 would also have reduced sensitivity to red compared to both subject 028 and 186 so his match midpoint would be closer to normal. This is exactly the phenomenon that the original version of the spectral proximity hypothesis was unable to explain, and led to the proposal that other mechanisms contribute to the loss of color vision.

The nearly perfect correlation between behavior and the predicted spectral separation between the underlying photopigments provides strong support for the spectral proximity hypothesis. Most of the variation in behavior can be accounted for simply by spectral proximity. It would be interesting to conduct a similar molecular genetic test of the spectral proximity hypothesis in protanomalous men.

5.4.1 What Distinguishes Normal from Anomalous Pigments?

The data in Figure 5.6 provide us with insight into the nature of the anomalous pigments that underlie deuteranomalous color vision. Detailed analysis of the visual pigment gene sequences underlying normal color vision have been carried out previously (Neitz et al., 1995a). Some of the same chimeric[3] L-pigment genes found in individuals

---

[3] Nathans et al. (1986a,b) originally used the term hybrid or fusion gene to refer to X-linked pigment genes that contained part M-pigment gene and part L-pigment gene sequence. Many dimorphisms occur among M- and among L-pigment genes as well as between M- and L-pigment genes. Thus, it is seems more appropriate to refer to "hybrid or fusion" genes simply as chimeric genes.

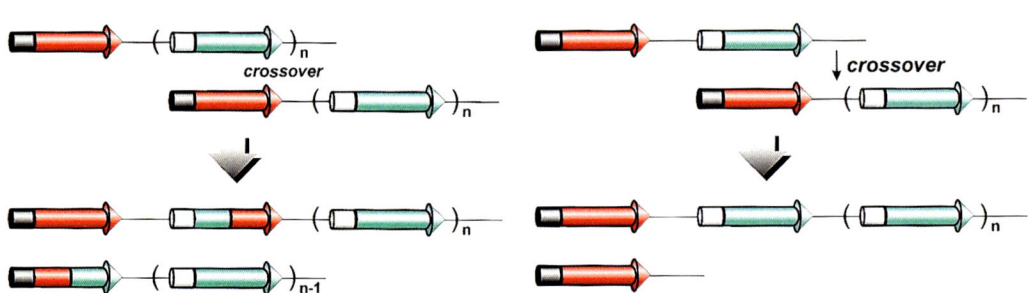

Fig. 5.8: Genetic mechanisms thought to produce the visual pigment gene arrays underlying congenital red-green color vision deficiencies. Red arrows indicate L-pigment genes, green arrows indicate M-pigment genes. The black versus white tails of the arrows indicate that the DNA sequences that flank the first gene in the array are unique to the first gene, but the sequences that flank the 5' end of the downstream genes are shared by all downstream genes.
(A) Two hypothetical X-chromosome photopigment gene arrays that underlie normal color vision (top) undergo *intragenic* recombination to produce two new arrays (bottom). The parental arrays are drawn as having a single L-pigment gene followed by a variable number of M-pigment genes, where n is any integer ≥ 1. One array structure, drawn here as having a single L-pigment gene, followed by a chimeric gene, followed by one or more M-pigment genes, is found in deutan and color-normal men. The other new array structure, which contains a chimeric gene first in the array, and may or may not be followed by M-pigment genes, has only been observed in protan men and female carriers of protan defects (Kainz et al., submitted).
(B) Two hypothetical gene arrays that underlie normal color vision (top) undergo *intergenic* recombination to produce two new arrays. One contains a single L gene, and no M genes, and underlies deuteranopia.

with deuteranomalous color vision are also found in men with normal color vision. Analysis of the L- and M-pigment genes expressed in retinas from male donors have revealed that of men who would be expected to have normal color vision because they express genes for three visual pigment classes, 10% express more than one L pigment gene (Strege et al., 1996; Sjoberg et al., 1998). In these men, the second L-pigment genes are chimeras identical to those found in some deuteranomalous men. Thus, the distinction between a "normal" L-pigment and a "deuteranomalous" pigment is fuzzy. That is, in some instances the two are identical.

Consideration of the genetic mechanisms believed to produce the visual pigment gene arrays underlying color vision defects serves to illustrate this point. The L- and M-pigment genes lie in a head-to-tail tandem array on the X-chromosome. Among men with normal color vision, the first gene in the array encodes an L-pigment (Neitz et al., 1996b). During cell division, the two X-chromosomes can misalign allowing a crossover to occur between an L- and an M-pigment gene. Intragenic crossovers of this sort produce two new X-linked pigment gene arrays, each containing a chimeric gene, as illustrated in Figure 5.8A. In this example, one array contains an intact L-pigment gene, one or more intact M-pigment genes, and a chimeric gene in which the front end derives from an M-pigment gene and the back end derives from an L-pigment gene. Exon 5 of this chimeric gene specifies Y277 and T285, and thus it encodes an L-pigment. The precise location of the crossover will determine the spectral peak of the chimeric pigment. This type of array structure is seen in men with normal color vision who express two L pigment genes – the "normal" L-pigment gene and the chimeric L-pigment gene (Neitz et al., 1996b; Neitz and Neitz, 1993; Sjoberg et al., 1997; 1998). It is also the type of structure seen in men with a deuteranomalous defect who, for reasons that remain mysterious, do not express any functional M-pigment but do express both the "normal" L-pigment gene and the chimeric one (Neitz et al., 1996a). Thus, the pigment encoded by the chimeric L-pigment gene can underlie either normal or deuteranomalous color vision.

The second product of the intragenic crossover shown in Figure 5.8A is an array in which the first gene is a chimera, and the downstream genes are typical M-pigment genes. Exon 5 of this chimeric gene specifies F277 and A285, and thus it encodes an M pigment. This type of chimeric gene in the first position in the array is the hallmark of a protan gene array (Kainz et al., 1997; 1998). The chimeric M-pigment gene encodes the protanomalous pigment, and its spectral peak is determined by the precise location of the crossover and the parent gene sequences.

Do the protanomalous pigments uniquely underlie protan defects, or are they also found in men with normal color vision? In a recent study addressing this question, we screened 150 male donor retinas looking for ones in which no L-pigment genes were expressed (Balding et al., 1997; 1998). Four such donors were found and three of them had and expressed more than one M-pigment gene suggesting that each had a protanomalous color vision defect. The fourth donor expressed a single M-pigment gene sequence suggesting he was a protanope.

Each of the three protanomalous donors had an X-linked visual pigment gene array structure that is uniquely characteristic of protanomalous men (Fig. 5.8A). Sequence analysis of the genomic genes and the genes expressed in the retinas revealed that the three men each expressed at least two distinct M-pigment genes. One of the expressed M-pigment genes corresponded in sequence to an M-pigment gene typically found in men with normal color vision. The other expressed gene was the chimeric gene that occupied the first position in the array, and encodes the putative protanomalous pigment. For all three men, the first gene in the array (the gene encoding the protanomalous pigment) was expressed at about twice the level of the downstream gene. The deduced amino acid sequence of the protanomalous pigment in each male indicated that it differs in sequence from M-pigments that have been found in men with normal color vision. These findings indicate that there are anomalous pigments that are unique to protan color vision defects.

5.4.2 What Distinguishes Photopigments Underlying Dichromacy from Normal Pigments?

Intragenic crossovers such as the one illustrated in Figure 5.8A produce a protanopic gene array if one of the parent arrays (the top array drawn in Fig. 5.8A) has only one M-pigment gene (n = 1). In this case, the crossover would produce an array with a single, chimeric gene which encodes an M-pigment. It can be seen from this that there is not necessarily any difference between protanopic and protanomalous pigments. As for the protanomalous pigments, the protanopic pigments will differ in amino acid sequence from the M-pigments found in color normal males if the crossover occurs downstream of the gene sequences that encode the polymorphic amino acid positions.

From spectral tuning studies we know that there is variation in the spectral positioning of M-pigments (see Fig. 5.5), which in turn predicts that there will be variation in the spectral positioning of protanopic pigments. In a recent study, electroretinographic (ERG) measures of the spectral sensitivity function and gene sequence analysis was done on 8 protanopes (Neitz et al., 1995b). Seven had similar spectral sensitivities which were best fit by a curve with a peak at 530 nm. The eighth was different, his pigment peaked at 537 nm. Sequence analysis of the underlying photopigment genes revealed that the seven who were similar each had a chimeric M-pigment gene in which exon 2 specified the long-shifting amino acid at position 116, but specified the short-shifting amino acids at all other spectrally active positions. The eighth protanope had a chimeric M-pigment gene which specified the long-shifting amino acids at positions 116, 180, 233, 236 and the short-shifting amino acids at the remaining relevant positions (see Figs. 5.3 and 5.4). Thus, results for these two types of protanopes indicate that the protanopic pigments differ in amino acid sequence from the M pigments found in color normal men, however the spectral sensitivities of these protanopic pigments are indistinguishable from those of M pigments underlying normal color vision (Jacobs and Neitz, 1993; Neitz et al., 1995b; 1989).

Deuteranopic gene arrays are thought to be produced by intergenic crossovers in which one product of the recombination event is an array from which all M-pigment genes have been deleted, as illustrated in Figure 5.8 B. Thus, deuteranopic pigments are the same L-pigments present in the normal population. We know from spectral tuning that there is variation in the spectral positioning of the L-pigments (see Fig. 5.5), and this leads to the prediction that there is variation in the spectral positioning of deuteranopic pigments. A study of dichromats confirms this prediction (Neitz et al., 1995b). Electroretinographic measurements of the spectral sensitivity functions from four deuteranopes revealed that two of the subjects had a pigment with λ_{max} of 563 nm, and the other two had λ_{max} of 558 nm. Molecular genetic analysis of the underlying cone pigment genes revealed that the two males with a pigment peaking at 563 nm had L-pigment genes that specified S180 (L-$_{S180}$ pigments), and the two males with a pigment peaking at 558 nm had L-pigment genes that specified A180 (L-$_{A180}$ pigments). Complete gene sequences were determined for one of each of the two types of deuteranopes, and the only spectrally active amino acid difference encoded by the genes was for the S/A 180 polymorphism. Also, the sequences of the deuteranope pigment genes were identical to those of L-pigment genes in color normal men.

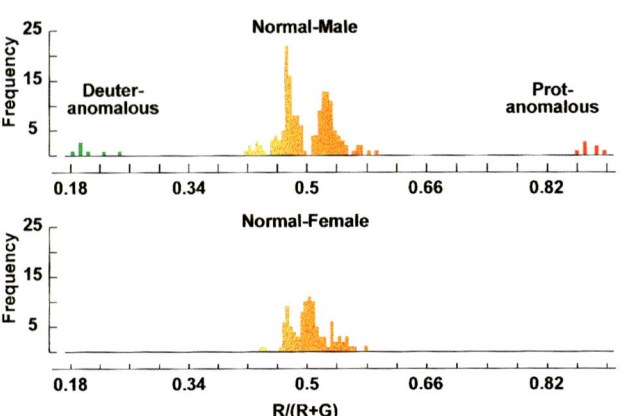

Fig. 5.9: Distribution of Rayleigh-match midpoints. The top histogram shows the distribution for males with normal, deuteranomalous and protanomalous color vision. The data for color vision deficient observers are shown to illustrate that although there is variation among men with normal color vision, all men classified as normal have Rayleigh matches that fall well within the normal range. The bottom histogram shows the distribution of Rayleigh-match midpoints for women with normal color vision. The color of the bars in the histogram illustrate the color of the red/green mixture that matches the standard orange as it would appear to a person whose match midpoint was 0.5 R/(R+G). That is, the red/green mixture set by a protanomalous appears red to an average normal observer, and that set by a deuteranomalous appears green. The matches made by men at the two extremes of normal set a match that appears orangish or greenish to a person who sets a match at 0.5.

Historically, the spectral sensitivity functions of "the deuteranope pigment" or "the protanope pigment" have been measured by averaging the results of the functions measured in a group of deuteranopes or a group of protanopes (Wyszecki and Stiles, 1982). One implication of the finding that there is variation in the spectral positioning of the pigments underlying both deuteranopia and protanopia is that the spectral sensitivity functions measured as an average of more than one individual are invalid.

5.5 Variation in Normal Color Vision

Another long-standing question is whether variation in spectral positioning of L- and M-pigments contributes to the significant variations in color matching that have been observed among individuals classified as having normal color vision. Neitz and Jacobs (1986, 1990) used a sensitive color matching assay to examine the magnitude and nature of individual variation in color matching among men and women with normal color vision. The distribution of the Rayleigh-match midpoints for 160 men and 100 women are shown in Figure 5.9. Winderickx et al. (1992) reported a similar distribution for the Rayleigh matches for color-normal men, as did Piantanida and Gille (1992). The matches for men in these studies appear to be multimodally distributed. The results of molecular genetic analysis of the L- and M-pigment genes of a representative subset of the men whose Rayleigh match data is shown in Figure 5.9 indicated a correlation between colour vision behavior and whether serine or alanine was specified at position 180 of the L- and M-pigment genes (Neitz et al., 1993). Neitz et al. suggested that most (83%) of the variation in normal color vision can be accounted for by variation in the spectral positioning of the L- and M-cone pigments.

Winderickx et al. (1992) examined L-pigment genes to investigate the relationship between the S/A 180 polymorphism and the Rayleigh match in 50 color-normal men. Indeed, whether an individual had a gene for L_{S180} versus L_{A180} strongly correlated to the amount of red light required in the Rayleigh match. They suggested that the S/A 180 polymorphism in L pigments underlies variation in normal color vision, and that this polymorphism in the M pigments does not contribute significantly to color vision variation.

From analysis of color-normal men we see that the frequency of genes for L_{S180} and L_{A180} are similar, being nearly equal. Most men have a gene for M_{A180}, but the frequency of genes for M_{S180} is lower (Neitz et al., 1995a; Winderickx et al., 1992). However, neither of these studies is likely to provide an accurate estimate of the frequency of the S/A180 polymorphism in L- and M-pigments in the population because the samples were small, and likely to be biased in the way they were selected. To get a better idea of the frequency of this polymorphism in L- and M-pigments, we sequenced the L- and M-pigment cDNAs from 130 male donors (Sjoberg et al., 1997; unpublished work). Each donor expressed both L- and M-pigment genes in the retina, and we took this as evidence that each was color normal. Of the expressed L-pigment genes, 51.5% specified L_{S180} and 48.5% specified L_{A180} (95% confidence limits ±8.5%). Of the expressed M-pigment genes, 93% were for M_{A180}, and 7% were for M_{S180} (95% confidence limits limits ±4.5%). If the contribution of this polymorphism to normal variation is directly related to the frequency at which the different alleles are expressed in the population, as one might anticipate, then one would predict that the polymorphism in L-pigments is responsible for a much larger portion of the variation.

From Figure 5.9 it can be seen that the majority of women make Rayleigh matches that fall intermediate between those made by the two largest groups of men. Is there a photopigment basis for this? From a theoretical standpoint, the answer is yes. As mentioned above, the frequency of genes for L_{S180} versus L_{A180} in the population of color-normal men is nearly equal. Females have two X-chromosomes. The probability that a woman will get both X-chromosomes with L_{A180} genes is 23.5% and the probability she will get both with L_{S180} genes is 26.5%. The probability that a woman will get one X-chromosome with an L-$_{S180}$ gene and one with an L-$_{A180}$ gene is almost exactly 50%). If, as theory predicts, half of the cells inactivate one X-chromosome and half inactivate the other, the heterozygous women will have approximately equal numbers of two spectral subtypes of L cone - L-$_{S180}$ and L-$_{A180}$. The distribution of Rayleigh matches in women (Fig. 5.9) shows that 28% of the women required a lower amount of red in the match, 20% required a higher amount, and 52% required an intermediate amount. If, as for men, the S/A180 polymorphism in L-pigments accounts for most of the variation in behavior, then we would predict that women in the group that requires the lesser amount of red will have L-$_{A180}$ genes on both X-chromosomes, those that require more red will have L-$_{S180}$ genes on both Xs and those that require an intermediate amount will have a gene for L-$_{A180}$ on one X-chromosome and a gene for L-$_{S180}$ on the other. We are in the process of testing these ideas.

Recent data from a study of visual pigment gene expression in the retinas from female donors provides some support for this idea (Kraft et al., 1998). We have looked at the visual pigment genes expressed in retinas from four female donors. All four women expressed both L- and M-pigment genes. Two of the four women express both a gene for L-$_{S180}$ and one for L-$_{A180}$. In both of these women, there is roughly equal expression of genes for L-$_{S180}$ and L-$_{A180}$. Based on these data, we hypothesize the distribution of L-, M- and S-cone types in the average female retina that is illustrated in Figure 5.10. This expression pattern is consistent with the idea that there is a photopigment basis for differences in the distribution of the Rayleigh match in men and women. Similar expression studies in males reveals that about 10% of men express more than one L-pigment gene (Strege et al., 1996; Sjoberg, et al., 1998). The difference is that in men, expression of one of the L-pigment genes usually predominates, representing about 75% or more of the expressed L-pigment genes (Neitz et al., 1996b; Strege et al., 1996, Sjoberg et al., 1998).

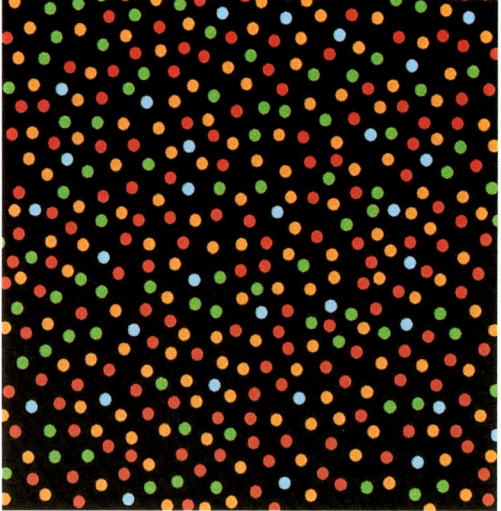

Fig. 5.10: Theoretical cone mosaic of a female. A representation of how the mosaic of cones might appear in a tiny patch of retina located at about 3 mm eccentric from the fovea. S-cones (colored blue) make up about 8% and M-cones (green) about 30% percent of the total. Evidence would suggest that about one-half of females have two spectrally different L-cone types (red and orange respectively). The two types are shown as being equal in number and randomly distributed as might be expected from random X-chromosome inactivation.

5.6 What Can Visual Pigment Gene Expression Tell Us about the Architecture of the Retina?

The three pigment hypothesis suggests that humans are trichromatic because there are three cone pigments in the retina (Brindley, 1970). What happens if there are more than three pigments? Does the person have an extra dimension of color vision? Historically, this question has been addressed in women known to be carriers of anomalous trichromacy (Jordan and Mollon, 1993; Nagy et al, 1981). The idea is that carriers have the unique potential for tetrachromacy because they will express the three normal pigments, in addition to an "anomalous" pigment. However, from a theoretical standpoint, and this is supported by a small study of expression in females, the majority of women are expected to have the photopigment basis for tetrachromacy. Given that in experiments to look for evidence of tetrachromacy in carriers, normal women serve as controls and they generally do not exhibit tetrachromacy, one might argue that this supports the idea that trichromacy is not a limitation of the number of spectrally distinct cone pigments.

Acknowledgements

The work from our laboratories reviewed here was supported by the National Institutes of Health, National Eye Institute grants EY09303, EY09620, and EY01931. It was also supported by Research to Prevent Blindness, Inc. by way of unrestricted grants to the Department of Ophthalmology at the Medical College of Wisconsin, a Career Development Award to M.N., and the James S. Adams Scholar Award to M.N. We would like to thank Phyllis Summerfelt for her assistance in preparing the figures and the manuscript.

References

Alpern, M. and Pugh, E. N. (1977). Variation in the action spectrum of erythrolabe among deuteranopes. Journal of Physiology, 266, 613–646.

Asenjo, A. B., Rim, J., and Oprian, D. D. (1994). Molecular determinants of human red/green colour discrimination. Neuron, 12, 1131–1138.

Balding, S. D., Sjoberg, S. A., Neitz, J., and Neitz, M. (1997). Cone opsin gene expression in men with colour vision defect. Investigative Ophthalmology and Visual Science (Supplement), 38, 14.

Balding, S. D., Sjoberg, S. A., Neitz, J., and Neitz, M. (1998) Pigment gene expression in colour vision defects. Vision Research, in press.

Brindley, G. S. (1970). *Physiology of the Retina and Visual Pathway.* London: Camelot.

Chan, T., Lee, M., and Sakmar, T. P. (1992). Introduction of hydroxyl-bearing amino acids causes bathochromic spectral shifts in rhodopsin: amino acid substitutions responsible for red-green colour pigment spectral tuning. Journal of Biological Chemistry, 267, 9478–9480.

Dartnall, H. J. A., Bowmaker, J. K., and Mollon, J. D. (1983). Human visual pigments: microspectrophotometric results from the eye of seven persons. Proceedings of the Royal Society of London B, 220, 115–130.

DeMarco, P., Pokorny, J., and Smith, V. C. (1992). Full spectrum cone sensitivity functions for X-chromosome-linked anomalous trichromats. Journal of the Optical Society of America A, 9, 1465–1476.

Donnelly, D., Findlay, J. B. C., and Blundell, T. L. (1994) Receptors and Channels, Vol. 2, (Harwood Academic Publishers), pp. 61–68.

Ibbotson, R. E., Hunt, D. M., Bowmaker, J. K., and Mollon, J. D. (1992). Sequence divergence and copy number of the middle- and long-wave photopigment genes in Old World monkeys. Proceedings of the Royal Society of London B, 247, 145–154.

Jacobs, G. H. and Neitz, J. (1993). ERG flicker photometric evaluation of spectral sensitivity in protanopes and protanomalous trichromats. In B. Drum (Ed.), *Colour Vision Deficiencies XI.* Dordrecht: Kluwer Academic Publishers.

Jameson, D. and Hurvich, L. M. (1956). Theoretical analysis of anomalous trichromatic colour vision. Journal of the Optical Society of America, 46, 1075–1089.

Jordan, G. and Mollon, J. D. (1993). A study of women heterozygous for colour deficiencies. Vision Research, 33, 1495–1508.

Kainz, P. M., Neitz, M., and Neitz, J. (1997). Molecular detection of female carriers of protan colour vision defects. Investigative Ophthalmology and Visual Science (Supplement), 38, S1015.

Kainz, P. M., Neitz, M., and Neitz, J. (1998) Genetic detection of femal carriers of protan defects. Vision Research, in press.

Kosower, E. M. (1988). Assignment of groups responsible for the "opsin shift" and light absorption of rhodopsin and red, green, and blue iodopsins (cone pigments). Proc. Natl. Acad. Sci. USA, 85, 1076–1080.

Merbs, S. L. and Nathans, J. (1992). Absorption spectra of the hybrid pigments responsible for anomalous colour vision. Science, 258, 464–466.

Merbs, S. L. and Nathans, J. (1993). Role of hydroxyl-bearing amino acids in differentially tuning the absorption spectra of the human red and green cone pigments. Photochemistry and Photobiology, 58, 706–710.

Nagy, A. L. (1982). Homogeneity of large-field colour matches in congenital red-green colour deficients. Journal of the Optical Society of America, 72, 571–577.

Nagy, A. L., MacLeod, D. I. A., Heyneman, N. E., and Eisner, A. (1981). Four cone pigments in women heterozygous for colour deficiency. Journal of the Optical Society of America, 71, 719–722.

Nathans, J., Piantanida, T. P., Eddy, R. L., Shows, T. B., and Hogness, D. S. (1986a). Molecular genetics of inherited variation in human colour vision. Science, 232, 203–210.

Nathans, J., Thomas, D., and Hogness, D. S. (1986b). Molecular genetics of human colour vision: the genes encoding blue, green, and red pigments. Science, 232, 193–202.

Neitz, J. and Jacobs, G. H. (1986). Polymorphism of the long-wavelength cone in normal human colour vision. Nature, 323, 623–625.

Neitz, J. and Jacobs, G. H. (1990). Polymorphism in normal human colour vision and its mechanism. Vision Research, 30, 620–636.

Neitz, J. and Neitz, M. (1994). Colour Vision Defects. In A. S. Wright & B. Jay (Eds.), Molecular Genetics of Inherited Eye Disorders. Chur: Harwood Academic Publishers.

Neitz, J., Neitz, M., and Jacobs, G. H. (1993). More than three different cone pigments among people with normal colour vision. Vision Research, 33, 117–122.

Neitz, J., Neitz, M., and Kainz, P. M. (1996a). Visual pigment gene structure and the severity of human colour vision defects. Science, 274, 801–804.

Neitz, M., Hagstrom, S. A., Kainz, P. M., and Neitz, J. (1996b). L and M cone opsin gene expression in the human retina: relationship with gene order and retinal eccentricity. Investigative Ophthalmology and Visual Science (Supplement), 37, S448.

Neitz, M. and Neitz, J. (1993). Individual males can express five different cone pigments. Investigative Ophthalmology and Visual Science (Supplement), 33, 911.

Neitz, M. and Neitz, J. (1995). Numbers and ratios of visual pigment genes for normal red-green colour vision. Science, 267, 1013–1016.

Neitz, M., Neitz, J., and Grishok, A. (1995a). Polymorphism in the number of genes encoding long-wavelength sensitive cone pigments among males with normal colour vision. Vision Research, 35, 2395–2407.

Neitz, M., Neitz, J., and Jacobs, G. A. (1995b). Genetic basis of photopigment variations in human dichromats. Vision Research, 35, 2095–2103.

Neitz, M., Neitz, J., and Jacobs, G. H. (1989). Analysis of fusion gene and encoded photopigment of colour-blind humans. Nature, 342, 679–682.

Neitz, M., Neitz, J., and Jacobs, G. H. (1991). Spectral tuning of pigments underlying red-green colour vision. Science, 252, 971–974.

Piantanida, T. P. (1976). Polymorphism of human colour vision. American Journal of Optometry and Physiological Optics, 53, 647–657.

Piantanida, T. P. and Gille, J. (1992). Methodology-specific Rayleigh-match distributions. Vision Research, 32, 2375–2377.

Pokorny, J. and Smith, V. C. (1977). Evaluation of a single pigment shift model of anomalous trichromacy. Journal of the Optical Society of America, 67, 1196–1209.

Pokorny, J. and Smith, V. C. (1982). New observations concerning red-green colour defects. Colour Research and Application, 7, 159–164.

Pokorny, J. and Smith, V. C. (1987). The functional nature of polymorphism of human colour vision. In C. o. Vision (Ed.), Frontiers of visual science: Proceedings of the 1985 symposium (pp. 150–159). Washington, D.C.: National Academy Press.

Regan, B. C., Reffin, J. P., and Mollon, J. D. (1994). Luminance noise and the rapid determination of discrimination ellipses in colour deficiency. Vision Research, 34, 1279–1299.

Sjoberg, S. A., Balding, S. D., Hoge, A., Lauer, C., Neitz, M., and Neitz, J. (1997). Structures of the L and M visual pigment genes expressed in normal colour vision. Investigative Ophthalmology and Visual Science (Supplement), 38, S14.

Sjoberg, S. A., Neitz, M., and Neitz, J. (1998) L pigment genes expressed in normal colour vision. Vision Resarch, in press.

Strege, S., Neitz, M., Kainz, P. M., and Neitz, J. (1996). Cone opsin gene expression in the retinas of two men with two different L-cone pigment genes. Investigative Ophthalmology and Visual Science (Supplement), 37, S338.

Weitz, C. J., Miyake, Y., Shinzato, K., Montag, E., Zrenner, E., Went, L. N., and Nathans, J. (1992a). Human tritanopia associated with two amino acid substitutions in the blue sensitive opsin. American Journal of Human Genetics, 50, 498–507.

Weitz, C. J., Went, L. N., and Nathans, J. (1992b). Human tritanopia associated with a third amino acid subsitution in the blue sensitive visual pigment. American Journal of Human Genetics, 51, 444–446.

Williams, A. J., Hunt, D. M., Bowmaker, J. K., and Mollon, J. D. (1992). The polymorphic photopigments of the marmoset: spectral tuning and genetic basis. EMBO Journal, 11, 2039–2045.

Winderickx, J., Battisti, L., Hibibya, Y., Motulsky, A. G., and Deeb, S. S. (1993). Haplotype diversity in the human red and green opsin genes: evidence for frequent sequence exchange in exon 3. Human Molecular Genetics, *2,* 1413–1421.

Winderickx, J., Lindsey, D. T., Sanocki, E., Distinguisher, D. Y., Motulsky, A. G., and Deeb, S. S. (1992). Polymorphism in red photopigment underlies variation in colour matching. Nature, *356,* 431–433.

Wyszecki, G. and Stiles, W. S. (1982). *Colour Science. Concepts and Methods, Quantitative Data and Formulae.* New York: Wiley.

6. Source Analysis of Color-Evoked Potentials in a Realistic Head Model Confirmed by Functional MRI

Walter Paulus, Renate Kolle, Jürgen Baudewig, Nora Freudenthaler, Mathias Kunkel, Michael Finkenstaedt and Hans-Heino Rustenbeck

6.1 Introduction

Electroencephalographic (EEG) activity recorded from the skull is an invaluable tool in clinical neurophysiology, for example, in supporting the diagnosis of epilepsy. In basic science it is used to record electrical activity generated by cerebral events. EEG changes induced by sensory stimuli, so-called evoked potentials (EP), reflect the activation of cortical areas to specific somatosensory, auditory or visual stimuli and can be best recorded close to the appropriate areas. These evoked potentials are usually much smaller than the spontaneous EEG activity. In order to detect them against the EEG background noise the EEG epochs after a sensory stimulus have to be averaged. The number of averages required depends on the signal-to-noise ratio, which in the case of visually-evoked potentials (VEP) requires some hundred averages. Due to the slow signal processing in the retina, VEPs have longer latencies than somatosensory or auditory evoked potentials. For foveal stimuli the cortex is activated at around 60 ms. VEPs to color stimulation differ from those after achromatic stimulation particularly in the early time range between 60 and 120 ms (Paulus et al., 1984). This is due to the different behavior of the receptive fields of color sensitive, so-called parvocellular cells (p-cells) in the retina. Parvocellular retinal ganglion cells terminate in the parvocellular layer of the lateral geniculate body in the thalamus of the brain. There are also magnocellular cells, terminating in the magnocellular layer, that are not involved in color vision. The receptive fields of all retinal cells consist of a receptive field center and antagonistic surround. In the case of a p-cell, the center consists of one cone, either blue, red or green and the surround of a mixture of these three cone types (Paulus and Kröger-Paulus, 1983). If these cells are stimulated by a homogeneous color stimulus, they will respond strongly, either by enhancing or by decreasing their spontaneous firing rate. With an achromatic stimulus, center and surround cones are excited equally and the antagonistic receptive field switching nullifies the net outcome. This explains why homogeneous color stimuli produce a prominent negativity of the visual cortex at 87 ms (N87), which is lacking with homogeneous achromatic stimuli (Paulus et al., 1986). With a chromatic stimulus, all cells covered by the stimulus respond vigorously, whereas in case of a luminance increment or decrement only the few units at the border of the stimulus are excited!

In order to isolate chromatic pathways for the investigation of color processing two important methodological aspects have to be kept in mind. 1). When looking for a pure color response it is necessary to use homogeneous color stimuli since in a combined color and pattern stimulus usually the pattern response dominates and occludes the color response. 2). Furthermore, the color stimulus should be exchanged with an equally-bright achromatic stimulus in order to avoid a contamination with a luminance onset stimulus.

With equally-bright (not equally-luminant) colors, the uniform color-specific surface negativity N87 can be recorded over the visual cortex (Oz) with an onset at around 60 ms with a clear occipital maximum (Paulus et al., 1984; Fig. 6.1). With a different type of equipment we have later confirmed these findings and have shown that the waveform of N87 is nearly constant regardless of the colors "red, green, blue or yellow" used for stimulation. In other words, different colors do not generate different EEG activity as long as they are matched for equal brightness. The N87 amplitude however increases with increasing color saturation (Paulus et al., 1988).

N87 can also be attributed to the decoding operation which has to be performed in the primary visual cortex for parvocellular activity which always transmits combined color and black-white luminance information (Paulus et al., 1986). Although, as already mentioned, p-cells play a major role in color perception, they also are – in parallel – heavily involved in discriminating high resolution black-white information. In order to be able to achieve this, the same p-cell encodes color information different from black-white border information (Paulus et al., 1986). These different aspects of information have to be decoded in the primary visual cortex, where we think N87 is the electrophysiological correlate of this decoding operation. Examples for a decoding operation may be seen in different behaviors of N87: It increases with an increase in luminance for red stimuli, it decreases for a luminance increase for green stimuli (Paulus et al., 1984). Improved methods of analysis have been developed in order to achieve a better understanding of these processes in the visual cortex.

At the beginning of this decade, advances in technology allowed a recalculation of the electrical generators within the brain from the EEG surface activity. This could be achieved by the use of dipole source analysis methods on the basis of multichannel recordings. These methods assume that the electrical activity measured at the skull surface can be used to reconstruct the electrical sources which in fact generate the surface activity and which cannot be measured directly by non-invasive methods. Basically, the program places single hypothetical dipoles into the brain and cal-

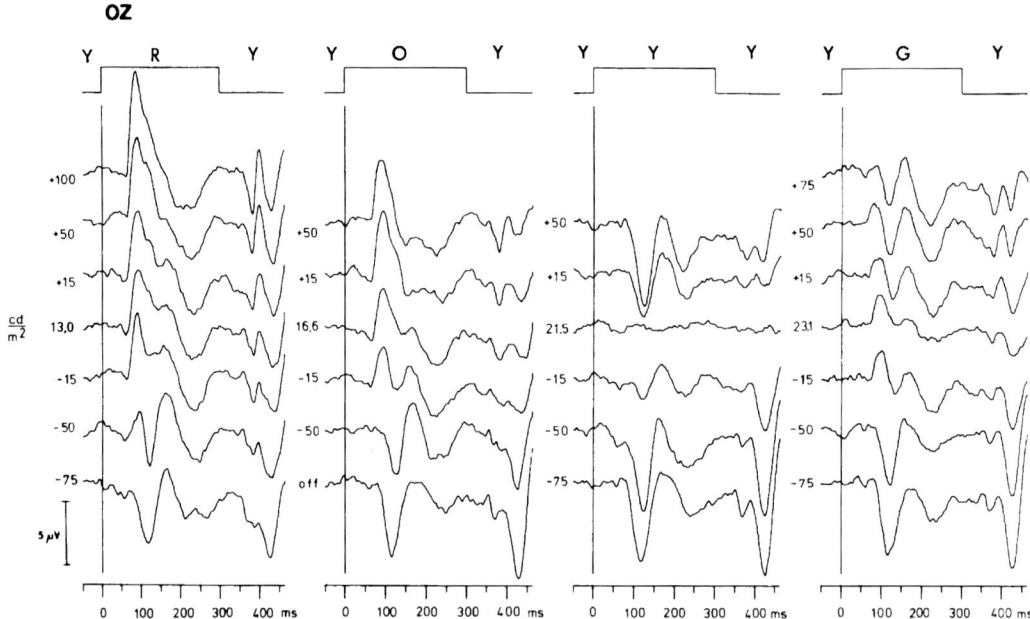

Fig. 6.1: Grand averages of VEPs from 10 subjects at the electrode site Oz. The middle row of traces (marked on the left by the actual test stimulus intensity in cd/m^2) represents the responses to subjectively equally-bright color stimuli. Color responses with additional luminance and decrements (marked in percentages at the left of each trace) are shown. All color stimuli are preceded and followed by the same yellow reference stimuli, as indicated at the top of each trace. Negativity is plotted upwards.
(Reprinted from: EEG and Clin. Neurophysiol., Vol. 58, Paulus W. et al., Colour and brightness components of foveal visual evoked potentials in man, pages 107–119 (1984), with kind permission from Elsevier Science Ireland Ltd., Bay 15 K, Shannon Industrial Estate, Co.Clare. Irland)

culates iteratively, how much of the surface activity is explained by the location and the orientation of that given dipole. It is then moved and rotated further unless an optimal decrease of the so-called residual variance is achieved. In other words, the program tries to explain as much as possible of the surface activity by as few dipoles as possible. Usually with three to five dipoles about 95% of surface EEG activity can be explained.

Resolution in space of the reconstructed generators increases with the number of recorded EEG channels. The first calculations were performed in a spherical head model. Originally we used 32 EEG channel recordings within this spherical head model and analyzed it by aid of the brain evoked sources analysis (BESA) software package. With this technique we were able to show that the N87 component can be attributed to the primary visual cortex (V1) (Plendl et al., 1995).

We have investigated higher stages of color processing by using color Mondrian stimuli, an abstract stimulus containing patches of different colors of different sizes without recognizable objects, closely resembling the paintings of Piet Mondrian (Plendl et al., 1993; Fig. 6.2 and 6.3). Again on the basis of 32 EEG channel recordings and in a spherical head model we could explain most of the electrical activity with a three dipole model. The first dipole was attributed to V1, the second to V2/V3 and the third tentatively to the fusiform and lingual gyrus (V4). The activity of the first dipole peaked at about 90 ms, the second at about 120 ms and the third at 160 ms. The main argument that the third source could be attributed to V4 was based on its perpendicular orientation at the base of the occipital cortex where V4 is to be expected and predicted from anatomy (Clarke and Miklossy, 1990; Fig. 6.4). Surprisingly, the dipole peaking at 160 ms did not differ after color and black-white Mondrian stimulation. This finding was basically confirmed a year later by Buchner et al. (1994). In a control experiment with motion stimuli the equivalent dipole to V4 changed its direction and rotates upwards and outwards

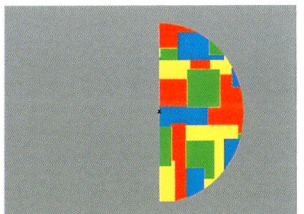

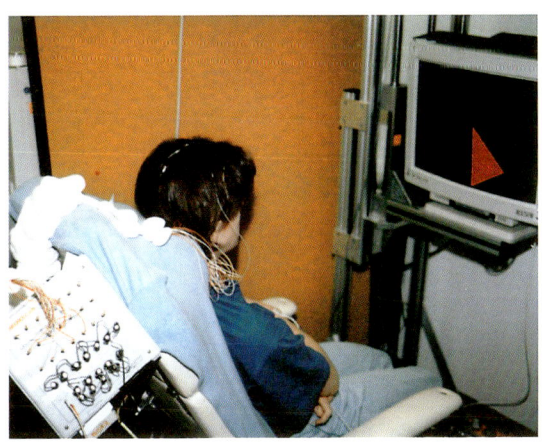

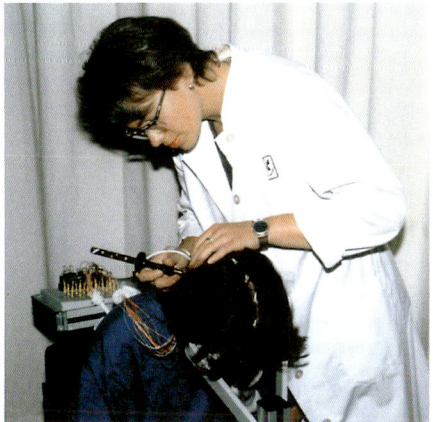

Fig. 6.2: A color Mondrian stimulus **(top)** and pictures of a subject being tested by VEP **(bottom, left)** and during the measuring of the exact positions of the electrodes using the optotrac system **(bottom, right)**.

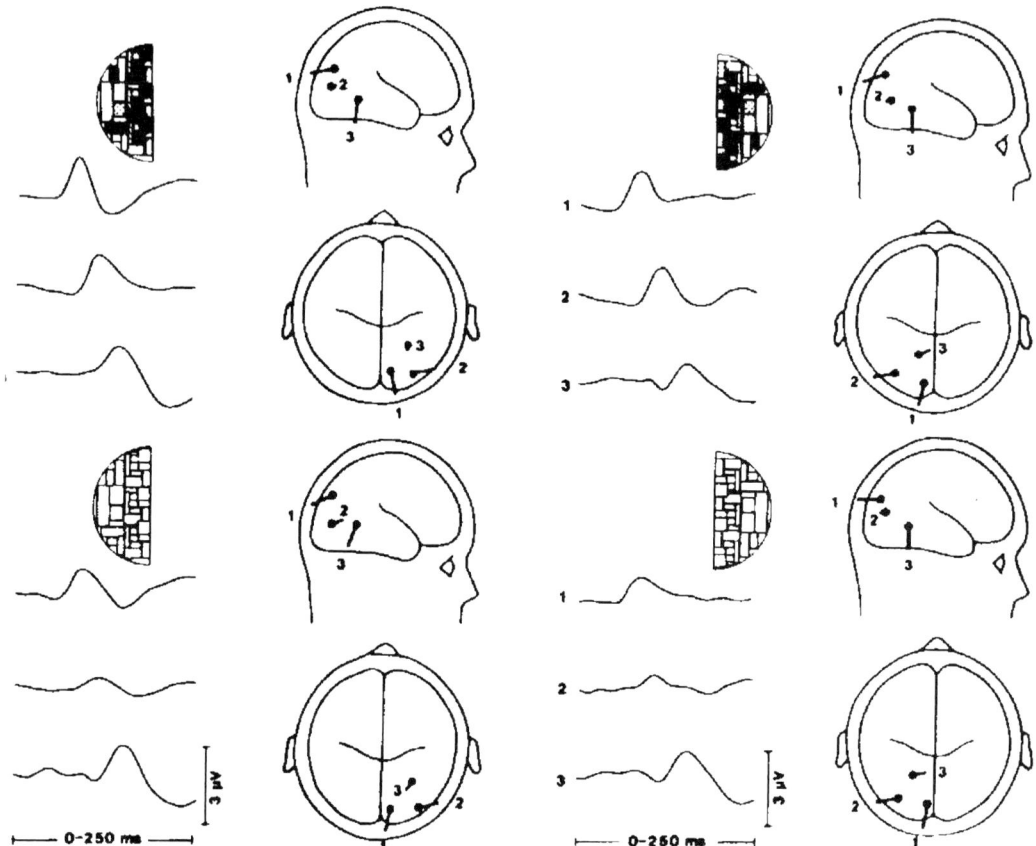

Fig. 6.3: Dipole sources in a spherical head model obtained for the colored (above) and colorless (below) Mondrian patterns presented in each half-field. The 3 dipoles explain 85–95% of the variance and are consistent with the origin of activity in V1, V2/3 and V4, respectively. There is little difference between the strength and character of dipole 3 for the colored and colorless stimuli. This shows that activity can be evoked anteriorly at the base of the occipital lobe (in the region of the fusiform and lingual gyri) by colorless patterned stimulation as well as by color.
(Reprinted from: Neuroscience Letters, Vol. 150, Plendl H. et al., The time course and location of cerebral evoked activity associated with the processing of color stimuli in man, pages 9–12 (1993), with kind permission from Elsevier Science – NL, Sara Burgerhartstraat 25, 1055 KV Amsterdam, The Netherlands)

(Probst et al.,1993), compatible with the location of V5 or MT in the human (Clarke and Miklossy, 1990).

It is however clear that particularly in the primary visual cortex these areas vary interindividually to a great extent (Brindley, 1972). Therefore more precise localization approaches have to take this variability into account by analyzing individual subjects. Recent advances in analysis methods allow source calculations in a realistic head model on the basis of magnetic resonance imaging (MRI). From the MR images the program knows the individual structures within each subject's head. Herewith the different surfaces of the cortex, the skull and the skin can be used for individual reconstruction of electrical activity in each subject's brain. With this method a rather precise localization of the individual sources can be achieved by superimposing electrical source activity onto the realistic individual MRI brain anatomy

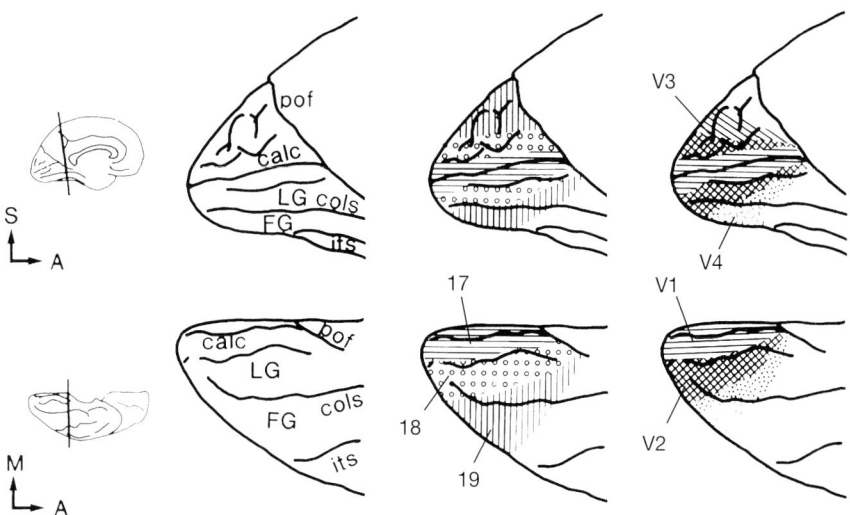

Fig. 6.4: Surface view of occipital cotex in man. Column 1 (from left) shows the left hemisphere from the medial (top) and inferior (bottom) aspects in man. The cortex posterior to the vertical line is represented in columns 2 (sulci and gyri), 3 (Brodmann's areas, 19) and 4 (visual areas according to newer terminology).
(After: Clarke S. and Miklossy J. (1990). Occipital cortex in man: organization of callosal connections, related myelo- and cytoarchitecture, and putative boundaries of functional visual areas. J. Comp. Neuro. 8, 298(2), 188–214, Fig.1, with permission from S. Clarke)

of the subject investigated (CURRY, Philips Inc., Hamburg).

The EEG methods described are particularly powerful in the time domain. Problems arise, if two sources are active at the same time, since their dipole fields may cancel each other or fuse to a pseudodipole. Newer functional imaging methods easily circumvent this problem. One widely used method is positron emission tomography (PET) which, however, inevitably exposes the subjects to some radioactivity. By this method, positron-emitting isotopes are used to" tag" molecules of a compound of interest which are introduced into the human body. These compounds are used to "trace" biological processes. After a given time, some of this atoms will decay and emit a positron. After collisions of these positrons with electrons, energy is liberated in the form of gamma rays which can be detected by a scanner. The density in the resulting images reflects the concentration of the positron-emitting probe in the tissue.

The method of the future for activation studies is probably functional magnetic resonance imaging (fMRI). Magnetic resonance imaging (MRI) makes use of the magnetic properties from the hydrogen nuclei. To perform MRI the individual lies in a scanner with a strong magnetic field inside. Using the different signals that the nuclei emit depending on their surrounding it is possible to visualize the human brain in consecutive sections in two-dimensional slices. The first successful application using MRI technology for detecting brain activity used contrast agents like gadolinium-DTPA. Nowadays fMRI is completely noninvasive: During brain activation blood flow and volume increase locally in the activated regions. So when comparing images acquired during stimulation and during a resting state it is possible to detect the areas of the brain that respond to the stimulus. The relation between oxyhemoglobin and deoxyhemoglobin, which changes in activated brain areas, works as an intrinsic contrast agent. The resulting contrast is called 'blood oxygen level dependent' (BOLD). A few advantages of fMRI are the excellent spatial resolution and the possibility to do repeated measurements on the same subjects. In this study we used

126   6. Source Analysis of Color-Evoked Potentials in a Realistic Head Model

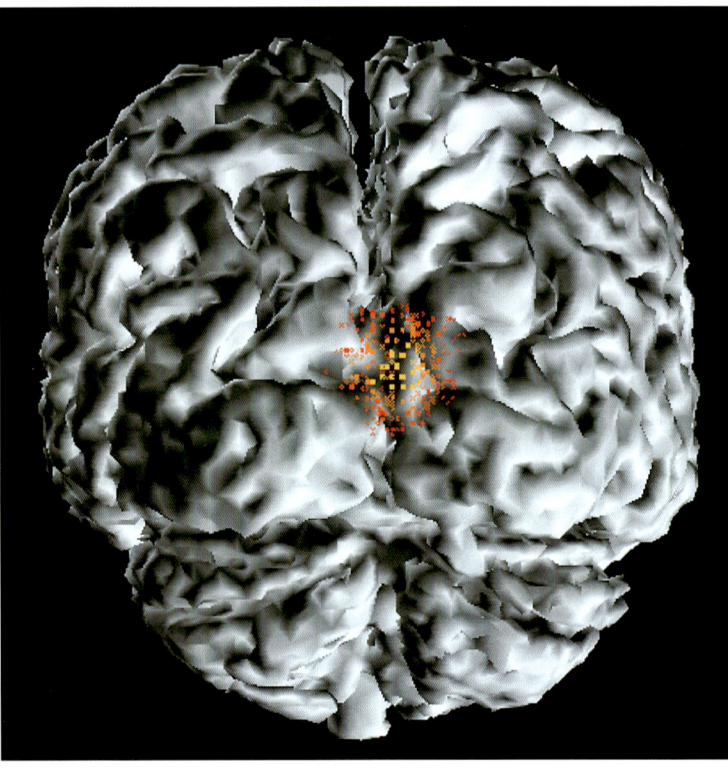

Fig. 6.5: Deviation scan of N87 after foveal stimulation in the human visual cortex. The colored dots represent those cortical regions which generate (with more than 90% likelihood) the electrical activity at the surface. The main activity is concentrated at the occipital pole, well in accord with the representation of the fovea in V1.

Fig. 6.6: Deviation scan at 160 ms in the human visual cortex after stimulation with a right lower red octant of 8° extent. The left lower figure represents the cortical area which generates the electrical activity at 160 ms with more than 90% likelihood; the middle lower figure represents the equivalent calculations with a threshold of 95%. The lower right part of the figure shows the equivalent dipole with a downward orientation.

DEVIATION SCAN / DIPOLE FIT

time: 160 ms after stimulus onset

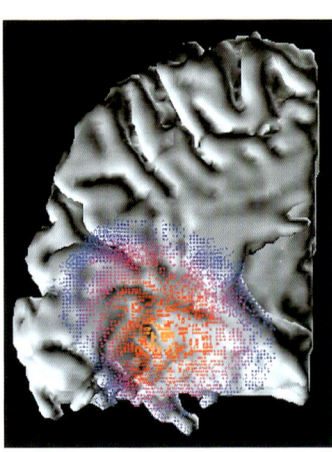

[threshold 90%]

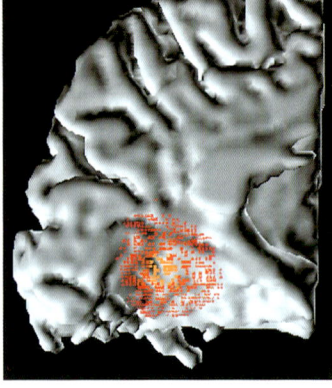

[threshold 95%]

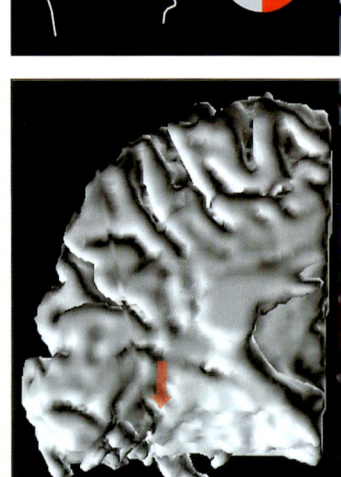

[dipole fit]

fMRI to confirm the findings of the EEG source analysis. The two methods complement each other; EEG data have excellent temporal resolution while fMRI has excellent spatial resolution.

6.2 Methods

The EEG was recorded from 64 channels, bandpass filtered between 3 Hz and 50 Hz. The electrodes were positioned according to the 10/10 system with a concentration over the occipital cortex. The exact position was measured by the optotrac system (Northern Digital, CDN) and transferred to the software package CURRY. An individual MRI (Siemens Vision) scan was obtained from the subject and transferred digitally into CURRY. Electrode position was superimposed onto the subject's skull. The reconstruction paradigm calculates the currents inside the head with boundary conditions. Two source models of a single moving dipole and of a deviation scan algorithm were performed to explain the measured data as well as possible. First, the single dipole model assumes that only one center is active with freedom in location, rotation and orientation. Secondly the deviation scan weights single dipole fits for current support points across the cortical surface. In order to obtain the specific structure of the cortex and the support points, the surface was segmented from a three-dimensional MRI data set. This calculation thus works in a realistic head model. In the spherical head model analysis program BESA, which we previously employed, the operator can choose to add additional test dipoles. In our present program this is not possible. Thus the analysis represents an objective result uninfluenced by the investigator's strategy. The results plotted in Figures 6.5 and 6.6 have been assessed by the straightforward application of the calculation algorithm.

In an independent session, we re-examined the

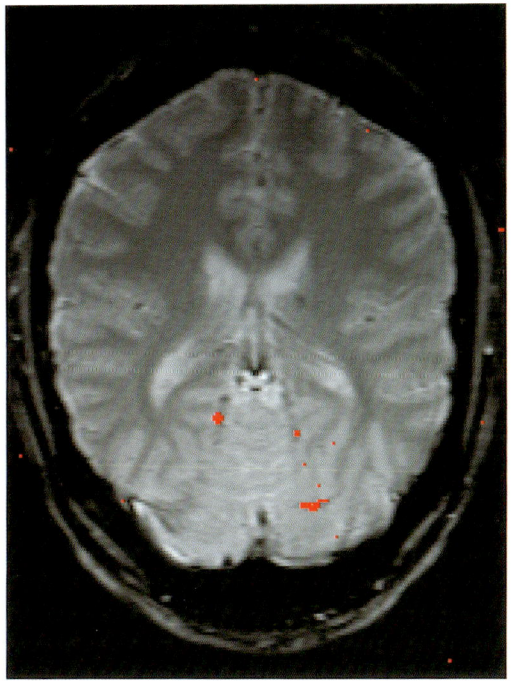

Colour Mondrian   Black-white Mondrian

Fig. 6.7: Functional MRI by using the FLASH technique. Stimulation was performed with a black-white Mondrian compared to a color Mondrian. Activation of secondary visual areas is present bilaterally in about the same region where the deviation scan localized the activity of the color-evoked potentials in Figure 6.5.

subject using fMRI. Visual stimulation was performed using a simple paradigm: closely in front of the subject's eyes we fixed a sheet of paper showing a black-white or color Mondrian. Then thirty-two images of a slice covering the visual cortex were acquired. This takes about four minutes or eight seconds per image. During one half of this time the subject was instructed to keep his eyes closed while during the other time the subject was instructed to look at the picture. In order to enhance the response the subject was instructed to blink at about 2 Hz while looking at the picture. In order to detect the BOLD contrast we use a pulse sequence called FLASH (fast low angle shot, Frahm et al 1993) with the following parameters: TR 63 ms, TE 30 ms, flip angle = 10°, slice thickness 4 mm, Field of View 250 cm^2, matrix size 256x256. The resulting time series were analyzed using a pixel-by-pixel analysis. Functional images were created using a pixel-by-pixel analysis by correlation of signal intensities with the stimulus protocol (Bandettini et al., 1993). Only pixels with high correlation coefficients (above 0.5) were assumed to be activated and were superimposed color coded onto a corresponding anatomical image (Fig. 6.7).

6.3 Results

In the first experiment we have focused our experimental design on stimulating V1 by reproducing the N87 component with the same stimulator and procedure as used by Paulus et al. (1984). Essentially, the subjects fixated centrally a 4° homogeneous yellow field with a luminance of 21.5 cd/m^2 which changed for 300 ms to a homogeneous red with a luminance of 26 cd/m^2. The same component N87 could be recorded again with a much more detailed spatial resolution. Figure 6.8 depicts the distribution of the electric field on the left side of the skull. The dipole source analysis algorithm calculates one main dipole as the main source, depicted in Figure 6.8 as a yellow arrow. On the right side the forward calculated field is projected onto the skull. It can be seen that there are deviations between measured (left) and calculated (right) field distributions particularly at the frontal cortex. These deviations show that there are additional sources of current.

Figure 6.5 represents a deviation scan of the data of Figure 6.8 onto the individual anatomy of the visual cortex of this subject. The red dotted areas represent the cortical gyri which generate

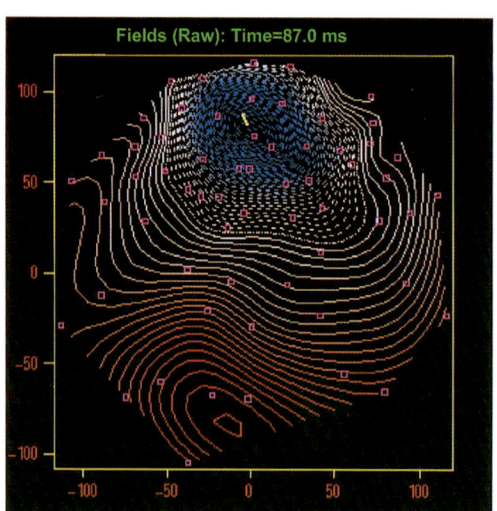 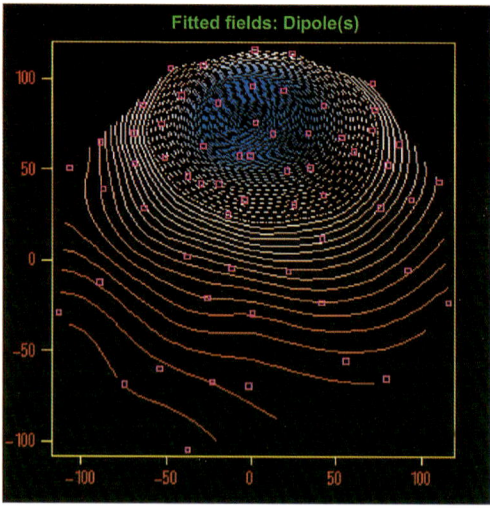

Fig. 6.8: left: Raw electric fields of N87 on the skull surface in arbitrary coordinates. The occiput is plotted at the top, the forehead at the bottom, right side of the skull on the left. The yellow dipole represents the orientation of the calculated dipole. The forward calculated field of this dipole is represented on the right. In particular, the frontal positivity remains unexplained and demonstrates the need for a more complex model.

(with a likelihood of more than 90%) the electrical generators of the surface activity. As can be seen, the activity originates at the occipital pole where the foveal representation of V1 is located.

Figure 6.6 demonstrates the corresponding calculations after stimulation with a lower right color octant using the field distribution 160 ms after stimulus onset. The lower left part shows the superposition of electrical activity onto the lingual and fusiform gyrus when the threshold is set to 90%, the lower middle part according to a threshold of 95%. The downward orientation of the equivalent dipole in the lower right part of the figure is the same as published by Plendl et al. (1993).

Figure 6.7 demonstrates the activation of primary and secondary visual areas when fixating a color Mondrian in the MRI. The plane of this MRI slice traverses the red dotted area in Figure 6.6.

6.4 Discussion

Multimodal imaging procedures allow the representation of cortically activated structures after color stimulation in a three-dimensional MRI reconstruction of the subject's brain. As predicted from anatomy, from PET studies (Lueck et al., 1989) and from earlier work in the spherical head model, N87 could be attributed to activation of V1 by CURRY. We were able to show by EEG source reconstruction and by functional MRI, that the generators of color-evoked potentials can be attributed to the lingual and fusiform gyrus, as was predicted earlier in a spherical head model (Plendl et al., 1993). Some tendency to more activation could be seen in the fMRI responses to color Mondrian stimulation when compared to black-white Mondrian stimulation. More work is necessary to elucidate the interindividual variability of the visual cortex, to demonstrate significant deviations between human and monkey visual system as predicted by other authors (Heywood et al., 1995) and to evaluate the distribution pattern of activation after different stimulation categories. This method seems to offer particularly promising results for studying differential cortical activation after different visual stimuli, e.g., when comparing color stimulation with stimulation with the category "face". According to clinical experience, cerebral achromatopsia (a syndrome in which the patient loses the ability to see colors after cortical damage) and prosopagnosia (a blindness for faces, a perceptual defect following a lesion of the posterior portion of the minor hemisphere) may occur together suggesting close by cerebral representation. We are quite optimistic that we will be able to show these relationships in the future by superimposing EEG and/or fMRI data onto the individual subject's anatomy.

We also hope to be able to contribute to questions concerning central color processing, particularly with respect to different aspects of color and luminance perception (Paulus and Kröger-Paulus, 1983; DeValois et al., 1993; Lennie et al., 1993).

6.5 Summary

We have recorded color-evoked potentials in order to trace sequential color processing stages in the visual system. In the first experiment, a foveal color coded component (N87) was recorded. In the second experiment, different segments (octants) of one hemifield were stimulated with homogeneous red in order to stimulate higher-order visual areas unilaterally. The EEG was recorded from 64 channels. A source analysis in a realistic head model was performed by using the individual MRI anatomy of the subject's brain by aid of the software package CURRY. In the first experiment we were able to trace the activity generated at 87 ms to V1 at the occipital pole and in the second experiment the activity at 160 ms to the fusiform and lingual gyrus. Activation of the latter areas was confirmed in the functional MRI by using a color Mondrian stimulus.

References

Bandettini P.A., Jesmanowicz A., Wong E. C. n and Hyde J. S. (1993). Processing strategies for time-course data sets in functional MRI of the human brain. Magn. Res. Med. *30*, 161–173.

Brindley G. (1972). The variability of the human striate cortex. J. Physiol. *225*, 1–2.

Buchner H., Weyen U., Frackowiack R. S. J., Romaya J., and Zeki S. (1994). The timing of visual evoked potential activity in human area V4. Proc. R. Soc. Lond. B. *257*, 99–104.

Clarke S. and Miklossy J. (1990). Occipital cortex in man: organization of callosal connections, related myelo- and cytoarchitecture, and putative boundaries of functional visual areas. J. Comp. Neuro. *8, 298(2)*, 188–214.

DeValois R. L. and DeValois K. K. (1993). A multistage color model. Vision Res. *33*, 1053–1065.

Frahm J., Merboldt K. D., and Hänicke W. (1993). Functional MRI of human brain activation at high spatial resolution. Magn. Res. Med. *29*, 139–144.

Heywood C. A., Gaffan D., and Cowey A. (1995). Cerebral achromatopsia in monkeys. Eur. J. Neurosci. *7*, 1064–1073.

Lennie P., Pokorny J., and Smith V. C. (1993). Luminance. J. Opt. Soc. Am. A. *10*, 1283–1293.

Lueck C. J., Zeki S., Friston K. J., Deiber M. P., Cope P., Cunningham V .J., Lammertsma A. A., Kennard C., and Frackowiack R. S. J. (1989). The color centre in the cerebral cortex of man. Nature *340*, 386–389.

Paulus W. and Kröger-Paulus A. (1983) A new concept of retinal color coding. Vision Res. *23*, 529–540.

Paulus W., Hömberg V., Cunningham K., Halliday A. M., and Rohde N. (1984). Color and brightness components of foveal color evoked potentials in man. EEG and Clin. Neurophysiol. *58*, 107–119.

Paulus W., Hömberg V., Cunningham K., and Halliday A. M. (1986). Color and brightness coding in the central nervous system: theoretical aspects and visual evoked potentials to homogeneous red and green stimuli. Proc. R. Soc. Lond. B. *227*, 53–66.

Paulus W., Plendl H., and Krafczyk S. (1988). Spatial dissociation of early and late color evoked components. EEG and Clin. Neurophysiol. *71*, 81–88.

Plendl H., Paulus W., Roberts I.G., Bötzel K. , Towell A. , Pitman J. R., Scherg M., and Halliday A. M. (1993). The time course and location of cerebral evoked activity associated with the processing of color stimuli in man. Neuroscience Letters *150*, 9–12.

Plendl H., Pröckl D., Schulze S., Mayer M., Bötzel K., and Paulus W. (1995) The cerebral generator of the color evoked component N87 of the visual evoked poten.tial: Localization by application of the regional source technique. In: B. Drum (Ed.) Color Vision Deficiencies XII, Kluwer, Dordrecht, 369–373.

Probst Th., Plendl H., Paulus W., Wist E. R., and Scherg M. (1993). Identification of the visual motion area (area V5) in the human brain by dipole source analysis. Exp. Brain Res. *93*, 345–351.

7. Wavelength Information Processing *versus* Color Perception: Evidence from Blindsight and Color-Blind Sight

Petra Stoerig

7.1 Introduction

The visual world of a person with normal vision is richly colored. The usefulness of color vision is easily demonstrated by comparing a color with a black-and-white photograph. A natural scene can immediately be grouped into friend and foe, into food and non-food, fruit and non-fruit on the colored one, and the fruits' ripeness is easily judged. In contrast, the mere detection of the fruit on the black-and-white photograph is a time-consuming task, with items having to be selected in serial search on the basis of brightness, reflection, and form. The advantage color vision must have brought about during evolution has transferred into modern life. Whether one is foraging in the market, retrieving one's car from a crowded parking lot, or choosing the best-matched sweater from one's wardrobe, color vision much facilitates the task (see Fig. 7.1).

How is it achieved? Every text book on vision explains that the color of objects is caused by the objects' dominantly reflecting light of a particular band of wavelengths. Newton's ingenious experiments showed that light consisted of rays that differ in their 'refrangability', and consequently in their disposition to exhibit this or that particular color (Newton, 1671/1953, p. 74). Day-active organisms have, to a different extent, learned to use the difference in refrangability, and have developed receptors which respond differentially to light of different wavelength.

Man and other primates, like rhesus monkeys who have a visual system and visual functions very much like ours (De Valois and Jacobs, 1968), have four types of receptors – three types of cone and one type of rod receptor. They differ in the absorption spectrum of their photopigment (see chapter 2), and together provide the input signal to the visual system that from the retinal processing stages on divides the incoming information about the distribution of light into different parallel channels or sub-systems. The rod system is specialized for vision at low luminance where different wavelengths excite the rod receptors to a different degree, with long wavelength stimuli requiring much more energy than blue-green stimuli whose wavelength lies at the peak of the rod absorption spectrum (see Fig. 7.2A). The second or broadband system receives its input from rods and cones; both middle- and long-wavelength cones contribute, but short-wavelength cones do, if at all, only to a minor extent (Lee et al., 1989). The receptoral input is reflected in the spectral sensitivity curve measured under conditions that favor the broadband system's physiological properties. The example shown in Figure 7.2B was measured with fast-flickering stimuli (45 Hz) presented at 30° eccentricity on a background of low photopic to mesopic luminance (0.1 cd/m^2). A smooth curve results which peaks in the 'green' range of the spectrum: the Vλ curve. Note the smooth decrease of sensitivity toward the short-wavelength ('blue') end of the spectrum. There is still some debate about the broadband system's possible contribution to color vision, and about the extent to which cells of this type are able to differentiate their response irrespective of relative luminance on the basis of chromatic information alone. However, the segregation of intensity and wavelength information clearly does not appear to be the broadband system's major domain.

The third or spectrally-opponent system receives input from all three cone types. These inputs get combined in a fashion that makes a color-opponent cell respond differentially to light

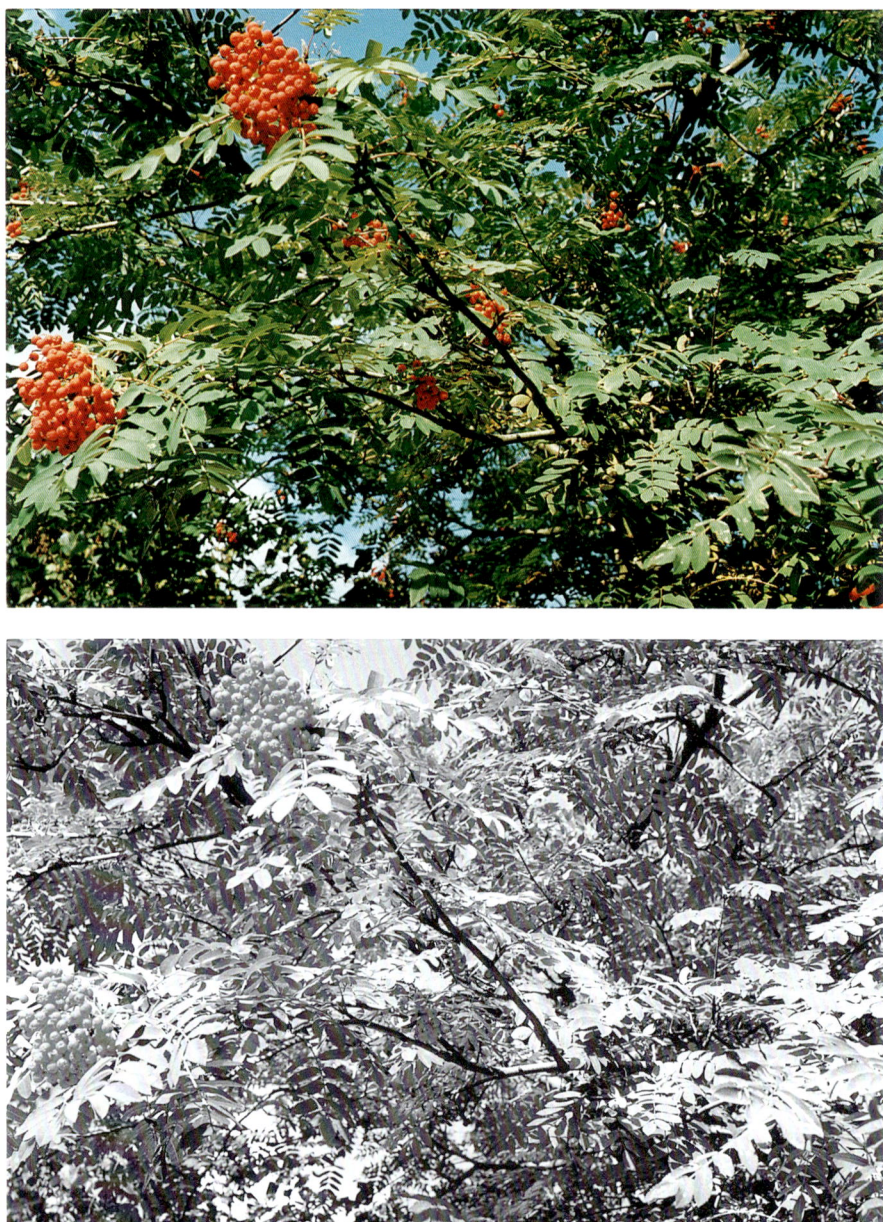

Fig. 7.1: Color helps to find the object of desire.

of different wavelength independent of variations in the intensity ratio of the two lights. The opponent organization is again reflected in the spectral sensitivity curve, which to favor this system is measured with large long stimuli on a white background of photopic luminance (Sperling and Harwerth, 1971; Snelgar et al., 1987). An example is given in Figure 7.2C. Note the minima and maxima in this bumpy curve that are displaced from the peak absorption of the pigments and reflect the opponent processes (Sperling and Harwerth, 1971). Together with the increase in

7.1 Introduction

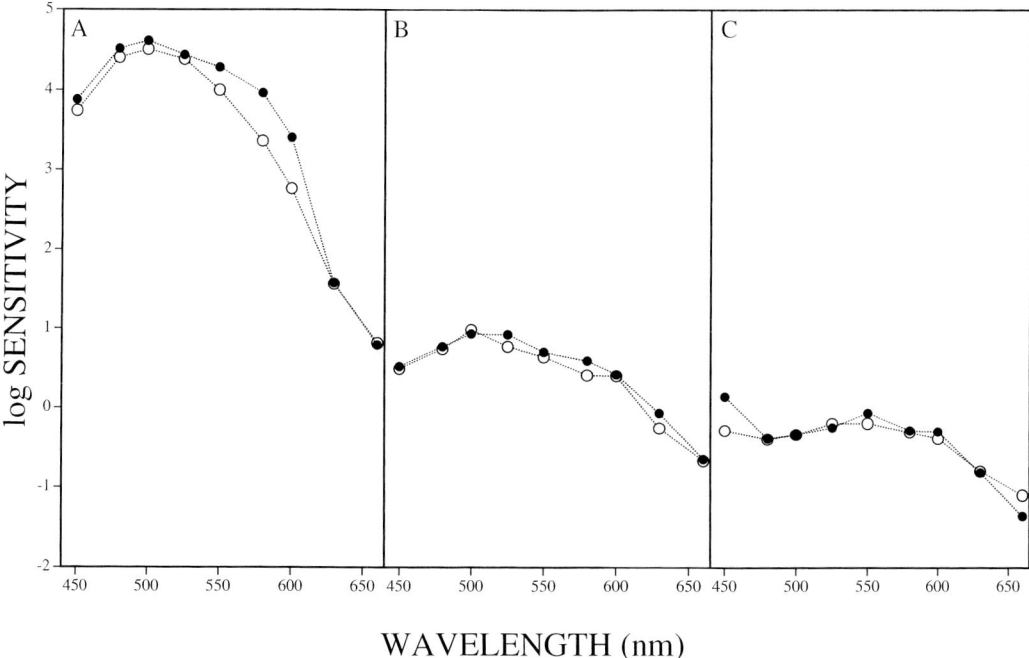

Fig. 7.2: Spectral sensitivity curves measured on the upper oblique meridians in a normal observer. Conditions were tailored to favor **(A):** the rod system: a background of scotopic luminance (0.0001 cd/m^2), and a 116', 200 ms stimulus presented at 10° eccentricity; **(B):** the broadband system: a low-photopic – mesopic background (and adaptation) of 0.1 cd/m^2, a 44', 45 Hz stimulus presented for 200 ms at 30° eccentricity; **(C):** the color-opponent system: a white adapting background of 32 cd/m^2 luminance, a 116', 200 ms stimulus presented at 10° eccentricity. All three curves are based on increment-threshold values which were determined by increasing the luminance of a stimulus of a particular wavelength in steps of 0.05 log units until that stimulus became detectable for the observer. Empty symbols: 135° meridian, nasal hemifield, filled symbols: 45° meridian, temporal hemifield.

sensitivity in the short wavelengths, these discontinuities distinguish the wavelength-opponent spectral sensitivity curve from the others. This system can process chromatic information independent of luminance, and is well suited to segregate the visual scene on that basis.

These systems are already segregated in the retina, and they remain largely so through the central processing stages. Note that they all use both wavelength and intensity information from the visual environment, but that only the wavelength-opponent system can use both types of information independently.

This brief account of the physiology of color vision, like the vast majority of everything that has been said about the topic, accounts for basic aspects of wavelength information processing. Does it equally well account for color vision? I want to argue that it does not, and that wavelength information processing is not the same as color perception. This can be demonstrated with the help of human patients who have lost color vision without having lost the ability to use wavelength information. The evidence I shall present stems mostly from patients with cortical blindness, and is complemented by evidence from patients with cortical color blindness. Thus, both groups of patients have lost color vision, the first because they have lost all phenomenal vision, the second because they have lost color vision selectively, while retaining conscious perception of other visual modalities, like motion and brightness, depth and form.

7.2 Wavelength Information Processing

7.2.1 Wavelength Information Processing in Cortical Blindness

Cortical blindness results from lesions that destroy or denervate the primary visual cortex. This structure is almost entirely buried on the medial side of the occipital lobes, and is topographically organized, with neurons in each part of the tissue responding to stimuli in a particular part of the visual field. A circumscribed destruction therefore causes a circumscribed visual field defect which due to the decussation of fibers in the optic chiasm is located in the contralesional visual hemifield. The field defect is perimetrically assessed and classified on the basis of its extent (a complete hemianopia affects an entire hemifield, a quadrantanopia only one quarter), its position in the field (to the left, to the upper right), and its density. Density, in contrast to the other two descriptors, refers not to spatial extent or position, but to the degree of visual loss. While stimuli presented within a relative field defect can be detected by the patient, provided they are of high contrast, transient, and fast-moving, stimuli presented within an absolute field defect are not seen at all. An absolute visual field defect is therefore characterized by an "absence of all and any sensation of light and color" (Wilbrand and Sänger, 1904, p. 353).

Despite the loss of all conscious vision caused by a total destruction or denervation of primary visual cortex, visual information from the cortically blind part of the visual field still enters the visual system. The part of the retina that corresponds to the lesion in primary visual cortex shows long-term transneuronal degeneration (van Buren, 1963; Cowey et al., 1989), but the surviving retinal ganglion cells continue to provide visual input to all known retinorecipient nuclei: the superior colliculus, the pulvinar, the three nuclei of the accessory optic system, the dorsal lateral geniculate nucleus (dLGN), the pregeniculate, the nucleus of the optic tract, the pretectum, and the nucleus suprachiasmaticus (see Cowey and Stoerig, 1991 for review). Physiological studies have shown that all nuclei that have so far been studied in this respect retain at least some visual responsivity after destruction of primary visual cortex (see Pasik and Pasik, 1982 for review). They send the visual information they receive from the retina either directly (dLGN, pulvinar nucleus) or indirectly (superior colliculus, pregeniculate nucleus) to the higher visual cortical areas. These surround the primary visual cortex, and extend forward into the parietal and temporal lobes of the cerebrum. At least the occipito-parietal cortical areas also remain visually responsive, as has been shown in monkeys (see Bullier et al., 1993 for review) and, using positron-emmission-tomography in man (Barbur et al., 1993). The functional visual subsystem that survives the destruction of primary visual cortex thus continues to process visual information from the cortically blind visual field.

Not surprisingly, this processing can also be demonstrated behaviorally. With experimental paradigms that circumvent the problem of the patient's inability to consciously see stimuli in the cortically blind field, visual responses can be elicited. The phenomenon of 'blindsight' (Weiskrantz et al., 1974) demonstrates that (and what) visual responses can be evoked when the phenomenal representation of the stimulus is lost.

The visual functions that make up blindsight and can be evoked from the cortically blind field can be grouped into three classes. The first is that of visual reflexes. While reflexes such as the pupil light reflex, the photic blink reflex, and optokinetic nystagmus can all be demonstrated after striate cortical destruction, neither one shows much wavelength selectivity. The pupil however constricts not only in response to an increase in luminance, but shows small differential responses to light of different wavelength. If monochromatic stimuli presented foveally are exchanged at isoluminance, systematic changes in pupil size can be observed (Saini and Cohen, 1979; Young and Alpern, 1980). As the pupil response in the periphery is largely rod dominated, Barbur and colleagues developed a technique to isolate the pupil's chromatic responses from the light reflex using a luminance masking technique. When a stimulus that consists of small checks of different

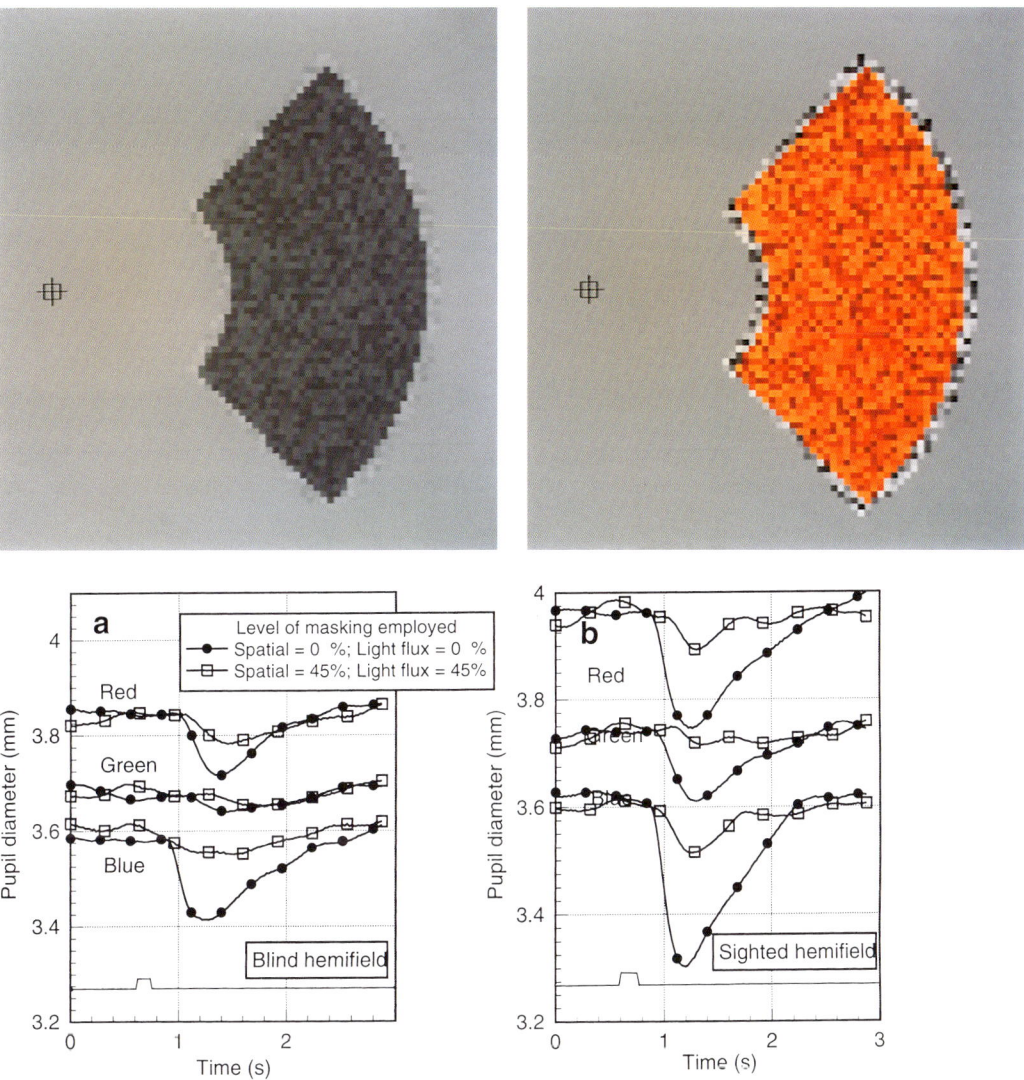

Fig. 7.3: The stimulus used to isolate the pupil response to spectral information. The grey squares are luminance-modulated in space and over time. The central stimulus field turns red (or blue, or green) while continuing to be luminance-modulated. The pupil traces demonstrate the effect of the masking; it markedly diminishes the response in both the normal and cortically impaired hemifields of the patient but does not abolish it entirely. (With kind permission from John Barbur).

luminance are individually luminance modulated over time, and turn red, green, or blue during presentation, is presented in the periphery of a normal hemifield, a reliable pupil wavelength response can be isolated (Barbur et al., 1995). When Barbur, Sahraie, Weiskrantz and I used the same stimulus in two hemianopic patients, the responses from the normal hemifield were essentially normal, while those from the cortically blind field showed less chromatic modulation in one patient (see Fig. 7.3), and as good as none in the other.

The next class of visual functions that remain in cortically blind visual fields is that of indirect implicit responses. In contrast to reflexive ones that can also be demonstrated in comatose patients, the indirect responses require the patient to both be conscious and to have some normal visual field which allows conscious vision. The normal field is necessary because these responses are demonstrated through the influence a stimulus in the blind field exerts on the response to a seen stimulus presented in the normal field. An example has been reported by Corbetta et al. (1990), who measured reaction times to a stimulus in the normal field, and showed it to be significantly altered through the presentation of a second stimulus in the blind field. An influence of chromatic information in the blind field has been indirectly demonstrated using a color-induction paradigm. A colored surround induces an apparent desaturated hue in the central white field, which can be seen in the after-image and depends on the colors used for the surround. Showing such a color-inducing pattern to a patient with an incomplete hemianopia, Pöppel (1986) found that the induced hue in the after-image depended not only on the seen colors, but also on the color of that part of the surround that was invisible to the patient because it fell into his blind field (see Fig. 7.4).

The third level of visual responses from a cortically blind field are those that require the patient to respond directly to a stimulus falling into the defective area. Because the patients cannot see stimuli within the absolute field defect, they have to be convinced to nevertheless try and guess whether a stimulus has been presented, where it has been presented, or which one of a limited number of stimuli has been presented. With forced-choice guessing paradigms, detection, localization, and discrimination of motion, direction, orientation, size, and stimulus luminance have been demonstrated (see Weiskrantz, 1990; Stoerig and Cowey, 1997 for recent reviews). Regarding wavelength information processing, Alan Cowey and I measured spectral sensitivity curves. We used dark- and light-adapted conditions to see whether we could find evidence for both rod and cone receptor function. Narrow-band stimuli (between 450 and 660 nm) were presented at corresponding positions in the normal and cortically blind hemifields of three patients. A Tübinger perimeter was used for the experiments. With the patient fixating a central fixation spot on a homogenous white background, a stimulus was presented in random alternation with blank trials; both stimulus and blank presentations were indicated with an identical sound emitted from the shutter. The patient's task was to guess upon each presentation whether or not a stimulus had been presented. Stimulus luminance was increased by 0.05 log units after each batch of presentations to find the minimum intensity at which the patient's detection was significantly different from chance. Measurements were compared with those from the corresponding retinal position in the normal hemifield.

The resultant curves from both hemifields show a normal Purkinje-shift, with the dark-adapted curve being narrowly tuned, peaking at 500–525 nm, and declining steeply in the long wavelengths, and the light-adapted curve being broadly tuned (see Figs. 7.5 A, B for examples).

In addition to the evidence for rod and cone function, measurements of spectral sensitivity under light-adapted conditions can differentiate

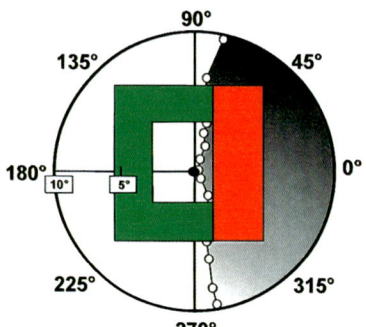

Fig. 7.4: A color-inducing stimulus presented partially inside the patient's cortically blind visual field (given in grey) caused the patient to report a different hue in the central square's after-image, depending on which color was presented. (Figure redrawn with kind permission from Ernst Pöppel).

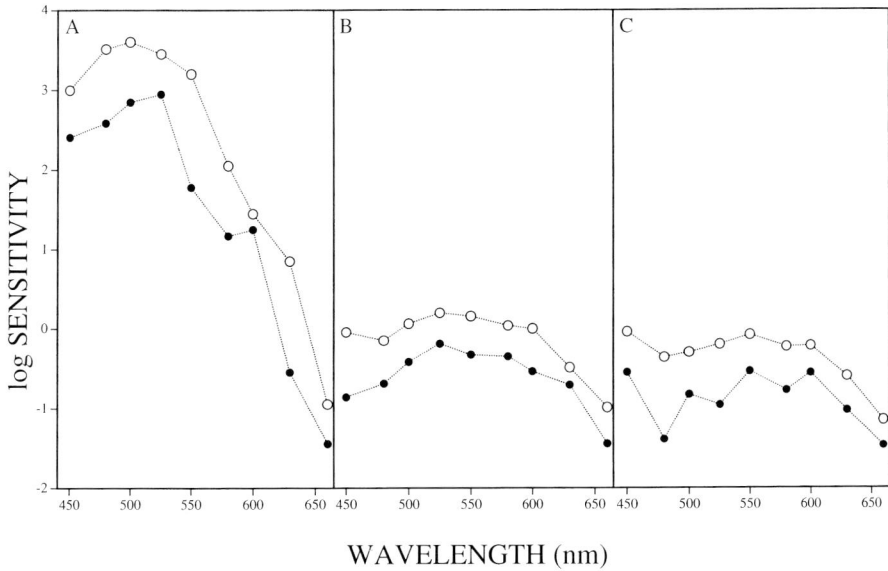

Fig. 7.5: Increment-threshold spectral sensitivity curves measured in patient B.R. who had a quadrantanopia to the upper left. The empty circles represent sensitivity for the normal nasal hemifield (10° eccentricity, 45° meridian); the filled circles the corresponding values from the cortically blind field (10°/135° meridian) which were determined with the use of two-alternative forced choice guessing. Note the relatively small difference in sensitivity. (A): 116′, 200 ms stimuli, background was set at 0.00001 cd/m². (B): 44′, 200 ms, 45 Hz stimuli, background 0.1 cd/m². (C): 116′, 200 ms stimuli, white background 32 cd/m². The curves' shapes indicate rod (A) and cone function (B/C) as well as broadband and chromatically-opponent processes (B/C). (Data in A and C from Stoerig and Cowey (1989)).

between broadband and chromatically opponent processes. When measured with large (116′), long (200 ms) stimuli presented on a white adapting background of 32 cd/m² to favor the chromatically-opponent system, the resultant curves from both hemifields show maxima at about 450, 550, and 600 nm and a minimum at 480 nm (Fig. 7.5C). These systematic discontinuities are hallmarks of chromatic opponency (Sperling and Harwerth, 1971). The curves that result from measurements using smaller (44′) flickering (45 Hz) stimuli presented at 10° eccentricity on a white adapting background of 0.1 cd/m² show a broad plateau of sensitivity between 500 and 600 nm and a slight decline toward both ends of the visible spectrum. The small increase in 'blue' sensitivity in the curve from the normal field probably indicates S cone intrusion (Fig. 7.5B). This increase is absent in the curves measured at 30 instead of 10° eccentricity (Fig. 7.2B), demonstrating that the conditions used here did favor but not isolate the broadband system. Together, the spectral sensitivity curves from the cortically blind hemifield show that it continues to be subserved not only by rod and cone receptors but by broadband and chromatically-opponent channels as well (Stoerig and Cowey, 1989; 1991).

The preservation of chromatically-opponent processes is further supported by the patient's ability to discriminate between stimuli of different wavelength. To eliminate discriminable cues that can arise from differences in effective brightness, the stimuli were set at luminances 0.5 log units above the previously established thresholds for statistically significant detection in each individual patient. Two-alternative forced-choice guessing was again used, with the patients verbally guessing upon each presentation which one of two stimuli of different color had been presented at a fixed position within the cortically blind field. The probability ratio for the two stimuli was systematically varied to trace out Receiver-Operating-Characteristic curves which provide a means to control for biases in the subjects' responses (Green and Swets, 1966; Stoerig et al., 1985). Red, green, yellow, and orange stimuli were used, with peak wavelength separation between 50 and 20 nm. The results (see Fig. 7.5 for example) showed that the patients were able to discriminate between the stimuli, albeit to a different extent (Stoerig and Cowey, 1992).

We tried to take these results, which agree with those of Stoerig (1987) and Brent et al. (1994), one step further by getting an estimate of wavelength discrimination thresholds. For that purpose, we measured wavelength discrimination as before, at corresponding positions in the normal and cortically blind hemifields, using stimuli from the middle part of the spectrum, with peak transmission between 553 and 600 nm, and peak separation from 47 to 7 nm. The results show that while wavelength discrimination thresholds in the periphery of the normal field are quite small, discriminability failing only at the smallest separation (553 vs 560 nm), they are increased in the field defect to 20–36 nm (Stoerig and Cowey, 1992).

Together, these results demonstrate that blindsight patients are able to use wavelength information in their cortically blind fields, although this information is not represented phenomenally: The patients do not see anything.

7.2.2 Wavelength Processing in Cortical Color Blindness

That wavelength information can be processed in the absence of color vision has also been shown with the help of patients who are cortically color blind. In contrast to cortical blindness that abolishes all phenomenal vision, cortical color blindness leaves the patient with a repertoire of phenomenal visual qualities other than that of color. A patient with dischromatopsia consciously sees the visual world, but its colors appear washed out; a patient with achromatopsia loses color vision altogether, seeing a monochromatic visual world in grayish shades. Often, this pathology is accompanied by additional visual deficits, for instance by a partial visual field defect or by a disturbance of form and object vision or recognition. The additional losses most probably arise from the lesion not being confined to the part of the lingual and fusiform gyri (which correspond to medial and lateral parts of the occipitotemporal gyrus) whose destruction abolishes color vision quite selectively

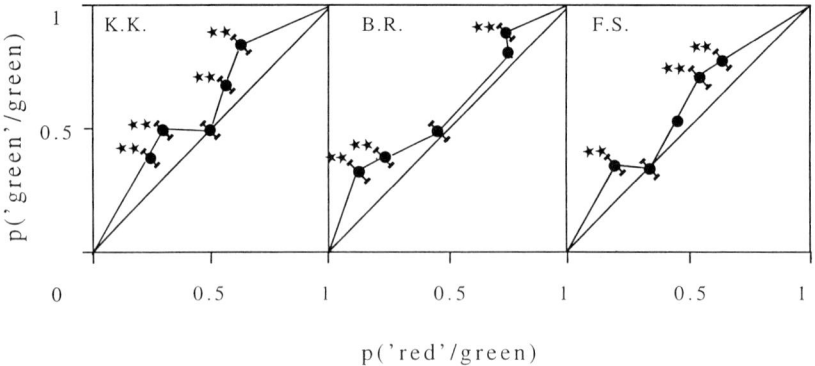

Fig. 7.6: Wavelength discrimination in three blindsight patients. Receiver-Operating-Characteristic curves were traced out by varying the probability ratio for red (600 nm) and green (550 nm) stimuli. Each ROC-point represents the result of 500 presentations. The area under the curve ($p_{(A)}$) is significantly different from 0.5 in all cases; asterisks indicate the significance level of the individual ROC-points (**: $p < 0.005$). (Data from Stoerig and Cowey (1992)).

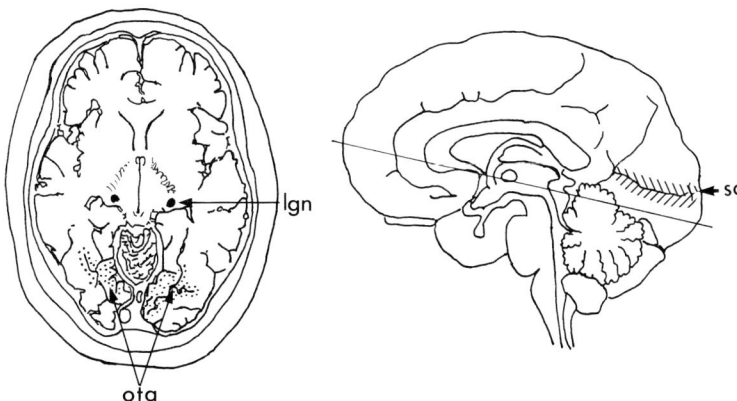

Fig. 7.7: A horizontal section through the human brain taken at the level indicated in the right-hand figure. The occipitotemporal gyrus (otg) – its lateral part is also called fusiform gyrus and its medial part lingual gyrus – is situated ventral to the calcarine sulcus (sc). The primary visual cortex lies on the banks of the calcarine, with the lower quadrant of the visual field represented on the upper bank and the upper quadrant on the lower bank. Because of its greater proximity to the lower bank, destruction of the occipitotemporal gyrus more commonly involves this part of primary visual cortex. The lateral geniculate nucleus appears on the same section (LGN).

(Meadows, 1974; Zeki, 1990). This cortical area which is needed for color vision and activated during stimulation with colored stimuli (Lueck et al., 1989), is situated at the base of the occipitotemporal cortex (see Fig. 7.7). As a consequence of the vicinity to the lower bank of the primary visual cortex, a lesion extending backward into the primary visual cortex will produce a quadrantanopia in the upper visual hemifield as well (Meadows, 1974); in contrast, more extensive lesions that destroy additional extrastriate visual cortical areas or their projections to the hippocampus (a sea horse shaped structure important for memory) can cause an agnosia in addition to the color blindness (Albert et al., 1979).

The latter is the case for patient M.S. who has been extensively studied by several groups (Mollon et al., 1980; Heywood et al., 1991; 1994). MS was 22 years old when an illness, presumed to be Herpes encephalitis, caused a cortical blindness to the left, and a cortical color blindness to the right. NMR-images show the extensive bilateral lesion which involves the 'color area' at the base of the left hemisphere (Heywood et al., 1991). The patient could not match, name, or sort colors, had an error score of 1245 in the Farnsworth-Munsell 100 hue test (a test where isoluminant colors have to be sorted, this score indicating random sorting), and made random matches when asked to adjust a mixture of 540 and 640 nm light to match 580 nm with a Nagel anomaloscope. Despite his complete failure at these and other tasks which classify him as totally color blind, the patient retained function of all three cone types (Mollon et al., 1980). Measurements of his increment threshold spectral sensitivity under appropriate conditions further indicated the presence of post-receptoral wavelength-opponent mechanisms (Heywood et al., 1991).

Despite his color blindness, the patient can make use of wavelength information: He could read the pseudo-isochromatic Ishihara-plates when they were presented at a distance of 2 m instead of at reading distance where he failed (Mollon et al., 1980). He showed a wavelength-specific motion after-effect: When tested in green light, the after-effect induced by 30 s exposure to a rotating textured disc presented in red light, was only 53% of its value when tested in the red light used for adaptation (Mollon et al., 1980). He could detect the border between adjacent color fields, such as red and green, no matter what their luminance ratio, although to him they both appeared the same shade of grey (Heywood et al., 1991). If the colors abutted one another, he could also pick out the odd color in a chromatic series, because, although all colors appeared the same shade of grey, he could detect an edge between them (Heywood et al., 1991). M.S.'s use of wavelength information was further demonstrated when Heywood et al. (1994) reported him to flawlessly discriminate between forms (squares and crosses) which were composed of small colored squares and seen against a surround of grey squares differing in luminance. In addition, the patient was presented with an isoluminant red-green sinewave grating that was phase shifted by 90°. In normal observers, such a stimulus produces the impression of (apparent) upward or downward motion which depends on information as to which bar is red, which green. Although in the absence of this information the direction of apparent motion is ambiguous, M.S. reported it correctly, demonstrating that "mysteriously, MS can detect the sign of color contrast without experiencing the colors" (Heywood and Cowey, 1998; see Fig. 7.7).

Presently, it has not been settled which cells, pathways, and cortical areas are responsible for the continued use of wavelength information. Both broadband (Heywood et al., 1991; Troscianko et al., 1996) and chromatically-opponent channels (Heywood et al., 1994) are being discussed. Independent of whether one or both systems are involved in the continued processing, it is obvious from the reports that wavelength information can be visually exploited in the absence of color vision.

Wavelength information can even be used by itself, as demonstrated by the cortically color-blind patient's ability to see a border between isoluminant red and green half-fields, an ability which is shared by broadband retinal ganglion cells (Lee et al., 1989). But the patient (and the cell) confounds luminance and wavelength information when both are available. His detection is based on salience and, in the case of form detection and discrimination, on border continuity, and can be abolished by conditions that eliminate those percepts. Heywood and colleagues (1994) conclude from their observation that "saturated chromatic and achromatic boundaries are conspicuously different to M.S. ... when they are of similar luminance contrast. Increasing the luminance contrast of the achromatic boundary renders the achromatic and chromatic boundaries perceptually similar." Therefore, "his contrast vision is mediat-

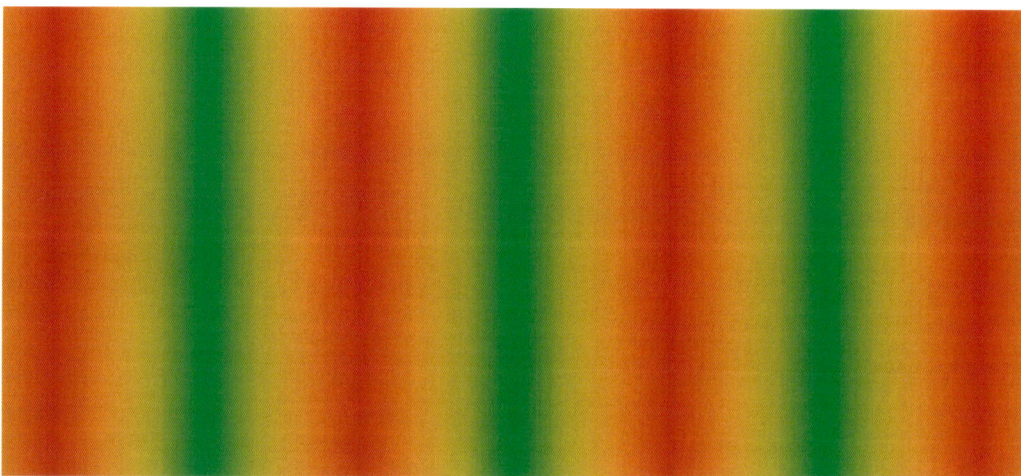

Fig. 7.8: Isoluminant red-green sinewave grating. Although unable to see the color of the bars the achromatopsic patient M.S. could correctly identify the direction of apparent motion that is produced by 90° phase shifts. (With kind permission from Charles Heywood).

ed by a mechanism that extracts color or luminance contrast without readily distinguishing between them" (p. 252). A similar effect can be demonstrated in blindsight patients whose detection of a stimulus, revealed by forced-choice guessing, can be much facilitated by adding wavelength to luminance information (Stoerig, 1987).

It follows that wavelength information helps solve visual tasks even when it is confounded with luminance. However, wavelength information processing is a long cry from color perception not only because it confounds the types of information, but because it is not phenomenal.

7.3 Segregation of Wavelength and Intensity Information and Constancy

De Valois and Jacobs (1984) define color vision by focussing on the necessity to unconfound luminance and wavelength information: "... what is meant (or should be meant) by saying that an individual has color vision is that he or she has the ability to respond *independently* to wavelength and to intensity differences" (p. 425).

In addition, the advantage of color vision owes much to color constancy which refers to our ability to identify colors under different illuminations. More precisely, it enables us to use spectral information for perceptual tasks such as image segregation and object identification despite considerable changes in the spectral composition of the illuminant(s). The spectral composition of daylight changes from sunrise to sunset; the spectral composition of tungsten light is quite different from that emitted by candles. Nevertheless, we can use spectral information and identify colors, if imperfectly, even under massively different illuminants, provided we are adapted and receive information from an array of reflecting surfaces. If information regarding the visual scene surrounding a particular object is artificially removed, our color identification fails (Land, 1977). In Figure 7.8, the effect of color constancy is illustrated by showing the remarkable difference a multi-colored display undergoes when illuminated

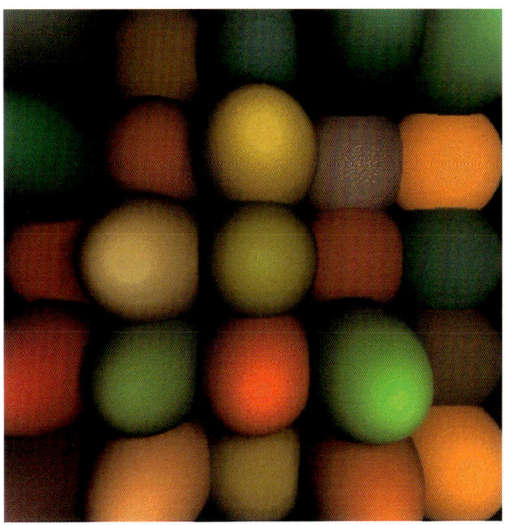

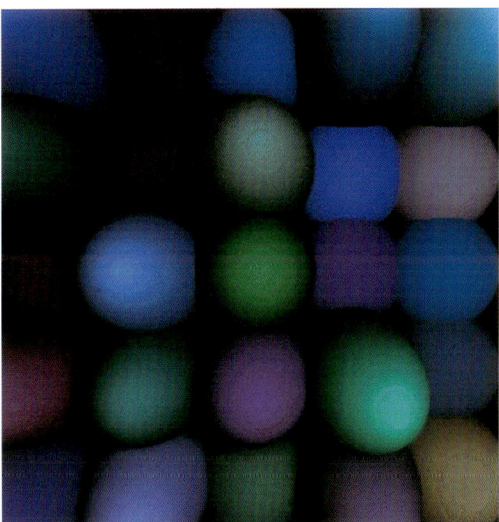

Fig. 7.9: Color constancy: The same array of computer-generated Munsell-paper covered eggs is shown under two different daylight illuminants (D40, CIE-coordinates x = 0.3823, y = 0.3838, above; D250, x = 0.2499, y = 0.2548, below). The massive shift in color appearance is largely (if imperfectly) compensated in human color constancy. It is achieved by comparison of the relative activity in the three cone receptor channels, adjustments for the adaptational state of the eye and the color signal of the background; in addition, it may use specular reflections and colored light cast by the objects in the scene. (With kind permission from Anya Hurlbert).

with different daylights: A person with color vision but without color constancy would see the displays about as different as they appear here.

Like size and form constancy, color constancy allows object identification despite constantly changing conditions: perspective, motion of oneself and of the seen object, depth, illumination, and the like. In the present context, this achievement is

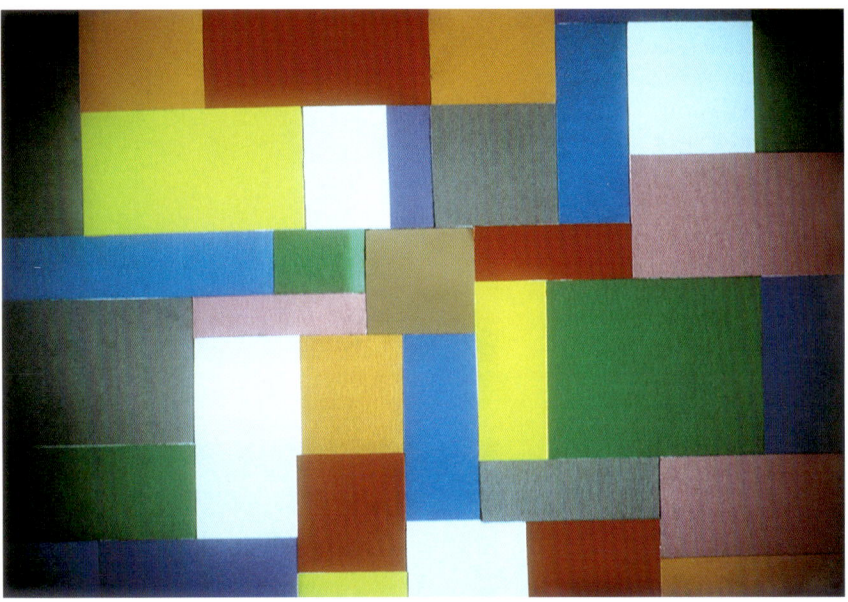

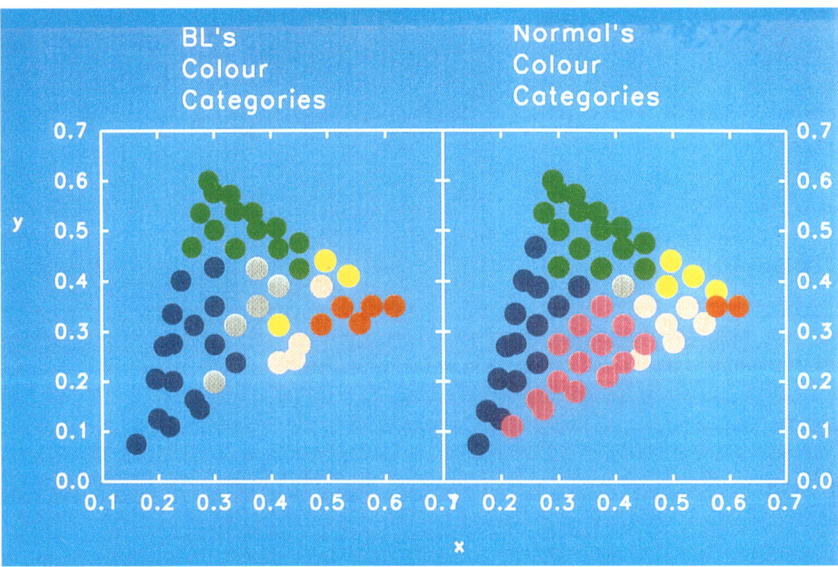

Fig. 7.10: Above: By varying the spectral composition of light falling onto a 'Mondrian' stimulus shown here under white light, color-constancy was assessed in the dyschromatopsic patient B.L.; it was found to be affected in tandem with his color vision. Below: Color categories (white light illumination) for the patient and a normal observer. (With kind permission from Keith Ruddock).

noteworthy because it enables us to use color for perceptual purposes such as image segmentation (see chapter 12) and object identification despite massive changes in wavelength information.

Can wavelength information be processed independent of intensity and in a manner that satisfies the requirements of constancy without being phenomenally represented as color? *Theoretically,* it is possible to conceive of 'wavelength' constancy and for that matter, of wavelength information processing largely independent from intensity information, without invoking the phenomenal perception of color. Man can conceive of highly complex mathematical and cognitive operations which appear without any qualitative dressing. Man can conceive of zombies, beings that are indistinguishable from us normal mortals but lack all experience, all qualia (see Metzinger, 1995 for recent discussion). The paradigm that qualia are functionally ineffective, inert, currently rules in both philosophy and neuroscience because there is no logical necessity for qualia. Therefore, on purely theoretical grounds, a complex form of wavelength information processing that is able to take into account all the relevant information about distribution of light, borders, reflections, and the like would suffice.

Practically or technically, the answer may also be Yes, albeit with a note of caution. There may indeed be a considerable number of algorithms that produce a relative independance of the assigned outputs from the spectral composition of the illuminant, provided they are fed sufficient information about wavelength distribution, borders, texture, specular reflections, and so forth (see Hurlbert, 1998; for a recent review). Quite successful constancy algorithms can and increasingly will thus be mathematically formulated and implemented in technical systems such as cameras and robots. Nevertheless, their conception depends in an important fashion on a biological system, namely the engineer who successfully mimicks his own color vision and constancy. Epistemologically, color was there before we knew the first thing about light being composed of different wavelengths of different 'refrangibility'.

Biologically, the question is empirical in nature: If color constancy depends on wavelength information processing and not on color perception, it could be preserved in cases of preserved wavelength information processing without color vision. If it depends on color vision, it should be abolished along with it. Recent evidence indicates that constancy depends on color vision: An investigation of color constancy mechanisms in a dyschromatopsic patient clearly demonstrated that constancy was affected in tandem with color perception (Kennard et al., 1995; see Fig. 7.9).

To complement this important first finding, studies of color constancy in the achromatopsic patient MS and in blindsight patients are currently underway. What little biological evidence there is at present indicates that constancy depends on color vision.

7.4 Color Perception

Although there is no logical necessity for colors, which are qualia or phenomenal representations with complex physiological underpinnings, there may still be a biological necessity. That it is possible to calculate a relatively constant designator on the basis of wavelength information (plus additional information about discontinuities etc.) does not indicate that biological organisms ever use a color constancy algorithm that is not based on color vision. If nature uses the phenomenal representation of wavelength information – color – to arrive at color constancy in man, it may well use a similar procedure in non-human organisms. Species as divergent as bees (von Frisch, 1964), gold fish (Ingle, 1985), pigeon (Thompson et al., 1992), and macaque monkeys (Wild et al., 1985) all display color constancy. In view of the similarity of our environment (which overrides the differences in ecological niches) and the concordant similarity in the visual equipment, one can argue that it is more likely that evolution has used similar means in different species, not qualia-dependance in one and qualia-independant algorithms in the others. In short, it is possible that in biological organisms there exists no processing of wavelength information that is independent of intensity information and that provides a designator largely independent of the wavelengths of the illuminant but is not phenomenal.

Color vision in the common sense of the word and as we know it is always phenomenal and thus conscious (Nelkin, 1996). As such it is distinct from wavelength information processing not only because it does not simply reflect the wavelength composition of a surface but because it is experienced in the thousands of shades we can tell apart. For an individual to possess color vision, he, she or it needs to have a phenomenal representation of light of different wavelength, a color experience.

Color vision serves three major visual tasks: It helps to detect visual objects, particularly in environments where many luminance levels render the use of luminance information alone insufficient. Like texture, contrast, and motion it is used for the segregation of the visual image. It contributes to the identification and recognition of visual objects.

Patients who lack the experience of color are also lacking in their performance regarding these tasks. Blindsight patients who in their cortically blind fields lack all phenomenal vision can detect and discriminate stimuli of different wavelength, but only in an unaware mode. In addition, this detection is rather limited: although it has not yet been tested formally, it seems unlikely that blindsight patients would be able to detect a target – defined by wavelength in this case – that was embedded in a visual environment. Existing clinical evidence strongly points to the phenomenal representation being prior to image segregation, because an inability to segregate an image into objects can be observed in patients who possess a full repertoire of phenomenal visual modalities, i.e., they can see color, brightness, texture, and motion, while a reverse disorder has never been described (Stoerig, 1996). Finally, object identification is possible only in an unconscious fashion (or better, in an unaware mode to indicate that the patient is of course conscious), if the object is not phenomenally represented. Implicit unaware recognition has repeatedly been reported. For instance, a patient with severe amnesia who is unable to remember ever having met an individual before, may nevertheless behave differently towards someone who has treated him in a friendly manner. Conscious recognition however appears impossible if the information is not presented phenomenally.

In addition, the blindsight patients do not consciously know that they have any visual information available. They experience themselves as only guessing whether or not something has been presented, and they cannot tell whether they have performed at chance level – for instance because the stimuli were presented on the natural blind spot which is receptor-free – or whether they have performed at 100% correct. In addition, they cannot consciously remember a stimulus that has been presented only to the blind field, and may simply be unable to use visual information processed solely in the unaware mode for any conscious intentional manipulation.

Patients with cerebral achromatopsia also use wavelength information in their color-blind visual fields. Under certain circumstances, an isoluminant red-green pattern will produce a phenomenal border between two half-fields of apparently similar greyness, or it will be used to infer information about (apparent) motion direction. Detection of a single colored square in an array of grey squares of similar size and different luminance however is impossible (Heywood et al., 1994). When conditions allow the patient to see a boundary which can be based on both luminance and chromatic information, this boundary can be used for image segregation; a cross or a large square become visible in the array, but the segregation into figure and ground depends on the phenomenal border. The same applies to object identification. The patient can identify a cross, can verbally and manually describe it, if he has those perceptual boundaries available. Identification based on color per color is absent, and I assume that information about the color of a stimulus cannot be consciously remembered (or otherwise consciously and intentionally accessed) if the stimulus has only been seen in the achromatopsic state or field.

Indeed, the uses wavelength without color can be put to seem rather limited. The patients' achievements appear remarkable and come as a surprise mainly because not only the cortically blind patients but the cortically color blind patients are visually disabled. M.S. describes his surroundings as grey, fails to identify surface colors, fails completely in a color sorting test. Another achromatopsic patient, described by Robert Boyle as early as 1688 (Mollon, 1989), was unable to distinguish by color the violets she wanted to gather, 'tho' she kneel'd in that place where they grew'.

Could it be that the patient's deficits are causally connected to the absence of color vision? That the quale, the experience is biologically necessary for the higher perceptual, cognitive, intentional functions? The currently ruling paradigm in both philosophy and neuroscience is that qualia simply do not have a function. They are regarded as mysterious addenda to cognitive and computational processes which could as well or better be explained without them. But maybe we should put this paradigm on the back-burner, not only because there exists a body of clinical evidence that does not agree with it, but also because it prevents us from asking whether any quale – color, pitch, pain, softness, or sweetness – serves a biological function. We'll only learn the answer if we put the question experimentally to biological organisms. To this purpose we can use a variety of approaches that include neuropsychological experiments on patients who have lost certain qualia, psychophysical experiments with paradigms that prevent information that still gets processed to become phenomenally represented in normal observers (see Kolb and Braun, 1995 for an example), behavioral experiments that assess in non-human animals the extent of higher perceptual and cognitive abilities which we know that man cannot perform without a phenomenal representation. Only by doing experiments of this kind will we learn whether qualia play a role, what role it may be, and hopefully how they come to play it: how a plain color comes to represent the staggering mathematical complexity that enters into its appearance.

Acknowledgements

It is a pleasure to thank Anya Hurlbert, Charlie Heywood, Keith Ruddock, and John Barbur for generously providing the figures that represent their work. Stephan Wirth and Erhardt Barth greatly helped with the processing of the figures. The Deutsche Forschungsgemeinschaft supported the work (Sto 206–4/2).

References

Albert, M. L., Soffer, D., Silverberg, R., and Reches, A. (1979). The anatomic basis of visual agnosia. Neurology 29, 876–879.

Barbur, J. L., Cole, V., Harlow, A., and Sahraie, A. (1995). Pupil colour and light reflex responses in the periphery of the visual field. Invest. Ophthalmol. Vis. Sci. 36 (4), 660.

Barbur, J. L., Watson, J. D. G., Frackowiak, R. S. J., and Zeki, S. (1993). Conscious visual perception without V1. Brain 116, 1293–1302.

Brent, P. J., Kennard, C., and Ruddock, K. H. (1994). Residual colour vision in a human hemianope: spectral responses and colour discrimination. Proc. R. Soc. Lond. B 256, 219–225.

Bullier, J., Girard, P., and Salin, P.-A. (1993). The role of area 17 in the transfer of information to extrastriate visual cortex. In: Cerebral Cortex, Vol.10, A. Peters and K. S. Rockland, eds. (New York: Plenum Press), pp. 301–330.

Corbetta, M., Marzi, C. A., Tassinari, G., and Aglioti, S. (1990). Effectiveness of different task paradigms in revealing blindsight. Brain 113, 603–616.

Cowey, A. and Stoerig, P. (1991). The neurobiology of blindsight. Trends Neurosci. 14, 140–145.

Cowey, A., Stoerig, P., and Perry, V. H. (1989). Transneuronal retrograde degeneration of retinal ganglion cells after damage to striate cortex in macaque monkeys: Selective loss of Pβ cells. Neuroscience 29, 65–80.

De Valois, R. L. and Jacobs, G. H. (1968). Primate color vision. Science 162, 533–540.

De Valois, R. L. and Jacobs, G. H. (1984). Neural mechanisms of color vision. In: Handbook of Physiology: The Nervous System Vol. III., I. Darien-Smith, ed. (Bethesda, MD: American Physiological Society), pp. 415–456.

Green, D. M. and Swets, J. A. (1966). Signal Detection Theory and Psychophysics, (New York: John Wiley).

Heywood, C. A. and Cowey, A. (1998). Cerebral achromatopsia. In: Case Studies in Cognitive Neuropsychology, G. Humphreys, ed. (Lawrence Erlbaum).

Heywood, C. A., Cowey, A., and Newcombe, F.

(1991). Chromatic discrimination in a cortically colour blind observer. Eur. J. Neurosci. *3*, 802–812.

Heywood, C. A., Cowey, A., and Newcombe, F. (1994). On the role of the parvocellular (P) and magnocellular (M) pathways in cerebral achromatopsia. Brain *117*, 245–254.

Hurlbert, A. C. (1998). Computational models of colour constancy. In: Perceptual Constancies. Why things look as they do. V. Walsh, J. Kulikowski, eds. (Cambridge: Cambridge University Press).

Ingle, D. J. (1985). The goldfish as a retinex animal. Science *227*, 651–654.

Kennard, C., Lawden, M., Morland, A. B., and Ruddock, K. H. (1995). Colour identification and colour constancy are impaired in a patient with incomplete achromatopsia asociated with prestriate cortical lesions. Proc. R. Soc. Lond. B *260*, 169–175.

Kolb, F. C. and Braun, J. (1995). Blindsight in normal observers. Nature *377*, 293–294.

Land, E. H. (1977). The retinex theory of color vision. Sci. Am. *237*, 108–128.

Lee, B. B., Martin, P. R., and Valberg A. (1989). Non-linear summation of M- and L-cone inputs to phasic retinal ganglion cells of the macaque. J. Neurosci. *9*, 3378–3415.

Lueck, C. J., Zeki, S., Friston, K. J., Deiber, M.-P., Cope, P., Cunningham, V. J., Lammerstsma, A. A., Kennard, C., and Frackowiak, R. S. J. (1989). The colour centre in the cerebral cortex of man. Nature *340*, 386–389.

Meadows, J. C. (1974). Disturbed perception of colours associated with localized brain lesions. Brain *97*, 615–632.

Metzinger, T. ed. (1995). Conscious Experience (Paderborn: Schöningh).

Mollon, J. D. (1989). "Tho' she kneel'd in that place where they grew...". The uses and origins of primate colour vision. J. Exp. Biol. *146*, 21–38.

Mollon, J. D., Newcombe, F., Polden, P. G., and Ratcliff, G. (1980). On the presence of three cone mechanisms in a case of total achromatopsia. In: Colour Vision Definiencies, Vol.5., G. Verriest, ed. (Bristol, England: Hilger) pp. 130–135.

Nelkin, N. (1996). Consciousness and the Origins of Thought. (Cambridge, England: Cambridge University Press).

Newton, I. (1671/1953). The new theory about light and colors. In: Newton's Philosophy of Nature: Selections from his Writings., H. S. Thayer, ed. (New York, London: Hafner).

Pasik, P. and Pasik, T. (1982). Visual functions in monkeys after total removal of visual cerebral cortex. Contributions to Sensory Physiology *7*, 147–200.

Pöppel, E. (1986). Long-range colour-generating interactions across the retina. Nature *320*, 523–525.

Saini, V. D. and Cohen, G. H. (1979). Using color substitution pupil response to expose chromatic mechanisms. J. Opt. Soc. Am. *69*, 1029–1035.

Snelgar, R. S., Foster, D. H., and Scase, M. O. (1987). Isolation of opponent-colour mechanisms at increment threshold. Vision Res. *27*, 1017–1027.

Sperling, H. G. and Harwerth, R. S. (1971). Red-green cone interactions in the increment-threshold spectral sensitivity of primates. Science *172*, 180–184.

Stoerig, P. (1987). Chromaticity and achromaticity: Evidence for a functional differentiation in visual field defects. Brain *110*, 869–886.

Stoerig, P. (1996). Varieties of vision: from blind processing to conscious recognition. Trends Neurosci. *19*, 401–406.

Stoerig, P. and Cowey, A. (1989). Wavelength sensitivity in blindsight. Nature *342*, 916–918.

Stoerig, P. and Cowey, A. (1991). Increment-threshold spectral sensitivity in blindsight. Brain 114, 1487–1512.

Stoerig, P. and Cowey, A. (1992). Wavelength discrimination in blindsight. Brain *115*, 425–444.

Stoerig, P. and Cowey, A. (1997). Blindsight in man and monkeys Brain. *120*, 535–559.

Stoerig, P., Hübner, M., and Pöppel, E. (1985). Signal detection analysis of residual target detection in a visual field defect due to a post-geniculate lesion. Neuropsychologia *23*, 589–599.

Thompson, E., Palacios, A., and Varela, F. J. (1992). Ways of coloring: comparative color vision as a case study for cognitive science. Behavioral and Brain Sciences *15*, 1–74.

Troscianko, T., Davidoff, J., Humphreys, G., Landis, T., Fahle, M., Greenlee, M., Brugger, P., and Philips, W. (1996). Human colour discrimination based on a non-parvocellular pathway. Current Biology *6*, 200–210.

van Buren, J. M. (1963). Trans-synaptic retrograde degeneration in the visual system of primates. J. Neurol. Neurosurg. Psychiatry *34*, 140–147.

von Frisch, K. (1964). Bees: Their Vision, Chemical Sense and Language. Cornell University Press, Ithaca NY.

Weiskrantz, L. (1990). Outlooks for blindsight: explicit methods for implicit processes. Proc. R. Soc. Lond., B 239, 247–278.

Weiskrantz, L., Warrington, E. K., Sanders, M. D., and Marshall, J. (1974). Visual capacity in the hemianopic field following a restricted cortical ablation. Brain 97, 709–728.

Wilbrand, H. and Sänger, A. (1904). Die Neurologie des Auges. Vol. III (Wiesbaden, Germany: J. F. Bergmann).

Wild, H. M., Butler, S. R., Carden, D., and Kulikowski, J. J. (1985). Primate cortical area V4 important for colour constancy but not wavelength discrimination. Nature 313, 133–135.

Young, R. S. L. and Alpern, M. (1980). Pupil responses to foveal exchanges of monochromatic lights. J. Opt. Soc. Am. 70, 697–706.

Zeki, S. (1990) A century of cerebral achromatopsia. Brain 113, 1721–1777.

8. Color Vision in Lower Vertebrates

Christa Neumeyer

8.1 Introduction

Karl von Frisch, famous for his discoveries in orientation, communication and sensory capacities of the honey bee, introduced a powerful behavioral training technique for investigating color vision in animals. He trained the minnow (*Phoxinus laevis*), a cyprinid fish, by providing a food reward, and was able to show for the first time that a lower vertebrate can discriminate all colors (red, green, blue, yellow) from various shades of grey (von Frisch, 1913). This was published even before his well known demonstration of color vision in the honeybee (von Frisch, 1914). With his experiments he disproved Carl von Hess's hypothesis that insects and lower vertebrates are completely color blind. Von Hess's conclusions were based on experiments using "reflexes" such as positive phototaxis as behavioral responses (von Hess, 1914). As we know today (see below), honeybees and cyprinid fishes do indeed behave as if they were color blind in some behavioral contexts, but not in contexts involving food acquisition as used by Karl von Frisch. Between 1920 and 1930 important results were obtained with training experiments with the minnow performed by students of Karl von Frisch and Alfred Kühn. Wolff (1925), for example, investigated wavelength discrimination in the spectral range between 300 nm and 800 nm. He showed (Wolff, 1925) that minnows possess three ranges of best discrimination ability (near 400 nm, 500 nm and 600 nm). He was even able to show that they see ultraviolet light, a result completely neglected until about 1980. Burkamp (1923) found that minnows and other fishes recognize a colored paper under colored illumination, and, thus, was already able to show color constancy. There are also early training experiments in reptiles: Wagner (1933) showed color discrimination in lizards, Wojtusiak (1933) demonstrated in turtles an excellent wavelength discrimination ability in three spectral ranges, and also showed ultraviolet vision. In amphibia, which are very difficult to train, it was shown that frogs and toads respond to ultraviolet light (Zipse, 1935). However, it has not yet been possible to measure wavelength discrimination.

In the attempts to understand the neural basis of human color vision, lower vertebrates, especially cyprinid fishes, have been important subjects. Because of the large cell size of their photoreceptors and neurons in their retinae, intracellular recordings were possible very early. The first recordings were performed by Svaetichin (1953). His "S-potentials" recorded from horizontal cells (originally believed to be cone responses) revealed so-called "color-opponent" properties showing depolarization in certain wavelength ranges and hyperpolarization in others. This type of "opponent" activity was exactly that property Ewald Hering had demanded to explain opponent colors and the four unique hues in human color vision. In the carp, Tomita (1963) recorded intracellularly from single cones and found three spectral types. The same result was obtained by microspectrophotometry, a method invented to measure the absorption spectra of the cone photopigments in situ (Marks, 1965). From that time on, the retina, especially that of cyprinid fishes and of the turtle *Pseudemys scripta elegans,* has been very intensively investigated. Compared with the retina of primates, it seems that important steps of information processing in color vision already occur on the peripheral level of the retina. This conclusion is based mainly on the finding that bipolar and ganglion cells in the retina of fishes show so-called double-opponent responses which are found in mammals only in the primary visual cortex (Daw, 1967; Kaneko and Tachibana, 1983).

The relatively easy access to retinal neurons in lower vertebrates and the possibility of performing behavioral training experiments, gives us the opportunity not only to investigate different aspects of color vision (as characteristics of the entire system), but also to investigate the cellular level. There is one animal, the goldfish, which is especially suitable as a subject. The goldfish, kept as a pet for at least a thousand years in China and Japan (Hervey and Hems, 1968/1981), can be easily tamed and also trained. Therefore, goldfish vision is best understood amongst all lower vertebrates.

8.2 Wavelength Discrimination in Lower Vertebrates

8.2.1 Goldfish

The way we measured wavelength discrimination in goldfish (and also in the turtle *Pseudemys scripta elegans*) is shown in Figure 8.1. Two test fields were presented to the animal freely swimming in a small (40 x 20 x 28 cm) tank. The test fields were illuminated with monochromatic light via fiber optics from the outside of the tank. The monochromatic light was adjusted to equal "animal-subjective" brightness, according to the spectral sensitivity functions measured under the same experimental conditions (Neumeyer, 1984). In Figure 8.2 the Δλ-function of the goldfish is shown, measured at first between 400 and 720 nm (Neumeyer, 1991), and later also between 300 and 400 nm (Fratzer et al., 1994).

There are three ranges of best discrimination ability: at about 610 nm, at 500 nm, and at 400 nm. In the range of maximal discrimination at 500 nm, a wavelength difference of 3–5 nm was sufficient for the goldfish to see a "just noticeable" difference. The ranges of best discrimination at 500 nm and 610 nm were roughly expected on the basis of the three cone types so far known from microspectrophotometry (Marks, 1965; Hárosi, 1976): in

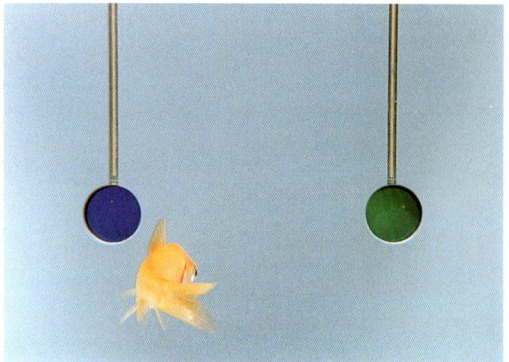

Fig. 8.1: Goldfish in training experiment.
The freely swimming goldfish has to decide between two testfields illuminated from the outside of the tank with monochromatic light of the same "goldfish-specific" brightness. The fish is trained on one wavelength by delivering a small amount of a food paste from the feeding tube at the test field. The second "comparison" testfield is illuminated with another wavelength. Discrimination ability is measured as the relative frequency with which the training wavelength is chosen. A bite or peck at one of the testfields is counted as a choice. To obtain the Δλ-function, the difference between training wavelength and the wavelength at which the threshold criterion of 70% relative choice frequency was reached, was calculated.
Foto: Jürgen Schramme

these spectral ranges the absorption functions of the short- and mid-, and of the mid- and long-wavelength photopigments, respectively, cross each other. The third range at 400 nm (although already found by Wolff, 1925!), however, was highly surprising. There were two possible explanations as shown in model computations (Neumeyer, 1986): the effect of a side maximum of the long-wavelength cone type (beta band), and the existence of a cone type (at that time unknown) maximally sensitive in the ultraviolet range. Additive color mixture experiments decided between these two possibilities (Neumeyer, 1985; 1992). They showed that the goldfish has not only three, but four cone types, the fourth being maximally sensitive in the ultraviolet range. This cone type was also deduced from measurements of spectral sensitivity in goldfish by Hawryshyn and Beauchamp (1985), and was demonstrated

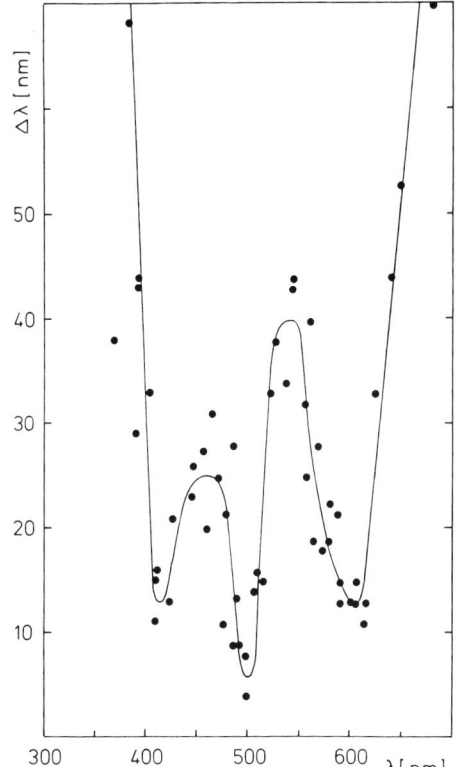

the outer segment (Fig. 8.3). In some amphibia and fishes, clear oil droplets only have been described.

Colored oil droplets act as cut-off filters for the light entering the outer segment of the cones where it is absorbed by the photopigment. As the short-wavelength and ultraviolet light is absorbed by most oil droplets, they alter the effective spectral sensitivity of the cones (Fig. 8.4), and, thus, oil droplets must have an effect on color vision. As photoreceptors and retinal neurons of some turtles are well investigated, it seemed especially promising to investigate the wavelength discrimination abilities of the turtle *Pseudemys scripta elegans*. In highly difficult experiments, Karin Arnold (Arnold and Neumeyer, 1987) succeeded in training three turtles, and obtained two complete $\Delta\lambda$-functions (Fig. 8.5). As in the goldfish, and also highly unexpectedly, three ranges of best discrimination ability were found at 400 nm, 500 nm, and at 600 nm.

As shown in additive color mixture experiments, the good discrimination at 400 nm is due to the

Fig. 8.2: Wavelength discrimination in goldfish ($\Delta\lambda$-function).
Small values of $\Delta\lambda$ (ordinate) stand for a high discrimination ability. Discrimination was highest in three spectral ranges (abscissa): 400, 500, and 610 nm. Wavelength discrimination was absent in the short- and long-spectral ranges (after Neumeyer, 1986, and Fratzer et al., 1994).

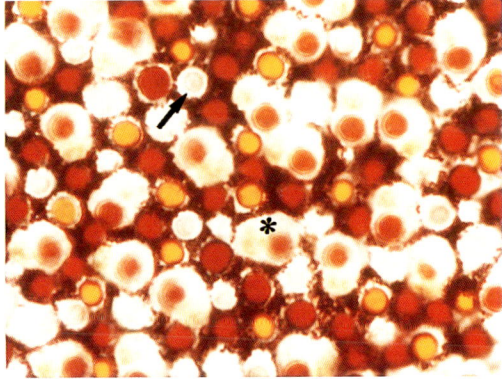

much later using microspectrophotometry by Bowmaker, et al. (1991). In other cyprinid fishes, evidence for the existence of ultraviolet cones came earlier (Avery et al., 1982; Hárosi and Hashimoto, 1983). Detailed color mixture experiments have shown that color vision in goldfish is tetrachromatic (Neumeyer, 1992).

8.2.2 Turtles

Many birds and reptiles possess brightly colored oil droplets in the inner segments of their cones just underneath the light-absorbing structures in

Fig. 8.3: Oil droplets in the retina of the turtle *Pseudemys scripta elegans*. Red oil droplets are most frequent, followed by orange and yellow ones. Clear oil droplets are relatively rare (arrow). There seem to be two types of clear oil droplets: with and without a high transmittance in the ultraviolet spectral range. One cone type in double cones (asterisk) possesses "pale green" oil droplets which also show a high transmittance in the ultraviolet range. Double cones do not seem to play a role in color vision (for references see Arnold and Neumeyer, 1987). Dark structures: pigment epithelium.
Foto: Teruya Ohtsuka

existence of an ultraviolet sensitive cone, which was only very recently found with microspectrophotometry (Govardovskiĭ, personal communication). As in goldfish, color vision in *Pseudemys* is tetrachromatic. Another unexpected finding was the fact that the turtles were entirely unable to discriminate wavelengths between 450 nm and 512 nm which is indicated by the high $\Delta\lambda$ values of 60–70 nm around 450 nm in Figure 8.5.

As shown in model computations (Arnold and Neumeyer, 1987), the gap in wavelength discrimination in the blue to blue-green range (between 450 and 520 nm) is a consequence of the yellow and red oil droplets which absorb all short-wavelength light entering the cones containing the mid- and long wavelength photopigments (Fig. 8.4). Wavelengths between 450 and 520 nm excite the short-wavelength cone type exclusively, causing an equal excitation ratio of the cone types and, thus, the same perceived hue. At first glance one might guess that this "wavelength discrimination gap" is a disadvantage for color vision. However, one has to take into consideration that color vision is not designed to "stare at the rainbow", as Victor Govardovskiĭ uses

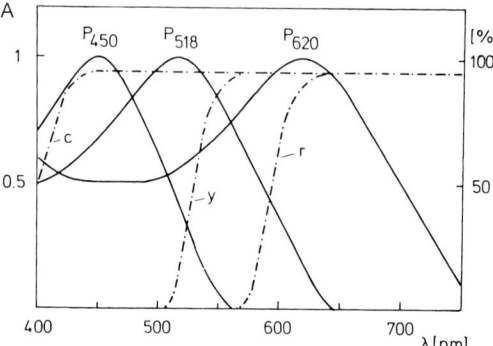

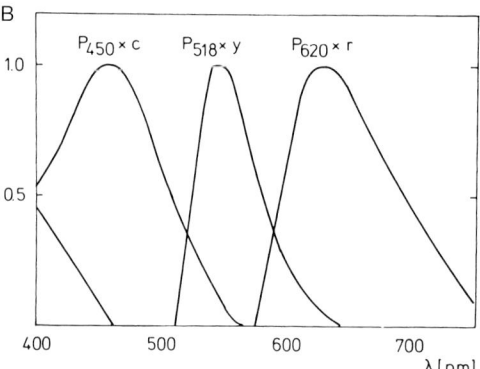

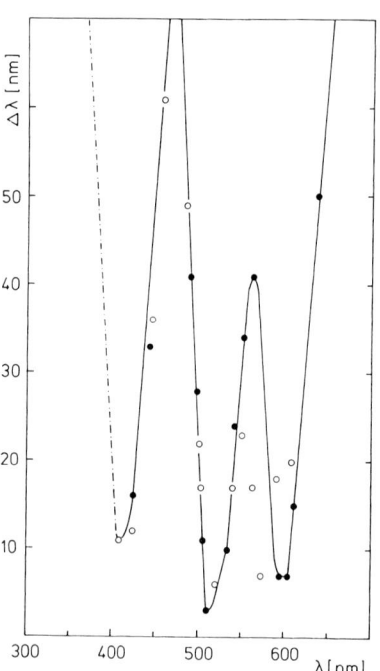

Fig. 8.4: Cone photopigments, oil droplets and effective cone sensitivity of the turtle *Pseudemys scripta elegans.*
A. Relative spectral absorbance of the cone photopigments identified so far (left ordinate scale). The three photopigment types are characterized by the peak wavelengths (continuous lines). Dashed lines: spectral transmission of the clear (c), yellow (y), and red (r) oil droplets (right ordinate scale). (After Neumeyer and Jäger, 1985).
B. Relative "effective" cone sensitivity functions obtained by weighting the photopigment absorption spectra with oil droplet transmission. The decreasing sensitivity slope between 400 and 460 nm indicates the ultraviolet cone type as concluded from wavelength discrimination and additive color mixture experiments. The functions explain the properties of wavelength discrimination of turtle S1 as shown in model computations. (After Arnold and Neumeyer, 1987).

Fig. 8.5: Wavelength discrimination ($\Delta\lambda$-function) of the turtle *Pseudemys scripta elegans.* Results from two turtles, S1 (dark), and S2 (open symbols). The stippled line is hypothetical (After Arnold and Neumeyer, 1987).

8.2 Wavelength Discrimination in Lower Vertebrates 153

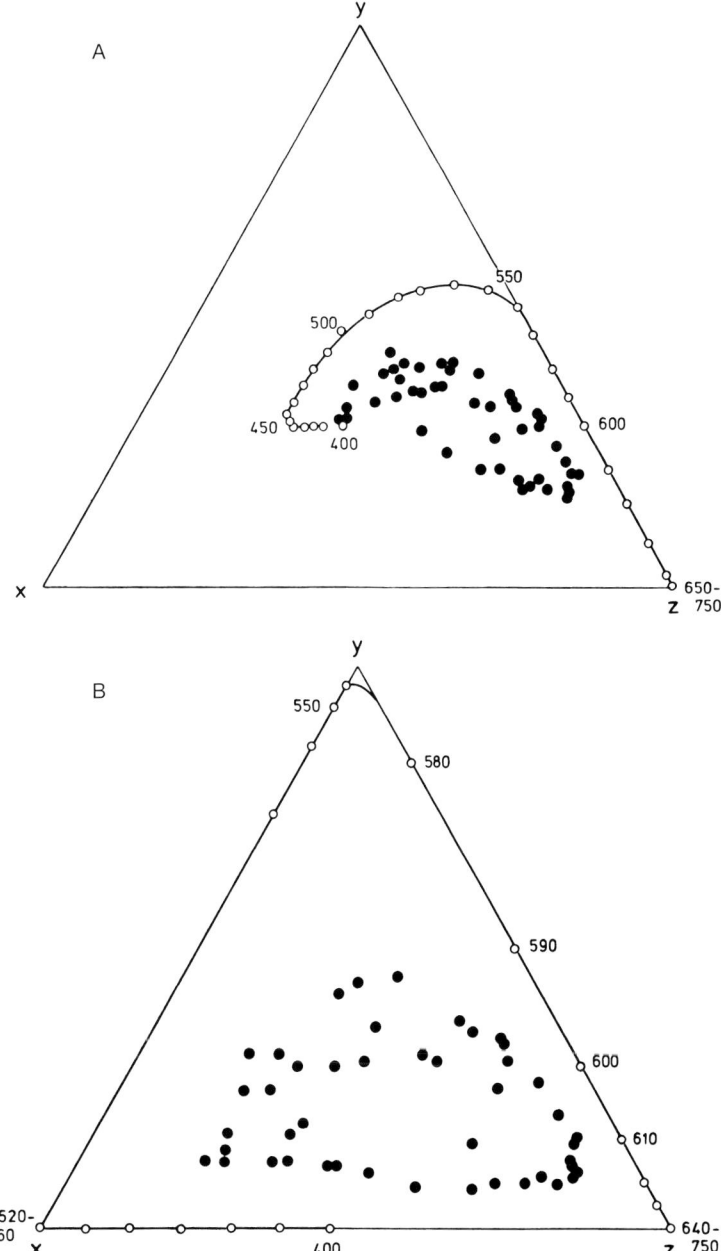

Fig. 8.6: Effect of object colors on turtle cones with and without oil droplets.
The color triangle in **A** is calculated on the basis of the turtle photopigments (from Fig. 8.5 A), the triangle in **B** on the basis of the "effective" cone sensitivity spectra which include the filter effect of the oil droplets (from Fig. 8.5 B). Each point in a triangle represents the relative values with which each of the three cone types is excited by the light reflected from the colored paper (black dots) or by spectral light (circles). The excitation of the UV-cone type is not taken into consideration. The corners x, y, z represent colors which excite exclusively the short-, mid-, and long-wavelength cone type, respectively.
For calculation of the color loci see Neumeyer (1980).

to say, but to discriminate object colors. Therefore, we asked whether the oil droplets would also impair discrimination of object colors. For that purpose, we calculated the color loci of about 50 differently colored papers (HKS papers) on the basis of cone types with and without oil droplets.

The results are shown in a presentation of the turtle color triangle (which does not take into account the ultraviolet cone type for simplicity) in Figure 8.6. The triangle in Figure 8.6A is calculated on the basis of the cone photopigments (Fig. 8.5A). Here, the loci of the spectral colors (open symbols) are located on the side between the corners "z" and "y" for wavelengths between 750 and 560 nm, indicating that the long- and the mid-wavelength cone types would be excited. The loci for wavelengths between 550 and 400 nm lie inside the triangle, indicating that these wavelengths excite all three cone types to certain degrees. The loci of the colored papers are rather close together, some even coincide. In Figure 8.6B, the loci are calculated for the same colored papers but on the basis of the "effective" cone sensitivity spectra from Figure 8.5B. Here, the loci of the spectral colors are found almost exclusively at the sides of the triangle, and the loci of the colored papers are distributed over a large area. Contrary to our expectation, the loci of blue and blue-green object colors do not coincide in one point (as do the loci of the spectral colors between 520 and 460 nm that are all located at the "x" corner) which would mean that they cannot be discriminated. Instead, they are more clearly separated than on the basis of the photopigments alone. Despite the fact that we do not know the meaning of a certain distance in the interior of the triangle, one has the impression that object colors are better separated, and, thus, better discriminable, than on the basis of the photopigments alone. The colored oil droplets certainly do not impair the discrimination of object colors. In goldfish, a similar effect was assumed to occur by neuronal inhibitory interactions between cone types of different spectral types (Neumeyer, 1986).

8.2.3 Amphibia

Color vision in amphibia is difficult to investigate because they cannot be trained easily. We used the European tiger salamander (*Salamandra salamandra*) to find out whether their color vision uses an ultraviolet cone type as goldfish and turtles, and whether their color vision is tri- or dichromatic. As a behavioral indicator we used a fixed action pattern which is released when the animal sees a moving prey. The animal then usually turns toward the object and snaps by flicking out its tongue. To elicit this response, we used a black "worm" dummy as shown in Figure 8.7 which moved slow-

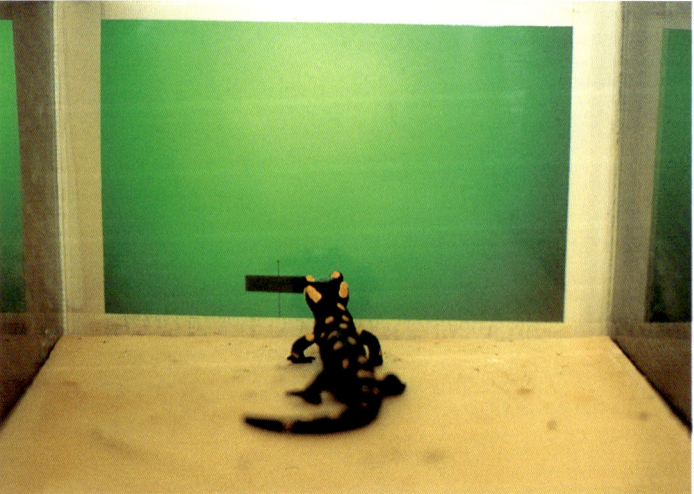

Fig. 8.7: *Salamandra salamandra* in experiment. The animal responds to a worm dummy (6 x 25 mm) moving at a speed of 6 mm/s. When the contrast between the monochromatically illuminated background and the dummy was high, the salamander turned its head, approached the screen and snapped by flicking out its tongue. As a measure of its reaction, we used the relative frequency of snapping related to the sum of turning movements and snapping responses. (From Przyrembel, Keller and Neumeyer, 1995).
Foto: Jürgen Schramme.

ly in front of a background illuminated with monochromatic light.

By varying the intensity we determined the number of quanta impinging on the screen that was just sufficient to elicit a response in the animal, and so measured a spectral sensitivity function. The result indicated maximal sensitivity in the range between 500 to 580 nm without pronounced maxima and minima (Przyrembel et al., 1995). A relatively high sensitivity (but 1–1.5 log units below the maximum) was also found in the ultraviolet range. However, measurements of chromatic adaptation under yellow illumination revealed that the sensitivity in the ultraviolet range was not independent of sensitivity in the mid-wavelength region. Thus, the existence of a separate ultraviolet photoreceptor type could not be concluded.

Color discrimination experiments were performed on a color monitor showing a moving colored worm dummy on a differently colored surround of the same salamander-specific brightness. The results indicate that salamanders are able to discriminate blue from green, and red from green, and, therefore, have most probably trichromatic color vision.

However, the existence of trichromatic color vision cannot be expected for all amphibia. Zipse (1935) already reported that some frogs and toads can see ultraviolet light rather well, and, in the american tiger salamander, *Ambystoma tigrinum*, four different cone photopigments, one with maximal absorption in the ultraviolet, have been found (Perry and McNaughton, 1991).

8.3 Color Constancy and Color Contrast

Biologically relevant colors are the colors of objects. The colors seen are caused by the light reflected by the surface. However, the spectral distribution of the reflected light impinging the eye is not only determined by the spectral reflectance properties of the surface but also by the spectral radiant flux of the illuminating light. The spectral composition of natural daylight changes considerably during the course of a day, and also depends on the filtering effects of clouds, forest canopy, water (for aquatic animals) and so on (Henderson, 1977; Kirk, 1983; Lythgoe, 1979; Endler, 1993). Therefore, if an animal uses color as a cue to recognize objects, it requires mechanisms compensating for the spectral changes of the illumination, and thus providing constancy. According to an idea of von Campenhausen (1986), the necessity to eliminate the spectral alterations of daylight could even have been the selective pressure for the generation of color vision during evolution. His experiments showed that an animal with one photoreceptor type only (for example a human being using rod vision) is unable to make correct lightness judgements whenever the spectral composition of the light changes. To detect changes in the spectral radiance, and to compensate for them, two photoreceptor types with different spectral sensitivities are required. This, however, is also the prerequisite condition for color vision.

Color constancy is best investigated in cyprinid fishes (for other animals see review by Neumeyer, 1998). Burkamp (1923) already showed that minnows and other fishes are able to recognize object colors under colored illuminations, a finding confirmed in the carp by Dimentman et al. (1972). In a famous experiment, Ingle (1985) showed color constancy in goldfish by using a Mondrian pattern. To analyze color constancy quantitatively in goldfish, we used a method first applied in the honeybee (Neumeyer, 1980; 1981). This method has the advantage that there is always a series of at least seven very similar but still discriminable colored papers (testfields) presented, amongst which the animal can choose that specific color which most resembles the color it has learned. The animal was trained on one medium color which turned out to be a very hard task for goldfish and experimenter: many weeks or even months had been required before the fish clearly preferred this training testfield amongst all the others. The training situation is shown in Figure 8.8.

In the experiments performed by Saskia Dörr, the goldfish was trained on a bluish gray testfield out of a series of 15 different bluish and yellowish testfields presented on a gray or a black background (Dörr, 1996; Dörr and Neumeyer, 1996). The training was performed under a white illumi-

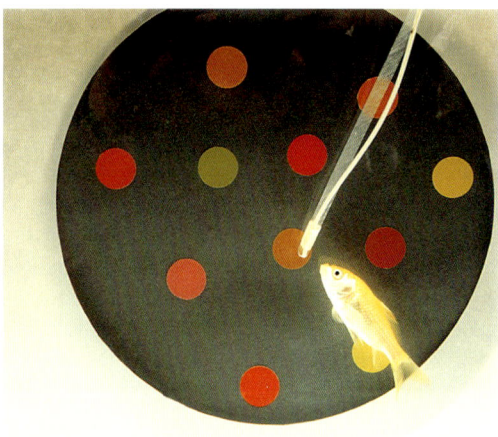

Fig. 8.8: Training procedure to show color constancy and color contrast. The goldfish is rewarded by a small amount of the food paste whenever it pecks at the training testfield (orange) shown together with similar reddish, orange and greenish testfields behind the tank. To measure color constancy, the setup is illuminated with white light during training, and with colored light during the tests. In the latter situation the fish are never rewarded. To measure color contrast, the testfields are presented on a grey background during training, in the test situation the background is changed to red or green, respectively. Foto: Guido Mangold.

and purple illuminations, i.e., for a direction in color space perpendicular to the direction in which the main changes of daylight (corresponding to the Planckian locus) occur.

Under these conditions also, color constancy was surprisingly good (Fig. 8.9 A). The color constancy effect was best when the testfields were

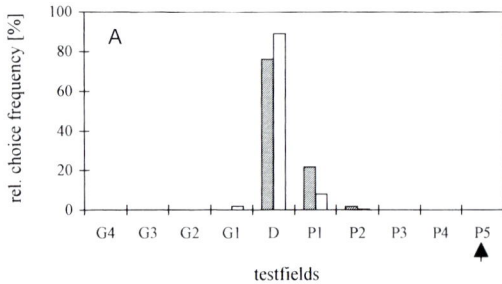
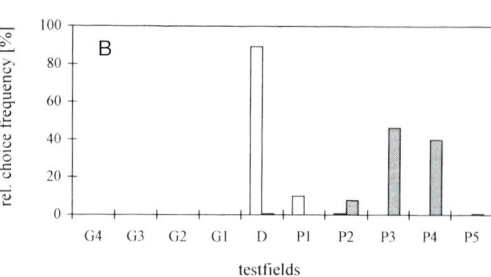

Fig. 8.9: Color constancy and simultaneous color contrast in goldfish.
A. Choice behavior of a goldfish in the color constancy experiment. Ordinate: relative choice frequency in %; abscissa: green (G4) to purple (P5) test field colors; D: greyish training color. The result of training under white light is indicated by the white bars. Under green illumination the choice frequency distribution (dark bars) is not changed. The testfields were presented with a grey surround. Testfield P5 (arrow) under green illumination stimulates the cone types in the same way as training testfield D under white training illumination (see text).
B. Choice behavior in simultaneous color contrast situation. White bars: choice frequency when the testfields are presented with grey surround (training situation); dark bars: testfields presented with purple surround. Here, goldfish preferred more purple testfields. This indicates that all testfields appeared more green with purple surround. With its choice of the purple testfields P3 and P4 the fish compensates for the color contrast effect.

nation. In the test for color constancy, the color of the illumination was changed to blue or yellow, everything else remaining the same. If color vision were determined by the cone excitation ratio only, i.e., if there were no color constancy, all the different test fields would appear to the fish "more" blue under a bluish illumination than under the white training light. Then, the fish would not recognize the training field, but should select a "more yellowish" test field which now stimulates its cone types in the same ratio as the training testfield did before under white illumination. (Which testfield has this property can be found by calculating the color loci of the testfields under the different illuminations.) A color constant goldfish, however, should always find his training field amongst all the different testfields. Saskia Dörr has shown that this is indeed the case within certain limits.

In another series of experiments we tested whether color constancy is also found for green presented on a medium grey background, not perfect with a black background, and over-compensated with a white background (Fritsch and Neumeyer, 1996). Surround size also played an important role which indicates that neuronal lateral interactions might be involved.

With the same method (Fig. 8.8), we also investigated simultaneous color contrast. Here, the goldfish were trained on one medium color while the entire series of nine green to purple testfields was presented on a grey background. In the test, the same testfields were shown on a purple or a green background, respectively. Here, the fish did not select their training field (which was also present) but a very different testfield. With its choice behavior (Fig. 8.9B shows one example) the goldfish indicated that the hues of all testfields have changed so that now the chosen testfield most resembled the training hue on a gray surround. As very small annular testfields were sufficient to cause color contrast, we concluded that lateral interactions and not chromatic adaptation is the main mechanism involved (Dörr and Neumeyer, 1997). Successive color contrast as found in the honeybee (Neumeyer, 1981) could not be shown in goldfish with our method (Dörr, 1996).

8.4 Color Vision and Other Visual Functions: Evidence for Parallel Processing of Visual Information

Spectral sensitivity functions in goldfish have been measured several times with very different results depending on the behavioral response used (Fig. 8.10).

Functions with a single maximum in the long wavelength range were obtained using the optomotor response (Fig. 8.10A), or the dorsal light reaction (b), whereas training methods (c and d) gave broad curves or even functions with three very pronounced maxima (e). The comparison of these functions and further investigations show that the term "spectral sensitivity" is misleading as it suggests that there is just one function. Actually

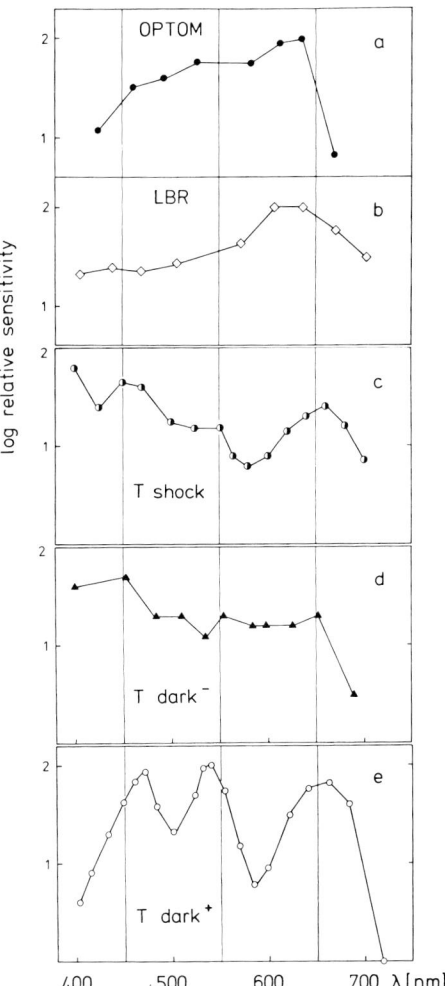

Fig. 8.10: Spectral sensitivity functions in goldfish. **a**: action spectrum of the optomotor response (after Cronly-Dillon and Muntz, 1965); **b**: action spectrum of the dorsal light reaction (after Powers, 1978); **c**: spectral sensitivity measured in a training experiment (classical conditioning using electro-shock) (after Beauchamp and Rowe, 1977); **d**: spectral sensitivity in training experiment (food reward, training on the illuminated testfield, comparison testfield: dark) (after Yager, 1967); **e**: spectral sensitivity in training experiment (food reward, training on the dark testfield, comparison testfield: illuminated) (after Neumeyer, 1984).

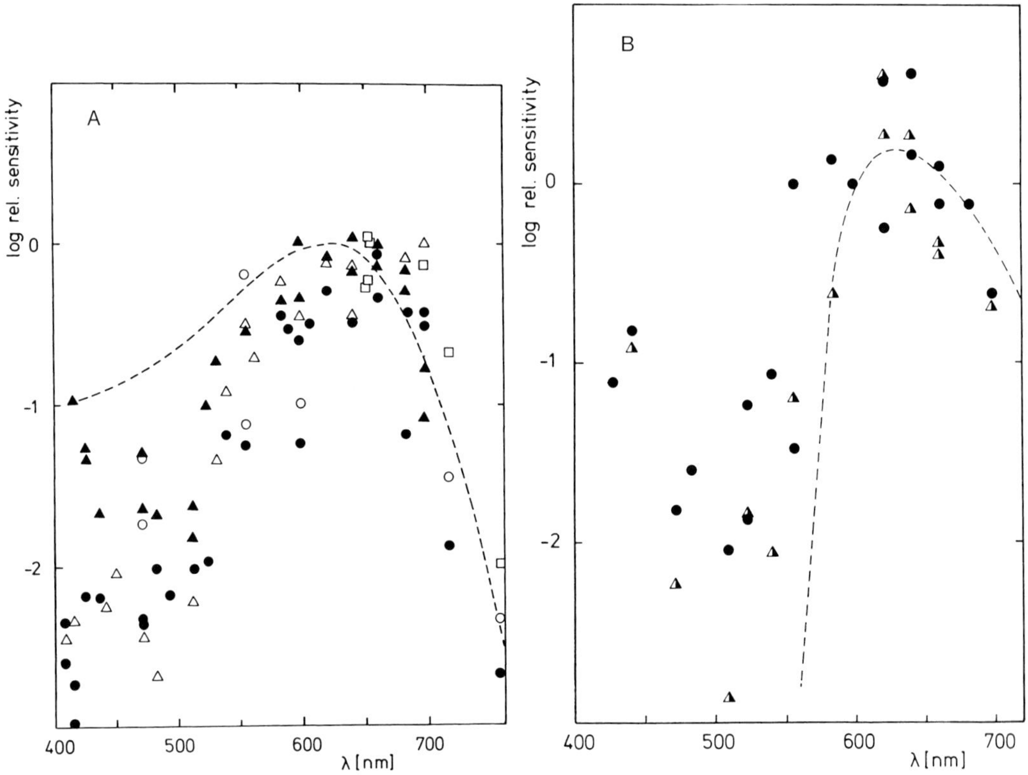

158   8. Color Vision in Lower Vertebrates

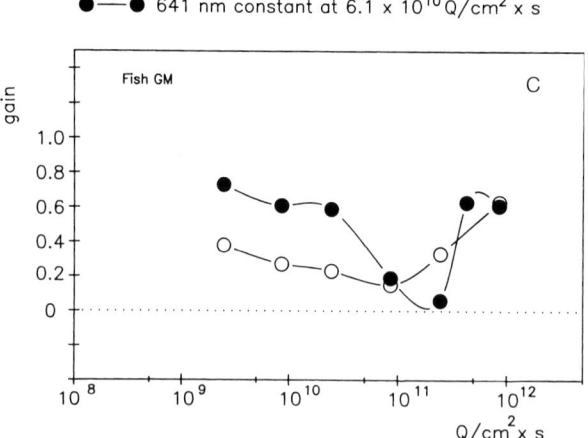

Fig. 8.11: Action spectra of the optomotor response in goldfish (**A**) and in the turtle *Pseudemys scripta elegans* (**B**). The dashed line in A represents the spectral sensitivity function of the long-wavelength cone type in goldfish. The comparison with the action spectrum indicates that the short wavelength flank is steeper than the cone sensitivity function. We assume that this is due to an inhibitory influence of the mid-wavelength cone channel (from Schaerer and Neumeyer, 1996). The dashed line in B shows the effective long wavelength cone sensitivity function combined with the red oil droplet (from Schaerer, 1993). **C:** optomotor response of one goldfish as an example in a red-green striped cylinder illuminated simultaneously by monochromatic red and green light. At a certain intensity of the red or green light, respectively, the response drops to zero. This result indicates that motion vision in the optomotor response is "color-blind" (from Schaerer, 1993).

one should speak of "action spectra" of different behavioral tasks which reflect the contribution of different cone types in different ways.

A re-investigation of the optomotor response in goldfish by Schaerer (1993) showed again a function with a single maximum in the long wavelength range (Fig. 8.11 A). This function can be regarded as the action spectrum of motion vision (wide field motion).

The comparison with the long wavelength cone sensitivity function (dashed line) indicates that motion vision measured with this behavioral method is mainly determined by the long-wavelength cone type. A similar result was obtained when the turtle *Pseudemys scripta elegans* was tested (Fig. 8.11 B). If only one cone type is involved in motion vision, the optomotor response should go to zero whenever an "isoluminant" red-green striped pattern is used. This is indeed the case as shown in Figure 8.11C. Motion vision in goldfish investigated using the optomotor response is "color blind" (Schaerer and Neumeyer, 1996). This seems to be a general principle of visual systems also found in the honeybee (Kaiser and Liske, 1974), and to some extent in humans as well.

The fact that the long-wavelength cone type in goldfish is (almost exclusively) involved in motion vision, and (together with the three other cone types) in color vision gives a first hint that both visual functions are processed in parallel, possibly already at a retinal level. That at least the long-wavelength cone information does indeed feed into different "channels" became evident from the following findings: 1.) Under reduced ("mesopic") light conditions of 1 lux, the long-wavelength cone type does not contribute to color vision any longer: red cannot be discriminated from green, and sensitivity in the long-wavelength range is reduced (Neumeyer and Arnold, 1989). However, if "brightness" detection is tested instead of color vision (by reversing the training procedure) under the same conditions of 1 lux, long-wavelength sensitivity is still high (Neumeyer et al., 1991). 2.) The tuberculostatic drug ethambutol impairs red-green discrimination by disturbing the contribution of the long-wavelength cone type, but does not affect the contribution of this cone type to "brightness" detection (Spekreijse et al., 1991). 3.) Dopamine seems to be important in bringing the retina into the light adapted state. When a D1-dopamine-receptor antagonist is injected into the eyes, trained goldfish are unable to discriminate red from green (Mora-Ferrer and Neumeyer, 1996). However, in the context of motion vision, also mediated by long-wavelength cones, the same drug does not impair long-wavelength sensitivity (Mora-Ferrer et al., 1995).

Thus, it seems that there is a functional dichotomy of the long-wavelength cone information: the contribution to color vision and to visual acuity (Neumeyer, in prep.) is affected in the mesopic state and by certain drugs, whereas the contribution to brightness, flicker and motion detection is not (Neumeyer and Schaerer, 1992). A parallel processing of color and shape on the one hand, and brightness and motion on the other hand seems to occur in primates also.

8.5 Color Perception

Tetrachromatic color vision as found in goldfish and turtles (and also in birds) including the ultraviolet range implies specific properties of color perception. In tetrachromatic color vision, all hues can be represented in a color tetrahedron which is the equivalent of the color triangle in a trichromatic color vision system (Neumeyer, 1991; 1992).

Ultraviolet is represented at the apex of the tetrahedron (Fig. 8.12). Which sensation an ultraviolet light will create we cannot know, but we may assume that it may be a fourth basic color (as it seems reasonable to assume that the number of basic colors corresponds at least to the number of photoreceptor types involved in color vision). More interesting is the question of how white light might be perceived by an animal with tetrachromatic color vision. White light has to include the ultraviolet range, and will stimulate all four cone types about equally. Thus, the corresponding color loci will be located in the interior of the tetrahedron (near "XW" in Fig. 8.12). If white light is perceived as "neutral" as in human color vision (which we do not know yet), we may ask how, for example, the goldfish perceives "our" white which does not contain ultraviolet. This color is represented by an area in the center of the triangle "x, y, z" of the tetrahedron. Such colors can be easily discriminated by goldfish from Xenon-white ("XW" in Fig. 8.12) as shown by Neumeyer (1992). But how will this "white without ultraviolet" be perceived? Certainly not as neutral. Perhaps it is perceived as a reddish-greenish-blue, a color containing three hues at once ("ternary" colors according to Thompson, Palacios and Varela, 1992)? Such colors (which we cannot picture) should also occur within the triangles "x, uv, y", "y, uv, z" and "x, uv, z" of the tetrahedron.

Another question which may also be asked about trichromatic color vision systems is whether there are more unique colors than cone types. In human color vision we have the perception of "yellow" between red and green, i.e., a color which excites the mid- and long-wavelength cone types about equally. Is this also true for the goldfish? Our experiments so far seem to indicate that colors appearing to us "yellow" are not seen by the goldfish as a unique color but as a perceptual mixture of "red" and "green" (Kitschmann and Neumeyer, 1996). It may also be asked whether there are unique hues in other spectral ranges such as around 500 nm, and 400 nm.

8.6 Summary

Color vision in goldfish (*Carassius auratus*) and in turtle (*Pseumdemys scripta elegans*) is tetrachromatic, and based on four different cones types (the fourth being an ultraviolet sensitive cone type). This was shown in training experiments (food reward) measuring the ability of wavelength discrimination and the properties of additive color mixture. Color vision in salamanders (*Salamandra salamandra*), however, seems to be trichromatic, as indicated by experiments using a fixed action pattern, the prey catching response. Color vision in turtles (and in birds) is especially remarkable because of the colored oil droplets located in the cones just underneath the outer segment. They act as cut-off filters and modify cone spectral sensitivity in the short wavelength range. They seem to be of advantage in the discrimination of object colors. Color vision in goldfish is investigated under many different aspects, and, thus, is best known amongst all lower vertebrates. Color constancy, for instance, was measured quantitatively for blue-yellow, and green-red illumination colors, and turned out to be highly effective. Simultaneous color contrast could be shown as well. Not all behavioral methods seem to be appropriate to investigate color vision. Using the optomotor response in goldfish, the action spectrum indicates the dominance of the L-cone type. Motion vision is "color-blind". Furthermore, there seems to be a parallel and separate processing of different visual functions, such as " color" and "acuity" on the one hand, and "motion", "flicker" and "brightness" on the other hand, similar to the properties of primate visual systems.

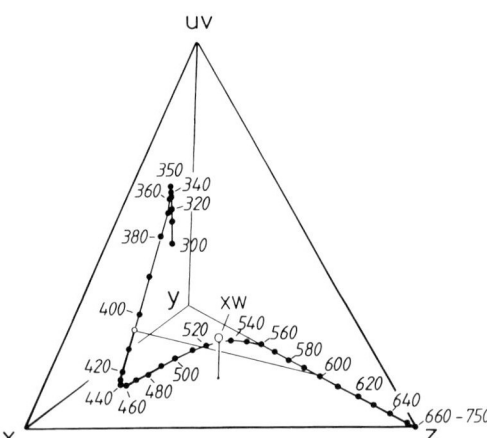

Fig. 8.12: Color tetrahedron of the goldfish. Each point in the tetrahedron represents the relative excitation values of the four goldfish cone types. The corners stand for the exclusive excitation of the UV, short-, mid-, and long-wavelength cone types, "uv", "x", "y", and "z", respectively. The line connecting the loci between 750 nm and 300 nm is the spectral locus. "X" represents the locus of the white light of a Xenon-arc lamp. This locus is near the line between 400 nm and 600 nm. These two wavelengths were found to be complementary colors for the goldfish (from Neumeyer, 1992).

Acknowledgements

The experimental work in goldfish, turtle and salamander was supported by Deutsche Forschungsgemeinschaft (Ne 215/3-9), and by the Human Frontier Science Program (PI: H. Spekreijse).

References

Arnold, K. and Neumeyer, C. (1987). Wavelength discrimination in the turtle *Pseudemys scripta elegans*. Vision Res. 27, 1501-1511.
Avery, J. A., Bowmaker, J. K., Djamgoz, M. B. A., and Downing, J.E.D. (1982). Ultra-violet sensitive receptors in a freshwater fish. J. Physiol. Lond. 334, 23P.
Beauchamp, R. D. and Rowe, J. S. (1977). Goldfish spectral sensitivity: a conditioned heart rate measure in restrained or curarized fish. Vision Res. 17, 617-624.
Bowmaker, J. K., Thorpe, A., and Douglas, R. H. (1991). Ultraviolet-sensitive cones in the goldfish. Vision Res. 31, 349-352.
Burkamp, W. (1923). Versuche über das Farbenwiedererkennen der Fische. Z. Sinnesphysiol. 5, 133-170.
Campenhausen, C. von (1986). Photoreceptors, lightness constancy and color vision. Naturwissenschaften 73, 674-675.
Cronly-Dillon, J. R. and Muntz, W. R. A. (1965). The spectral sensitivity of the goldfish and the clawed toad tadpole under photopic conditions. J. Exp. Biol. 42, 481-493.
Daw, N. (1967). Goldfish retina: organisation for simultaneous color contrast. Science 158, 942-944.
Dimentman, A. M., Karas, A. Y., Maximov, V. V., and Orlov, O. Y. (1972). Constancy of object color perception in the carp (*Cyprinus carpio*). Pavlov J. Higher Nerv. Act. 22, 4, 772-779 (in Russian).
Dörr, S. (1996). Quantitative Untersuchungen zur Farbkonstanz beim Goldfisch. Thesis, Mainz.
Dörr, S. and Neumeyer, C. (1996). The goldfish – a color constant animal. Perception 25, 243-250.
Dörr, S. and Neumeyer, C. (1997). Simultaneous color contrast in goldfish – a quantitative study. Vision Res. 37, 1581-1593.
Endler, J. A. (1993). The color of light in forests and its implications. Ecological Monographs 63, 1-27.
Fratzer, C., Dörr, S., and Neumeyer C. (1994). Wavelength discrimination of the goldfish in the ultraviolet spectral range. Vision Res. 34, 1515-1520.
Frisch, K. von (1913). Weitere Untersuchungen über den Farbensinn der Fische. Zool. Jahrb., Abt. f. Zool. und Physiol. 34, 43-68.
Frisch, K. von (1914). Der Farbensinn und Formensinn der Biene. Zool. Jahrb., Abt. Allg. Zool. Physiol. 35, 1-182.
Fritsch, J. and Neumeyer, C. (1996). Colour constancy in goldfish - influence of surround size and reflectance. In: Göttingen Neurobiology Report 1996. N. Elsner and H.-U. Schnitzler (eds.) (Stuttgart: G. Thieme).
Govardovskiĭ, V I. (1983). On the role of oil drops in colour vision. Vision Res. 23, 1739-1740.
Hárosi, F. I. (1976). Spectral relations of cone pigments in goldfish. J. Gen Physiol. 68, 65-80.
Hárosi, F. I. and Hashimoto, Y. (1983). Ultraviolet visual pigment in a vertebrate: a tetrachromatic cone system in the dace. Science 222, 1021-1023.
Hawryshyn, C. W. and Beauchamp, R. (1985). Ultraviolet photosensitivity in goldfish: an independent u.v. retinal mechanism. Vision Res. 25, 11-20.
Henderson, S. T. (1977). Daylight and its spectrum. (2nd edn. Bristol, England: Hilger)
Herter, K. (1950). Über simultanen Farbkontrast bei Fischen. Biol. Zentralblatt 69, 283-300.
Hervey, G. F. and Hems, J. (1968, 1981). The goldfish. (London, Boston: Faber and Faber).
Hess, C. v. (1914). Die Entwicklung von Lichtsinn und Farbensinn in der Tierreihe. (Wiesbaden: J. T. Bergmann).
Ingle, D. J. (1985). The goldfish as a retinex animal. Science 227, 651-654.
Kaiser, W. and Liske, E. (1974). Die optomotorische Reaktion von fixiert fliegenden Bienen bei Reizung mit Spektrallichtern. J. Comp. Physiol. 89, 391-408.
Kaneko, A. and Tachibana, M. (1983). Double color-opponent receptive fields of carp bipolar cells. Vision Res. 23, 381-388.
Kirk, J. T. O. (1983). Light and photosynthesis in aquatic ecosystems. (Cambridge: Cambridge University Press).
Kitschmann, M. and Neumeyer, C. (1996). Do goldfish perceive "yellow" between "red" and "green"? In: Göttingen Neurobiology Report 1996. N. Elsner and H.-U. Schnitzler (eds.) (Stuttgart: G. Thieme).
Liebman, P. A. and Granda, A. M. (1971). Microspectrophotometric measurements of visual pig-

ments in two species of turtle, *Pseudemys scripta* and *Chelonia* mydas. Vision Res. *11,* 105-114.

Lipetz, L. E. (1985). Some neuronal circuits of the turtle retina. In: The visual system. A. Fein and J. S. Levine, eds. (New York: Alan R. Liss).

Lythgoe, J. N. (1979). The ecology of vision. (Oxford: Clarendon Press).

Marks, W. B. (1965). Visual pigments of single goldfish cones. Journal of Physiology *178,* 14–32.

Mora-Ferrer, C., Dechent, P., and Neumeyer, C. (1995). Dopamine affects motion perception in goldfish. Investigative Ophthalmology and Visual Science *36* (Supp.), S 57.

Mora-Ferrer, C. and Neumeyer, C. (1996). Reduction of red-green discrimination by dopamine D1 receptor antagonists and retinal dopamine depletion. Vision Res. *36,* 4035–4044.

Neumeyer, C. (1980). Simultaneous colour contrast in the honeybee. J. Comp. Physiol. *139,* 165–176.

Neumeyer, C. (1981). Chromatic adaptation in the honeybee: successive color contrast and color constancy. J. Comp. Physiol. *144,* 543–553.

Neumeyer, C. (1984). On spectral sensitivity in the goldfish. Evidence for neural interactions between different "cone mechanisms". Vision Res. *24,* 1223–1231.

Neumeyer, C. (1985). An ultraviolet receptor as a fourth receptor type in goldfish colour vision. Naturwissenschaften *72,* 162–163.

Neumeyer, C. (1986). Wavelength discrimination in the goldfish. J. Comp. Physiol. *158,* 203–213.

Neumeyer, C. (1991). Evolution of colour vision. In: Vision and visual dysfunction, Vol. 2, J. Cronly-Dillon (ed.). (Houndsmills: Macmillan), pp. 284–305.

Neumeyer, C. (1992). Tetrachromatic color vision in goldfish: evidence by color mixture experiments. J. Comp. Physiol. A *171,* 639–649.

Neumeyer, C. (1998). Comparative aspects of colour constancy. In: Visual constancy: why things look as they do. V. Walsh and J. Kulikowsky, eds. (Cambridge: Cambridge University Press) (in press).

Neumeyer, C. and Jäger, J. (1985). Spectral sensitivity of the freshwater turtle *Pseudemys scripta elegans*: evidence for the filter effect of colored oil droplets. Vision Res. *25,* 833–838.

Neumeyer, C. and Arnold, K. (1989). Tetrachromatic color vision in the goldfish becomes trichromatic under white adaptation light of moderate intensity. Vision Res. *29,* 1719–1727.

Neumeyer, C., Wietsma, J. J., and Spekreijse, H. (1991). Separate processing of "color" and "brightness" in goldfish. Vision Res. *31,* 537–549.

Neumeyer, C. and Schaerer, S. (1992). Two separate pathways in the processing of L-cone type information in goldfish: color and acuity vs. brightness and flicker. Invest. Ophthal. Vis. Sci. *33,* 703.

Perry, R. J. and McNaughton, P. A. (1991). Response properties of cones from the retina of the tiger salamander. J. Physiol. *433,* 651–687.

Powers, M. K. (1978). Light-adapted spectral sensitivity of the goldfish: a reflex measure. Vision Res. *18,* 1131–1136.

Przyrembel, C., Keller, B., and Neumeyer, C. (1995). Trichromatic color vision in the salamander (*Salamandra salamandra*). J. Comp. Physiol. A *176,* 575–586.

Schaerer, S. (1993). Die Wellenlängenabhängigkeit des Bewegungssehens bei Goldfischen (*Carassius auratus*) und Schildkröten (*Pseudemys scripta elegans*) gemessen mit der optomotorischen Reaktion. Thesis, Mainz.

Schaerer, S. and Neumeyer, C. (1996). Motion detection in goldfish investigated with the optomotor response is "color blind". Vision Res. *36,* 4025–4034.

Spekreijse, H., Wietsma, J. J., and Neumeyer, C. (1991). Induced color blindness in goldfish: a behavioral and electrophysiological study. Vision Res. *31,* 551–562.

Svaetichin, G. (1953). The cone action potential. Acta Physiol. Scand. *29* (Suppl. 106), 565–600.

Thompson, E., Palacios, A., and Varela, F .J. (1992). Ways of coloring. Behavioral and Brain Sciences *15,* 1–74.

Tomita, T. (1963). Electrical activity in the vertebrate retina. J. Opt. Soc. Amer. *53,* 49–57.

Wagner, H. (1933). Über den Farbensinn der Eidechsen. Z. Vergl. Physiol. *18,* 378–392.

Wojtusiak, R .J. (1933). Über den Farbensinn von Schildkröten. Z. Vergl. Physiol. *18,* 393–436.

Wolff, H. (1925). Das Farbunterscheidungsvermögen der Ellritze. Z. Vergl. Physiol. *3,* 279–329.

Yager, D. (1967). Behavioural measures and theoretical analysis of spectral sensitivity and spectral saturation in the goldfish, Carassius auratus. Vision Res. *7,* 707–727.

Zipse, W. (1935). Können unsere einheimischen Frösche und echten Kröten ultraviolettes Licht sehen? Zool. Jahrb. *55,* 487–524.

9. Color Vision: Ecology and Evolution in Making the Best of the Photic Environment

Peter G. Kevan and Werner G. K. Backhaus

9.1 Introduction

"The primary necessity which led to the development of the sense of colour was probably the need of distinguishing objects much alike in form and size, but differing in important properties, such as ripe and unripe, or eatable and poisonous fruits, flowers with honey [i.e., nectar] or without, the sexes of the same or closely allied species. In most cases the strongest contrast would be the most useful, especially as the colours of objects to be distinguished would form but minute spots or points when compared with the broad masses of tint of sky, earth, or foliage against which they would be set."

So wrote the co-founder of modern evolutionary theory, Alfred Russel Wallace over a century ago (Wallace, 1878, p. 243; 1891, p. 411). Our essay places his ideas into a modern framework of evolution, ecology, and neurobiology.

First, it is important to explore the photic environment from a palaeontological viewpoint, and with respect to the biotic evolution of an oxygenated atmosphere on earth. The consequences of oxygenating the atmosphere prior to 400 million years ago were major and must have changed the nature of daylight, especially in attenuating ultraviolet light. Whether or not color vision existed for the marine animals of the time is unknown, but the possibility is discussed briefly from viewpoints of habitats and phylogeny.

Color vision in arthropods is mostly trichromatic, with the stimulating wavebands of light which might look "ultraviolet", "blue" and "green" to the respective species, as it is in vertebrates for which the stimulating wavebands might appear "blue", "green", and "red" as in the case of human color vision. The existence of color vision systems with four photoreceptor spectral types (tetrachromacy) in both groups present some fascinating problems about why such a complex color vision system should have arisen, and how it works. For the reader's convenience, wavelengths are denoted in the following by the names of the colors they cause in human perception.

The ideas expressed by Wallace are employed to develop an ecological and evolutionary argument, based mainly on the light reflecting properties of flowers and the species-specific color information derived by flower visiting animals. Flowers are of interest to insects and birds, both with well developed appreciations of the colors of objects around them, and we suggest that, through evolutionary events the trichromatic colour spaces of insects and of birds both became filled, as far as physically and chemically possible on the part of the plants, with floral colors in at least some ecological communities. Thus, for the flowers to assume distinctiveness to pollinators, a situation favored by natural selection because of the greater reliability and efficiency of intra-specific (constant) pollen transfer and so reproductive output by the plants, color shifts would be favored for flowers of some members of competing guilds of plants. This phenomenon may be thought of as character displacement and directional or disruptive selection (Kevan and Baker, 1984). This process would cause a filling of the color space for the guild of pollinators available. However, escape from that guild could occur if floral colors changed to embrace another color space of a different pollinator guild. Thus, flowers in the insect trichromatic color space could fill also the bird trichromatic color space by emphasising "red" (e.g., the larkspur, *Delphinium nudicaule*, Guerrant 1982).

The evolutionary obverse to the above concerns

visual systems. It is assumed here, for the purpose of floral and pollination biology, that trichromacy is the plesiomorphic condition (common original attribute) for both insects and birds. One may use analogous arguments to those presented for floral colors, and as expressed by Wallace, to suggest that flower foragers with greater abilities to discriminate colors would be able to forage more efficiently. This may be especially important to flower and fruit-feeding animals which have high energy requirements and other activities to which to attend (e.g., birds and butterflies in mate-finding, courtship, territoriality, predator avoidance, etc.). Thus, tetrachromatic color vision systems might be favored if they allow for ready discrimination of colored objects also of interest to potentially competing trichromatic organisms, such as other insects or other birds (see 9.8).

9.2 Palaeontological Record

It is likely that even the first metazoan (multicellular) animals of late Proterozoic or Precambrian time (ca. 600 Million years ago), mostly Cnidaria-like (jellyfish and their relatives) (Norris, 1989; Seilander, 1989) were able to distinguish photic signals of different wavelengths. Image processing and possibly color vision must have originated somewhat later with the first animals with complex eyes perhaps early in Cambrian time (ca. 570 Million years ago). By mid-Cambrian there existed an astounding diversity of invertebrates (Gould, 1989), including arthropods (the Phylum of animals including centipedes, millipedes, insects, crustacea, spiders, mites, scorpions, and others, especially the now extinct Trilobites with sophisticated compound eyes (Levi-Setti, 1993)) had become common. Although it is unknown whether or not these ancient animals had color vision, it is known that compound eyes are well constructed for separating photic stimuli of differing wavelengths, as in modern day arthropods (Menzel, 1979). Evidence for the antiquity for arthropods' being able to distinguish lights of different wavelengths may be inferred from Cambrian times when the Mandibulata (modern examples being Crustacea and Insecta) and Chelicerata (modern examples being horse-shoe crabs, spiders, and scorpions) were already evolutionarily separated. Both major groups have peaks of sensitivity in the ultraviolet and green parts of the spectrum, and the mandibulates also in the blue (Menzel, 1979; Menzel and Backhaus, 1991; Chittka, 1996).

Camera eyes, as in chordates (cartilaginous and bony fish) and cephalopods (nautiloids and their relatives) are represented in late Cambrian and Ordovician (ca. 500 million years ago) times and may also have had capabilities in color vision. There is no reason to assume achromacy because these organisms were restricted to marine habitats. Light in the visual spectrum (from ultraviolet to red, ca. 360 nm to 750 nm) penetrates well into sea water (Morel, 1974; Kishino, 1994) even though local conditions create much variability in the underwater photic environment (Munz and McFarland, 1975). Even so, the evolution of color vision may have come later. It is difficult to know how bottom dwelling organisms, such as the earliest fish and arthropods would benefit from color vision. Indeed, McFarland and Munz (1975) have argued that color vision in fish arose in the Silurian (ca. 418 million years ago) and was favored by free-swimming habits which required greater optical appreciation of surroundings. The argument can be extended to embrace invertebrates, in particular, arthropods. The free-swimming cephalopods of today do not seem to have color vision (Wells, 1978; Menzel, 1979), a paradox considering how colorful these animals can be, and how they can change color to match their substrates or even when threatened.

During Ordovician time (to about 430 million years ago) the diversity of life in the sea expanded greatly and most modern Phyla (major taxonomic units of organisms sharing fundamental patterns of organization and a common descent) are represented in the fossil record. Throughout the early history of life on earth, oxygen must have been produced by photosynthetic unicells and plants (Cloud, 1978, Schopf, 1983) and was in sufficient quantities in the seas to support animal respiration by early Cambrian time. However, up until Silurian time the atmosphere is believed to have contained slowly increasing, but perhaps little free oxygen (Robinson, 1991). At about that time, though, the photic environment of the earth must have changed greatly as oxygen built up in the atmosphere (Birkner and Marshall, 1965; Cloud, 1978; Robinson, 1991), being produced by plants too rapidly to be precipitated from the seas by oxygen fixing microbes and removed from the atmosphere by biotic and physical oxidative processes (Garrels et al., 1976; Robinson, 1991). Robinson (1991) suggests that oxygen levels rose to over 30% of the atmosphere into the Carboniferous, about 300 Million years ago. The prime consequences were that short-wave ultraviolet light reaching the earth's surface from the sun was attenuated as the atmosphere became oxygenated. Protected from ultraviolet radiation in an oxygenated atmosphere, aerobic organisms could become terrestrial. From that time, we assume that levels of oxygen and ozone have remained more or less in stasis, being in balance with carbon dioxide through photosynthesis, respiration, and bio-physical-chemical processes of oxidation after the Carboniferous (Garrels et al., 1976; Robinson, 1991). The spectral quality of daylight (Fig. 9.1) has remained more or less the same (see Henderson, 1977) and color vision accords with it.

9.3 Daylight and Color Vision

In general, within visual spectra, "ultraviolet" is the least represented (has the lowest intensity), and "blue" the most. A useful standard based on daylight measurements is the normlight function D65 (because of the related color temperature of a black body radiator of about 6,500 K; see e.g., Wyszecki and Stiles, 1982). That standard is a close approximation of daylight and so is ecologically relevant despite the attenuation of ultraviolet by various natural fluctuations in the atmosphere which are expected to effect the quality of natural light throughout the day, under cloud, in shade, and so on. Daylight is often described in terms of relative power across the spectrum (e.g., Henderson, 1977), but for color vision, it is the quantum emissions at each wavelength that matter.

Because the energy of a quantum of light is inversely proportional to its wavelength, the conversion is simple. Figure 9.1 presents the quantum flux of representative daylight.

In terrestrial arthropods, the relative sensitivities of the different spectral classes of photoreceptors are proportional to the inverse of the adaptation light. Thus in honeybees and other species of insects for dark as well as for daylight adapted eyes, sensitivity to ultraviolet is about 4–6- or more-fold that to other parts of the spectrum (Daumer, 1956; Kevan, 1970, 1978, 1983; v. Helversen, 1972; Laughlin, 1976; Menzel, 1979; Backhaus and Menzel, 1987; Menzel and Backhaus, 1991). This effect is especially manifest in the attractiveness of ultraviolet light in insect phototaxis (Kevan, 1979a; Menzel, 1979). It has been suggested that the high level of responsiveness to ultraviolet light reflects the insects' taking it as indicating the open environment in escaping enclosures (Laughlin, 1976).

Many vertebrates are insensitive to ultraviolet light, which is filtered from the retina by the optical humours, pigments and the lens. The relative sensitivities of the three types of cone cells in many vertebrates, and by which light appears blue, green, and red for us, are quite similar (Thompson 1995; Neitz and Neitz, see chapter 5) by comparison with rather more separated and discrete sensitivity curves in the photoreceptors, "ultraviolet", "blue" and "green", of many arthropods (Menzel, 1979). Some arthropods have an additional photoreceptor for red (long-wave) light (e.g., some bees (Hymenoptera), Menzel, 1990; Menzel and Backhaus, 1991) or even up to two additional photoreceptors (e.g., butterflies (Lepidoptera), Arikawa et al., 1987). Some vertebrates (e.g., various fish, Bowmaker and Kunz, 1987; Neumeyer, 1985), amphibia and reptiles (Neumeyer, see chapter 8, birds; Goldsmith, 1980; Bowmaker, 1980; Bennett et al., 1996, rodents; Jacobs et al., 1991) have an additional ultraviolet sensitivity (see Goldsmith, 1991; Jacobs, 1992). The full and ultimate reasons for tetrachromacy (Goldsmith, 1990, 1994; Neumeyer, 1991; Bennett and Cuthill, 1994; Thompson, 1995) are not ecologically understood, but presumably are important in the lives of these animals (cf. Wallace, 1878, 1891).

9. Color Vision: Ecology and Evolution in Making the Best of the Photic Environment

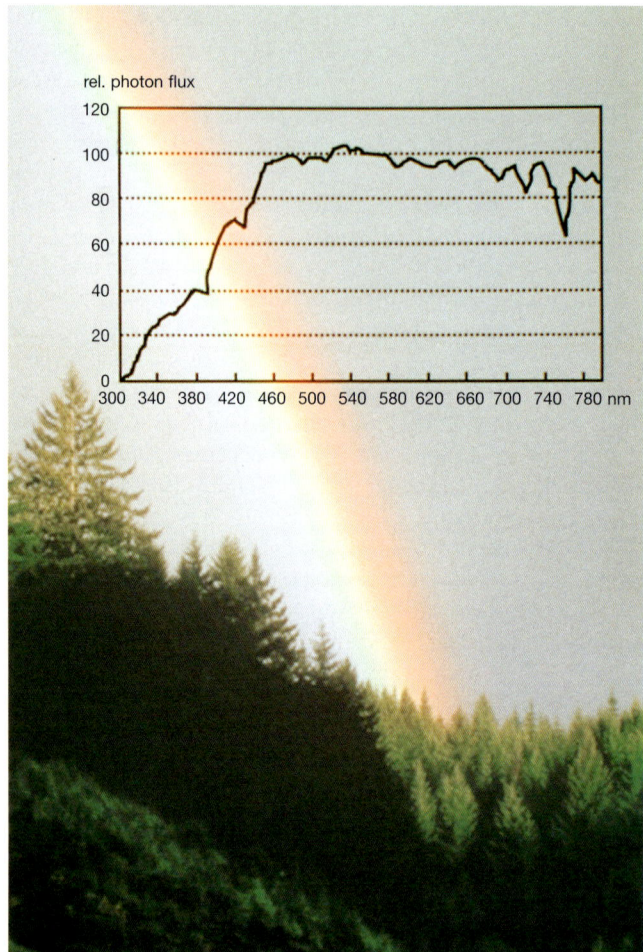

Fig. 9.1: Daylight and its spectrum (normalight D65) in terms of the relative quantum flux (see Henderson 1977).

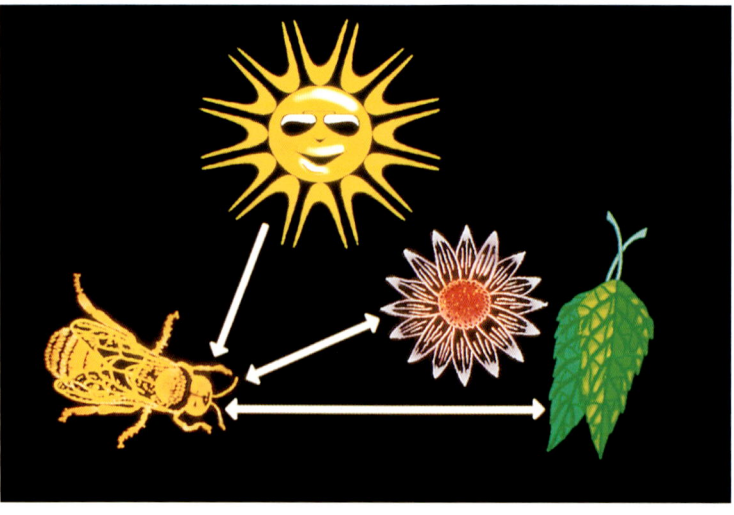

Fig. 9.2: Components of illumination, the photic environment, and color vision. Daylight is reflected from vegetation (a background) and from objects of interest to animals with color vision (a flower to a bee) and is perceived by the animal. Color vision and color discrimination involves integration of all components of the photic environment (see also Kevan, 1975, 1983; Menzel, 1990).

Noteworthy is the fact that the flowers which provide nectar to butterflies are often especially reflective in the red part of the spectrum (Müller, 1883; Proctor and Yeo, 1973) *vis à vis* flowers that attract the attention of trichromatic insects. Fruits sought after by tetrachromatic birds reflect ultraviolet (Burkhardt, 1982).

9.4 Colorimetry

The measurement of light reflected by objects of importance to animals must be made according to their spectral sensitivities and the natural photic environments in which they live. Thus, and because UV light is depauperate in natural lights (Fig. 9.1), one can not use, for example, CIE definitions for the human eye of "white" when discussing insect color vision and colorimetry. The definition of a "white looking surface" as having equiproportionate reflectance across the light spectrum of the illuminant (e.g., daylight) visible to the sensor in question, and that of a "colored looking surface" as reflecting only certain parts of this spectrum, has served well in an ecological context. This allows for simple representations of colors as dots in color triangles representing the light intensities reflected by the respective surfaces (Daumer, 1956; Kevan 1972, 1978, 1983). However, that system is rather too simple for accurate denotation of colors seen by the insects. Spectral sensitivity as well as the adaptation state of the photoreceptors has to be taken into account. Furthermore, it has been found that background reflectance surrounding the colored object and ambient light have profound influences on color discrimination in insects (Neumeyer, 1980, 1981; Backhaus and Menzel, 1987; Backhaus,1992a; Dittrich, 1995a,b). Thus, adaptation of the photoreceptors to background light and ambient light must be taken into account as well. Color-Opponent Coding (COC) as the neuronal mechanism for color vision in honeybees (Kien and Menzel, 1977; Backhaus, 1991, 1993; Backhaus, see chapter 2) explains well their observed abilities and limitations in color discrimination. The COC color space is based on the interplay of the spectral intensity distribution of the photic environment (e.g., daylight), the spectral reflectance of the objects and the background, the transduction process as also responsible for adaptation, and the spectral sensitivities of the photoreceptors. This system seems to have wide applicability to insects, especially Hymenoptera (Backhaus and Menzel, 1987; Menzel and Backhaus, 1991; Peitsch et al., 1994).

When considering floral colors to trichromatic bees, the background reflectance of leaves or ground is dull and more or less uniform reaching from ultraviolet to yellow-green (Kevan, 1972, 1978, 1983; Chittka et al., 1994). Thus, neutral (grey) backgrounds can be used as approximations of natural ones in behavioral experiments (see Backhaus et al., 1987; Backhaus, 1992a; Dittrich, 1995a,b) and the COC system can be used to predict the outcomes and explain the results of experiments in which honeybees are tested for their capabilities to discriminate colored targets from backgrounds and from each other (Backhaus, 1993; Giurfa et al., 1994, 1995, 1996).

In vertebrate color vision, the dimensions of brightness (lightness, dark to dazzling) and two chromaticness dimensions of colors (aspect of color different from brightness, German: Farbart, e.g., hue and saturation) are important components (Wyszecki and Stiles, 1982) of discrimination (Burnham et al., 1963; Thompson, 1995) and psychophysical measurement of colors (Wright, 1969) as is brought out in other chapters of this book. Because of the way spectral reflectance information is gathered and processed by the insect eye and brain, brightness is not used for color vision (only the two dimensions of chromaticness) even though it is in other behavioral contexts, in which the honeybee appears to be color blind (no chromaticness information used), as for example, in the case of natural phototaxis (open space response) when the bee is escaping from an enclosure (v. Hess, 1913) or when leaving the feeding place (Menzel and Greggers, 1985). Also in the case of optomotor or large field movement response (Kaiser and Liske, 1974; Kaiser et al., 1977) as well as in visual scanning behavior in front of vertical gratings and flight orientation towards horizontal and vertical gratings (Lehrer et al., 1985; Srinivasan and Lehrer, 1988), the bee also appears to be color blind. As in the case of color vision, the choice behavior is not mediated by a brightness system, to which all three photoreceptor spectral types would contribute, but exclusively by the green contrast coded in the green receptor. This is also the case for small object detection as has been shown now in experiments in which the decision point was fixed for the honeybees at certain distances to the targets. Also object detection depends in general on the color difference of the object from the background. Only if the objects are too small for color vision, object detection depends exclusively on the green contrast (Lehrer and Bischof, 1995; Giurfa et al., 1996). In the experiments by Giurfa et al. (1996) using a Y-maze with retractable back walls, vertically presented colored targets which had both color and green contrast (e.g., yellow or blue) with the background (grey) could be detected at minimum angle subtended at the eye of 5°, but when only color contrast was present (e.g., with brown) in the target against the background, the angle was about 15°. When green contrast and color contrast were both lacking (e.g., rose-pink), the bees failed to find the target.

From the foregoing it can be understood why it has been pointed out that the many studies in which ultraviolet reflections of flowers have been examined *in vacuo* are inadequate (Kevan, 1979b) because these provide information on only one photoreceptor to anthophilous (flower visiting) insects. The information content of such analyses is even less than those made using human perception of color which provides information on the other two photoreceptor spectral types combined. Data from both approaches are difficult to interpret ecologically and functionally. The value of appropriate trichromatic colorimetry for appreciation of color differences to animals with different systems of trichromacy has been emphasized by several scientists (Daumer, 1958; Kevan, 1972, 1978, 1983; Backhaus and Menzel, 1987; Backhaus, 1991, 1993; Menzel and Backhaus, 1991; Chittka and Menzel ,1992; Chittka et al., 1994; Menzel and Shmida, 1993; Kevan et al., 1996) and several graphical representations for different purposes were explored (see Backhaus, chapter 2).

9.5 Color Spaces

The color spaces used for insect vision have ranged from color wheels to various triangular forms. The COC color space provides for a physiologically adequate description of color vision by honeybees. It describes their neuronal color-opponent coding (COC) system and their color-choice behavior in training experiments as well as allowing for the derivation of subjective color differences by the city-block metric (Backhaus and Menzel, 1987; Backhaus et al., 1987, Backhaus, 1991; see Backhaus, chapter 2). Backhaus (1991) has developed recent approaches by allowing a precise means of plotting the loci of colors and of measuring distances between them by the city-block metric (Backhaus and Menzel, 1987, Backhaus et al., 1987; see Backhaus, chapter 2). The distances between color loci are measured by the same subjective scale (COC units) throughout the space, so eliminating the non-linearity of the distances between loci in different parts of triangles which represent colors by relative light intensities or relative photon fluxes absorbed in the three photoreceptor spectral types. Chittka (1992) has derived a trivariant color diagram with a Euclidean metric (color hexagon) from the COC color space for the honeybee, comparable to an earlier developed photoreceptor model of color vision (Backhaus and Menzel, 1987; Backhaus, 1992b; see Backhaus, chapter 2), with the aim to describe color vision of other insects (mostly bees, Peitsch et al., 1994). All color circles, triangles, and hexagons used are trivariant, i.e., are related to three photoreceptor spectral types (or primary lights). This provides for six broad color categories, the boundaries of which are defined by the dominant wavelengths of the primary lights used for light mixtures (e.g., Daumer 1956) or the maximum sensitivity of the photoreceptors, and the half-way (50%) boundaries inbetween (e.g., Backhaus and Menzel, 1987; Chittka, 1992; Menzel and Shmida, 1993; Fig. 9.3). Daumer (1956, 1958) referred to "UV-yellow" as "bee-purple", named by analogy to human color-naming because the color combines the shortest and longest wavebands of visible light for bees, *vis à vis* blue-red for human beings. Kevan (1972) extended and harmonized the analogy so that "yellow-green" was termed "insect-red", blue was "insect-green", and ultraviolet was "insect-blue". Chittka (1992) and Menzel and Shmida (1993) have used a symbolic color-naming system involving the letters, UV, B, G, etc. (Fig. 9.3). Most recently, Backhaus (see chapter 2) discusses five elementary color names based on the bee-subjective COC diagram: "UV", "violet", "green", "yellow", and achromatic "grey". Only one achromatic elementary color, "grey", is postulated because color vision of the bee has no brightness dimension, i.e., the bee does not discriminate "black" and "white" in color training experiments. As in the case of human color vision, intermediate colors can be described by a combination of the respective elementary colors, e.g., "yellow-green" or "UV-yellow" (bee-purple).

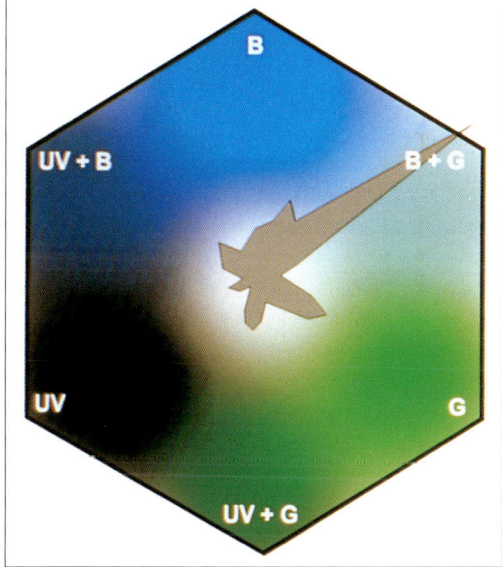

Fig. 9.3: A color hexagon (after Chittka, 1992) based on the color opponency space (Backhaus, see chapter 2), with ultraviolet depicted as black, blue as blue, and green (also yellow-green) as green (color classes are related to the spectral sensitivity of the three photoreceptor types, UV, B, G). Objects with equiproportionate reflectances in those three wavebands for trichromatic insects are neutrally colored (depicted as white) (see Kevan, 1975, 1983). The grey shape represents the relative numbers of floral colors in each color class (e.g., Blue + Green denoted as B + G) (for details see Chittka et al., 1994).

For general ecological and evolutionary discussion, the color names are used as designations and the form of the color space does not influence more general conclusions. For specific ecological and evolutionary analysis of colorimetric data (such as are needed to measure and understand the differences in colors of flowers, for example, as they age, in closely related species, in species competing for pollinators, in model and mimic pairs of species, and so on) accurate and precise measurements of reflectance spectra are required.

When using a simple triangle for plotting insect (bee) *versus* human trichromaticity coordinates of floral colors, the available color space is much fuller for the former. For human beings, many flowers have similar colors which cluster in the yellow, white, pink, and pale blue parts of the triangle. For insects, the individual loci for blossoms of different species within a community of flowering plants are more discrete and spread throughout the triangle except for the ultraviolet sector (Kevan, 1972, 1978, 1983) (Fig. 9.4a–d). This same trend has been shown for floral colors in a more general sense (Chittka et al., 1994) (Fig. 9.4e).

Further, it is worth noting that the greatest abundance and diversity of floral colors falls in the region where insects have the greatest abilities to distinguish between wavelengths of light, i.e., between about 360 and 520 nm (Menzel and Backhaus, 1991) with especially highly developed discriminability at about 400 nm and 500 nm (honeybee: v. Helverson, 1972; Menzel, 1979; Backhaus and Menzel, 1987; Menzel and Backhaus, 1991). The greatest abundance of flowers (33%) are colored in the blue-green part of the spectrum around 500 nm (Fig. 9.3 and 9.4) which corresponds to the waveband of greatest color discrimination in insects. The wavebands of highest discrimination correspond to those at which at least one of the photoreceptors shows greater changes in membrane potential per unit change in wavelength (Backhaus and Menzel, 1987; Backhaus, 1992b; Backhaus, see chapter 2). By analogy, one would expect that flowers which reflect light into one or two photoreceptor types at the most discriminated wavelengths, would have color loci in those color categories with the greatest degrees of discriminability for small variations within them.

170   9. Color Vision: Ecology and Evolution in Making the Best of the Photic Environment

The color space for human beings, and other trichromatic vertebrates, is also well described by a triangular diagram, even though lightness adds an additional dimension to produce a color solid (see Wright, 1969; Wyszecki and Styles, 1982). The problem with representation of tetrachromatic spaces is clear. It is simpler for insects for which brightness is not a factor in color vision (i.e., the tetrachromatic color space is three dimensional in this case (see Menzel and Backhaus, 1991), but has added complexity for vertebrates for which it is fourdimensional (Thompson et al., 1992; Thompson, 1995; Neumeyer, see chapter 8). We have made no attempt to illustrate tetrachromatic color spaces, except through stacking of the two trichromatic spaces represented only as simple triangles or hexagons (see Fig. 9.6a, b).

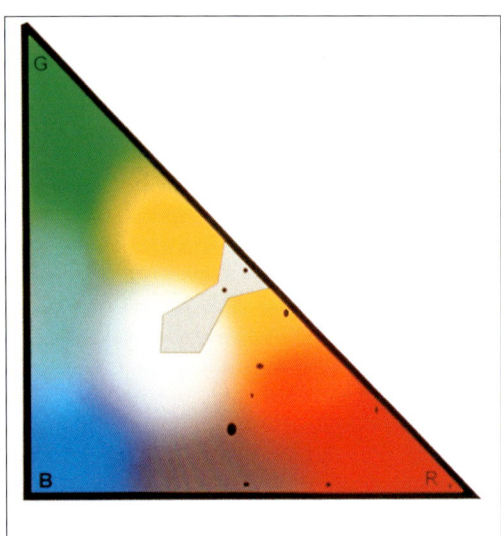

a

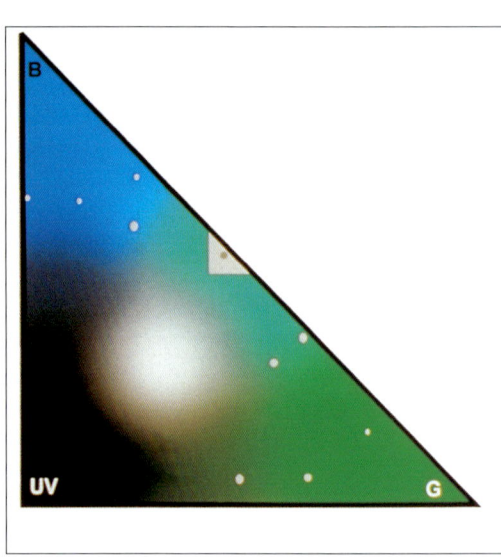

b

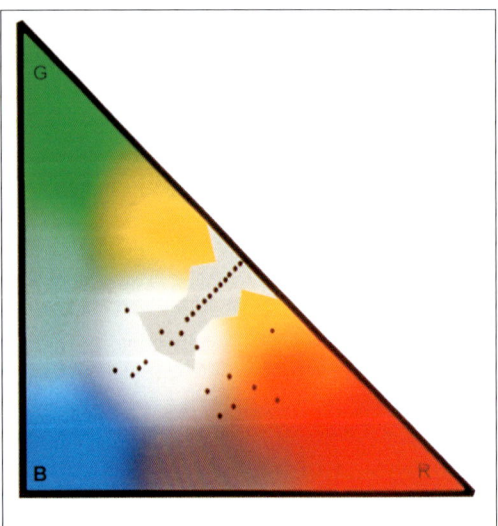

c

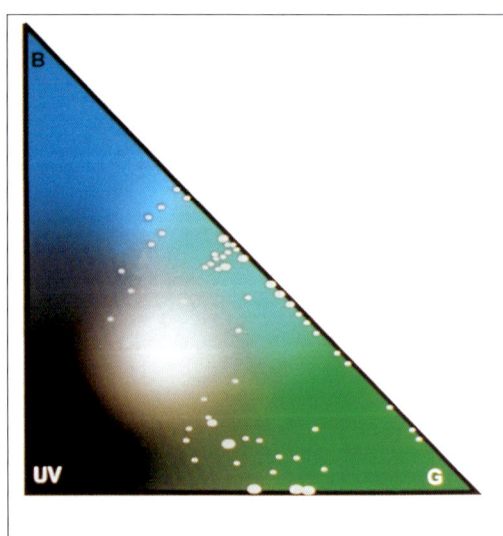

d

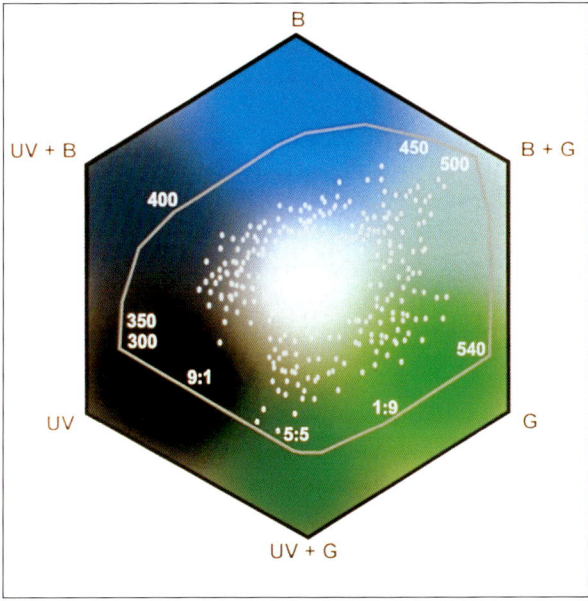

e

Fig. 9.4: The diversity of floral colors presented in a simple triangular trichromatic color space with respect to human and insect color vision. **a, b** are for flowers of the Canadian High Arctic (from Kevan, 1970, 1972) and **c, d** are for flowers of the weedy flora of Eastern North America (from Mulligan and Kevan, 1973). Spots indicate, by their size, the color loci of flowers of one, two, or three species of plants. The shapes indicate, by their widths, the numbers of species of plants with flowers having a color locus along the center line of the shape. The greater diversity and discreteness of the colors in the insect's color space *vis à vis* the human color space is clear, as is the greater area of the space occupied by floral colors for insects. **e** shows the diversity and discreteness of the floral colors examined by Chittka et al. (1994). In all spaces, the center is the point of equiproportionate reflectance in the appropriate wavebands for color vision in insects and human beings. For insects, natural backgrounds (soil, vegetation, etc.) tend to fall at the center of the space (Kevan, 1972; Mulligan and Kevan, 1973; Chittka et al., 1994). The paucity of loci in the ultraviolet sectors of the insect's color spaces is noteworthy and discussed in the text.

9.6 Evolution of Floral Colors and Color Vision

All in all, studies of ecological assemblages of floral colors have shown that the individual floral colors are more distinctive to insects than they are to human beings, a characteristic which would offset constraints caused by the former's lesser visual acuity (Kevan, 1978, 1983; Chittka et al., 1994; Dafni et al., 1997). Extending those ecological community findings, one may surmise that, throughout evolutionary time, the color space for insects has become more and more filled with floral colors according to the model of Kevan and Baker (1984). That model presents the interplay of competition of plants for pollinators and flower visitors for floral resources with the mutualistic benefits for both partners in the relationships. The model predicts increasing specialization of both partners though co-evolutionary processes involving character displacement (e.g., divergence in colors of flowers of two taxa of plants) and greater reliability in foraging by pollinators and gene flow for plants. The greater the pollinators' abilities to discriminate between flowers, the greater the probability of their finding resources and the more likely it is that intra-specific pollen flow results;

i.e., the Darwinian advantage of floral constancy would operate. Floral constancy is the tendency of pollinators to visit flowers of the same species of plant during a foraging trip (Thompson, 1983) and abets reproductive success of both pollinators (through greater efficiency in foraging) and their plants (through more, and more reliable, intraspecific pollen flow) (Waddington, 1983; Nuboer, 1986).

The ecological relationships between color vison systems of pollinating insects and spectral properties of flowers are subject to ongoing investigations by population genetical simulations, based on the models of the neuronal color-opponent coding (COC) system and the color choice behavior of the honeybee and a model of spectral reflectance of flowers (Backhaus and Breyer, 1995; Backhaus et al., 1996; Pielot and Backhaus, 1996; Pielot et al., in prep.). It turned out in these simulations that mutation of the physiological parameters and selection of the fittest individuals results in a dynamical system which is indeed self-optimizing because of the reciprocal adaptation, i.e., the parameters of both systems are best possibly tuned to each other. Nevertheless, the individual parameters do not reach stable end-states, but fluctuate finally without selection pressure, whereby both the systems remain constantly well adapted (best fitness) to each other. These results show up evolutionary possibilities under the most restrictive constraints of co-adaptation between pollinators and plants. Whether one of these possibilties has indeed been realized by the evolution which actually took place, has to be further investigated.

Therefore, it is interesting to step back to the evolution of angiosperms (flowering plants) and pollinators. Kevan et al. (1975) suggested that even some of the earliest terrestrial arthropods of Devonian time (about 360 Million years ago) visited sporangia of early vascular plants to feed. The sporangia of extant club-mosses and horestails are often colored differently (pale to yellow) from the vegetative parts of the plants. Spores of Carboniferous plants have been found on the bodies (mouthparts and thoraces) of some of the huge fossil insects of the time (Kukalova-Peck, personal communication). The earliest fossil bees are of Triassic age (about 200 Million years ago) (Hasiotis et al., 1995) and appear to predate the first definitive flowering plants of Cretaceous time (about 100 Million years ago). Moreover, it has been suggested that among the earlier Mesozoic Cycadoidea (primitive trees resembling some palms) were species which produced flower-like structures which attracted spore dispersing insects (Leppik, 1960). Their colors are not known but many extant cycads have sporangia which are pale in color and rely on insects to disperse microspores of one plant to the megaspores of another and so promote fertilization (Farrera, personal communication).

Spore dispersal by insects, as considered above, is not true pollination because such microspores are not multicellular (microgametophytes), as are pollen grains. Nevertheless, the fauna which thrived before the true flowering plants probably had behaviors functional later in true pollination already entrenched (Kevan and Baker, 1983). Indeed, Labandeira and Sepkowski (1993) indicate that the evolution of flowering plants had no influence on the diversification of insect families and feeding types. It is generally thought that the earliest pollinators associated with the earliest flowers were beetles (Coleoptera), flies (Diptera) and possibly bees and that the flowers were achlorophyllous (lacking chlorophyll) and so were probably yellowish-white (as in etiolated vegetation growing in the dark) (Willemstein, 1987). Floral scent, rather than color, may have been the more important floral cue to pollinators. Such flowers would likely have had strong green contrast against the vegetation, as well as color contrast through ultraviolet absorption. Osche (1983) suggested that yellow pigmented anthers and pollen optically signalled foraging pollinators to food, primarily pollen, in early angiosperms. Through evolutionary time, some pigments presumably became more concentrated in the reproductive structures and intensified their colors and green contrast with respect to the vegetation. It is worth noting that these pigments probably arose as protective pigments for photosynthesis (Demmig-Adams and Adams, 1996) or for chromosomes, or both. Carotenoids, with colors ranging from pale (xanthophylls) to intense yellow (carotenes) in intracellular plastids, were probably accompanied by flavonoids (anthocyanins,

Fig. 9.5: Composite and semi-diagramatic representation of the spectrally relevant components of flowers. The large white arrow represents incoming natural light (daylight) and the four differently colored arrows represent reflections in the four wavebands of light comprising trichromacy for insects (arrows: ultraviolet = black, blue, and green) and for human beings (arrows: blue, green, and red) and for tetrachromacy (all four arrows). Zone A represents green vegetation with green chloroplasts, the organelles containing chlorophyll, in the cells' cytoplasm (depicted as pale green). On the underside of the leaf, the closable stomata, which allow for gas exchange with the atmosphere, are presented. Zone B represents etiolated vegetation with few chloroplasts and many yellow chromoplasts. Zone C represents vegetation which appears silvery white because of the large air spaces between the cells beneath the epidermis. Zone D demonstrates the way in which the bright shiny yellow (plus ultraviolet) color of buttercups are generated from reflections from the oil rich epidermal cells underlain with cells rich in reflective starch granules (white). Zone E represents the common situation for yellow flowers which absorb blue light and, often ultraviolet (*) by flavonoids, but reflect other wavebands by the carotinoids. Zones F and G are similar to Zone E, except that physical structures, here epidermal papillae, are also involved in reflection and refraction of light, including ultraviolet (F) or not (G). Zone H represents the effects of chromoplasts with orange and red reflecting pigments (carotenoids). Zones I, J and K represent the colors of petals influenced by anthocyanins dissolved throughout the cytoplasm. These may cause blue (I), purple to mauve and rose (J), to red (K) colors of flowers, but without reflecting ultraviolet unless special structures are also present (as in Zone F). Zone L represents white colored flowers, with cytoplasmic pigments (anthoxanthins) which do not reflect ultraviolet. Zone M represents translucency in petals.

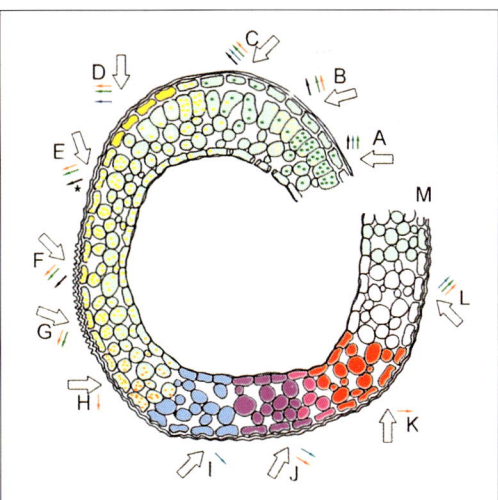

anthochlors, and flavonols) in cytoplasmic vacuoles. Combinations of these, and minor chemical changes in them, have allowed for the versatility of absorptions and reflections of natural light (see Fig. 9.5). The anthocyanins are particularly interesting as they allow for blue and red colors (Scogin, 1983; Guerrant, 1982).

The color space, one can imagine, would have become increasingly occupied by colors of reproductive structures and of floral colors radiating from pale yellow to bright yellow and, by changes in the types of anthocyanins and their chemical make-up, to blues as diversification of the flora dependent on insects for pollination or spore transfer took place and the fauna co-evolved and diversified as well.

The anthocyanins and carotenes also allow for coloration in red, which is considered to be an advanced floral trait by botanists. Red sensitivity is known in a variety of insects, including butterflies and bees (see above). Flowers looking reddish to human beings are associated mainly with pollination by butterflies and birds (Faegri and van der Pijl, 1978). Both groups, as well as bees, are considered to be evolutionarily advanced. Thus, from the color space associated with trichromatic insects, the color space for tetrachromatic insects, and later birds, could also become occupied by loci of floral colors through co-evolutionary mutualistic diversification.

Recently, Chittka (1996) posed the question "Does bee color vision predate the evolution of flower color?" His answer, not surprisingly, given the information above, is that this is most likely the case. The color vision systems of arthropods appear to be conservative because the investigated taxa show only smaller fluctuations of the spectral positions of the ultraviolet and blue maximum sensitivity. However, some special cases seem to

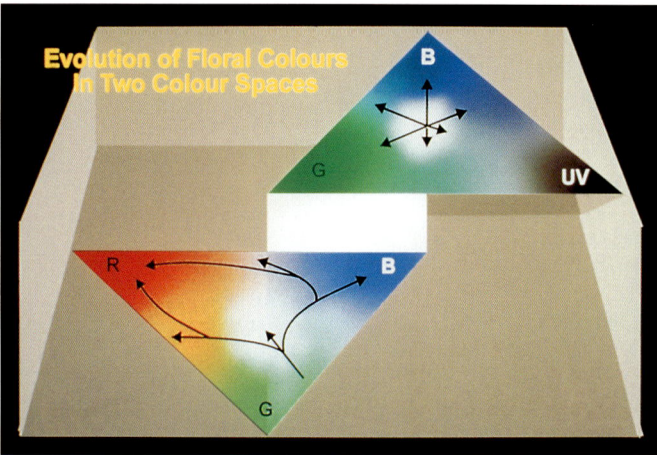

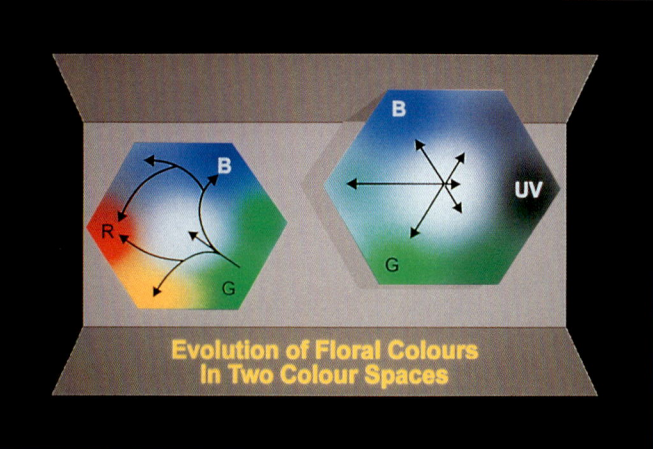

Fig. 9.6: The evolution of floral colors in two trichromatic color spaces (ultraviolet, blue, green; blue, green, red) presented in a triangle a) and in a hexagon b). It is supposed that the original color contrast for the reproductive parts of plants against the green vegetation came about by yellowing (etiolation) and emphasis of reflectance from yellow, carotenoid, pigments. Thus, chromatic and green contrast would arise, making the parts highly visible to insects. The evolutionary trend in the higher placed space of both a) and b) radiates from the neutrally colored center to the periphery in the direction of the green receptor's sensitivity. Many plants also contain anthocyanic pigments in the protoplast of leaf cells. These tend to be bluish. Thus, in the absence of chlorophyll, a trend in coloration into the blue-green area is indicated. Many flowers in this part of the insect's color space appear white to human beings. Flowers lacking carotenoid pigments, but with anthocyanins (flavonoids), also evolved and entered the blue part of the color spaces. Generally, it is considered that yellow is a relatively unspecialized floral color but blue is advanced (see Kevan, 1983). Ultraviolet is absorbed by flavonoids and its reflection is caused mostly by physical properties of floral cells. Thus, the interplay of physical and chemical characteristics allows for a wide diversity of floral colors, with constraints in ultraviolet reflective properties (see Fig. 9.4). The ultraviolet part of the spaces are not well occupied by color loci, although ultraviolet absorbing parts are. The major influence of ultraviolet in floral colors is in combination with yellow (i.e., in the waveband of the green receptor of insects' eyes) and have been termed bee- or insect-purple (Daumer, 1958, Kevan, 1972 et seq.).

It is assumed that vertebrate pollination arose from insect pollination. The main classes of floral pigments, carotenoids, and flavonoids, evolved to embrace red reflectances (e.g., Guerrant, 1982) as presented in the

exist in addition, for examples, those of the shorter wavelength peak for the ultraviolet receptor of the alpine bumble bee, *Bombus jonellus*, living in a bright and ultraviolet-rich environment versus the reverse shift in *Mellipona quadrifasciata* which lives beneath the canopy of tropical forests (Menzel, 1990). The green receptor shows some consistent difference between higher taxa, and bees have the maximum sensitivity for the green receptor shifted at least about +10 nm to 530–556 nm. Chittka (1996) rejects the hypothesis that insect photoreceptors are "tuned to code for particular objects, such as flowers in the case of bees," but in an earlier paper (Chittka et al., 1993) he points out that the system of color vision in bees is optimal for the detection of floral colors. The shift in peak sensitivity of the long waveband sensor to longer wavelengths merits consideration and cannot be dismissed because other possibly non-anthophilous insects related to bees share the feature as probably pleisiomorphic. Examination of the spectral reflectance curves of a large diversity of flowers (Chittka et al., 1994) reveals that peak sensitivity at 520 nm corresponds to about half the maximum spectral reflectance from yellow flowers. A peak sensitivity of 535 nm, however, corresponds closely to the asymptotic (maximum) level of reflectance. That has important consequences for perception of green contrast and for color discrimination, especially with ultraviolet mixtures as in "bee- or insect-purple" (Daumer, 1958; Kevan, 1983) or UV+G-B (Menzel and Shmida, 1983; Chittka et al., 1994) flowers. Tuning of the spectral receptor arrays in relation to behavioral ecology in foraging and mate recognition has been proposed for butterflies (*Lycaena* spp.) (Bernard and Remington, 1991).

Although ultraviolet reflections from flowers would impart especially discriminable colors to them, the paucity of flowers which actually reflect in the ultraviolet sectors of the color spaces (Fig. 9.3 and 9.4) suggests that there is general difficulty of synthesizing pigments, or producing structures, that do reflect it. The flowers that reflect ultraviolet (mostly yellow, blue and red, Chittka et al., 1994; Kevan et al., 1996) do so by specialized epidermal structures (Kugler, 1963) rather than pigments. Almost no white (to human beings) flowers reflect ultraviolet. This may be an evolutionary consequence of the fact that such flowers would be colorimetrically dysfunctional by their chromatic similarity to their darker backgrounds, showing only brightness contrast, and so would be difficult for insects to detect (Kevan et al., 1996) coupled with possible physico-chemico problems in ultraviolet reflection (see above). As an aside, it is worth noting that variability in the long-waveband receptors is also greater than in the short and medium wavebands in vertebrates. This may be related to foraging (color vision), escape (phototaxis), and object recognition (green receptors) in general (see Thompson, 1995).

9.7 Color Patterns in Flowers

Kevan (1983) has pointed out that the color patterns in flowers, often called nectar guides because they are involved in the orientation of pollinators to nectar rewards (as well as to pollen and the reproductive structures) within the flowers, seem to follow some general rules (Kevan, 1983; Dafni and Kevan, 1996). It seems that the shorter wavelengths of light are reflected from the periphery, or background color of the petals. Thus, some blue-reflecting (including pinky-purple and white) flowers have yellow centers (as in forget-me-nots) and yellow flowers that reflect ultraviolet do so from the outer ring of color. Lunau (1992, 1993)

---

lower placed spaces. The paths for the evolution of floral colorations with respect to trichromacy in vertebrates branch from the green area (vegetation), but, and more importantly as implied by the descending grey wall linking the triangular spaces (too difficult to present within both diagrams a) and b), branch from the floral colors in the green and blue parts of both spaces into the red. Thus, flowers which stimulated insects' blue and green receptors have evolved convergently and stimulate the red receptor of vertebrates (e.g., hummingbirds) and some insects (e.g., butterflies). Red, as a floral color, is considered to be highly advanced. Tetrachromacy can take advantage of the combined trichromatic spaces.

has suggested that pollinators (namely bumblebees, *Bombus* spp.) innately respond to increasing color purity in moving centripetally on approach to and on flowers. However, there is more to the story than meets the eye.

As has been pointed out, the vegetation or other backgrounds against which flowers bloom are more or less neutrally colored in the insects' color spaces, so that most floral colors are of greater purity than the background. In addition, to the fact that producing ultraviolet reflecting structures and pigments is difficult for plants to produce (see above), Kevan et al. (1996) have argued that the rarity of "insect-white" flowers has to do with the fact that brightness is not perceived in color discrimination by insects (Backhaus, 1991) so that insect-white flowers are not especially chromatically different from a gray background and would not be perceived through color discrimination. It is indeed very difficult if possible at all to train honeybees to learn to associate reward with insect-white targets on achromatic backgrounds (Hertz, 1937 a,b; Englander, 1941). Population genetical simulations of co-evolution of color vision systems of pollinating insects and spectral properties of flowers (see above) showed that no brightness systems develop during co-evolution, also in the case of polychromatic color vision systems (Pielot and Backhaus, 1997a).

The Color-Opponent Coding system of color vision has the interesting property of making any background color into a neutral standard against which the color of an object is viewed (see Backhaus, chapter 2 and Fig. 9.2). Thus, as a bee approaches a multicolored flower, it first sees the flower, in relation to the background, as a single color represented by the average effect (reflectance and area) of the colors present. Thus, a flower which is "yellow-ultraviolet" peripherally and "yellow" centrally would first appear as "yellow-ultraviolet", but more yellow that the periphery itself. Once the bee is close enough to, and looks long enough at the flower, the COC model predicts that the "yellow-ultraviolet" periphery becomes the background for the flower's smaller center and the chromatic difference between the center and the periphery is perceived. If that hypothesis is correct, it is possible for the center of the flower to be the same color as the vegetation because centripetally arranged chromatic differences would be preserved. Thus, colored flowers with greenish centers, of which there are many, might appear effectively colored and with nectar guides visible to insect visitors.

There is, however, the matter of the role of green contrast in profoundly affecting the size over which colored targets can be seen (Giurfa et al., 1996, and above). Thus, we hypothesize that finely dissected and small nectar guides have both green and color contrast against the background coloration of their petals, but nectar guides lacking green contrast would have to be large to be effective. That appears to be the case, but has still to be experimentally tested and a thorough survey of floral colorations must be made. There are many "yellow-ultraviolet" flowers which have "yellow-ultraviolet" reflecting nectar guides. These guides do not show green contrast with respect to "yellow-ultraviolet" and almost all are presented as large, bull's eye patterns or large patches (see Daumer, 1958; Kevan, 1972; Mulligan and Kevan, 1973; Beidinger and Barthlott, 1993; Burr and Barthlott, 1993) rather than as discrete and fine radiating lines or small spots which are visible to human beings (e.g., "blue"-reflecting flowers with "yellow" and other colorated guides).

All that accords with the finding that both chromatic and green contrast are needed for greatest detectability. Anthers could act as signals only when presented against vegetation or specially colored bracts (see Osche, 1983). The ultraviolet patterns associated with some floral buds, which expose the back (abaxial) sides of petals prior to anthesis, could serve to camouflage them by causing a small average chromatic difference with the vegetational background and lack of green contrast (see example in Eisner et al., 1973).

Given all the constraints associated with floral coloration and insect vision, the combinations of colors for easy discrimination by insects are limited. The flower's average color must have both chromatic and green contrast against the general backdrop of the environment (which, by application of COC, is neutral), then the inner colors of the nectar guides on the flowers are similarly constrained for maximum effect, but large patterns lacking green contrast can be effective because the insect would be already on, or very close to, the flower by the time the chromatic difference could be discriminated. In the centres of open, bowl-shaped flowers, the pistils are often exposed and greenish, and chromatic contrast would suffice, especially with tactile (Kevan and Lane, 1985) and chemosensory (Lex, 1954; Bolwig, 1954; Dobson, 1987) cues available to the flower visitor. Thus, the explanation for the ordering of the arrangements of colors of nectar guides presented by Lunau (1992, 1993) can be better understood, not in terms of color purity *per se*, but in relation to the rules set forth by Kevan (1983; Dafni and Kevan, 1996).

9.8 Trichromacy and Tetrachromacy

A major advance in color vision capability must have come about through tetrachromacy and it must be assumed that Wallace's "necessity" (1878) applies. The issue of trichromacy and tetrachromacy also deserves mention because there appear to be some correlates with the breadth of the visual spectrum.

Trichromatic color vision spans daylight over about 300 nm and tetrachromacy spans an extra 100 nm. General constraints on the band widths of greatest sensitivity of the photoreceptors involved in color vision may be hypothesized, even though there is much overlap especially at wavelengths at which the receptors are less sensitive (Menzel and Backhaus, 1991 for insects; Neitz and Neitz, see chapter 5; Lee, see chapter 3). The nature of the photosensitive pigments and cellular function work in concert to make the greatest waveband-specific sensitivity of the photoreceptors mostly about 100–150 nm wide. That being the case, and that a standard shape of spectral sensitivity of photoreceptors (Dartnall, 1953; Ebrey and Honig, 1977; Maximov, 1988; Stavenga et al., 1993) can be used to approximate sensitivity functions, may be, at least with the help of additional optical devices as filtering pigments, colored lenses etc., that approximate sensitivity functions of about 50–70 nm bandwidth for 50% or better sensitivity can be derived. The similarities in spectral sensitivity functions for insects and other invertebrates are exemplified in extensive reviews (Menzel, 1979; Menzel and Backhaus, 1991). If the foregoing is valid, then the information gathered by spectrally overlapping sensors would be maximal for one sensor per ca. 100 nm. Vorobyev (in preparation) has calculated that for the ca. 300 nm bandwidth for color vision, color discriminability is much less for dichromats than for trichromats, but the addition of a fourth sensor produces only a small gain in color discriminability. For a ca. 400 nm bandwidth of color vision, trichromacy is much less effective in color discrimination than is tetrachromacy, but pentachromacy results in little relative improvement. Thus, even though pentachromacy has been reported in butterflies (Arikawa et al., 1987), it seems that the different trichromatic and similar tetrachromatic systems of color vision use the available daylight spectrum from ultraviolet to red each in their best possible way (for model calculations of wavelength discrimination of tri-, tetra-, and pentachromatic color vision systems (see Menzel and Backhaus, 1991; Goldsmith, 1994).

One may conjecture that the addition of other spectral sensors to improve color discrimination in existing systems of color vision would require the existing sensors to shift and become narrower. The amazing arrays of at least 11 sensors in mantis shrimps (Cronin and Marshall, 1989; Cronin et al., 1994) begs the question that returns us to the quotation from Wallace at the start What is it in the environment of these creatures that they need to discriminate so exactly to be competitive in the Darwinian sense? Predator detection and avoidance has been indicated as a role for the ultraviolet receptor in these shrimps (Cronin et al., 1994). Although this same question has been partially answered in regard to tetrachromacy and frugivory in birds and primates (Gauthier-Hion et al., 1985) and to flower visiting in some insects, the link between ecology and color discrimination in many tetrachromatic vertebrates remains to be investigated (see Bennett and Cuthill, 1994; Bennett et al., 1996; Neumeyer, see chapter 8). It may be that some of the spectral sensitivity maxima and associated cells do not have a role in image processing *per se*, but are related to wavelength specific behaviors and are not part of color vision (see Menzel and Backhaus, 1991; Goldsmith 1994). Population genetical simulations of co-evolution of polychromatic (six photoreceptors and five COC neurons) color vision systems of pollinating insects based on the COC model for the honeybee and spectral reflectance of flowers (see above) show indeed that the number of photoreceptor types tend to reduce to oligochromatic systems (Pielot and Backhaus, 1997b).

9.9 Conclusions

Palaeontological and phylogenetic evidence indicates that color vision has existed probably for at least half a billion years. The sorts of sensors that comprise color vision systems accord with the most energetic, uniform, and stable parts of the daylight spectrum from near ultraviolet to red (Henderson, 1977) and the range of spectral sensitivity maxima extends from 320 nm to 630 nm (Menzel, 1979). There appear to be some generalities with respect to the bandwidths over which spectral sensors operate so that they mostly have a half-band width of about 50–70 nm in which they show the highest sensitivity. The numbers of sensors (three or four) accord with requirements for greatest discriminability and fewest sensors.

Linking the fine-tuning of color vision and sensor types must be done with care and with the photic environment, reflectance of objects of interest, and of the backgrounds against which they appear, in mind. The question of why there are not more sensors, but with narrower band sensitivities, may be the effect of the nature of rather broad spectral reflectances from natural objects, such as vegetation, flowers, fruits, other animals, sky, and the ground. Presumably achromatic and dichromatic vision can be understood in terms of the lesser needs of animals with such vision in discriminating colors. The remarkable arrays in mantis shrimps (see above) (Cronin and Marshall, 1989) and tetrachromacy in many vertebrates are not yet understood in ecological terms (Bennett and Cuthill, 1994; Goldsmith, 1994; Thompson, 1995). Thus, although color vision systems mostly seem to make the best of natural photic environments and are attuned to the perception of a wide variety of objects of importance, and their backgrounds, the hypotheses that fall from all that provide a diverse landscape of research opportunities in physiology, genetics, neurobiology, behavior, ecology, evolution and philosophy as explanations for ultimate functionality are sought.

Acknowledgements

We thank Rainer Pielot for helpful comments on the manuscript. We extend special thanks to Sheila MacLeod for her extensive assistance in preparing the illustrations for this chapter. We gratefully acknowledge support from the Natural Sciences and Research Council of Canada (NSERC), the Deutscher Akademischer Austauschdienst (DAAD) to P. Kevan, and the Deutsche Forschungsgemeinschaft (DFG) to W. G. K. Backhaus. P. G. K. is most grateful to Prof. Randolf Menzel and his team for opportunity and encouragment given for research at FUB.

References

Arikawa, K., Inokuma, K., and Eguchi, E. 1987. Pentachromatic visual system in a butterfly. Naturwissenschaften *74*, 297–298.

Backhaus, W. 1991. Color opponent coding in the visual system of the bee. Vision Research *31*, 1381–1397.

Backhaus, W. 1992a. The Bezold-Brücke effect in the color vision system of the honeybee. Vis. Res. *32*, 1425–1431.

Backhaus, W. 1992b. Color vision in honeybees. Neuroscience and Biobehavioral Reviews *16*, 1–12.

Backhaus, W. 1993. Color vision and color choice behavior of the honey bee. Apidologie *24*, 309–331.

Backhaus, W. 1997. Color sensations in honeybees? In: John Dalton's Colour Vision Legacy. eds. C. Dickinson, I. Murray, and D. Carden, 567–589. Taylor & Francis, London.

Backhaus, W. and Breyer, J. 1995. Simulation of coevolution of color vision systems of pollinating insects and spectral reflectance of flowers. In: Proceedings of the 4th International Congress of Neuroethology, Cambridge, England, *276*. Thieme, Stuttgart.

Backhaus, W., Gerster, U., Buckow, H., Pielot, R., Breyer, J., and Becker, K. 1996. Physiological Simulations of Neuronal Color Coding in Honeybees. In: Bionet '96. Bio-Informatics and Pulspropagating Networks – Selected Contributions, 3rd Workshop November 14–15, 1996, Berlin, pp. 24–32., GFAI, Berlin.

Backhaus, W. and Menzel, R. 1987. Color distance derived from a receptor model for color vision in the honeybee. Biological Cybernetics *55*, 321–331.

Backhaus, W., Menzel, R., and Kreißl, S. 1987. Multidimensional scaling of color similarity in bees. Biological Cybernetics *56*, 293–304.

Bennett, A. T. D. and Cuthill, I.C. 1994. Ultraviolet vision in birds: What is its function? Vision Research *34*, 1471–1478.

Bennett, A. T. D., Cuthill, I. C., Partridge, J. C., and Maier, E. J. 1996. Ultraviolet vision and mate choice in zebra finches. Nature *380*, 433–435.

Bernard, G. D. and Remington, C. L. 1991. Color vision in *Lycaena* butterflies: Spectral tuning of receptor arrays to behavioral ecology. Proceedings of the National Academy of Sciences U.S A. *88*, 2783–2787.

Berkner, L. V. and Marshall, L. C. 1965. On the origin and rise of oxygen concentration in the earth's atmosphere. Journal of Atmospheric Science *22*, 225–261.

Biedinger, N. and Barthlott, W. 1993. Untersuchungen der Ultraviolettreflexion von Angiospermenblüten I. Tropische und subtropische Pflanzenwelt *86*, 1–122.

Bolwig, N. 1954. The role of scent as a nectar guide for honey bees on flowers and an observation on the effect of colour on recruits. British Journal of Animal Behaviour *2*, 81–83.

Bowmaker, J. K. 1980. Birds see ultraviolet light. Nature *284*, 306.

Bowmaker, J. K. and Kunz, Y. W. 1987. Ultraviolet receptors, tetrachromatic colour vision and retinal mosaics in the brown trout (*Salmo trutta*): age dependent changes. Vision Research *27*, 2101–2108.

Burkhardt, D. 1982. Birds, berries, and UV: a note on some consequences of UV vision in birds. Naturwissenschaften *69*, 153–157.

Burkhardt, D. 1989. UV vision: a bird's eye view of feathers. Journal of Comparative Physiology *164*, 787–796.

Burkhardt, D. and Maier, E. 1989. The spectral sensitivity of a passerine bird is highest in the UV. Naturwissenschaften *76*, 82–83.

Burnham, R. W., Hanes, R. M., and Bartleson, J. C. 1963. Color: A guide to basic facts and concepts. John Wiley & Sons, New York and London. 249 pp.

Burr, B. and Barthlott, W. 1993. Untersuchungen zur Ultraviolettreflexion von Angiospermenblüten II. Magnoliidae, Ranunculidae, Hamamelididae, Caryophyllidae, Rosidae. Tropische und subtropische Pflanzenwelt *86*, 1–193.

Chittka, L. 1992. The colour hexagon: A chromaticity diagram based on excitations as a generalized representation of colour opponency. Journal of comparative Physiology A. *170*, 533–543.

Chittka, L. 1996. Does bee color vision predate the evolution of flower color? Naturwissenschaften *83*, 136–138.

Chittka, L. and Menzel, R. 1992. The evolutionary adaptation of flower colours and insect pollinators' colour vision. Journal of Comparative Physiology A. *171*, 171–181.

Chittka, L., Shmida, A., Troje, N., and Menzel, R. 1994. Ultraviolet as a component of flower reflections, and colour perception of Hymenoptera. Vision Research *34*, 1489–1508.

Chittka, L., Vorobyev, M., Shmida, A., and Menzel, R. 1993. Bee colour vision – the optimal system of the discrimination of colours with three spectral receptor types? In: K. Wiese, F. G. Gribakin, A. V. Popov, and G. Renninger (eds). Sensory Systems of Arthropods. Birkhauser Verlag, Basel, Switzerland. pp. 211–218.

Demming-Adams, B. and Adams, W. W. 1996. The role of xanthophyll cycle carotenoids in the protection of photosynthesis. Trends in Plant Science *1*, 21–26.

Cloud, P. 1978. Cosmos, Earth, and Man: A Short History of the Universe. Yale University Press, New Haven and London. 372 pp.

Cronin, T. W. and Marshall, N. J. 1989. Multiple spectral classes of photoreceptors in the retinas of gonodactyloid stomatopod crustaceans. Journal of Comparative Physiology A. *166*, 267–275.

Cronin, T. W., Marshall, N. J., Quinn, C. A., and King, C. A. 1994. Ultraviolet photoreception in mantis shrimp. Vision Research *34*, 1443–1449.

Dafni, A. and Kevan, P. G. 1996. Floral symmetry and nectar guides: ontogenetic constraints from floral development, colour pattern rules and functional significance. Botanical Journal of the Linnaean Society *120*, 371–377.

Dafni, A., Lehrer, M., and Kevan, P. G. 1997. Spatial flower parameters and insect spatial vision. Biological Reviews *72*, 239–282.

Dartnall, H. J. A. 1953. The interpretation of spectral sensitivity curves. British Medical Bulletin *9*, 24–30.

Daumer, K. 1956. Reizmetrische Untersuchungen des Farbensehens der Bienen. Zeitschrift für vergleichende Physiologie *38*, 413–478.

Daumer, K. 1958. Blumenfarben wie sie die Bienen sehen. Zeitschrift für vergleichende Physiologie *41*, 49–110.

Dittrich, M. 1995a. Time course of color induction in the honeybee. Journal of Comparative Physiology A. *177*, 207–217.

Dittrich, M. 1995b. A quantitative model of successive color induction in the honeybee. Journal of Comparative Physiology A. *177*, 219–234.

Dobson, H. E. M. 1994. Floral volatiles in insect biology. In: E. A. Bernays, ed. Insect-Plant Interactions, Volume 5, pp. 47–81. C.R.C. Press, Boca Raton.

Eisner, T., Eisner, M., and Aneshansley, D. 1973. Ultraviolet patterns on rear of flowers: basis of disparity of buds and blossoms. Proceedings of the National Academy of Sciences U.S.A. *70*, 1002–1004.

Engländer, H. 1941. Die Bedeutung der weißen Farbe für die Orientierung der Bienen am Stand. Archiv für Bienenkunde *22*, 516–549.

Faegri, K. and van der Pijl, L. 1978. The Principles of Pollination Ecology (3rd rev. ed.). Pergamon Press, Oxford, New York, etc.

Garrels, R. M., Lerman, A., and Mackenzie, F. T. 1976. Controls of atmospheric O_2 and CO_2: Past, present, and future. American Scientist *64*, 306–315.

Gautier-Hion, A., Duplantier, J.-M., Quris, R., Feer, F., Sourd, C., Decoux, J.-P., Dubost, G., Emmons, L., Erard, C., Hecketsweiler, P., Moungazi, A., Roussilhon, C., and Thiollay, J.-M. 1985. Fruit characters as a basis for fruit choice and seed dispersal in a tropical forest vertebrate community. Oecologia *65*, 324–337.

Giurfa, M., Nuñjes, J.A., and Backhaus, W. 1994. Odour and colour information in the foraging choice behaviour of the honeybee. Journal of Comparative Physiology A. *175*, 773–779.

Giurfa, M., Backhaus, W., and Menzel, R. 1995. Colour and angular orientation in the discrimination of bilateral symmetric patterns in the honeybee. Naturwissenschaften *82*, 198–201.

Giurfa, M., Vorobyev, M., Kevan, P. G., and Menzel, R. 1996. Detection of coloured stimuli by honeybees: minimum visual angles and receptor specific contrasts. Journal of Comparative Physiology A. *178*, 699–709.

Goldsmith, T. H. 1972. Invertebrate visual pigments. In: Dartnall H. J. A. (ed.) Photochemistry of Vision. Volume VII/1 Handbook of Sensory Physiology. Springer Verlag, Berlin, Heidelberg, New York. pp. 685–719.

Goldsmith, T. H. 1980. Hummingbirds see near ultraviolet light. Science *207*, 786.

Goldsmith, T. H. 1990. Optimization, constraint, and history in the evolution of eyes. Quarterly Review of Biology *65*, 281–322.

Goldsmith, T. H. 1994. Ultraviolet receptors and color vision: evolutionary implications and a dissonance of paradigms. Vision Research *34*, 1479–1487.

Gould, S. J. 1989. Wonderful Life: The Burgess Shale and the Nature of History. W. W. Norton, New York.

Guerrant, E. O. 1982. Neotenic evolution of *Delphinium nudicaule* (Ranunculaceae): a hummingbird-pollinated larkspur. Evolution *36*, 699–712.

Helversen, O. von 1972. Zur spektralen Unterschiedsempfindlichkeit der Honigbiene. Journal of Comparative Physiology *80*, 439–472.

Henderson, S. N. 1977. Daylight and its Spectrum (2nd ed.). John Wiley and Sons, New York.

Hertz, M. 1937a. Versuche über das Farbensystem der Bienen. Naturwissenschaften *25*, 492–493.

Hertz, M. 1937b. Beitrage zum Farbensinn und Formensinn der Biene. Zeischrift für vergleichende Physiologie *24*, 413–421.

Hess, V. von 1913. Experimentelle Untersuchungen über den angeblichen Farbensinn der Bienen. Zoologisches Jahrbuch (Physiologie) *34*, 81–106.

Jacobs, G. H. 1992. Ultraviolet vision in vertebrates. American Zoologist *32*, 544–554.

Jacobs, G. H., Neitz, J., and Deegan, J. F. H. 1991. Retinal receptors in rodents maximally sensitive to ultraviolet light. Nature *353*, 655–666.

Kaiser, W. and Liske, E. 1974. Optomotor reactions of stationary flying bees during stimulation with spectral light. Journal of Comparative Physiology A. *89*, 391–408.

Kaiser, W., Seidel, R., and Vollmar, J. 1977. Spectral sensitivities of behavioural patterns in honey bees. Journal of Comparative Physiology A. *122*, 27–44.

Kevan, P. G. 1970. High Arctic insect-flower relations: The inter-relationships of arthropods and flowers at Lake Hazen, Ellesmere Island, N. W. T.,

Canada. Ph. D. Dissertation, University of Alberta, Edmonton, Alberta, Canada.

Kevan, P. G. 1972. Floral colours in the High Arctic with reference to insect flower relations and pollination. Canadian Journal of Botany 50, 2289–2316.

Kevan, P. G. 1978. Floral coloration, its colorimetric analysis and significance in anthecology. In: Richards, A. J. (ed.) The Pollination of Flowers by Insects. Linnaean Society Symposium No. 6, pp. 51–78.

Kevan, P. G. 1979a. The spectral efficiency of phototaxis some High Arctic Diptera. Journal of Arctic and Alpine Research 11, 349–352.

Kevan, P. G. 1979b. Vegetation and floral colours revealed by ultraviolet light: Interpretational difficulties for functional significance. American Journal of Botany 66, 749–751.

Kevan, P. G. 1983. Floral colours through the insect eye: What they are and what they mean. In: C. E. Jones and R. J. Little (eds.) Handbook of Experimental Pollination Biology. Scientific and Academic Editions, Van Nostrand and Company, New York. Chapter 1, pp. 3–25.

Kevan, P. G. and Baker, H. G. 1983. Insects as flower visitors and pollinators. Annual Review of Entomology 28, 407–453.

Kevan, P. G. and Baker, H. G. 1984. Insects on flowers: Pollination and floral visitations. In: C. B. Huffaker and R. C. Rabb (eds.) Insect Ecology. J. Wiley and Sons, New York. Chapter 21, pp. 607–631.

Kevan, P. G., Chaloner, W. G., and Savile, D. B. O. 1975. Interrelationships of early terrestrial arthropods and plants. Palaeontology 18(A), 391–417.

Kevan, P. G., Giurfa, M., and Chittka, L. 1996. Why are there so many and so few white flowers. Trends in Plant Science 1, 280–284.

Kevan, P. G. and Lane, M. A. 1985. Flower petal microtexture is a tactile cue for bees. Proceedings of the National Academy of Sciences of the U.S.A. 82, 4750–4752.

Kien, J. and Menzel, R. 1977. Chromatic Properties of interneurons in the optic lobes of the bee. II. Narrow band and colour opponent neurons. J. Comp. Physiol. 113, 35–53.

Kishino, M. 1974. Interrelationships between light and phytoplankton in the sea. In: Ocean Optics (R. W. Spinrad, K. L. Carder, and M. J. Perry (eds)). Oxford University Press, Oxford and New York. pp. 73–92.

Kugler, H. 1963. UV-Musterungen auf Blüten und ihr Zustandekommen. Planta 59, 296–329.

Labandeira, C. C. and Sepkowski, J. J. Jr. 1993. Insect diversity in the fossil record. Science 261, 310–315.

Laughlin, S. B. 1976. The sensitivities of dragonfly photoreceptors and the voltage gain of transduction. Journal of Comparative Physiology 111, 221–247.

Lehrer, M., Wehner, R., and Srinivasan, M.V. 1985. Visual scanning behaviour in honeybees. Journal of Comparative Physiology A. 157, 405–415.

Leppik, E. E. 1960. Early evolution of flower types. Lloydia 23, 72–92.

Levi-Setti, R. 1993. Trilobites. The University of Chicago Press, Chicago and London. 342 pp.

Lex, T. 1954. Duftmal an Blüten. Zeitschrift für vergleichende Physiologie 36, 212–234.

Lunau, K. 1992. A new interpretation of flower guide coloration: absorbtion of ultraviolet enhances colour saturation. Plant Systematics and Evolution 181, 51–65.

Lunau, K. 1993. Interspecific diversity and uniformity of flower colour patterns as cues for learned discrimination and innate detection of flowers. Experientia 49, 1002–1010.

McFarland, W. N. and Munz, F. W. 1975. Part III: The evolution of photopic visual pigments in fishes. Vision Research 15, 1071–1080.

Menzel, R. 1979. Spectral sensitivity and colour vision in invertebrates. In: H. Autrum (ed.) Invertebrate Photoreceptors. Vol VII/6A Handbook of Sensory Physiology. Springer Verlag, Berlin, Heidelberg, New York. pp. 503–580.

Menzel, R. 1990. Color vision in flower visiting insects. Internationales Büro Forschungszentrum Jülich GmbH, Jülich, Germany. 16 pp.

Menzel, R. and Backhaus, W. 1991. Colour vision in insects. In: P. Gouras (ed.) Vision and Visual Dysfunction. The Perception of Colour. Macmillan Press, London. pp. 268–288.

Menzel, R. and Greggers, U. 1985. Natural phototaxis and its relationship to colour vision in honeybees. Journal of Comparative Physiology A. 141, 389–393.

Menzel, R. and Shmida, A. 1993. The ecology of flower colours and the natural colour vision of insect pollinators: The Israeli flora as a study case. Biological Reviews 68, 81–120.

Mollon, J. D. 1989. "Tho' she kneel'd in that place where they grow …" The uses and origins of primate colour vision. Journal of Experimental Biology 146, 21–38.

Morel, A. 1974. Optical properties of pure water and pure sea water. In: Optical Aspects of Oceanography (N. G. Jerlov and E. S. Nielson, eds). Academic Press, London and New York. pp. 1–24.

Mulligan, G. A. and Kevan, P. G. 1973. Color, brightness and other floral characteristics attracting insects to the blossoms of some Canadian weeds. Canadian Journal of Botany *51,* 1939–1952.

Müller, 1883. Die Befruchtung der Blumen durch Insekten und die gegenseitigen Anpassungen beider. Wilhelm Engelmann Verlag, Leipzig, 478 pp.

Munz, F. W. and McFarland, W. N. 1975. Evolutionary adaptations of fishes to the photic environment. In: Handbook of Sensory Physiology. Volume VII/5. The Visual System in Vertebrates. pp. 193–274.

Neumeyer, C. 1980. Simultaneous color contrast in the honeybee. Journal of Comparative Physiology A. *139,* 165–176.

Neumeyer, C. 1981. Chromatic adaptation in the honeybee: successive color contrast and color constancy. Journal of Comparative Physiology A. *144,* 543–553.

Neumeyer, C. 1985. An ultraviolet receptor as a fourth receptor type in goldfish colour vision. Naturwissenschaften *72,* 162–163.

Neumeyer, C. 1991. Evolution of colour vision. In: Cronley-Dillon, J. R. and R. L. Gregory (eds.) Evolution of the Eye and Visual Systems: Vision and Visual Dysfunction. Volume 2 pp. 284–305. Macmillan and Company, London.

Neumeyer, C. 1992. Tetrachromatic color vision in goldfish: Evidence from color mixing experiments. Journal of Comparative Physiology A. *171,* 639–649.

Norris, R. D. 1989. Cnidarian taphonomy and affinities of the Ediacara biota. Lethaia *22,* 381–393.

Nuboer, J. F. W. 1986. A comparative view of colour vision. Netherlands Journal of Zoology *36,* 344–380.

Osche, G. 1983. Optische Signale in der Coevolution von Pflanzen und Tier. Berichte Deutsche Botanische Gesellschaft *96,* 1–27.

Pielot, R. and Backhaus, W. 1996. Simulation of co-evolution of tri- and tetrachromatic color vision systems of pollinating insects and spectral reflectance of flowers. In: Brain and Evolution. Proceedings of the 24th Göttingen Neurobiology Conference, eds. N. Elsner & H.-U. Schnitzler, 320. Thieme, Stuttgart.

Pielot, R. and Backhaus, W. 1997a. Brightness coding does not develop in simulations of co-evolution of polychromatic color vision systems of insects and spectral reflectance of flowers. In: Neurobiology: From Membrane to Mind. Proceedings of the 25th Göttingen Neurobiology Conference, eds. H. Wässle and N.Elsner. Thieme, Stuttgart.

Pielot, R. and Backhaus, W. 1997b. Polychromatic color vision systems tend to reduce to oligochromatic systems in simulations of co-evolution of neuronal color coding in pollinating insects and spectral reflectance of flowers. Verhandlungen der Deutschen Zoologischen Gesellschaft. *90,* 310.

Peitsch, D., Fietz, A., Hertel, H., de Souza, J., Ventura, D. F., and Menzel, R. 1994. The spectral input systems of hymenopteran Insecta and their receptor-based colour vision. Journal of Comparative Physiology A. *170,* 23–40.

Polyak, S. 1957. The Vertebrate Visual System. Chicago University Press, Chicago.

Proctor, M. and Yeo, P. 1973. The Pollination of Flowers. Collins, London. 418 pp.

Robinson, J. M. 1991. Phanerozoic atmospheric reconstruction: a terrestrial perspective. Palaeogeography, Palaeoclimatology, Palaeoecology *97,* 51–62.

Schopf, J. W. (ed.) 1983. Earth's Earliest Biosphere: Its Origin and Evolution. Princeton University Press, Princeton, N. J. 543 pp.

Scogin, R. 1983. Visible floral pigments and pollination. In: C. E. Jones and R. J. Little (eds.) Handbook of Experimental Pollination Biology. Scientific and Academic Editions, Van Nostrand and Company, New York. Chapter 7, pp. 160–172.

Seilander, A. 1989. Vendozoa: organismic construction in the Proterozoic biosphere. Lethaia *22,* 229–239.

Srinivasan, M.V. and Lehrer, M. 1988. Spatial acuity of honeybee vision and its spetcral properties. Journal of Comparative Physiology A. *162,* 159–172.

Stavenga, D. G., Smits, R. P., and Hoenders, B. J. 1993. Simple exponential functions describing the absorbance bands of visual pigment spectra. Vision Research *33,* 1011–1017.

Thompson, E., Palacios, A., and Varela, F. J. 1992. Ways of coloring: Comparative color vision as a case study for cognitive science. Behavioral and Brain Sciences *15,* 1–74.

Thompson, E. 1995. Colour Vision: A Study in Cognitive Science and the Philosophy of Perception. Routledge, London and New York. 354 pp.

Waddington, K. D. 1983. Floral-visitation-sequences by bees: Models and experiments. In: C. E. Jones and R. J. Little (eds) Handbook of Experimental Pollination Biology. Scientific and Academic Editions, Van Nostrand and Company, New York. Chapter 23, pp. 461–473.

Wallace, A. R. 1878. Tropical Nature and other Essays. Macmillan and Company, London. 356 pp.

Wallace, A. R. 1891. Natural Selection and Tropical Nature. Macmillan and Company, London. 492 pp.

Wehner, R. 1981. Spatial vision in arthropods. In: H. Autrum (ed.) Invertebrate Photoreceptors. Vol VII/6C Handbook of Sensory Physiology. Springer Verlag, Berlin, Heidelberg, New York. pp. 183–194.

Wells, M. J. 1978. Octopus: Physiology and Behaviour of an advanced Invertebrate. Chapman and Hall, London. 417 pp.

Willemstein, S. C. 1987. An evolutionary basis for pollination ecology. Leiden Botanical Series *10*, 425 pp.

Wright, W. D., 1969. The Measurement of Colour. Adam Hilger Ltd., London. 340 pp.

Wyszecki, G. and Stiles, W. S. 1982. Colour Science: Concepts and Methods, Quantitative Data and Formulae. 2nd Edition. John Wiley & Sons, New York, 950 pp.

III Psychology and Philosophy

10. The Perception of Blackness: An Historical and Contemporary Review

Vicki J. Volbrecht and Reinhold Kliegl

10.1 Introduction

Historically, the perception of blackness has spirited a lively debate as to its actual validity as a 'real' perception (e.g., Ward, 1905, 1916; Titchener 1916a,b) and its place in theories of color vision (e.g., Neifeld, 1924; Ladd-Franklin, 1925; Lemmon, 1925; Michaels, 1925; Venable, 1925; Rich, 1926; Luh, 1930). Yet, despite the years of heated discussion on blackness, this perception has become an integral part of Hurvich and Jameson's (1957) opponent-process theory of color vision and Heggelund's (1974a,b; 1992) bidimensional theory of achromatic vision and has sparked a relatively recent flurry of scientific investigation into the neural processes mediating the perception of blackness (e.g., Werner et al., 1984; Cicerone et al., 1986; Fuld et al., 1986; Kulp and Fuld, 1989; Volbrecht and Werner, 1989; Volbrecht et al, 1989; 1990; Shinomori et al., 1994; 1997).

This chapter provides an historical and contemporary survey of theoretical and empirical work on the perception of blackness, including the accepted as well as the controversial aspects of blackness. The first place to commence the discussion of blackness is with the theories of Helmholtz and Hering, each an exemplar of the differing perspectives on blackness. The long-reaching impact of these two theories will be recognized in the review of other color vision theories (e.g., Ladd-Franklin, Müller, Hurvich and Jameson, Heggelund), psychophysical research on blackness, and physiological findings.

10.2 The Phenomenology of Blackness

How did the perception or the sensation of blackness become a source of controversy? Basically, the discord arose over the two different views on the physical conditions required to elicit the perception of blackness. In particular, one group believed blackness was the outcome of the *absence* of light while the other group credited blackness to the *presence* of light. Since the nineteenth century, these two diverse concepts are best exemplified in the color vision theories of Helmholtz (1867/1962) and Hering (1878, 1920/1964).

Helmholtz wrote in his Handbuch der Physiologischen Optik (1867):

Das Schwarz ist eine wirkliche Empfindung, wenn es auch durch Abwesenheit allen Lichts hervorgebracht wird. Wir unterscheiden die Empfindung des Schwarzen deutlich von dem Mangel aller Empfindung. Ein Fleck unseres Gesichtsfeldes, von welchem kein Licht in unser Auge fällt, erscheint uns schwarz, aber die Objekte hinter unserem Rücken, von denen auch kein Licht in unser Auge fällt, ... erscheinen uns nicht schwarz, sondern für sie mangelt alle Erfahrung (pp. 109 ff).[1]

According to Helmholtz, black was the result of the complete absence of light; but it was not the

---

[1] English translation: "Black is a real sensation, even if it is produced by the entire absence of light. The sensation of black is distinctly different from the lack of all sensation. A spot in the field of view which sends no light to the eye looks black; but no light comes to the eye from objects that are behind our back, whether they are dark or bright, and yet these objects do not look black - there is simply no sensation so far as they are concerned."

same as the absence of sensation. Black was a *true* sensation. This notion that blackness resulted from the lack of light stimulation was not original to Helmholtz. Aristotle and/or his students (1967) had much earlier proposed this as one condition under which blackness could be perceived and Goethe (1810/1970) had iterated the same idea. Likewise, this view of blackness also did not terminate with Helmholtz and his theory of color vision. Others (e.g., Schopenhauer, 1905; Troland, 1921; Ladd-Franklin, 1922a, 1925) also supported the perception of blackness originating from zero light stimulation.

Ewald Hering was not persuaded by Helmholtz's reasoning. He argued that the perception of blackness could not occur from the absence of light stimulation since closing one's eyes did not produce a perception of blackness but rather one of gray, referred to as Eigengrau. Instead, he (Hering, 1874) proposed:

> Gleichwohl ist es eine Thatsache der alltäglichen Erfahrung, welche ich jedoch noch nirgends besonders betont gefunden habe, *dass die eigentliche schwarze Empfindung erst unter dem Einfluss des äussern Lichtreizes zu Stande kommt,* wie ja auch die weisse Empfindung für gewöhnlich durch objectives Licht hervorgerufen wird; nur mit dem Unterschiede, dass sich die weisse Empfindung unter dem directen, die schwarze aber unter dem indirecten Einflusse des Lichtreizes entwickelt, nämlich durch den sogenannten simultanen oder successiven Contrast. (p. 97)[2]

Thus, according to Hering, blackness was the result of the indirect influence of light from spatial (simultaneous) and/or temporal (successive) contrast. An object could reflect a large quantity of light and be perceived as red, green, blue, yellow, or white; but if this same object was surrounded and/or preceded by more intense stimulation, it would begin to appear black. As the intensity of the contrasting stimulus increased, the object would become blacker until at some luminance level the object would appear completely black to the observer.

Gelb (1929/1955) elegantly demonstrated Hering's ideas by using a smooth black disk and a single light source. The light source, which was hidden from view, illuminated only the disk but none of the surrounding fixtures in the environment. When the black disk was observed under these conditions, it appeared white and *not* black. When a piece of white paper, which reflected much more light than the black disk, was imposed into the scene such that it covered a portion of the disk, the disk suddenly appeared black.

This relationship between spatial contrast and blackness was more recently demonstrated with a complex stimulus. Wright (1980, 1981), using a slide of van Eyck's painting, "The Arnolfini Marriage," separated the chromatic and achromatic components to create a new slide containing only the chromatic information and a print containing only the achromatic information. When the chromatic slide was projected onto the white-black print, the color of the original slide was restored; but when the chromatic slide was projected onto a black background, the blackness components of the painting were not reproduced. The luminance contrast captured in the achromatic print was required to restore the color of black to the painting. Both Gelb's and Wright's demonstrations once again illustrated that the perception of blackness was due to light stimulation and not a lack of light stimulation.

Hering was by no means the first person to report the perception of blackness under conditions of contrast. Chevreul (1839/1883), who was Director of Dyes for the Royal Manufactures at Gobelins, received complaints on the quality of the black used in their tapestries: the black appeared quite dull or lackluster. Chevreul noted that to achieve a perceptually "good" black the threads next to the black area needed to reflect more light than the black threads. Goethe

---

[2] English translation: "It is a matter of everyday experience (which, however, I have not found especially emphasized anywhere) *that the genuinely black sensation arises only under the influence of external light stimuli* just as the sensation of white is usually evoked by objective light. The difference is that the sensation of white develops under direct influence of light whereas the sensation of black does so under indirect influence, namely the so-called simultaneous or successive contrast."

(1810/1970) and Helmholtz (1867/1962) also wrote about blackness induction under conditions of temporal and spatial contrast, but neither attributed blackness perception to the physical light conditions of contrast. Because of the failure to acknowledge the importance of light in the perception of blackness, Hering (1874) remarked:

> Wenn man alle diese Thatsachen bedenkt, muss man sich wundern, wie man die Empfindung des Schwarzen als diejenige definieren konnte, welche der ruhenden, nicht durch Licht gereizten Netzhaut eigenthümlich ist. Gerade das Auge, welches vor jedem äusseren Lichtreize sorgfältig ... geschützt wurde, ... empfindet durchaus kein Schwarz, sondern hat Empfindungen, welchen man eine ziemlich bedeutende Helligkeit zuschreiben muss ... (p. 98)[3]

These differing opinions as to the physical conditions necessary to create blackness highlight one of the important theoretical distinctions between Helmholtz and Hering, although it was not the only one. Other differing theoretical conceptualizations between the two men are elaborated below and traced to contemporary research endeavors.

10.2.1 Helmholtz: Trichromatic Theory of Color Vision

While Helmholtz is probably given the most credit for the trichromatic theory of color vision, he was not the first to postulate such a theory (see Balaraman, 1962; Weale, 1957). In fact, he did not originally believe that a trichromatic theory could adequately explain the perception of color (see Hurvich and Jameson, 1949; Sherman, 1981). Unhindered by his initial misunderstanding, Helmholtz incorporated the ideas of Young (1802/1970; 1845/1970) and Maxwell (1860) to develop his universally recognized theory of color vision.

Following from Newton (1730/1979), Helmholtz realized that the correspondence between the various wavelengths of light and color perception, such as experienced with a rainbow, was achieved solely within the organism; it was *not* the rays of light that were colored and produced the various color perceptions. He, therefore, proposed the existence of three types (violet, green, and red) of retinal nerve fibers or receptors. Each fiber class was differentially sensitive to wavelengths of light ranging from approximately 400 nm to 700 nm, with the violet-coding fibers maximally sensitive to the short wavelengths, the green-coding fibers maximally sensitive to the middle wavelengths, and the red-coding fibers maximally sensitive to the long wavelengths. An alternative model would have been to assume one nerve fiber sensitive to one particular wavelength of light in the visible spectrum; however, color-matching experiments (Maxwell, 1860; Helmholtz, 1867/1962) revealed three mechanisms were sufficient to account for color perception.

Within this tri-receptor model, different color sensations were the outcome of the relative strengths with which these three fiber types were activated by physical light. Since these fibers were assumed to have a direct connection to the cortex, stimulation of one or a combination of these fibers generated the various psychological experiences of color. In particular, equal activation of all three fiber types created the sensation of whiteness. The blackness sensation occurred when none of the fibers were stimulated by light.

10.2.2 Hering: Opponent-Process Theory of Color Vision

Whereas Helmholtz's theory was guided by the physics of light, Hering's theory was strongly influenced by the phenomenological experience of color. Hering (1920/1964) observed that when the different hues were arranged in a circle there were a great number of bichromatic mixtures but none of these mixtures could be described as yellow-blue or red-green. Hering (1888/1897, 1920/1964)

---

[3] English translation: "All things considered, one wonders how the sensation of black could be defined as the one which is peculiar to the resting retina, not stimulated by light. It is exactly the eye protected carefully from any external stimulus of light which does not sense any black but has sensations that must be attributed to a considerable amount of brightness."

argued that this mutual exclusivity between yellow-blue and between red-green had its origin in neurophysiologically-based chemical processes of the visual system. He interpreted this perceptual constraint as evidence for an antagonistic relation between the chemical processes mediating yellow and blue and similarly red and green. He, therefore, proposed the existence of two chromatic-opponent processes (red-green and blue-yellow); each process had an excitatory and inhibitory component, which Hering referred to as assimilation and dissimilation. These two antagonistic processes struggled to maintain a state of equilibrium in the visual system, although under most normal viewing conditions there was usually an imbalance. The vast array of chromatic perceptions, therefore, arose from the degree of imbalance within the opponent processes.

Hering realized, however, that besides the chromatic component or hue of a color, there was also an achromatic component. A third chemical or visual process was needed to describe this added dimension of color. He, therefore, proposed a white-black chemical process and also viewed it as antagonistic. He based this inference on the reciprocal relation observed between black and white under conditions of spatial and temporal contrast, but not on mutual exclusivity since there was a continuous transition from white to black passing through the various shades of gray (i.e., gray could be described as white-black – see Quinn et al., 1985).

Nonetheless, it was assumed that when dissimilation was greater than assimilation, white was perceived; but when assimilation was greater than dissimilation, black was seen. Furthermore, the metabolic activity evoked by a light stimulus in one particular area of the visual system did not affect just that area but also influenced the chemical activity in surrounding and succeeding visual areas, but in the opposite direction. This property could easily explain color perceptions created by simultaneous and successive contrast, in particular that of black which only occurred under contrast conditions.

Hence, if the intensity of a white annular light increased around a center stimulus, dissimilation of the affected areas of the visual field would increase and at the same time this activity would induce assimilation into the surrounding areas of the visual field. If this surround induced more assimilation into the center such that it canceled or inhibited the dissimilation already present in that visual area, the center would appear black. Under conditions of temporal contrast, a white inducing stimulus would generate dissimilation in the visual area excited by it. After termination of the white stimulus, the process of assimilation would dominate over dissimilation in an attempt to restore the system to a state of equilibrium. Before equilibrium would be reached, a black afterimage would be perceived.

Of course, Helmholtz, as his historical exposition attests, was familiar with contrast phenomena and the perception of blackness under such conditions. Unlike Hering, he did not use these perceptual experiences to structure his theory of color vision. His theory focused on physical parameters of stimuli to explain and predict color perception. Such an emphasis proved cumbersome in trying to account for some of the more complex color perceptions encountered in everyday life, especially those not directly linked to physical stimuli. To compensate for this limitation, Helmholtz suggested retinal fatigue to explain successive contrast and unconscious inference to account for simultaneous contrast.

The basic premise of the retinal fatigue hypothesis was that certain receptor types exposed to particular wavelengths of light became fatigued such they were selectively suppressed and unable to respond immediately to succeeding light stimulation of the same or similar wavelengths. For example, a white object reflecting wavelengths across the entire visible spectrum would suppress all three receptor types. When the object was removed or the light extinguished, the fatigued receptors would be unable to respond to any light; consequently, the perception of blackness.

The retinal fatigue hypothesis could not be applied to conditions of simultaneous contrast since color induction in these circumstances was immediate and the retinal mechanisms did not have time to become fatigued (Chevreul, 1839/1883). Instead, Helmholtz (1867/1962) proposed that a person perceiving any object in a complex scene formed an unconscious judgment of its color. The final perceived color was determined by correcting mentally for lighting conditions causing the induction. The more practice people had in these cognitive operations, the less contrast influenced their perception and the better able they were to judge the 'true' color of an object despite the viewing conditions. It was the lack of experience with the involuntary inferences that led to the perception of induced colors in simultaneous contrast.

This unconscious correction for illumination was challenged by Gestalt psychologists (e.g., Katz, 1930/1935) as inadequate to explain such contrast phenomena as the Gelb effect (discussed above; for an earlier criticism of this explanation see also Hering, 1887). Even with complete knowledge about the experimental set-up, people still could not correct their perception of blackness when the white paper was introduced.

10.2.3 Criticism and Other Theories

The color vision theories of Helmholtz and Hering, although probably the most well known and debated, were not necessarily accepted by their peers or colleagues. The theory of Helmholtz was acknowledged to provide the best and most feasible account of color mixture (Troland, 1921; Rich, 1926). While this was its forte, it was also its limitation in that it relied on the parameters of physical stimuli to predict the outcome of color appearance. Such an emphasis introduced problems in that the physical causes of the gray sensation were assumed to be the same as the physical causes of the red, green, and violet sensation combined; and from this premise, one could easily conclude that the gray sensation was the "coincidence of the sensations red, green, and blue" (Franklin, 1893; p. 477), rather than a separate sensation. This argument also applied to Helmholtz's assumption about the sensation of white arising from stimulation of all three classes of nerve fibers and proved to be even more troublesome since a person missing the green class of fibers still perceived white like a color-normal person (Franklin, 1983). Even von Kries, presumably one of Helmholtz's most well-known students, expressed doubt about Helmholtz's theory when he wrote in his commentary of the 1924 English edition of Physiological Optics: "To begin with, it may be regarded as certain that there actually is a reciprocal physiological action as Hering supposed, especially with respect to luminosity contrast"(p. 300).

The strength of Hering's (1878, 1920/1964) theory was his explanation of achromatic sensations (Mach, 1906/1959; Rich, 1926), but at the same time it was also his discussion of the white-black chemical process that presented some difficulties. The major problem was that the sensations of black and white were not mutually exclusive as were the chromatic-opponent pairs (Mach, 1906/1959; Troland, 1921; Ladd-Franklin, 1922a). Furthermore, Hering did not offer a reason for this discrepancy or the seemingly special status assigned to the white-black process (McDougall, 1901a); and it was, therefore, questioned whether a special process for blackness was really necessary (McDougall, 1901b). At the same time, though, Hering's physiological explication of simultaneous contrast with dissimilation and assimilation seemed more parsimonious than Helmholtz's speculations about unconscious inference (Franklin, 1893); and Helmholtz's fatigue hypothesis for successive contrast could not explain the presence of afterimages with closed eyes (McDougall, 1901c), Hering's could.

Other Theories: Ladd-Franklin and Müller

Ladd-Franklin offered her evolutionary or developmental theory of color vision as an alternative to Helmholtz's and Hering's theories. According to Ladd-Franklin, there originally existed only one photosensitive substance in the retina which, when stimulated by light, signaled the perception of whiteness. Over the evolutionary process this substance differentiated into blue and yellow molecules, so when either was separately activated, the perception of blue or yellow followed. When both were simultaneously activated, the perception of whiteness ensued. The yellow molecules separated into red and green molecules in the last evolutionary stage. Light stimulation of one or any combination of these molecules produced the chromatic and white sensations.

Because Ladd-Franklin viewed black as a nonlight sensation, she did not integrate the sensation of blackness with the other color sensations into her evolutionary theory. Rather, she led the reader to conclude that blackness resulted from the inactivation of the red, green, and blue molecules. This aspect of her theory spawned a series of papers criticizing, defending, or elaborating her position on blackness (e.g., Troland, 1921; Neifeld, 1924; Michaels, 1925; Lemmon, 1925; Venable, 1925; Rich, 1926; Luh, 1930).

Due to their stance on blackness, neither Helmholtz's nor Ladd-Franklin's theory of color vision could readily account for the experience of Eigengrau. Müller (1896, 1897) developed a theory that attempted to overcome this problem and improve on Hering's theory. Müller's theory was also one of the first to distinguish between retinal and cortical activities in the visual pathway; Hering had not been so clear in this structural distinction with his opponent processes.

Müller (1896, 1897) suggested the presence of three reversible or antagonistic chemical reactions in the retina: white-black, red-green, and blue-yellow. If light caused a white reaction in the retina, it initiated an opposing reaction to neutralize the white reaction and return the retina to a state of equilibrium. The reverse occurred during a black reaction. Similar reciprocal processes were assumed to exist for the red-green and blue-yellow pairs.

In the cortex, there existed an endogenous white process and an endogenous black process that were also antagonistic with each other and dominated over the weaker chromatic excitations. The active retinal processes determined which of the cortical processes were in an excited state. If a white reaction dominated the retina, the white-black balance was disturbed, causing the white excitation in the cortex to increase and signal the perception of whiteness. Similarly, if a black reaction prevailed in the retina, it increased the black excitation in the cortex to signal the sensation of blackness. Lastly, if the black and white reactions in the retina were in equilibrium, Eigengrau was perceived.

Besides the color theories of Ladd-Franklin and Müller, many other theories of color vision were proposed (e.g., McDougall, 1901 a,b,c; Schopenhauer, 1905; see Parsons, 1915, and Boring, 1942). Most of these theories assumed that blackness resulted from the absence of light and/or the absence of neural activity. But despite this plethora of theories, the influence of the theories of Helmholtz and Hering surpassed the others.

Contemporary Theories: Hurvich and Jameson and Heggelund

In the scientific community Helmholtz's theory received far greater attention than Hering's. There also were a number of attempts to combine the theories of Helmholtz and Hering (e.g., Ladd-Franklin, 1916, 1922a,b; Franklin, 1893; Hartridge, 1948), but the most important experiments to clarify the connection between both theories were the zone theories of von Kries (1905) and Schrödinger (1925). Nevertheless, and especially in the United States, it was not until Hurvich and Jameson's (1957) work in the 1950's that an interest in Hering's work was rekindled. Hurvich and Jameson incorporated the idea of three receptor types from Helmholtz (1867/1920) with Hering's (1878, 1920/1964) assumption of three opponent processes and suggested a model whereby neural signals from the photoreceptors combined to produce an opponent response in another neural unit further along the visual pathway. In general, as Figure 10.1 illustrates, they proposed that outputs from the short- and long-wavelength photoreceptors combined at a postreceptoral level to interact antagonistically with output from the middle-wavelength receptors. This interaction generated a red-green opponent response. Likewise, there was a postreceptoral site at which the neural signals from the middle- and long-wavelength photoreceptors opposed signals from the short-wavelength receptors. This particular activity produced a blue-yellow opponent response. Similar to the idea of Helmholtz, the perception of whiteness was attributed to the additive combination of all three cone signals at a later site in the visual pathway. The perception of blackness was assumed to be the consequence of all three receptor types in close spatial and/or temporal proximity signaling inhibition, and this inhibition from each receptor type also merged at a later neural site in the visual pathway. Together, then, activation of the three receptor types in a similar manner, either excitatory or inhibitory, defined the white-black opponent process.

This general theoretical framework proved to be quite economical in that it included the three variables necessary to explain color matching and the four chromatic (red, green, yellow, blue) and two achromatic (black, white) variables necessary to explain color appearance. Moreover, psychophysical measures of the chromatic-opponent response functions from a hue cancellation task (Jameson and Hurvich, 1955) could be reasonably fitted by the theoretical equations that described the relationship between the cone inputs and the response outputs for the chromatic-opponent processes (Hurvich and Jameson, 1955, 1957; Romeskie, 1978; Werner and Wooten, 1979); however, a similar experimental verification was not obtained for the achromatic processes.

Hurvich and Jameson (1957) equated, rather arbitrarily, the responsivity of whiteness to a photopic luminosity function as operationalized by a spectral sensitivity curve measured on a white background (Hurvich and Jameson, 1953). The blackness response function was assumed to have the inverse shape of the whiteness function "since the strength of the black contrast response is directly related to the magnitude of either the surrounding or the preceding whiteness or brightness" (p. 389, Hurvich and Jameson, 1957). The problem with these assumptions about the response functions for the white-black process was that neither function was based on a perceptual criterion (e.g., whiteness or blackness). Although it might be assumed that the stimuli appeared "whitish" at threshold on a white background, the authors noted that the stimuli sometimes appeared chromatic, especially at the short and long wavelengths (Hurvich and Jameson, 1953).

Heggelund (1974a,b; 1992) formulated a theory concerned solely with the achromatic processes and conducted some provocative, albeit not conclusive, experiments to support his postulations. Heggelund, first, disregarded both Helmholtz's unidimensional view that achromatic colors represented a continuum of different intensities of white and Hering's bidimensional view that black and white were opponent. Rather, Heggelund acknowledged that there were mutually exclusive achromatic perceptions if one considered both surface (object) and film (aperture) colors.

Heggelund proposed that the color terms black, gray, and white were often used to describe the colors of objects in the visual field (surface colors) while the terms luminous (clear) and white were often used to describe the colors of lights in the visual field (film colors). Most investigators (e.g., Katz, 1930/1935; MacLeod, 1932; Evans, 1949) conceded that there was a qualitative difference between achromatic colors in the object and aperture modes but did not attempt to account for these differences in one theoretical model. Heggelund suggested such an inclusive model by proposing that luminous and black were opponent since both colors could not be seen simultaneously in the

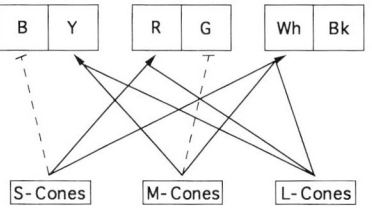

Fig. 10.1: Representation of Hurvich and Jameson's opponent-process model of color vision. The three cone types are short-wavelength-sensitive (S-cones), middle-wavelength-sensitive (M-cones), and long-wavelength-sensitive (L-cones). The three opponent processes are blue-yellow (B/Y), red-green (R/G), and white-black (Wh/Bk). The solid lines denote excitation and the dashed lines inhibition to represent the opponency among the cone signals. Cone inputs to the black process are not represented since black is the result of the three cone types in close spatial and/or temporal proximity signaling inhibition.

same place (i.e., luminous was only perceived in aperture mode and black only in surface mode). Black and white were, however, orthogonal to each other and could be seen at the same time in the grayness of a surface; and luminous and white were orthogonal to each other since both could be seen together in a luminous white of a light. From his experiments, Heggelund (1974b, 1992, 1993) concluded that the strength and quality of black were related to contrast while the strength and quality of whiteness were related to local luminance values.

10.3 Historical Review

10.3.1 Induction Experiments

The first psychophysical measures of the chromatic-opponent response functions were obtained in 1955 (Jameson and Hurvich, 1955); however, it was not until 1984 (Werner et al., 1984) that response functions based on a perceptual criterion of complete blackness were reported. Because the perception of blackness resulted from spatial and/or temporal contrast, an experimental procedure incorporating contrast stimuli was required to measure the blackness component of the achromatic process (i.e., a hue cancellation based on the direct influence of light and on mutual exclusivity could not be used). Oddly, contrast experiments had been used for years to study spatially-induced brightness/darkness (e.g., Hess and Pretori, 1894/1970; Wallach, 1948; Heineman, 1955), but none had directly investigated blackness-induction thresholds.

In the spatial induction studies of brightness contrast, a broadband ("white") test field was presented at the same time as a broadband ("white") inducing field. The actual stimulus configuration varied among studies. Some used a circular test field surrounded by an annular inducing field; others used a rectangular test field contiguous with a rectangular inducing field positioned on one side or two opposing sides. Since the stimulus parameters were quite easy to manipulate, they readily permitted the study of test and inducing field luminance (Diamond, 1953), area (Diamond, 1955, 1962), configuration (Horeman, 1963), and separation from each other (Leibowitz et al., 1953) on spatially-induced brightness/darkness. Regardless of their particular emphasis, these studies showed that as the intensity of the inducing field increased, the test field became darker until a point was reached where the test field appeared completely black.

Other investigators extended the spatial induction paradigm by adding chromatic test and/or inducing fields and measuring spectral sensitivity functions for different achromatic response criteria. For example, one study measured thresholds for gray (Evans, 1967) and then expanded the work to examine the threshold between gray content and apparent fluorescence (Evans and Swenholt, 1969), while another group investigated the just-noticeable darkening of a test field (Mount and Thomas, 1968). Results from Evans (1967) and Mount and Thomas (1968) disclosed that luminance was the sole factor determining thresholds for gray and a just-noticeable darkening; spectral compositions of the stimuli were irrelevant. The threshold between gray and apparent fluorescence, however, revealed a chromatic influence. None of these studies, however, looked at the effects of chromatic stimuli on a perceptual criterion of complete blackness.

Fewer studies have examined the effects of temporal contrast on achromatic perception, although many spatial contrast studies contained an inherent temporal contrast component due to long viewing times of the experimental stimulus that permitted successive eye movements over the stimulus. Nonetheless, Hering (1878) demonstrated that blackness could be temporally induced by superimposing one stimulus on another and subsequently removing it, and Creed (1931) used the same procedure to study achromatic afterimages. Others (e.g., Jacobs and Gaylord, 1967; Wooten, 1984) introduced chromatic stimuli and presented an inducing field at a particular intensity level for a specific period of time. Upon termination of the inducing field, a test field was shown in the same spatial location as the inducing field and chromatic induction effects were measured, but no achromatic effects. Another group of researchers modified this design so that the preceding stimulus was either annular in shape (e.g., Kitterle, 1972, 1975) or two half fields separated by a specific gap (Kinney, 1962). After termination of the inducing field, the test field was either presented in the location of the center of the annulus or the gap between the two half fields. Both researchers observed changes in brightness due to the contrast; however, test field placement introduced simultaneous contrast into a successive contrast paradigm.

10.3.2 Blackness-Induction Experiments

Blackness-induction experiments have fallen into two groups: those that have investigated the color appearance of stimuli under conditions of spatial and temporal contrast and those that have measured spectral sensitivity functions of achromatic processes under conditions of spatial and temporal contrast. While these studies have not always arrived at the same conclusions, they have increased our understanding of the white-black process and its role in the visual system.

Color-Naming Studies

Quinn et al. (1985) investigated Hering's (1878, 1920/1964) premise that black and white, but not gray, were the elemental achromatic sensations. In other words, gray was not a necessary color term since it could be described as a blackish white or a whitish black. Observers in their study viewed a perceptually white (i.e., devoid of hue) test center surrounded by a perceptually white annulus at varying intensity levels and described the test center by assigning percentages to the color terms black, white and/or gray. Each test session varied as to which of the three or combination of the three terms could be used by the observer. Results from their study supported Hering's claim as to the elemental nature of black and white, and the non-elemental nature of gray. This study also showed that as the intensity of the surround increased, the percent of whiteness required to describe the test center decreased, while the percent of blackness increased. None of the test centers were specified as 100% black, but the highest surround intensity (3.5 log troland) was most likely insufficient to induce complete blackness into the 2.2 log troland test center.

At the same time Fuld and Otto (1985) were studying the effects of spatial contrast on monochromatic lights. Similar to Quinn et al. (1985), a perceptually white (i.e., unique white) annulus surrounded a monochromatic test center. They noted that as the intensity of the surround increased, the percent of whiteness decreased; at the higher intensity levels, percentages were assigned to blackness such that at the highest surround level the monochromatic stimulus was sometimes described as completely black. Also, a test center was rarely perceived as containing both a black and white component at the same time; it was either a whitish chromatic perception or a blackish chromatic perception. According to Fuld and Otto (1985), this later observation seemed to suggest that Hering's white-black process was indeed antagonistic and similar to that of the chromatic-opponent processes, especially when a strong hue component was present with an achromatic component.

It was not until a few years later that this was applied to the study of the temporal induction of blackness (Volbrecht et al., 1989). Unlike the two previous spatial induction studies, the inducing fields for this study were an observer's unique blue, unique green, unique yellow, and unique white. The test stimulus, also called the reference field, was an observer's unique white. Both the inducing and test stimuli were the same size. After the inducing field was presented for five seconds, the reference field was immediately presented for 400 ms in the same spatial location.

Figure 10.2 presents the color-naming data of one observer for each of the four inducing fields. As surround intensity increased, the percent of whiteness (open circles) decreased while the percent of blackness (solid circles) increased until the test stimulus was described as 100% black. When the blackness-response functions of this observer were compared across the four inducing fields (bottom panel), a pattern of convergence was observed, such that the same illuminance level was

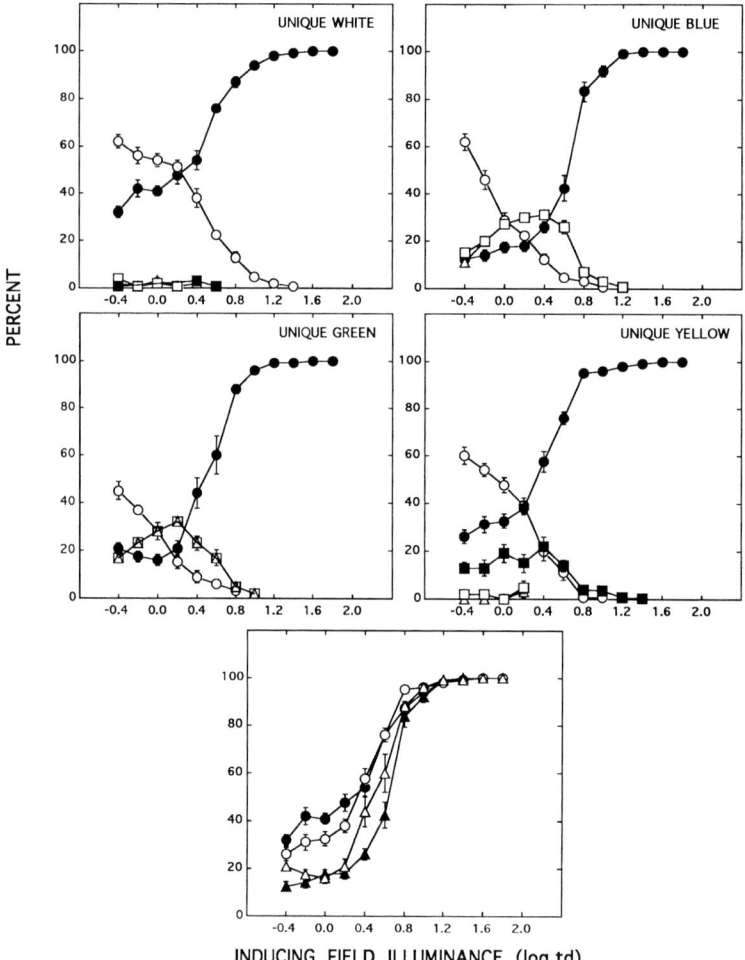

Fig. 10.2: Color-naming functions are shown for one observer (LA). In each panel, mean percent color is plotted as a function of inducing field illuminance. The top four panels represent a different inducing field (unique white, unique blue, unique green, unique yellow), and different symbols denote different color terms: black (solid circles), white (open circles), blue (solid squares), yellow (open squares), red (open triangles). Error bars denote ±1 standard error of the mean. The bottom panel replots the black response functions from each of the four top panels. Different symbols denote the different inducing field conditions: unique white (solid circles), unique blue (solid triangles), unique green (open triangles), unique yellow (open circles). After Volbrecht et al. (1989).

required to induce 100% blackness regardless of the spectral content of the inducing field. The same pattern was seen for all observers in this study and for the two test intensity levels. It was, therefore, concluded that illuminance and not chromaticity of the inducing field was the key determinant for the threshold of 100% blackness. This finding was also verified by Shinomori and colleagues (1994) in a color-naming study of spatially-induced blackness.

The color-naming studies did not resolve many questions about mechanisms related to the neural processes underlying the perception of blackness. Rather, they piqued further curiosity as to the nature of the specific processes responsible for blackness perception. Because of the laborious procedure of color naming, the measurement of spectral sensitivity functions of the achromatic processes provided a quicker and more intensive alternative by which to explore these neural processes, in particular the threshold for complete blackness.

Spectral Sensitivity Studies

The first study to measure systematically a spectral sensitivity function based on a perceptual criterion of complete blackness was by Werner et al. (1984). In their spatial induction experiment, observers viewed a circular, broadband ("white") test center separated from a monochromatic annulus by a dark gap. The observers adjusted the intensity of the monochromatic surround until the test center "just turned black, its contour disappeared, and the central field became indistinguishable from the dark surrounding gap that separated it from the annulus" (p. 982–983). The spectral sensitivity of blackness was assumed to be inversely related to the intensity of the monochromatic annuli required to render the field completely black.

Data from one observer in this study are presented in Figure 10.3. The figure shows that this observer's blackness-induction function (solid circles) is similar to his heterochromatic flicker photometry (HFP) function (open circles). HFP is defined by an operation that minimizes flicker between a monochromatic light and a standard light presented in counterphase. The HFP response function represents an individual's photopic luminosity function and is believed to be mediated by the additive input of the M- and L-cone signals (Vos and Walraven, 1979; Schnapf et al., 1987; Lee et al., 1988). Because the HFP function is not influenced by the chromaticity of experimental stimuli, the similarity between the blackness-induction and HFP functions implies that the illuminance of the monochromatic annulus, and *not* its chromaticity, is responsible for blackness induction. Also, the close fit between the two functions suggests that the additive input of the M and L cones may mediate blackness induction.

The work of Cicerone et al. (1986) further substantiated the finding from Werner et al. (1984). Cicerone and colleagues showed that changing the spectral composition of the center stimulus from 5500K to 480, 500, 580 or 660 nm did not alter the spectral sensitivity function of blackness; it was still inversely related to an individual's HFP function.

The one limitation to the Werner et al. (1984) and Cicerone et al. (1986) studies was that they did not measure an individual's brightness function and compare it to the blackness-induction function. Unlike the luminosity function, the brightness function requires an observer to equate two fields of different chromaticities in brightness and is known to represent the influence of antagonistic chromatic processes (Guth et al., 1969; Ikeda et al., 1982; Yaguchi and Ikeda, 1983; Nakano et al., 1988), as shown by Sloan's (1928) notch at approximately 580 nm. Kulp and Fuld (1989) argued that some of the blackness data from Werner et al. (1984) showed the presence of a notch at 580 nm (e.g., the blackness curve in Fig. 10.3). Kulp and Fuld also questioned the presence

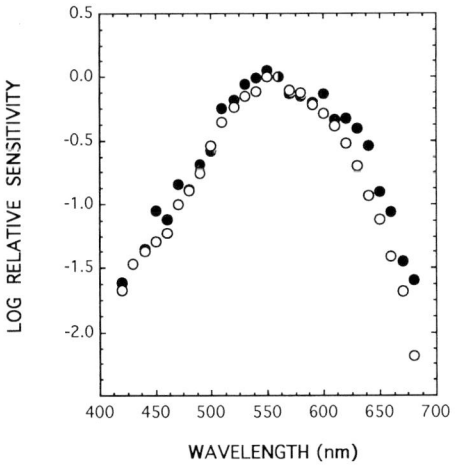

Fig. 10.3: Log relative sensitivity for blackness induction (solid circles) and HFP (open circles) are plotted as a function of wavelength (nm) for one observer (RK). Both curves have been normalized to 560 nm. After Werner et al. (1984).

of the gap and whether observers were actually setting a criterion of complete blackness or setting a minimally distinct border (MDB) between the center stimulus and the gap. Previous work (Wagner and Boynton, 1972) demonstrated that an MDB criterion yielded a spectral sensitivity function quite similar in shape to that of an HFP function.

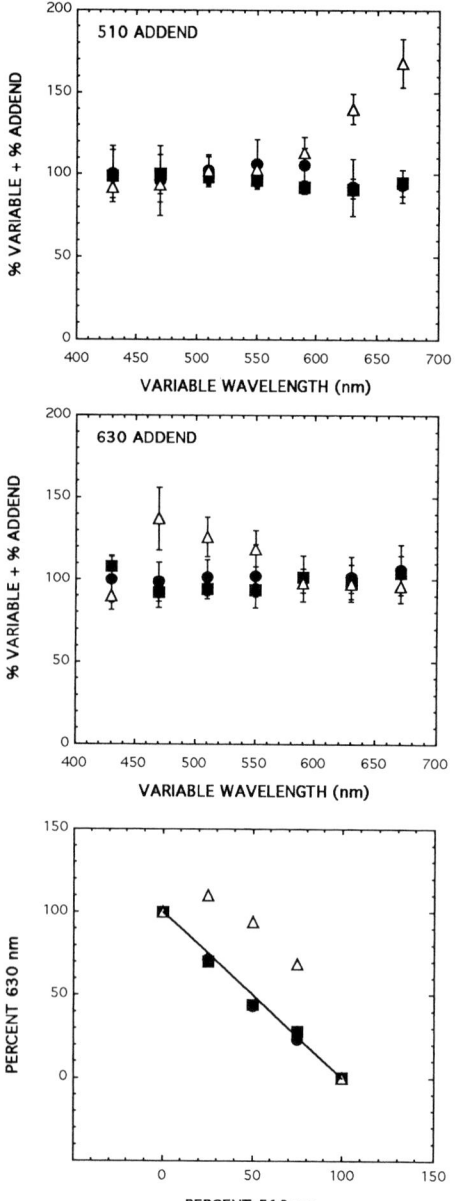

Kulp and Fuld (1989), therefore, repeated the spatial induction experiments. Two different induction functions were measured: for one, the radiance of the monochromatic annulus was increased until the broadband "white" test center appeared black and for the other the radiance of the annulus was increased until the edge between the test center and gap disappeared. HFP and brightness-matching functions were also obtained for each observer. In general, it was difficult to differentiate whether an individual's HFP or brightness-matching function better fit the induction data from either condition. Part of this problem can be attributed to the fact that HFP and brightness-matching functions under certain experimental conditions can be very similar in shape to each other (e.g., Ives, 1912a; Sperling and Lewis, 1959; Volbrecht and Werner, 1989). Unfortunately, this study did not directly compare the two induction functions to each other to determine if both perceptual criteria yielded the same function.

Although the difference among the shapes of the three functions seems quantitatively quite small, they are theoretically quite significant. As discussed above, the HFP function represents the additive input of the cone signals, whereas the brightness function represents nonadditive interactions among the cone signals. It was assumed that if the blackness-induction function was better described by either the HFP or brightness function, the same neural mechanism mediating that function was also mediating the blackness-induction function. Because, at times, it was difficult to distinguish any differences among the three func-

Fig. 10.4: Additivity results for spatially-induced blackness (solid circles), HFP (solid squares), and brightness matching (open triangles) are shown for one observer (VV). In the top two panels mean percent of light in a variable and addend (510 nm in top panel, 630 nm in middle panel) mixture is plotted as a function of the variable wavelength (nm). Error bars denote +/–1 standard error of the mean. The bottom panel shows the mean percent light at 630 nm plotted as a function of the mean percent light at 510 nm. The diagonal line represents complete additivity. After Volbrecht et al. (1990).

tions, later studies (e.g., Volbrecht et al., 1990; Shinomori et al., 1997) took a more stringent approach by subjecting spatially-induced blackness to tests of additivity.

Volbrecht et al. (1990) tested for additivity in the blackness induction, HFP, and brightness-matching functions. Although it had been demonstrated that HFP was additive (e.g., Ives, 1912b; Guth et al., 1969) and brightness was nonadditive (e.g., Tessier and Blottiau, 1951; Yaguchi and Ikeda, 1983; Nakano et al., 1988), the additivity (nonadditivity) patterns for these two functions were utilized as a template by which to judge the additivity data from the induction of complete blackness. In one set of additivity experiments, two addends (510 nm and 630 nm) were used. The addend was reduced by 70% and a series of wavelengths, called variable wavelengths, from 430 to 670 nm in 40 nm steps were one-by-one superposed on the addend. Observers adjusted the intensity of the variable wavelength until the criterion response was achieved. Results from this study are presented for one observer in the top two panels of Figure 10.4. While the brightness-matching data (open triangles) show flagrant violations of additivity (i.e., deviations from 100%), neither the HFP (solid squares) nor the blackness-induction (solid circles) data show signs of additivity failure. When 510 nm and 630 nm were combined in different proportions for the three different psychophysical tasks, blackness induction and HFP again showed no violations of additivity (see Fig. 10.4, bottom panel). The data confirmed the earlier studies from Werner et al. (1984) and Cicerone et al. (1986) and once again suggested that blackness was mediated by additive input from the cones and determined by the luminance of a stimulus and not its spectral composition.

These findings and conclusions from the spatial induction studies were further strengthened by the temporal induction study of blackness (Volbrecht and Werner, 1989). Observers' blackness-induction functions appeared to be better fitted to their HFP functions than their brightness-matching functions and temporally-induced blackness did not deviate from additivity. Likewise, as Figure 10.5 reveals, the difference in induction paradigms did not seem to affect the shape of the blackness functions. Also shown in Figure 10.5 are spectral sensitivity measurements of spatially-induced blackness obtained from a protanope, a dichromat known to be missing the long-wavelength-sensitive photopigment. As expected, his blackness-induction function (solid circles) was narrower than that of the color normals and basically indistinguishable from that of his HFP function (open circles), suggesting mediation of both functions by the M cones.

Altogether the evidence from studies of spatially and temporally-induced blackness supported the hypothesis that blackness was mediated by the additive combination of cone signals such as Hurvich and Jameson (1957) proposed in their opponent-process theory of color vision. The picture, however, became a bit muddied by Fuld and colleagues (1986). Unlike the other studies, this study measured the spectral sensitivity function for a perceptual criterion based on equal white-

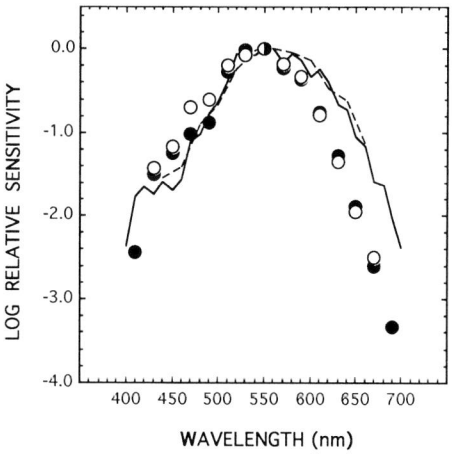

Fig. 10.5: Log relative sensitivity is plotted as a function of wavelength (nm). The solid line is the blackness-induction function from one color-normal observer (VV) measured under conditions of temporal contrast. The dashed line is the blackness-induction function for the same color-normal observer measured under conditions of spatial contrast. The closed circles represent the blackness-induction function for one protanope (KK) measured under conditions of spatial contrast. The open circles represent the protanope's HFP function. The data have been normalized to 550 nm. After Volbrecht and Werner (1989).

black. In their experiment, a "white" xenon annulus surrounded a series of monochromatic, circular test stimuli, each equated to the same illuminance level. Observers ignored the chromatic content of the center stimulus and increased the intensity of a dim annulus until reaching a threshold between predominantly white and equal white-black. They then continued to increase the illuminance of the annulus until reaching a second threshold between equal white-black and predominantly black. From the studies using a blackness criterion, it might be predicted that the equal white-black point would occur at the same annular illuminance level. This was not the case. The function resembled what would be expected from a brightness function, indicating a nonadditive chromatic influence.

For a number of years, the difference between the blackness-induction studies and the equal white-black study were attributed to differences in the response criteria (Fuld et al., 1986; Volbrecht et al., 1989; Volbrecht et al., 1990). It was assumed by these experimenters that the blackness criterion tapped into the black component of the achromatic process while the equal white-black criterion conveyed the interaction of both achromatic processes. Although the black-response function was assumed to be the inverse of the white-response function (Hurvich and Jameson, 1957), the spectral sensitivity of the white-response function had never been formally measured using a perceptual criterion of whiteness. It was easy to conclude that the two response criteria were mediated by different neural processes.

Unfortunately, during discussions of response criteria, another critical feature was ignored, namely differing stimulus parameters. Shinomori et al. (1994) in their color-naming study compared not only the spatial blackness-induction studies and the white-black study but earlier studies and reported that, in general, a stimulus duration of 500 ms or less showed functions dependent only on the illuminance of the stimuli (e.g., Werner et al., 1984; Cicerone et al., 1986; Volbrecht et al., 1990), while durations of 2 s or more showed achromatic functions with a chromatic contribution (e.g., Fuld et al., 1986; Evans and Swenholt, 1969). Using a 2 s stimulus duration and a circular, "white" test field surrounded by a monochromatic annulus, Shinomori and colleagues found that the slope of the blackness-induction function from a color-naming task did not change as a function of annular wavelength. Rather, the function was contingent on the luminance of the surround.

What Shinomori et al. (1994) did not investigate, though, was a fundamental difference in the spectral content of the inducing and test fields. The blackness-induction studies utilized a monochromatic annulus while the equal white-black study used a broadband "white" annulus. Shinomori et al. (1997), therefore, experimentally pursued this difference. In their study, blackness-induction functions were measured under two conditions: monochromatic annulus surrounding a "white" center and a "white" annulus surrounding a monochromatic center. In both conditions, observers adjusted the monochromatic stimulus until the center just turned black. They found that these two conditions were the crucial determinants as to whether a blackness-induction function was influenced by the chromaticity of a stimulus. As Figure 10.6 shows, when the annulus was monochromatic (solid circles), the blackness-induction

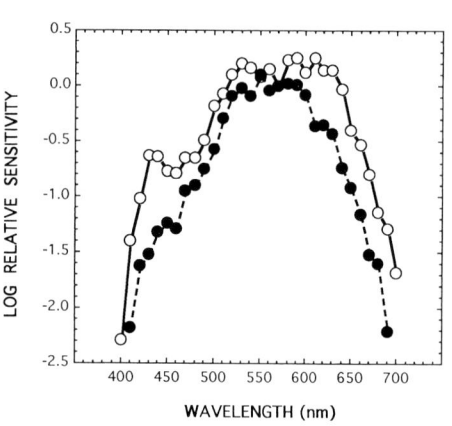

Fig. 10.6: Log relative sensitivity is plotted as a function of wavelength (nm) for one observer (KS). Solid circles represent the blackness-induction function obtained with a monochromatic annulus and a broadband ("white") center. Open circles represent the blackness-induction function obtained with a broadband ("white") annulus and monochromatic center. Both curves were normalized to 550 nm. After Shinomori et al. (1997).

function was only determined by the luminance of the surround, as indicated by the unimodal function; however, when the annulus was broadband (open circles), the blackness-response function revealed a chromatic contribution, as evidenced by the three distinct peaks in the function and a dip at approximately 580 nm. As further confirmation, additivity tests were conducted with the monochromatic center/"white" annulus configuration. Failures of additivity were readily observed. It was concluded that the blackness-induction functions represented an interaction among achromatic signals from the annulus and both achromatic and chromatic-opponent signals elicited from the test center.

From this study (Shinomori et al., 1997), a more comprehensive model of spatially-induced blackness has emerged. A schema of this model is presented in Figure 10.7. This model describes the neural response functions arising from the center and annulus and how they combine to give the experience of blackness. The first stage of the model represents the excitation of the three cone types (S, M, L) from the center stimulus, whose signals can be combined in one of four ways [L+M, L-2M, 2M-L, S-(M+L)], and excitation of two cone types (M, L) from the annulus, whose signals are additively combined. At the second stage, M/L opponent signals arising from the test center are rectified in the cortex such that only one of the two M/L opponent processes is active at a time. The signals originating from the center continue on to stage three, where an S-(M+L) signal interacts in an opposing manner with the rectified output. After a logarithmic transformation of the signals from both the center and the surround, the signals from both are subtractively combined to create the neural output necessary to perceive blackness.

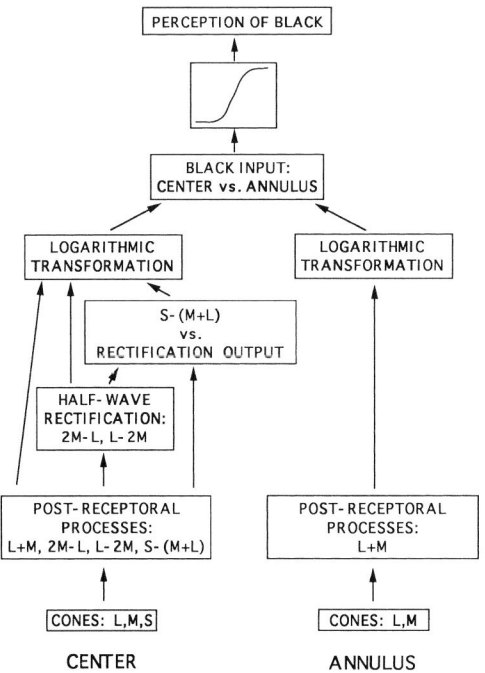

Fig. 10.7: Schematic representation of Shinomori et al.'s (1997) model of blackness. L, M, S denote long-wavelength-sensitive, middle-wavelength-sensitive, and short-wavelength-sensitive cones, respectively.

10.4 Physiological Mechanisms

The early theorists on the perception of blackness speculated on the mechanisms contributing to color vision and several years later physiological evidence emerged to support and at times contradict their theories. For example, Helmholtz's nebulous nerve fibers were identified as three cone receptors, each differentiated by the photopigment it contained and classified by the peak sensitivities of their absorption spectra - short-wavelength sensitive (S), middle-wavelength sensitive (M), and long-wavelength sensitive (L; Brown and Wald, 1963; Bowmaker and Dartnall, 1980; Schnapf et al., 1987). Neural mechanisms further along the visual pathway have not, however, shown similar response functions as the cones.

Hering, on the other hand, surmised that there were neural mechanisms displaying antagonistic behavior, although it was never completely clear if he believed these mechanisms to exist in the retina, in the cortex or both. Electrophysiological recordings have disclosed spatially antagonistic achromatic and chromatic mechanisms in both the retina and cortex (De Valois et al., 1966; Wiesel and Hubel, 1966; Livingstone and Hubel, 1984).

Of particular interest for achromatic processing are the broadband cells which have a spectral response function in both the center and surround (the surround being the inverse of the center response function) that are similar in shape to those obtained with humans for HFP and blackness induction. It has further been demonstrated at the ganglion cell level that most of these cells receive input from the M and L photoreceptors and a small set receive input from all three cone types – albeit very weak input from the S cones (de Monasterio and Gouras, 1975; de Monasterio, 1978). In addition, the magno cells have been directly linked to HFP responses (Lee et al., 1988).

Categorically, the broadband cells are commonly divided into two groups: on-center/off-surround and off-center/on-surround. The on-center cells respond to increments of light and can be thought of as white+/black-cells since optimal activity for these cells occurs when a white spot appears on a black background. The off-center cells, however, respond to decrements of light, showing the greatest excitatory activity when a black spot appears on a white background, and can be referred to as black+/white- (DeValois and DeValois, 1975). It would appear that these two cell types could explain the experience of all achromatic perceptions.

The problem is how to explain the recent model of Shinomori et al. (1997) which implies a more complex interaction between both the achromatic and chromatic channels in the perception of black. While it is often easier to think of the white-black process as completely separate from the chromatic-opponent processes, cells may multiplex both types of information (De Valois and De Valois, 1975; Lennie, 1984; Ingling and Martinez-Uriegas, 1985). Perhaps, it is better to think not in terms of achromatic and chromatic pathways but rather in terms of on-channels to signal increments of light and off-channels to signal decrements of light, which includes both achromatic and chromatic responsive cells (Schiller, 1984; Schiller, 1992). The problem, however, in relating the past physiological findings to this current theory of blackness is that none of the past physiological studies have been guided by this current psychophysical theory or have directly investigated blackness. It is probably better to wait and use this theory to drive future physiological studies, rather than casually implicate an unrelated neural process in blackness perception.

10.5 Conclusion

While it is easy to speculate as to the initial impact of a theory, it is much more difficult to predict its long-lasting contribution. Two color vision theorists from the nineteenth century, Helmholtz and Hering, have certainly influenced the direction and interpretation of past and current color vision theories and research. In this chapter only one domain of their theories was explored, namely the perception of blackness. As evidenced above, the theory of Hurvich and Jameson (1957) drew from the ideas of both theorists with a strong emphasis on Hering's views of blackness. The psychophysical studies of blackness also followed the Hering tradition, and the physiological studies point to the use of Helmholtz and Hering's ideas to interpret their experimental findings. The problem arises when others propose different ideas. For example, while Heggelund acknowledges the idea of opponency, he does not follow the ideas of Hering. In fact, he has charted new territory by attempting to explain color appearance in both the surface and aperture modes. Also, the new model of Shinomori and colleagues (1997) deviates from the original concepts of Helmholtz, Hering, and Hurvich and Jameson. One can only wonder what the impact of these new ideas will have on future research, especially in physiology. Will some retinal and cortical cells be classified as luminous +/black? Or will physiologists develop their own visual theories and guide the psychophysical study of blackness?

References

Aristotle (1967). De coloribus. (T. Loveday & E. S. Forster Trans.) In: The works of Aristotle, Vol. 6, W.D. Ross ed. (London: Oxford University Press), pp. 791–799.

Balaraman, S. (1962). Color vision research and the trichromatic theory: A historical review. Psychological Bulletin 59, 434–448.

Boring, E. G. (1942). Sensation and perception in the history of experimental psychology. (New York: Appleton-Century-Crofts, Inc.).

Bowmaker, J. K. and Dartnall, H. J. A. (1980). Visual pigments of rods and cones in a human retina. Journal of Physiology 298, 501–511.

Brown, P. K. and Wald, G. (1963).. Visual pigments in human and monkey retinas. Nature 200, 37–43.

Chevreul, M. E. (1883). The principles of harmony and contrast of colors. (C. Martel, Trans.) (London: George Bell and Sons). (Original work published 1839).

Cicerone, C. M., Volbrecht, V. J., Donnelly, S. K., and Werner, J. S. (1986). Perception of blackness. Journal of the Optical Society of America A 3, 432–436.

Creed, R. S. (1931). The after-image of black. Journal of Physiology 73, 247–266.

de Monasterio, F. M. (1978). Properties of concentrically organized X and Y ganglion cells of macaque retina. Journal of Neurophysiology 41, 1394–1417.

de Monasterio, F. M. and Gouras, P. (1975). Functional properties of ganglion cells in the rhesus monkey retina. Journal of Physiology 251, 167–195.

De Valois, R. L. and De Valois, K. (1975). Neural coding of color. In: Handbook of perception, E. C. Carterette and M.P. Friedman eds. (New York: Academic Press), pp. 117–166.

De Valois, R. L., Abramov, I., and Jacobs, G. H. (1966). Analysis of response patterns of LGN cells. Journal of the Optical Society of America 56, 966–977.

Diamond, A. L. (1962). Simultaneous contrast as a function of test-field area. Journal of Experimental Psychology 64, 336–345.

Diamond, A. L. (1955). Foveal simultaneous contrast as a function of inducing-field area. Journal of Experimental Psychology 50, 144–152.

Diamond, A. L. (1953). Foveal simultaneous brightness contrast as a function of inducing- and test-field luminances. Journal of Experimental Psychology 45, 304–314.

Evans, R. M. (1967). Luminance and induced colors from adaptation to 100-millilambert monochromatic light. Journal of the Optical Society of America 57, 279–281.

Evans, R. M. (1949). On some aspects of white, gray, and black. Journal of the Optical Society of America 39, 774–779.

Evans, R. M. and Swenholt, B. K. (1969). Chromatic strength of colors, III. Chromatic surrounds and discussion. Journal of the Optical Society of America 59, 628–634.

Franklin, C. (1893). On theories of light-sensation. Mind 2, 473–489.

Fuld, K. and Otto, T. A. (1985) Color of monochromatic lights that vary in contrast-induced brightness. Journal of the Optical Society of America A 2, 76–83.

Fuld, K., Otto, T. A., and Slade, C. W. (1986). Spectral responsivity of the white-black channel. Journal of the Optical Society of America A 3, 1182–1188.

Gelb, A. (1955). Colour constancy. In: A source book of Gestalt psychology, W. D. Ellis ed. (New York: The Humanities Press Inc.), pp. 196–209, (Original work published 1929).

Goethe, A. (1970). Theory of colours. (C. L. Eastlake, Trans.) (Cambridge, MA: MIT Press), (Original work published 1810).

Guth, S. L., Donley, N. J., and Marrocco, R. T. (1969). On luminance additivity and related topics. Vision Research 9, 537–575.

Hartridge, H. (1948). Recent advance in color vision. Science 108, 395–404.

Heggelund, P. (1974a). Achromatic color vision I: Perceptive variables of achromatic colors. Vision Research 14, 1071–1079.

Heggelund, P. (1974b). Achromatic color vision II: Measurement of simultaneous contrast within a bidimensional system. Vision Research 14, 1081–1088.

Heggelund, P. (1992). A bidimensional theory of achromatic color vision. Vision Research 32, 2107–2119.

Heggelund, P. (1993). Simultaneous luminance contrast with chromatic colors. Vision Research 33, 1709–1722.

Heinemann, E.G. (1955). Simultaneous brightness induction as a function of inducing- and test-field luminances. Journal of Experimental Psychology 50, 89–96.

Helmholtz, H. v. (1962). Handbook of physiological optics. J. P. C. Southall, ed. and trans., (New York: Dover), (Original work published 1867).

Hering, E. (1964). Outlines of a theory of the light sense. (L. M. Hurvich and D. Jameson, Trans.) (Cambridge, MA: Harvard University Press), (Original work published 1920).

Hering, E. (1897). Theory of functions in living matter. Brain 20, 232–258. (Original work published in 1888).

Hering, E. (1887). Über die Theorie des simultanen Contrastes von Helmholtz. Pflügers Archiv für die gesammte Physiologie des Menschen und der Tiere *40*, 172–191.

Hering, E. (1878). Zur Lehre vom Lichtsinne. (Vienna: Carl Gerolds Sohn).

Hering, E. (1874). Über die sogenannte Intensität der Lichtempfindung und über die Empfindung des Schwarzen. Sitzungsberichte der Kaiserlichen Akademie der Wissenschaften *69*, 84–104.

Hess, C. and Pretori, H. (1970). Quantitative investigation of the lawfulness of simultaneous brightness contrast. (H. R. Flock and J. H. Tenney, Trans.) Perceptual and Motor Skills *31*, 947–969. (Original work published 1894).

Horeman, H.W. (1963). Inductive brightness depression as influenced by configurational conditions. Vision Research *3*, 121–130.

Hurvich, L. M. and Jameson, D. (1949). Helmholtz and the three-color theory: An historical note. American Journal of Psychology *62*, 111–114.

Hurvich, L. M. and Jameson, D. (1953). Spectral sensitivity of the fovea. I. Neutral adaptation. Journal of the Optical Society of America *43*, 485–494.

Hurvich, L. M. and Jameson, D. (1955). Some quantitative aspects of an opponent-color theory. II. Brightness, saturation, and hue in normal and dichromatic vision. Journal of the Optical Society of America *45*, 602–616.

Hurvich, L. M. and Jameson, D. (1957). An opponent-process theory of color vision. Psychological Review *64*, 384–404.

Ikeda, M., Yaguchi, H., and Sagawa, K. (1982). Brightness luminous-efficiency functions for 2° and 10° fields. Journal of the Optical Society of America *72*, 1660–1665.

Ingling, C. R. and Martinez-Uriegas, E. (1985). The spatiotemporal properties of the r-g X-cell channel. Vision Research *25*, 33–38.

Ives, H. E. (1912a). Spectral luminosity curves obtained by the equality of brightness photometer and the flicker photometer under similar conditions. Philosophical Magazine *24*, 149–188.

Ives, H.E. (1912b). Distortions in spectral luminosity curves produced by variations in the character of the comparison standard and of the surroundings of the photometric field. Philosophical Magazine *24*, 744–751.

Jacobs, G. H. and Gaylord, H. A. (1967). Effects of chromatic adaptation on color naming. Vision Research *7*, 645–653.

Jameson, D. and Hurvich, L. M. (1955). Some quantitative aspects of an opponent-colors theory. I. Chromatic responses and spectral saturation. Journal of the Optical Society *45*, 546–552.

Katz, D. (1935). The world of colour. (R.B. MacLeod and C. W. Fox, Trans.) (London: Kegan Paul, Trench, Trubner and Co., Ltd.). (Original work published 1930).

Kitterle, F. L. (1972). The effects of simultaneous and successive contrast on perceived brightness. Vision Research *12*, 1923–1931.

Kitterle, F. L. (1975). The effects of inducer duration on successive brightness contrast. Vision Research *15*, 273–275.

Kinney, J. A. S. (1962). Factors affecting induced color. Vision Research *2*, 503–525.

Kries, J. von (1905). Die Gesichtsempfindungen. In: Handbuch der Physiologie des Menschen, Vol. 3, W. Nagel, ed., (Braunschweig:Vieweg), pp. 109–282.

Kulp, T. D. and Fuld, K. (1989). Black spectral responsivity. Journal of the Optical Society of America A *6*, 1233–1238.

Ladd-Franklin, C. (1916). On color theories and chromatic sensations. Psychological Review *23*, 237–249.

Ladd-Franklin, C. (1922a). Tetrachromatic vision and the development theory of color. Science *55*, 555–560.

Ladd-Franklin, C. (1922b). Practical logic and color theories. Psychological Review *29*, 180–200.

Ladd-Franklin, C. (1925). The theory of blackness. American Journal of Physiological Optics *6*, 453–454.

Lee, B. B., Martin, P. R., and Valberg, A. (1988). The physiological basis of heterochromatic flicker photometry demonstrated in the ganglion cells of the macaque retina. Journal of Physiology *404*, 323–347.

Leibowitz, H., Mote, F. A., and Thurlow, W. R. (1953). Simultaneous contrast as a function of separation between test and inducing fields. Journal of Experimental Psychology *46*, 453–456.

Lemmon, V. W. (1925). A modification of the Ladd-Franklin theory of color vision. American Journal of Physiological Optics *6*, 449–452.

Lennie, P. (1984). Recent developments in the physiology of color vision. Trends in Neuroscience *7*, 243–248.

Livingstone, M. S. and Hubel, D. H. (1984). Anatomy and physiology of a color system in the primate visual cortex. Journal of Neuroscience *4*, 309–356.

Luh, C. W. (1930). 'Practical Logic' and Ladd-Franklin's black. Psychological Review *37*, 267–270.

MacLeod, R. B. (1932). An experimental investigation of brightness constancy. Archives of Psychology *21*, 5–102.

Mach, E. (1959). The analysis of sensations. (C. M. Williams and S. Waterlow, Trans.) (New York: Dover), (Original work published 1906).

Maxwell, J. C. (1860). On the theory of compound colours, and the relations of the colours of the spectrum. Philosophical Transactions of the Royal Society *150*, 57–84.

McDougall, W. (1901a). IV. Some new observations in support of Thomas Young's theory of light- and colour-vision (I). Mind *10*, 52–97.

McDougall, W. (1901b). IV. Some new observations in support of Thomas Young's theory of light- and colour-vision (II). Mind *10*, 210–245.

McDougall, W. (1901c). IV. Some new observations in support of Thomas Young's theory of light- and colour-vision (III. Conclusion). Mind *10*, 347–382.

Michaels, G. M. (1925). Black: A non-light sensation. Psychological Review *32*, 248–250.

Mount, G. E. and Thomas, J. P. (1968). Relation of spatially induced brightness changes to test and inducing wavelengths. Journal of the Optical Society of America *58*, 23–27.

Müller, G. E. (1896). Zur Psychophysik der Gesichtsempfindungen. Kapitel 2. Zeitschrift für Psychologie und Physiologie der Sinnesorgane *10*, 321–413.

Müller, G. E. (1897). Zur Psychophysik der Gesichtsempfindungen. Kapitel 4. Zeitschrift für Psychologie und Physiologie der Sinnesorgane *14*, 1–76.

Nakano, Y., Ikeda, M., and Kaiser, P. K. (1988). Contributions of the opponent mechanisms to brightness and nonlinear models. Vision Research *28*, 799–810.

Neifeld, M. R. (1924). The Ladd-Franklin theory of the black sensation. Psychological Review *31*, 498–502.

Newton, I. (1979). Opticks. (New York: Dover), (Original work published 1730).

Parsons, J. H. (1915). An introduction to the study of colour vision. (Cambridge, England: University Press).

Quinn, P. C., Wooten, B. R., and Ludman, E. J. (1985). Achromatic color categories. Perception & Psychophysics *37*, 198–204.

Rich, G. J. (1926). Black and grey in visual theory. American Journal of Psychology *37*, 123–128.

Romeskie, M. (1978). Chromatic opponent-response functions of anomalous trichromats. Vision Research *18*, 1521–1532.

Schiller, P. H. (1992). The ON and OFF channels of the visual system. Trends in Neuroscience *15*, 86–92.

Schiller, P. H. (1984). The connections of the retinal on and off pathways to the lateral geniculate nucleus of the monkey. Vision Research *24*, 923–932.

Schnapf, J. L., Kraft, T. W., and Baylor, D. A. (1987). Spectral sensitivity of human cone photoreceptors. Nature *325*, 439–441.

Schopenhauer, A. (1905). Über das Sehn und die Farben: Eine Abhandlung von Arthur Schopenhauer. In Schopenhauer's Sämmtliche Werk Vol. 3, (Leipzig: Inselverlag). pp. 675–779.

Schödinger, E. (1925). Ueber das Verhältnis der Vierfarben- zur Dreifarbentheorie. Sitzungsbericht der Wiener Akademie der Wissenschaften, Mathematisch-naturwissenschaftliche Klasse *134*, 471–490.

Sherman, P. D. (1981). Colour vision in the nineteeth century. (Bristol: Adam Hilger).

Shinomori, K., Nakano, Y., and Uchikawa, K. (1994). Influence of the illuminance and spectral composition of surround fields on spatially induced blackness. Journal of the Optical Society of America A *11*, 2383–2388.

Shinomori, K., Schefrin, B. E., and Werner, J. S. (1997). Spectral mechanisms of spatially-induced blackness: Data and quantitative model. Journal of the Optical Society of America A *14*, 372–387.

Sperling, H. G. and Lewis, W. G. (1959). Some comparisons between foveal spectral sensitivity data obtained at high brightness and absolute threshold. Journal of the Optical Society of America *49*, 983–989.

Sloan, L. L. (1928). The effect of intensity of light, state of adaptation of the eye, and size of photometric field on the visibility curve. Psychological Monograph *38*, 1–87.

Tessier, M. and Blottiau, F. (1951). Variations des caraceristiques photometriques de l'oeil aux luminances photopiques. Revue d'Optique *30*, 309–322.

Titchener, E. B. (1916a). A note on the sensory character of black. Journal of Philosophy: Psychology and Scientific Method *13*, 113–121.

Titchener, E. B. (1916b). A further word on black. Journal of Philosophy: Psychology and Scientific Method *13*, 649–655.

Troland, L. T. (1921). The enigma of color vision. American Journal of Physiological Optics *2*, 317–337.

Venable, W. M. (1925). The Ladd-Franklin theory of color vision. American Journal of Physiological Optics *6*, 521–526.

Volbrecht, V. J. and Werner, J. S. (1989). Temporal

induction of blackness II. Spectral efficiency and tests of additivity. Vision Research 29, 1437–1455.

Volbrecht, V. J., Werner, J. S., and Cicerone, C. M. (1990). Additivity of spatially induced blackness. Journal of the Optical Society of America A 7, 106–112.

Volbrecht, V. J., Werner, J. S., and Wooten, B. R. (1989). Temporal induction of blackness I. Color appearance. Vision Research 29, 1425–1436.

Vos, J. J. and Walraven, P. L. (1971). On the derivation of the foveal receptor primaries. Vision Research 11, 799–818.

Wallach, H. (1948). Brightness constancy and the nature of achromatic colors. Journal of Experimental Psychology 38, 310–324.

Wagner, G. and Boynton, R. M. (1972). Comparison of four methods of heterochromatic photometry. Journal of the Optical Society of America 62, 1508–1515.

Ward, J. (1905). Is 'black' a sensation? British Journal of Psychology 1, 407–427.

Ward, J. (1916). A further note on the sensory character of black. British Journal of Psychology 8, 212–221.

Weale, R. A. (1957). Trichromatic ideas in the seventeenth and eighteenth centuries. Nature 179, 648–651.

Werner, J. S., Cicerone, C. M., Kliegl, R., and Dellarosa, D. (1984). Spectral efficiency of blackness induction. Journal of the Optical Society of America A1, 981–986.

Werner, J. S. and Wooten, B. R. (1979). Opponent chromatic mechanisms: Relation to photopigments and hue naming. Journal of the Optical Society of America 69, 422–434.

Wiesel, T. N. and Hubel, D. H. (1966). Spatial and chromatic interactions in the lateral geniculate body of the rhesus monkey. Journal of Neurophysiology 29, 1115–1156.

Wooten, B. R. (1984). The effects of successive chromatic contrast on spectral hue. In: Sensory experience, adaptation, and perception, B. R. Wooten and L. Spillmann, eds. (Hillsdale, NJ: Lawrence Erlbaum Associates Publishers), pp. 471–494.

Wright, W. D. (1980). The perception of blackness. Die Farbe 28, 161–166.

Wright, W. D. (1981). The nature of blackness in art and visual perception. Leonardo 14, 236–237.

Yaguchi, H. and Ikeda, M. (1983). Subadditivity and superadditivity in heterochromatic brightness matching. Vision Research 23, 1711–1718.

Young, T. (1970). On the theory of light and colors. In: Sources of color science, D.L. MacAdam, ed. (Cambridge, MA: MIT Press), p. 51, (Original work published 1802, 1845).

11. Basic Color Terms and Basic Color Categories

Clyde L. Hardin

Twenty-five years have passed since the publication of Brent Berlin and Paul Kay's influential book, *Basic Color Terms* (1969). After it appeared, there was a flurry of critiques, responses, and further studies. When the work became enshrined in the textbooks, most people took the issue of the nature and implications of basic color term usage to be settled. Strangely enough, exactly what was supposed to have been settled depended on whom you consulted. On the left wing were the unreconstructed cultural relativists who maintained that the Berlin and Kay findings were an artifact of their methods, and that these were riddled with dubious assumptions. On the right wing were the nativists who found the Berlin-Kay picture totally persuasive.

As usually turns out to be the case, the truth lies between these extreme views. Although the Berlin and Kay position was significantly modified in subsequent years, many of its basic tenets have proved to be quite robust, supported by various bits of independent evidence. Nonetheless, there are many important questions that remain unresolved. If the grand multilayered story that the Berlin Kay work suggests can be completed in its most essential details, it will connect perception, thought, and culture. At the center of the story is the experience of color and its representation in individual consciousness. One branch of the story reaches downward into human biology and the organization of the nervous system. The other branch reaches outward into language and social interaction. Doubtless there will in time be many such stories, but at the present juncture in the history of science, this one is the only viable candidate. There are numerous gaps and holes between levels and within levels. All the same, there is enough on the table to suggest that holes can be filled and links forged.

Here is how the original story went. Berlin and Kay were struck by how easily common color terms could be translated between languages from places as diverse as Tahiti and Mesoamerica. But if, as cultural relativists had suggested, languages divide color space arbitrarily, and moreover, shape the way that their speakers perceive colored objects, how is this possible? To investigate the question, Berlin and Kay proposed criteria to separate the basic from the non-basic color terms of a language. Basic terms are to be those that are *general* and *salient*. A term is general if it applies to diverse classes of objects and its meaning is not subsumable under the meaning of another term. A term is salient if it is readily elicitable, occurs in the idiolects of most informants, and is used consistently by individuals and with a high degree of consensus among individuals. To determine the references of the basic color terms of a language, Berlin and Kay used a rectangular array of Munsell color chips of maximum available chroma, vertically ordered in ten equal lightness steps, and horizontally ordered by hue, each column differing from its neighbors by a nominal 2.5 Hue steps. (The array was essentially a Mercator projection of the outer skin of the Munsell solid.) The test array was covered by transparent acetate, and each informant was asked, for each basic color term, to mark with a grease pencil (a) the best example, or *focus* of the color, and (b) the region of chips that could be called by the color term. Figure 11.1 illustrates the naming of all of the chips of the Berlin-Kay array by a 35-year-old male English speaker. 'Plus' signs represent the focal examples chosen by this speaker for each of the basic color categories.

The investigation on which *Basic Color Terms* was based used native-speaking informants in the

San Francisco Bay Area for 20 languages, supplementing this limited field study with a literature search on 78 additional languages. The *synchronic* results were that languages vary in numbers of basic color terms, from a minimum of two terms (Papuan Dani) to a (probable) maximum of eleven, Russian and Hungarian being possible exceptions. But no matter how many basic color terms languages might have, their foci tend to cluster reliably in relatively narrow regions of the array, whereas boundaries are drawn unreliably, with low consistency and consensus for any language.

The *diachronic* conclusion was that if languages were ordered according to numbers of basic color terms, the sequences of *encodings* of basic color terms were tightly constrained (the conception of successive steps as encodings was subsequently changed by Berlin and Kay). For example, if a language has two basic color terms (a "Stage I" language) those terms will encode black and white. If it has three ("Stage II"), those terms will encode black, white, and red. If it has four ("Stage III"), the terms will be for black, white, red, and either yellow or green. The entire sequence comprises seven stages and eleven basic color terms. Berlin and Kay interpreted these as stages in an evolutionary sequence, and it is this interpretation that has occasioned the greatest controversy. The nature of the stages and the rules that govern their development are the points of the Berlin-Kay theses that have been most revised by their authors.

The early emergence of black, white, red, yellow, green, and blue, along with the clustering of the focal examples of each of these terms readily suggests an interpretation in terms of Hering's opponent-process theory. This reading of the matter was strengthened when McDaniel (1972) showed that when experimental subjects were asked to match their respective focal choices of red, yellow, green, and blue Munsell color chips with monochromatic lights, they chose lights of unique hue. Evidence for the view that hue categories based upon the perception of four elementary Hering hues are conceptually more fundamental than the other hue categories comes from hue-naming experiments with human adults. That the primacy of these Hering hue categories is biologically rather than linguistically based has been argued for by the congruence between adult human color-naming data and color categorization by human infants as well as other primates. Let us consider these points in turn.

A typical hue-naming experiment asks subjects to look at spots of monochromatic light and describe them with a restricted set of hue names prescribed by the experimenter. They are instructed to estimate the percentage of the specified hue that they see in the stimulus. Subjects tend to be quite reliable in performing this task. Sternheim and Boynton (1966), along with later investigators, used an estimation procedure to determine the minimum number of hue terms necessary to describe the spectrum completely. The requirement for a stimulus to be described completely was that the percentage estimate of component hues add up to 100. A total component estimation of less than 100 per cent over a spectral range was interpreted as meaning that another hue term was required, whereas if every portion of the spectrum could be specified in terms of 100 per cent totals of the permitted hues, the names of those hues were taken to constitute a descriptively sufficient set for that spectral portion. Thus the term 'orange' proves to be unnecessary, since subjects are able to describe stimuli that look orange entirely in terms of yellow and red, whereas if the terms 'orange' and 'green' are permitted but 'yellow' forbidden, yellow-looking stimuli will not be describable as a combination of orange and green. English speakers find the hue names 'red', 'yellow', 'green' and 'blue' prove to be both necessary and sufficient to describe any spectral stimulus.

Hue naming as we have so far described it relies upon language. What about creatures without language? Do they find some categorizations of color continua more natural than others? Four-month human infants know precious little English, and they cannot describe what they see. Nevertheless, by watching their eye fixations one can tell whether they see two stimuli as similar or different. Infants will lose interest in a stimulus that looks similar to its predecessor, but continue looking at a stimulus that they regard as different from what went before. By exposing infants to sequences of colored lights whose dominant wavelengths are 20 nm apart, and recording their eye movements, Bornstein, Kessen and Weiskopf (1976) were able to map out their spectral color categories. These proved to line up rather well with the spectral categories of adults that are mapped with color-naming procedures. Using a rather different subject pool, Sandell, Gross, and Bornstein (1979) trained macaques to respond differentially to colored papers that human beings would see as good representatives of their categories, and then presented them with randomized sequences of colored papers that did not match the training stimuli. Their response rates changed markedly as the stimuli crossed human red-yellow-green-blue category boundaries, and were not sensitive to minor variations from monkey to monkey in the actual values of the training stimuli.

All of this suggests that categorization is in an important respect prior to language. This is consistent with what we know about certain brain-damaged people, who can pass color-vision tests as well as produce color names (see chapter 7). Though they are unable to apply the color names to objects correctly, they are able to sort colored yarns correctly. However, it may well be the case that the categories available to these people are a function of their past experience with language and with socially influenced color-sorting experiences. We would like to know if there is a set of default categories that members of our species and our closest cousins bring into the world. The infant data suggest that there is, and that these default categories are based upon the Hering primaries.

The very success of the nativist argument puts a significant burden on visual and cognitive scientists. It is one thing to note with satisfaction that basic infant hues are basic Hering hues. It is quite another to give an account of why there are eleven Berlin-Kay categories but only six Hering categories, why some derived categories such as purple are basic but others such as chartreuse are not, and why the categories are so uneven in size and placement. When one examines the color space in three dimensions rather than just looking at the outer skin, as Berlin and Kay did, the problems are even more pronounced.

Working independently of each other and using different color-order systems and different methods, Boynton and his collaborators in the United States (Boynton and Olson, 1987; Uchikawa and Boynton, 1987) and Sivik and Taft (Sivik, 1985; Sivik and Taft, 1991) in Sweden asked subjects to name samples drawn from the whole color space. Their determinations of the sizes and locations of the eleven Berlin and Kay categories are quite comparble, although they used different methods.

Boynton and Olson (1987), using separately presented samples from the Optical Society of America's Uniform Color Space (OSA) asked their English-speaking informants to name the samples with monolexical terms, but put no further restrictions on what those terms were to be. After each informant named each of the 424 color chips, presented in random sequence on two separate occasions, Boynton and Olson assessed the consistency with which each subject named the chips as well as the extent of agreement, or consensus, among informants. During the trials, response latency between each presentation and the production of the name was covertly measured. Boynton and Olson found that each of these three salience measures – consistency, consensus, and response time – neatly separated the chips named by Berlin and Kay's eleven basic color terms from all of the others. Uchikawa and Boynton repeated the procedure with native speakers of Japanese with essentially the same results. Later data gathered from testing English-speaking two and four-year old children and a four-year old Japanese child were consistent with these findings.

The Boynton work raises several intriguing issues. Here is one of them. Although all three of the salience measures separate basic from non-basic color terms, none of them distinguishes between the terms for the Hering primaries and the terms for the other basic colors. Corbett and Davies (1997) looked at a number of linguistic as well as salience measures that would not only discriminate basic from non-basic color terms, but also distinguish between the Hering primaries and the other basic terms. The only procedure that they found that reliably made this latter distinction was to ask people to list the color terms that first come to mind. The Hering primaries almost always get mentioned first. Why do the other techniques fail to establish such a difference among the primary and derived basics? Boynton is inclined to say that none of the basic colors is more fundamental than the rest, and that whatever native neural machinery makes for color classifications, the category-generating mechanisms for orange are on a par with those for red and yellow. Here is a direct quotation: "I feel it reasonable to suppose that there may be eleven categorically-separate varieties of activity, corresponding to each of eleven kinds of color sensations that are identified by the eleven basic color terms" (Boynton, 1997). And this from the man who helped bring us the Sternheim-Boynton color-naming technique that established that red and yellow are more basic than orange!

A second problem has to do with the large differences in size between the regions of color space that are called 'red' or 'yellow' and the ones that are called 'blue' or 'green'. The latter, but not the former, are found at all lightness levels. To this one might appropriately respond that we call light reds 'pink' and dark – or, more accurately, *blackened* – yellows 'brown'. Now many people will hesitate to say that a brown is *just* a blackened orange or yellow, for brown looks to have a very different quality from those two. Indeed, Fuld, Werner and Wooten (1983) found some evidence to support the conclusion that brown might be an elemental color. Although Quinn, Rosano, and Wooten (1988), by running a careful Sternheim-Boynton procedure, were subsequently able to show that brown is none other than blackened yellow, the subjective impression remains that there is something special about brown. Its appearance of strong qualitative difference from yellow distinguishes it from other blackened colors, most of which resemble their parent hues. Blackened blues continue to look blue, blackened greens, i.e., olive greens, continue to look green. Only oranges and yellows seem to lose the parental connection when blackened. I would suggest that we have here an important phenomenal fact that has not been fully accounted for.

Another question has to do with the absence of basic terms for two regions of binary hue that are marked by such non-basic terms as 'chartreuse' and 'lime' on the one hand, and 'aqua' and 'turquoise' on the other. If one takes a simple-minded look at the basic opponent-colors scheme, one finds no reason to expect that the yellow-green binaries and the green-blue binaries would be less salient than the yellow-red binaries that we call 'orange' and the red-blue binaries that we call 'purple'. And yet, Berlin and Kay tell us that there are many languages with basic terms for orange and purple, but not a single one with a basic term for either chartreuse or turquoise.

'Chartreuse' is not the most common of words. Many people think that it falls between pink and purple. Suppose, however, that one had a group of people who knew how to use the term correctly. Would their use of the term be closely analogous to their use of 'orange'? Several years ago, Beare and Siegel (1967) had shown that in color-naming experiments when 'yellow' and 'red' were permitted but 'orange' forbidden, subjects would fully describe the spectral range around 590 nm in terms of 'red' and 'yellow', in complete accordance with the findings of Sternheim and Boynton. But if 'orange' were permitted in addition to 'red' and 'yellow', the ranges of both of these latter terms would be sharply constricted, and neither name would ever be used to describe a 590 nm stimulus. In similar fashion, in using the OSA chip set, Boynton never found a case in which a chip was called 'yellow' on one occasion and 'red' on another, by either the same or different subjects, whereas many chips were called 'red' on one occasion and 'orange' on another.

Miller (1997) explored the comparative uses of 'orange' and 'chartreuse' by using a forced-choice color-naming procedure in which the available hue names were 'red', 'yellow', 'green', and 'blue' along with 'orange' and 'chartreuse'. All of Miller's subjects were told that chartreuse is "a greenish-yellow or yellowish-green about halfway between green and yellow." They viewed monochromatic lights ranging from 430 to 660 nm, and "were instructed that after a warning tone they would receive a hue term and then must push one of two buttons indicating whether the hue is 'present' or 'absent'." The resulting identification functions for the six hue terms are good matches for the curves obtained in the more usual hue-naming experiments. However, the functions for 'chartreuse' and 'orange' relate quite differently to their neighbors. 'Orange' shows the expected behavior, restricting the ranges of 'red' and 'yellow', whereas 'chartreuse' seems essentially redundant, 'yellow' and 'green' behaving in the *presence* of 'chartreuse' much the way that 'red' and 'yellow' behave in the *absence* of 'orange'. Taken with the Berlin and Kay data, this suggests a difference between the binaries that we would not have expected from the opponent scheme alone.

We have seen that there are several lines of evidence to support Berlin and Kay's distinction between basic and non-basic color terms, with six of the basic terms having as their referents the Hering primaries. The color categories that these six pick out appear to have a prototypic structure, with the foci for the most part positioned where visual science would have expected them to be, the generalization from the prototypic instances being achieved by mechanisms held in common by members of our species and our animal cousins. It is reasonable to expect that visual science will have a central role to play in explaining the details of color category organization, although it seems clear that our understanding of the color-vision system is not yet fully up to the task. But it also seems clear that although *perceptual* mechanisms can account for the saliences in our experience, *cognitive* mechanisms must be invoked to explain how and why certain of these saliences are seized on and exploited, while others play a minor role.

This becomes all the more apparent when we direct our attention to the processes by which color categories receive cultural elaboration and expression. We have every reason to suppose that human visual systems function the same way in almost everyone almost everywhere, whereas the stock of basic color terms varies from place to place and time to time. This is, as Berlin and Kay themselves came to see, not just a matter of labels coming to be attached to pre-existent categories, but of a development of the categories themselves.

Kay and McDaniel (1978) proceeded to reconceive the developmental scheme as the successive division of macro-categories into smaller categories focused on the Hering primaries, and then the partition of the Hering categories into the other basic, or "derived" categories plus narrower versions of the Hering six. They suggested thinking of the macro-categories as fuzzy-set unions of the Hering categories, and of the derived categories as rescaled fuzzy-set intersections of pairs of the Hering six. The developmental scheme they proposed is illustrated in an idealized fashion in Figure 11.2. For an intuitive reference, compare the schema for Stage 7 with Figure 11.1c.

Stage I systems (of which Dani is the only attested example) are followed by systems of the Stage II type, with three categories: a white category, a (red plus yellow) category, and a (black plus green plus blue) category. According to Kay and McDaniel, there were two types of four-term systems. Stage IIIa had a (white), a (red plus yellow), and a (green plus blue) and a black category. Stage IIIb had a white, a red, a yellow, and a (green plus blue plus black) category. One could, they suggested, think of Stage IIIa as having resulted from the (green plus blue plus black) category of Stage II splitting into (green plus blue) and black. One could think of Stage IIIb as having resulted from the (red plus yellow) category of Stage II splitting into separate red and yellow categories.

In the transition from IIIa to IV, the (red plus yellow) category splits into separate red and yellow categories. In the transition from IIIb to IV, (black plus green plus blue) splits into black and (green plus blue), often referred to as 'grue'. Passing from Stage IV to Stage V, grue splits into green and blue, producing a system with exactly one basic color term for each of the Hering fundamentals. After Stage V, derived terms, based on fuzzy-set intersection, make their first appearance, and this process continues until the Stage VII languages such as contemporary English have developed. Hereafter, we shall call all of this "the Kay-McDaniel sequence" and the sequence plus the fuzzy-set interpretation "the Kay-McDaniel theory". The virtues of the Kay-McDaniel theory were recently set out by Kay (personal conversation):

"As far as color *per se* is concerned the neurology that is devoted to strictly to color yields as output only the six Hering fundamentals. Then, the other categories, derived like orange, or composite like (black or green or blue), are dependent on the interaction of the strictly color-devoted circuitry with some kind of general cognitive circuitry that has to do with some kind of general category-forming operations that are not restricted to color. One way to interpret the Kay and McDaniel story is, then, that after you get the six Hering primaries, the color story is over, and you enter general psychology, a general cognitive psychology, as it operates on color stuff, but using psychological processes that may operate on other stuff besides color."

Two caveats are in order here. First, as we shall shortly see, there are reasons to wonder whether it is indeed the case that color science would have nothing else to contribute to the story. For instance, where else should we turn to find out why the warm category always divides before the cool category? Visual salience is surely needed in addi-

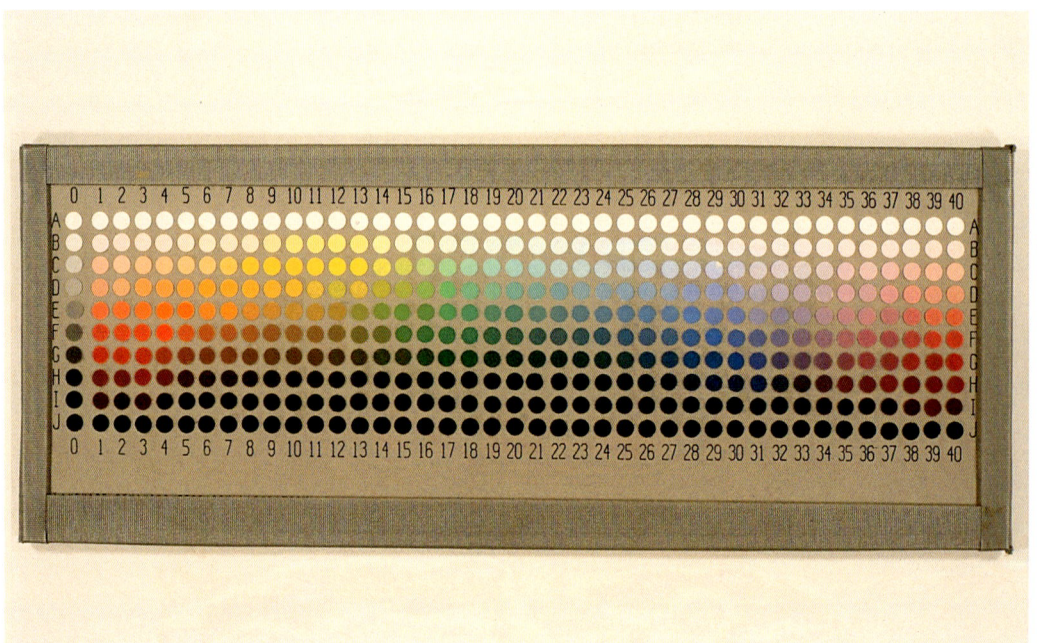

Fig. 11.1 a: This is a photograph of the minature Munsell color array that was used in field trials of the World Color Survey for indicating informants' choices of focal referents of color terms. Color-naming trials used standard-sized Munsell chips of the same designations as those in the array. Those chips were presented individually in randomized order.

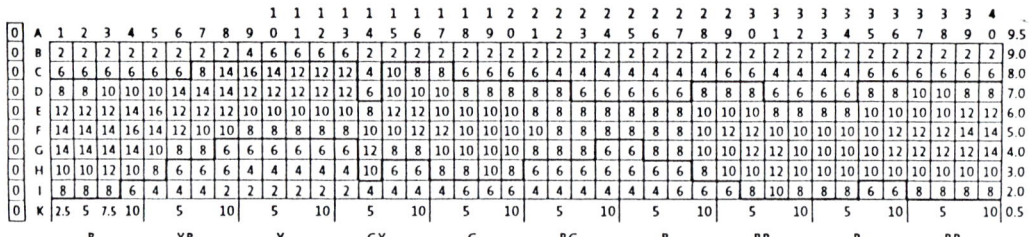

Fig. 11.1 b: This figure gives the specifications of the Munsell color chips that were used in the array pictured in Figure 11.1 and as color-naming stimuli. On the left and at the top are the designations that are printed on the field array. The corresponding Munsell specifications for Hue are given at the bottom, and the specifications for Value appear on the right. The numbers within each cell specify the Munsell Chroma. Heavy lines distinguish Chroma at /6 and below from /8 and above. The left column represents the achromatic Value scale, all of whose chips have a Munsell Chroma of 0. (Courtesy of Robert MacLaury.)

11. Basic Color Terms and Basic Color Categories 213

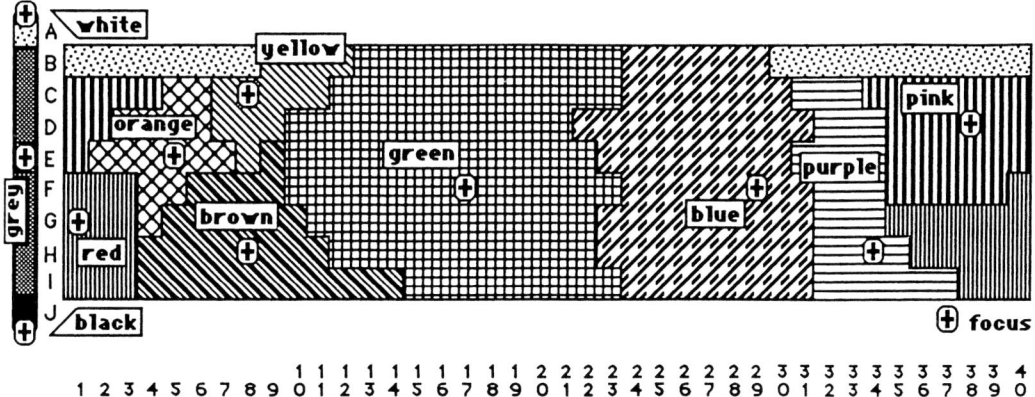

Fig. 11.1c: Color-naming of the Berlin-Kay Munsell array by an English-speaker (see text). (Courtesy of Robert MacLaury).

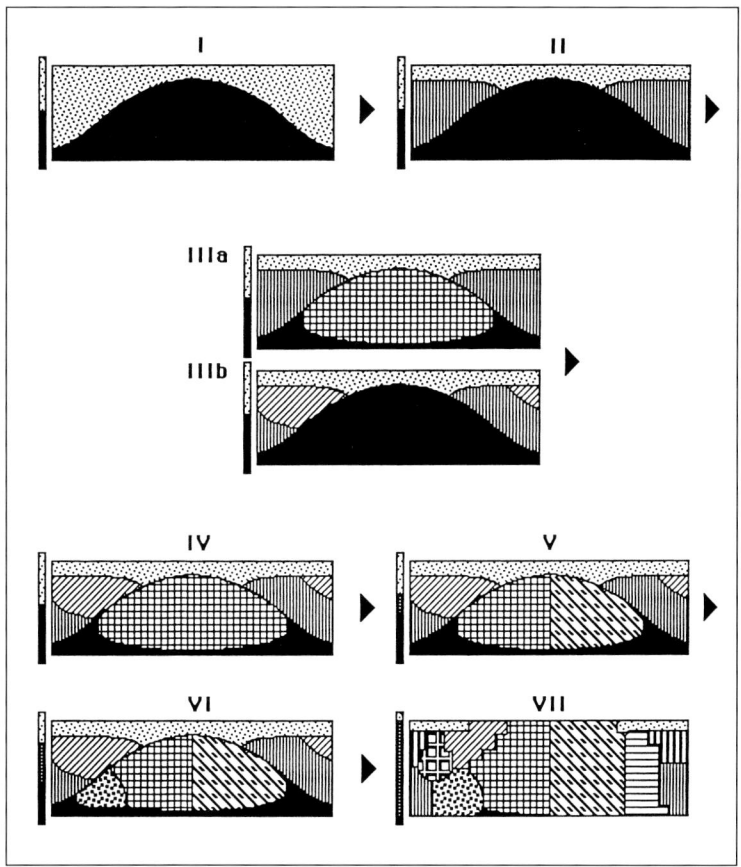

Fig. 11.2: Schematic representation of the Kay-McDaniel sequence (see text). (Courtesy of Paul Kay and Robert MacLaury).

tion to general cognitive processes. Secondly, it is not clear that fuzzy logic alone will be able to do all the work that Kay and McDaniel ask of it. Orange is a case in point. According to fuzzy logic, a theory that permits graded set membership, since orange is the product (along with a scaling factor) of red and yellow, focal orange should be an example of both red and yellow, yet Boynton found no case in which a chip was called both 'red' and 'yellow'. Here, it is important to distinguish between the color category to which a colored sample is assigned and the hue components that can be distinguished in that sample. Samples called 'red' can have a distinct yellow hue component in them – a fact marked in English by the 'ish' suffix – without anyone's being inclined to label the samples as 'yellow'. Depending upon instructions, subjects can be driven to respond either to an overall category established by the dominant hue, or to the admixed hue. Someone who is asked to affix to a sample a monolexemic color word of her choice will likely respond quite differently from one who is presented with the same sample with the instruction, "Yellow: yes or no." To ask how *the* orange category is formed from *the* red category and *the* yellow category without relativizing the question to the task demand or without making the category-component distinction can easily lead to confusion. Beyond that, the fuzzy-logic model would suggest that the behavior of orange and chartreuse should be the same, but Miller's study indicates the contrary. Such considerations call the Kay-McDaniel *theory* into question, but leave the Kay-McDaniel *sequence* intact – for the moment at least.

In the 1970s, while the Kay-McDaniel theory was being hatched, Berlin, Kay and Merrifield were planning the ambitious World Color Survey. Protestant evangelists, dispatched to the most remote regions of the world, were instructed in color term elicitation, interviewing techniques, and the use of a standard randomized array of Munsell color chips as well as a miniaturized color sample array. The objective was to gather data in the field from a wide variety of languages, with 25 monlingual informants for each language (Kay et al., 1991). In addition to their efforts, and those of several other workers, MacLaury (1997) conducted a wide-ranging Mesoamerican Color Survey, using the WCS methods as well as some innovations of his own. Altogether, there is now analyzed data on 111 exotic languages. The new data have required substantial complications to the Kay-McDaniel sequence (Kay et al., 1997).

I shall have nothing particular to say about these complications, save for two remarks. The first is that the results from some of the languages in which there seem to be very broad categories embracing mid-lightness yellow, green, and blue cease to be quite so puzzling when the categories are seen as marking distinctions primarily in brightness or lightness rather than in hue. MacLaury (1992) has suggested a separate brightness sequence for some languages that later merges with Kay-McDaniel hue sequences. This would correct a bias in the Berlin-Kay tradition so far in favor of hue categories that has been pointed out from the beginning by Hickerson (1971) and others. As Casson (1997) tells us, "The eight Old English terms that survived and evolved into basic color terms were brightness terms that had minor hue senses (except red and green, which had major hue senses)."

My second comment is that the basic color vocabularies of the great majority of languages are consistent with the Kay and McDaniel sequence. The exceptions to it are striking and interesting, but they are few. There are solid independent reasons for taking it to be describing an historical process. Historical linguists have performed several reconstructions of earlier states of present-day languages, proto-Mayan, proto-Polynesian, and Anglo-Saxon for example, and have generally found the roots of their basic color terms to be in accord with the Kay-McDaniel sequence. And some of the WCS interviews are best interpreted as marking languages in transition from an earlier to a later stage, with the speakers who use a new basic term tending to be younger than those speakers who do not use the new term. It is of no small interest that in virtually all cases linguistic forms that undergo development in time devolve as well as evolve. According to linguistic typologist Greville Corbett (oral communication), there are just two known counterexamples to this: numeral systems and systems of basic color terms.

There remain the questions of what drives the

evolution of basic color terms, and what, beyond the resources of fuzzy-set logic, constrains the patterns of basic color term development. The answer or, more likely, answers to the first question lie at least in part within the domain of social theory. Some authors see the development of basic color terms as related to social complexity, though what one is to understand by "social complexity" is a question that is bound to be provocative. Others link the development to color technology.

More to the point of our concerns here is to identify the sources of constraint in the development of basic color terms. Why do the Dani divide color space into a warm-light (mola) region and a dark-cool (mili) region? An answer that occurs to us all is implicit in the gloss itself: the colors called 'warm' and the colors called 'cool' seem to form natural resemblance classes. The division is robust, and the same cross-modal semantic labels are reliably used in different languages: Sivik and Taft (1990, 1991) have determined this for English, Swedish, Russian, and Croatian. An interesting question here is whether red and yellow on the one hand, and blue and green on the other, are lumped together because of their association with warmth and coolness respectively, or whether there are intrinsic resemblances that are marked by the associational terms. If, as I suspect, the second opinion, is correct, there is an important phenomenal fact to be accounted for, and not much in the way of currently available resources to do the accounting. (It is interesting to notice that Hering gave red and yellow positive values, and green and blue negative values. This assignment of sign to chromatic valence has persisted to the present, although it is now officially viewed as only conventional). An important first step in exploring this matter was undertaken by Katra and Wooten (1996), who found that subjects' ratings of color chips as "warm" or "cool" closely tracked their opponent-response functions.

Another striking feature of the Kay-McDaniel sequence, to which the World Color Survey provides no exceptions, is the invariable tendency of the "warm" macrocategory to divide before the "cool" macrocategory. There are many languages, particularly in mesoamerica, which have basic categories for red, yellow, and white, along with an intact "grue" – green plus blue – category. There are, on the other hand, no languages with separate basic terms for green and blue that retain an undifferentiated red plus yellow category. MacLaury has remarked in conversation that this would be readily explained if green were more similar to blue than red is similar to yellow. I know of no study that has established this to be so, though it is certainly interesting to observe that people seem to argue more frequently about whether a given sample is "really" blue rather than green than whether it is "really" red rather than yellow. And we have already noted the rather striking fact that green and blue cover large areas of phenomenal color space whereas the "warm" region is differentiated much more finely into red, yellow, orange, pink, and brown. Just why any of this is so is, I think, quite mysterious. It seems to me that once more language is tracking visual saliences, the nature of which has scarcely been explored by visual science.

The chief features of the Berlin-Kay synchronic findings and the chief trends of the Kay-McDaniel sequence are real and robust. They cry out for fuller explanation. Psychophysicists need to establish the detailed character of the visual saliences that underly basic color categories and macro-categories, and ask how biological mechanisms might account for those saliences. Cognitivists need to ask about the dynamics that propel the development of color categories, and whether those dynamics are operative in the formation of other kinds of basic experiential categories as well. There is a lot of work here for everybody.

Discussion and Summary

Although the details of the Berlin-Kay evolutionary sequence have been criticized by many scholars, and the sequence substantially revised, particularly by Kay and McDaniel, the basic claims have been confirmed, and those claims invite interpretation in terms of innate perceptual and cognitive mechanisms. That the mechanisms are indeed innate is supported by both infant and chimpanzee studies of color naming, which are consistent with color naming by adult native speakers of European languages, as studied by Boynton, Sivik, and others. The location of the foci of basic color terms and the order of their appearance in the Berlin-Kay evolutionary sequence indicate that the six Hering elementary colors have a central role to play. However, there are many features of the data and theory that are not explained by an appeal to simple opponent-process models. These include the naming of some but not all binary colors by basic terms, the failure of many salience tests to distinguish between Hering basic terms and the other basic color terms, the strikingly unequal size and distribution of basic color categories, and the early-stage formation and subsequent asymmetrical dissolution of macro-categories, such as "warm-light" and "cool-dark" in languages that have but few basic color terms. The invariability of some of these sequences-e.g. the warm categories always break up into red and yellow categories before the cool categories are resolved into green and blue-suggests that they derive from biologically-based perceptual saliences. Some very preliminary-though provocative-work has been done to investigate these questions. One experiment seems to tie the warm-cool division to the levels of opponent-channel activation, and another suggests that color categorizations by individuals may replicate the Berlin-Kay sequence. All of these questions cry out for further investigation. Psychophysicists need to establish the detailed character of the visual saliences that that underly basic color categories and macro-categories, and ask how biological mechanisms might account for those saliences. Cognitivists need to ask about the dynamics that propel the development of color categories, and whether those dynamics are operative in the formation of other kinds of basic experiential categories as well. At stake is the possibility of framing a coherent account of how a piece of language is fitted to perception. Potentially, it is a story that reaches all the way from neurobiology to human culture; it is the only such story that now lies within our grasp.

References

Beare, A. C. and Siegel, M. H. (1967). Color name as a function of wavelength and instruction. Perception and Psychophysics *2(11)*, 521–527.

Berlin, B. and Kay, P. (1969). Basic Color Terms: Their Universality and Evolution. Berkeley: University of California Press.

Bornstein, M. H., Kessen, W., and Weiskopf, S. (1976). The categories of hue in infancy. Science *191(4223)*, 201–202.

Boynton, R. M. and Olson, C. X. (1987). Locating basic colors in the OSA space. Color Research and Application *12*, 94–105.

Boynton, R. M. (1997). Insights Gained from Naming the OSA Colors. In: C. L. Hardin and L. Maffi (eds.) Color Categories in Thought and Language. Cambridge: Cambridge University Press.

Casson, R. W. (1997). Color Shift: Evolution of English Color Terms from Brightness to Hue. In: C. L. Hardin and L. Maffi (eds.) Color Categories in Thought and Language. Cambridge: Cambridge University Press.

Corbett, G. and Davies, I. (1997). Establishing basic color terms: Measures and techniques. In: C. L. Hardin and L. Maffi (eds.) Color Categories in Thought and Language. Cambridge: Cambridge University Press.

Fuld, K., Werner, J. S., and Wooten, B. R. (1983). The possible elemental nature of brown. Vision Research *23(6)*, 631–637.

Hardin, C. L. (1988). Color for Philosophers: Unweaving the Rainbow. Indianapolis: Hackett Publishing Company.

Hardin, C. L. and Maffi, L. (eds.) (1997). Color Categories in Thought and Language. Cambridge: Cambridge University Press.

Heider [Rosch], E. (1972a). Universals in color naming and memory. Journal of Experimental Psychology *93(1)*, 10–20.

Heider [Rosch], E. (1972b). Probabilities, sampling and the ethnographic method: The case of Dani colour names. Man *7*, 448–466.

Hickerson, N. (1971). Review of Basic Color Terms: Their Universality and Evolution, by B. Berlin and P. Kay. International Journal of American Linguistics *37*, 257–270.

Katra, E. and Wooten, B. (1996). Perceived lightness/darkness and warmth/coolness in chromatic experience. Submitted for publication.

Kay, P. and McDaniel, C. K. (1978). The linguistic significance of the meanings of basic color terms. Language *54*, 610–646.

Kay, P., Berlin, B., and Merrifield, W. R. (1991). Biocultural implications of systems of color naming. Journal of Linguistic Anthropology *1*, 12–25.

Kay, P., Berlin, B., Merrifield, W. R., and Maffi, L. (1997). Color naming across languages. In: C. L. Hardin and L. Maffi (eds.) Color Categories in Thought and Language. Cambridge: Cambridge University Press.

MacLaury, R. E. (1992). From brightness to hue: An explanatory model of color-category evolution. Current Anthropology *33*, 137–186.

MacLaury, R. E. (1997). Color and Cognition in Mesoamerican Languages: Constructing Categories as Vantages. Austin: University of Texas Press.

McDaniel, C. K. (1972). Hue perception and hue naming. Unpublished B. A. Thesis, Harvard University.

Miller, D. (1997). Beyond the Elements: Investigations of Hue. In: C. L. Hardin and L. Maffi (eds.) Color Categories in Thought and Language. Cambridge: Cambridge University Press.

Quinn, P. C., Rosano, J. L., and Wooten, B. R. (1988). Evidence that brown is not an elemental color. Perception + Psychophysics *43(2)*, 156–164.

Sandell, J. H., Gross, C. G., and Bornstein, M. H. (1979). Color Categories in Macaques. Journal of Comparative and Physiological Psychology *93*, 626–35.

Sivik, L. (1985). Mapping of color names in NCS. Proceedings of the 5h Congress of the AIC, Monte Carlo, Monaco.

Sivik, L. (1997). Color systems for cognitive research. In: C.L. Hardin and L. Maffi (eds.) Color Categories in Thought and Language. Cambridge: Cambridge University Press.

Sivik, L. and Taft, C. (1991). Cross-cultural studies of color meaning. Proceedings of AIC-conference on Color and Light '91, Sydney.

Sternheim, C. E. and Boynton, R. M. (1966). Uniqueness of perceived hues investigated with a continuous judgmental technique. Journal of Experimental Psychology *72*, 770–776.

Uchikawa, K. and Boynton, R. M. (1987). Categorical color perception of Japanese observers: Comparison with that of Americans. Vision Research *27*, 1825–1833.

12. Color Perception: From Grassmann Codes to a Dual Code for Object and Illumination Colors

Rainer Mausfeld

12.1 Introduction

Among the many different attributes of visual experiences the attribute of color appears to be the most enigmatic with respect to our attempts to deal with it theoretically. Unlike shape for instance, color does not seem to be part of a physico-geometrical description of the physical worlds. Color rather seems to be a product of the organism's visual system; it appears to be of a subjective nature. Though the concepts of 'subjective' and 'objective' resist any clear-cut definition, it is obvious that color cannot be entirely internal, like emotional states, since under normal conditions color experiences are tied in a lawful way to properties of the physical world. This Janus-facedness of color has not only made color an important target for epistemological inquiries into the relation between the 'external world' and its 'internal representation', but has also made color perception a field of paradigmatic interest for investigations into fundamental aspects of the cognitive sciences. Color perception encompasses the entire gamut of levels, from neural transduction to linguistic classifications and conscious percepts, with which the cognitive sciences are concerned.

Its unique blend of physics, neurophysiology and phenomenology makes color science particularly rewarding for studies of foundational and conceptual issues of perception. What properties does the perceptual coding of physical features of the environment exhibit? What kind of internal structure does the perceptual system impose on the sensory input? How can the achievements of color perception be characterized in terms of the adaptive coupling of the organism to its environment? What kind of physical regularities does the visual system take advantage of in pursuing its functional goals?

Such questions can only be successfully dealt with if one clearly distinguishes different levels of description and analysis: the physical description of perceptually relevant aspects of the physical environment, the phenomenological description, the description of functional achievements and descriptions of neural processing. The notion of a color code, as advanced by Krantz (Suppes et al., 1989, p. 256 ff.), is a particulary helpful tool for separating these levels in color research and for understanding their interrelation. It allows the conflation of physical, phenomenological and neurophysiological aspects to be avoided and the following questions to be distinguished from one another:

- what kind of psychological relations are referred to? (e.g., metamerism, color cancellation measures, thresholds, color appearances, assessment of 'object colors')
- what is the underlying physical structure? (e.g., physical structure of 'lights', physical structure of 'natural lights' and 'ecological surfaces')
- how can codes with certain properties (e.g., codes for metamerism, codes for unique colors, codes that are illumination independent) be constructed on the basis of the joint psycho-physical structure?

In this chapter I will try to provide an introductory and abbreviated outline of different psychophysical perspectives in color research from a purely psychophysical and functionalist point of view. In order to bring out the basic theoretical elements more clearly I shall, in an intuitive and implicit way, employ the formal notion of a color code and sketch along these lines the Grassmann theory of primary color coding, schemes for opponent color-coding, codes for accounting for spatial and temporal context, and the computational perspective developed in the context of color constancy. This outline then serves as the background for the discussion of some general topics, such as phenomenology and attributes of color, and conceptual problems, like the measurement device conception of color perception. Finally, I shall give the outlines of a new perspective on color perception that is inspired by ethology. According to this perspective, which considers the parsing of the sensory input in terms of, e.g., 'objects', 'surfaces', and 'events' to be determined by an innately fixed categorization process, color is not regarded as simply representing a specific set of physical attributes of the environment, like surface spectral reflectances, but rather is understood as part of the very format, as it were, of the perception instinct that couples our perceptuo-motorial system as a whole to its environment. The celebrated phenomena that show the dialectic relationship of light and object in color perception – which in present-day computational approaches is misrepresented and over-idealized as the 'problem of color constancy' – are, according to this view, an inseparable part of our *form of perception*, rather than a computational achievement of estimating natural surface reflectance functions on the basis of certain sensory inputs. If the perceptual categories of 'illumination color' and 'object color', which are the mold into which the internal coding of color is fitted, are internally constituted by a few 'representative' physical features, then these physical characteristics could be instantiated by an otherwise highly reduced stimulus. Such 'minimal' stimuli would then suffice to trigger internal perceptual achievements, like the segregation of 'object' and 'illumination' information, whose complexity far exceeds that of the triggering stimulus. Two problems of perceptual theory, though related, have to be distinguished here (referring to two different units of analysis, viz., the individual in a specific context and the evolving species). The first is to understand the nature of the internal 'semantics' of the perceptual categories of 'lights' and 'objects' for a given organism. The second problem refers to evolutionary processes during which the internal semantics originated: what physical properties of the environment gave rise in evolutionary history to the structure of these perceptual categories? This second problem is part of a general evolutionary perspective on the universal structure of color perception, as advanced by Shepard (1992; 1994).

12.2 Elementaristic vs. Ecological Perspectives in Color Research

In research on color perception we can schematically distinguish two different kinds of theoretical perspectives: an elementaristic psychophysical (and often neurophysiological) perspective focusing on 'front end' color coding, and a functional perspective emphasizing complex perceptual achievements like color constancy or the perception of shadows or illumination.

The starting points for the elementaristic psychophysical perspective are elementary achievements like color matching, color discrimination etc. and their temporal and spatial coding properties. Typical stimuli used here are decontextualized colors, i.e., mere color and light patterns that are not embedded into a natural scene. It is well known that this perspective proved to be fruitful for our understanding of elementary neural color codes.

On the other hand, the functionalist perspective which became intimately connected with a computational approach to color perception takes as its starting point complex achievements of the visual system, like color constancy. The corresponding stimuli are complex 'scenes' that are physically described in terms of complex achievement-related concepts, i.e., in terms of 'surface', 'specular highlights', 'shadows', 'transparency' etc.

Whereas the elementaristic psychophysical perspective only employs elementary spatio-temporal light patterns as such without relating them to perceptual categories or interpretations in terms of environmental entities, the computational perspective takes the perceptual classification of the environment, i.e., the furniture of the physical world as perceived by the organism, as given and attempts to establish computational mechanisms that allow properties of the theoretically predetermined environment to be reconstructed from the sensory input. In the theoretical language of the elementaristic perspective the stimulus is described in terms of elementary physical variables, whereas the computational approaches tend to describe the input by employing perceptual categories of the output. (The different spirits of these two perspectives is mirrored in the different kinds of apparatus typically employed for experimental investigations, namely Maxwellian viewing systems, as shown in Figure 12.1, vs. complex spatio-temporal patterns on CRT screens.)

Thus, the elementary psychophysical perspective only deals with processes like sensory transduction, filtering, signal-noise analysis etc. without addressing the problem of how elementary perceptual categories, like surface, object and light, are constructed. On the other hand, the computational perspective takes these perceptual categories for granted and uses them right from the beginning for the physical description of the scene. But the physical and the perceptual categories of, say, 'illumination', 'surface', 'object' and 'motion' do not coincide, and the existence of the physical entity is not only not sufficient, but not even necessary for the corresponding percept (think of an object on a CRT screen or in a virtual reality setting). Neither of these perspectives (or combinations thereof) thus deals explicitly with the core problem of how elementary perceptual categories, like 'surface', 'object', 'illumination color' or 'object color' come about. It is this aspect that I shall address in the final section.

Theories on the internal coding of color – both within an elementary and within an ecological perspective – are only weakly and often only very indirectly linked to appearances of color. Yet observations about color appearances usually provide the starting point and motivation for investigations of color coding. Since the question of attributes of color is a far less trivial and settled question than is suggested by the current color term orthodoxy of 'hue', 'brightness' and 'saturation', I shall briefly outline in the next section

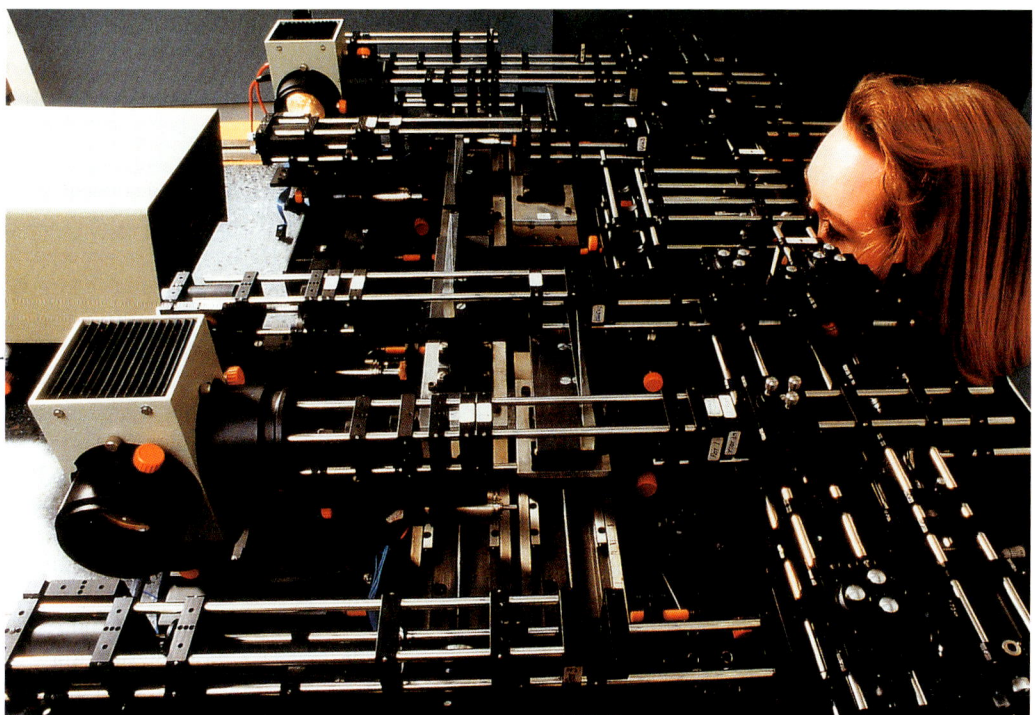

Fig. 12.1: The Kiel micro-optic Maxwellian-view system.

some of the conceptual intricacies involved in the issues of assessing attributes of color (without dealing with the many empirical intricacies in the complex phenomenology of color appearances).

12.3 Attributes of Color

The great variety of nuances of color appearances that natural scenes offer us can only be made accessible for perceptual judgments and linguistic concepts by processes of abstraction and categorization. Color terms gradually emerged in the process of cultural evolution. From Homer's emphasis on forms of light, such as brightness, luster, and the changeability of colors, to the subsequent and continuing interest in the proper color of objects and in color as such, there has been a culturally shaped progression toward an increasingly abstract color vocabulary. Thus, the building-up of a color terminology is a cultural achievement that from the very beginning of human culture mirrors not only the significance of certain biologically important objects, but to an increasing extent the invention and cultural role of coloration techniques and dyeing-processes. Our abstract color terms mostly derive from either concrete objects (like red, which in all Indo-European languages seems to be derived from the Sanskrit word for blood, rudhira, e.g., erythros, ruber, ruadh, rot, rouge, rosso) or from material properties, e.g., shining, glossy, speckled, dull, drab, resplendent (see Marty, 1879; Hochegger, 1884; Waetzoldt, 1909). Our conscious awareness is of objects and their material character, whereas color appearances only seem to be a kind of medium we are reading through, as it were, in the visual system's attempts to functionally attain the biologically significant object. Therefore cognitive processes of similarity classification and abstractive categorization are necessary for a linguistic description of color experiences. This achievement of an abstractive categorization entails the Janus-facedness of color with respect to its objective and subjective aspects, mirrored by the incoherence of our everyday concept of color, which hovers between two quite different meanings of color, namely (objective) color patches and (subjective) color experiences.

Whereas properties of the brain certainly restrict and predetermine the possible kinds of categorization and linguistic comprehension of perceptual experiences, there is to date no compelling evidence that the coupling of color experiences to linguistic categories is in a specific way predetermined by properties of internal coding (cf., Frumkina, 1984; for alternative viewpoints see chapter 1 and 11). Though the basic perceptual categories of bright and dark (which have become metaphorically linked to several culturally significant dichotomies) may have influenced linguistic categories, there does not seem to be a fixed set of natural kinds for linguistic color concepts. Biologically and functionally crucial aspects of the perceptuo-motorial system do not map in a natural and direct way to language, but have to be 'reconstructed' by conscious cognitive activity. Our linguistic grip on color experiences is based on a categorization process that is primarily shaped by contingent properties of the environment (like kinds of biologically significant objects and the availability of natural dyes), by the cultural context and the degree of linguistic abstraction achieved. Though there have been several attempts to show that this process of categorization is determined by certain internal properties of color coding (e.g., Ratliff, 1976), no convincing evidence so far could be provided for such a claim. If the construction of a color terminology is first of all a cultural achievement, it does not come as a surprise that scientific insights into the nature of internal color coding have since the last century themselves reciprocally influenced the way we categorize and classify colors. From the invention of the 'basic color attributes' hue, saturation and brightness and the ideas on an internal opponent organization of color to color-order systems, like the Munsell or DIN system (which are used for industrial processes that require standards and norms for referring to colors), the way we talk about color is continuously changing. Therefore it is hardly an exaggeration to say that "'color' did not mean to the Greeks what it means to us" (Irwin, 1974, p. 14). Color terms are the product of a culturally shaped abstraction process. "The Homeric

Greek had not yet learned to think in abstract terms. 'What is color?' is a question they would never have formulated, let alone been able to answer." (Irwin, 1974, p. 22)

If we look at standard textbooks on color perception we find the following kind of description of color attributes, which is usually regarded as a natural, unique and complete classification for describing color appearances:

brightness: "the attribute of a visual sensation according to which a given stimulus appears to be more or less intense" (Note the ambiguity of the concept 'intense' in this description.)

hue: "the attribute of a color perception denoted by blue, green, yellow, red, purple, and so on"

saturation: "the attribute of a visual sensation which permits a judgment to be made of the degree to which a chromatic stimulus differs from an achromatic stimulus regardless of their brightness" (Wyszecki and Stiles, 1982, p. 487).

The received, but misguided idea that these attributes adequately characterize color appearances amounts to downplaying the complex phenomenal structure of color experiences (for linguistic evidence of their inadequacy see Frumkina, 1984, p. 24). These attributes were, in the wake of Helmholtz, derived from the corresponding physical operations of selecting a wavelength, increasing light intensity and diluting a light stimulus with white light. The elementary color attributes were thus taken from elementary physical operations (furthermore the fact of trichromacy of elementary color coding is incorrectly taken as evidence that color appearances can completely be described by three perceptual variables). Many writers in the early literature were aware of that. For instance, Hering rejected the concept of saturation altogether as a mixing-up of perceptual and physical aspects. He preferred the (reciprocal) concept of veiling (*"Verhüllung"*) of color (Hering, 1920, p. 40). And Stumpf, who considered the problem of color attributes to be a problem of the ability and the conditions for an isolating abstraction (*"Fähigkeit und Bedingungen der isolierenden Abstraktion"*, Stumpf, 1917, p. 8), dismissed 'saturation' as a color attribute completely (*"Sättigung können wir nicht als Attribut anerkennen"*, Stumpf, 1917, p. 86). He conceived saturation to be a cognitive abstraction and a cognitively added relation capturing the approximation of a color to its ideal. In a similar vein, the concept of saturation was rejected by many others, among them Katz and G. E. Müller, who spoke instead of forcefulness (*"Eindringlichkeit"*), and K. Bühler, who spoke of intensity of colors. Another interesting case is the perceptual category of achromatic appearances, which being a highly complex – and up to now poorly understood – perceptual achievement within color perception is from a physicalistic perspective misconceived as a simpler case than color perception proper. Even for achromatic colors, as is well known since Hering, at least a bidimensional account is necessary, as can be witnessed by appearances like luminous grey.

Von Kries, a pupil of Helmholtz, was aware of such problems but he preferred to trade psychological arbitrariness for an apparent precision of color concepts that results from their strong tie to physical operations. He remarked that a division of color appearances in terms of hue, saturation and brightness "does not claim to be a natural one; without much ado we can regard it as a completely arbitrary one. Such a description is, however, a completely rigorous one, since it only refers to objective properties of the light that causes the corresponding appearances" (von Kries, 1882, p. 6)[1].

In the history of perceptual psychology, the physicalistic trap of slicing the nature of perception along the joints of elementary physics is one of the most seductive and misleading ideas. The problematic nature of attempts to parse perceptual phenomena according to categories derived from elementary concepts and operations of physics has

---

[1] "Diese Gliederung macht keinen Anspruch darauf, eine naturgemässe zu sein; wir können sie vor der Hand als eine ganz willkürliche betrachten. Sie ist aber eine vollkommen strenge, da sie sich an die objective Beschaffenheit desjenigen Lichtes hält, welches die betreffende Empfindung hervorzurufen vermag.".

been discussed since the beginnings of perceptual theory again and again. The conception of the perceptual system as a kind of measuring device which 'informs' the organism about the physical input, along with the idea that elementary physical variables, like intensity and wavelength of light, are connected with elementary perceptual variables, like brightness and color, is an important (mostly implicitly employed) metaphor, which itself is a legacy of the way we separated physical and psychological aspects in the philosophical history of the field and which has governed our thinking in the study of perception since. Along with this *measurement device conception of perception* (cf., Mausfeld, 1993) comes the idea that there are atoms of perception, as it were, that are strongly tied to these elementary physical variables: namely the sensations from which perceptions – as something referring to the external world – are constructed.

Because of the difficulties in keeping apart the physical and psychological aspects of the investigation of color and in not succumbing to the stimulus error, Katz (1911, p. 29) remarked: "The most important rule for describing color phenomena is: what vagueness they have needs to be described as such; particularly in this respect there is a dangerous temptation to adulterate the description by perspectives borrowed from physics."[2]

The problem of how to deal theoretically with the complex phenomenology of color has not been squarely met by current theories of color perception. This is not only testified by the vexing problem of the dimensionality of color codes: Since Hering, Katz, Gelb and others, indications have been accumulating that color appearances cannot be represented by a three-dimensional color code. As Niederée (1996) rigorously showed, even in center-surround configurations the dimensionality of color codes must be greater than three if one is willing to accept the topological assumptions which, at least implicitly, underlie almost all models of color coding. Though this formal argument for the inappropriateness of three-dimensional color codes is based on the traditional view on center-surround stimuli, it is consonant with the perspective to regard center-surround configurations as minimal stimuli for triggering a dual code for 'object' and 'illumination' colors.

12.4 Early Color Coding and the Elementaristic Approach

12.4.1 Newton and Helmholtz's Approach to Color Perception

Newton regarded color as an intrinsic property or disposition of light alone and he tied the concepts of refrangibility and color together. Newton found the basic fact of what we call *metamerism* – namely that there are lights (i.e., wavelength compositions) that can be physically different but are perceptually indistinguishable – and was aware of the existence of extraspectral hues. He considered (psychologically simple) white light to be physically complex, namely composed of all different lights. One important insight of his is that the ends of the spectrum have something in common perceptually, which led him to provide a metric for specifying color mixtures: his famous center-of-gravity principle. Newton meant this model to be more than just a pictorial representation of his ideas; the model is a quantitative scheme to account for the results of color mixture (and in fact it is the first quantitative model in psychophysics).

Helmholtz started from this model – with some misunderstandings in the beginning that were clarified by Maxwell and Grassmann. Helmholtz's goal was to investigate the nature of (in his words) "terminal processes that are responsible for the dependency of visual experiences on light stimuli." He developed the basic experimental paradigm for investigating basic principles of color perception, connected psychophysical findings with neurophysiological conjectures and provided the fundamentals of a theory of early color coding.

---

[2] "Darf ich die, wie mir scheint, wichtigste Regel für die Beschreibung von Farbphänomenen nennen, so ist es diese: was an den Farbphänomenen unbestimmt ist, verlangt auch als solches beschrieben zu werden; gerade in dieser Beziehung ist die Gefahr groß, daß die Beschreibung durch der Physik entlehnte Betrachtungsweisen verfälscht wird."

However, there is one aspect that this theory does not address at all, namely the appearance of color (it only deals with metamerism, i.e., equality of appearances).

12.4.2 The Young-Helmholtz Theory and Grassmann's Laws

The Young-Helmholtz theory is based on some simple experimental findings in certain viewing conditions: if a small spot of light – typically of the size of about 2° visual angle – is presented in an otherwise dark visual field, the psychological relation of metamerism, denoted by $\equiv$, is found to be unaffected by the physical operations of superimposing lights (corresponding to the addition of spectral energy densities), denoted by $\oplus$, and changing intensity of lights, denoted by $*$.

This means that if A and B are perceptually indistinguishable lights (*metameric lights*), i.e., $A \equiv B$, with spectral energy distributions $E_A(\lambda)$ and $E_B(\lambda)$ and if the same light C with energy distribution $E_C(\lambda)$ is added pointwise to each of these lights (*"additive color mixture"*), i.e.

$$E_{A \oplus B}(\lambda) = E_A(\lambda) + E_B(\lambda),$$

then the following relations ("Grassmann laws") hold

$$A \oplus C \equiv B \oplus C$$
$$t * A \equiv t * B$$

Thus, metamerism is (to a large extent) preserved under addition and scalar multiplication of lights.

Together with the trichromacy of color matching and the uniqueness of trichromatic matches, this gives rise to a triple of linear codes that represent metamerism in the following sense. Let $<L, \oplus, *>$ be the qualitative physical structure of lights (where L is the set of lights identified with their spectral radiant energy distributions). Then a mapping $\varphi = (\varphi_1, \varphi_2, \varphi_3)$ exists which maps the qualitative physical structure $<L, \oplus, *>$ homomorphically (i.e., linearly) into the three-dimensional real vector space, such that $A \equiv B \Leftrightarrow \varphi(A) = \varphi(B)$.

Thus, the physical structure

$$<L, \oplus, *>$$

and the psychological structure

$$<L, \equiv>$$

neatly interact to yield the psychophysical structure

$$<L, \oplus, *, \equiv>.$$

The empirical validity of the Grassmann laws makes the psychological relation (a congruence relation with respect to the physical operations $\oplus$ and $*$).

The mapping φ will be called a *Grassmann code*. It is not unique, but there exists a whole family of such codes, which are linearly related. Among these are the mappings that represent the physiological receptor codes and the mapping (X, Y, Z) that leads to CIE color space.

The visual system thus constructs equivalence classes on the set of physical lights, which from a physical point of view amounts to coarsening the physical description. How perceptual equivalence classes are factored out of the infinite-dimensional physical description is described by the Grassmann laws. These laws make it possible to numerically represent colors in a convex cone in three-dimensional real vector space, which leads to the conception of a three-dimensional color space, whose elements are described by a color code $\varphi = (\varphi_1, \varphi_2, \varphi_3)$ in this vector space. Classes of metameric lights can then be identified with color appearances.

These Grassmann codes representing metamerism constitute the (purely) psychophysical core of the Newton-Young-Helmholtz theory of color vision (Grassmann, 1853; Schrödinger, 1920; Suppes et al., 1989, ch. 15). As already mentioned above, the notion of a Grassmann code for metamerism does not refer to specific attributes of color (as opposed to color codes referred to in opponent-color theory).

The Grassmann structure of color coding constitutes the core not only of the Young-Helmholtz theory of color vision but of all other theories of color perception, such as opponent-color theory, industrial systems for specifying color, computational theories of color constancy, etc. Since it is often wedded to tacit additional assumptions and interpretations that go beyond its content, some remarks may be useful.

1. The Grassmann structure only refers to lights, and not to the color of objects. Though light is the medium for assessing the color of objects, much more complex perceptual mechanisms are involved when the stimulus consists of perceived objects and lights.

2. The only psychological relation involved in the Grassmann structure is metamerism. Therefore only those formal properties of the vector space of equivalence classes of lights can be given an empirical interpretation that are based on the relation of metamerism together with the two physical operations. These are only those that are invariant under linear transformations. Thus the vector space has no empirically meaningful scalar product, and Euclidean distances between vectors cannot be interpreted as color similarities or indices of color discriminability. This can be easily seen from the fact that the vector space distance between two colors does not change when the same color is added to both of them; if this third color is, for instance, a very bright one, the psychological distance between the colors will be reduced, however. How to construct a color space in which, in addition to the psychological relation of metamerism, other psychological relations like similarity and discriminability are represented is still an unsolved problem of what Schrödinger called higher color metrics (*"höhere Farbmetrik"*).

3. The idealized and theoretical relation of metamerism – which, for instance, implies strict transitivity of color matches – can only be related to the empirical relation of metameric matches, if (at least implicitly) the usual vector space topology is taken into account. Thus the Grassmann structure needs to be supplemented by topological aspects. Judgmental fluctuations are then taken to lie within a neighbourhood of the 'true' point, and small variations in the physical variables are assumed to lead to small variations in the color appearance (there are no jumps in color appearance). Grassmann (1853, p. 72) and Schrödinger (1920, p. 415 f.) therefore explicitly included continuity assumptions in their formulations.

4. The Grassmann structure does not refer to color appearances (except for the distinguishability-indistinguishability aspect)! In particular, it does not represent equality or inequality of color attributes like hue, saturation, and brightness. The ratio of the length of two vectors does not correspond to a ratio of brightnesses, and a line in Grassmann space does not necessesarily correspond to a constant hue. The Bezold-Brücke shift of hues under changes of intensities of lights does not contradict properties of the Grassmann structure.

5. The well-known nonlinearities of neural coding do not call into question the validity of the linear color representation of the Grassmann theory. First of all, they do not refer only to the Grassmann theory itself (the empirical validity of which is a purely psychophysical question), but to the Grassmann theory cum neurophysiological linking propositions. Secondly, even if the usual linking proposition – discussed below – is assumed, namely that two lights are metameric, if they result in the same number of photopigment isomerizations for each of the three univariant types of receptors, any strictly monotonic transformation of this process will preserve the linear representability of the structure.

12.4.3 Opponent-Color Theory

Since Leonardo da Vinci and, later, Goethe, Aubert and Mach 'red' and 'green', and 'blue' and 'yellow' have been regarded as psychologically basic and principle colors. Goethe, who considered polarity to be one of the basic principles underlying color experiences (for an account of Goethe's metatheoretical principles on which his approach to color is based, see Mausfeld, 1996) provided central ideas and observations – notably on afterimages, simultaneous contrast and colored shadows – upon which opponent-color theory came to be based.

For Hering, who took up central principles of Goethe's approach, already the local color code is intrinsically determined by the entire spatio-temporal excitation of the retina. Phenomenologically Hering started from the observation that certain color experiences have the property of being unitary and that pairs of color experiences that exhibit this property are perceptually incompatible. The three perceptual attributes that constitute a distinguished coordinate system for color attributes are the bipolar or opponent pairs: redness/greeness, yellowness/blueness, and whitness/blackness. Hering developed together with a wealth of ingenious experiments – a theoretical account of color coding that was based on such an opponent character of the phenomenal structure of color. His ideas were taken up and further developed by G. E. Müller and others, and more recently by Jameson and Hurvich (see Jameson and Hurvich, 1972), who systematically employed an experimental technique, color cancellation, that was invented by Hering and used by Brückner (1927). The technique of color cancellation allows the determination of the amount of redness in a reddish color by the amount of a standard green that has to be added to bring the color to equilibrium with respect to the redness-greenness attribute. Thus this technique combines judgments of opponent attributes with the additive structure of the set of lights and allows a version of opponent-color theory to be formulated that refers to configurations consisting only of a single spot of light.

12.4.3.1 Color Codes Representing Opponent-Color Attributes

As a neurophysiological theory, opponent-color theory basically states that the color signals for a homogeneous stimulus emerging from the three types of primary receptors are combined at a second level in some specific way to form three types of channels, denoted here by Q_{r-g}, Q_{b-y} and Q_{w-bl}, associated with the 'red-green', 'blue-yellow' and 'white-black' opponent color codes, respectively. This, then, is related to the psychophysical concept of *unique colors* by means of the linking hypothesis that unique colors are determined by the respective zero points of the two chromatic (neurophysiological) codes. For instance, a 'red-green equilibrium', i.e., $Q_{r-g} = 0$, corresponds to colors that are neither reddish nor greenish, i.e., to either a unique blue, a unique yellow, or a white color appearance. (In addition, positive and negative values of Q_{r-g} are taken to correspond to color appearances containing a reddish and greenish component, respectively.)

This condition allows the introduction of pairs of chromatic opponent codes Q_{r-g} and Q_{b-y} (using the same notation again) in purely psychophysical terms. The essential qualitative relations involved are (in addition to metamerism and the basic physical attributes) the psychological predicates U_i (i = 1, 2), where $U_1(A)$, $A \in L$, means the stimulus A being psychophysically in red-green equilibrium, i.e., appearing neither greenish nor reddish, and $U_2(A)$, that A appears neither bluish nor yellowish. The corresponding psychophysical opponent-color theory deals with the qualitative laws governing the interplay of these relations with the relations/operations of the Grassmann structure.

Since the beginnings of opponent-color theory, the meaning of the corresponding types of color codes has undergone various changes, with its interpretation to the present day vacillating between referring to the idea of a 'neural code' vs. a 'psychophysical code', and here in turn between 'perceptual codes' or more abstract ones. Of course, the meaning of such a system of codes may vary with the experimental paradigm and theoretical framework adopted.

12.4.3.2 Relating Grassmann and Opponent Codes

If one considers a system of opponent codes $Q(A) = (Q_{r-g}(A), Q_{y-b}(A), Q_{w-bl}(A))$ as neural codes, it is natural to ask how they are related to primary receptor codes, i.e., to a Grassmann code ϕ. A corresponding question can be asked if the opponent codes are considered as purely psychophysical ones (i.e., in terms of qualitative relations and laws concerning properties of phenomenological relations and their interplay with physical ones). It turns out that from this perspective, triples of opponent codes may simply be chosen among the family of Grassmann codes, provided certain qualitative assumptions in addition to unitariness and incompatibility of attributes – are fulfilled. These conditions have to do with the requirement that cancellation measurements be independent of the choice of the equilibrating light, which imposes the restriction that cancellation equivalences yield one-dimensional Grassmann structures. This implies the condition of scalar invariance (of unique colors), i.e., the closure of the class of unique colors under change of intensity. Furthermore, the additive complement of, say, unique green must be unique red, i.e., each unique green can be made achromatic by an addition of unique red.

A corresponding rigorous measurement theoretic analysis of the relation of primary and opponent codes was given by Krantz (see Suppes et al., 1989, chap. 15). This result could also have been stated in such a way that under the above conditions a system of opponent codes can be achieved from a fixed Grassmann code by linear transformations. The operation of color cancellation then yields a linear representation in the vector space derived from the three-dimensional Grassmann structure of metameric color matching, i.e.

$$Q_{r\_g}(A) = \Sigma_{i=1,2,3}\ c_{1,i} \cdot \varphi_i(A)$$

$$Q_{y\_b}(A) = \Sigma_{i=1,2,3}\ c_{2,i} \cdot \varphi_i(A)$$

$$Q_{w\_bl}(A) = \Sigma_{i=1,2,3}\ c_{3,i} \cdot \varphi_i(A)$$

which, under the above assumptions, neatly connects primary and opponent-color coding (in the experimental situation of a single small light spot in an otherwise dark visual field).

A re-coding of primary color codes into opponent-color channels can be understood as a decorrelation of receptor signals that proves to have interesting formal properties from the perspective of efficient and reliable information transmission in the visual system (Buchsbaum and Gottschalk, 1983).

However, the simplicity and beauty of the exactly defined version of opponent-color theory characterized above is in conflict with empirical evidence. For instance, observations have been reported that
- a mixture of unique green and unique red appears yellowish
- a mixture of unique yellow and unique blue appears reddish
- desaturating a spectral unique blue makes it appear reddish
- a unique white is not intensity invariant.

Because of this and other empirical results, the concepts of 'opponent color', 'complementary color', and (successive or simultaneous) 'contrast color' do not coincide, nor do the concepts of 'unique color' and 'intensity invariant color'.

Up to now, attempts to formulate a clear-cut and empirically adequate theory of opponent-color coding have met with little success. There is no coherent and empirically satisfying theory to account for our introspective observations that give rise to the intuition about an opponency of color coding. The field of corresponding research is rather strewn with highly experiment-specific models of opponent coding that are hardly compatible with each other.

There are several other attempts at modelling second or higher-order chromatic mechanisms based not on color cancellation but instead on other kinds of psychological relations, which suggest the existence of a great variety of higher-order color mechanisms. For instance, Krauskopf, Williams and Heeley (1982) investigated changes in chromatic thresholds in chromatically modulated fields and found 'cardinal directions' in color space corresponding to a luminance channel, a red-green channel and an S-cone axis, the last being clearly distinct from the axis defining the set of colors that were in equilibrium for the red-green channel.

12.4.4 Relating Psychophysical and Neurophysiological Color Codes

The color codes considered so far are based on only two psychological relations, namely metameric matches and color cancellation (though the motivation that leads to singling out these psychological relations refers to a much richer set of observations). Now the question arises whether the purely psychophysical color codes obtained from color matches and color cancellation techniques can be interpreted in terms of neural codes, i.e., neural mechanisms.

Current neurophysiological theories of color vision assume two major stages of the primary encoding of color: the first stage refers to the activity of three types of univariant receptors, the second stage to the subsequent integration and reorganization of this activity by cells with spectrally and spatially-opponent response characteristics.

12.4 Early Color Coding and the Elementaristic Approach

These two stages of neural encoding are taken to correspond psychophysically (i.e., with respect to psychological relations) to the two types of color codes discussed above. There is, however, a logical gap between quantitative psychophysical notions of color codes that refer only to psychological relations on the one hand, and the neurophysiological interpretations of these codes in terms of neural codes on the other. Usually, these different interpretations of the term 'code' are simply conflated in vision research parlance. Accordingly, the 'linking propositions' that have to be invoked to bridge this gap are usually not spelled out explicitly.

The linking proposition that has had the greatest appeal in color science since Helmholtz is one that relates the psychophysical code for metameric matches to a corresponding neural code in terms of primary receptors and gives the purely psychophysical concept of metamerism an interpretation in neurophysiological terms based on the idea that among codes for metamerism one can single out certain color codes that in some sense characterize the output of three types of receptors. Psychophysical opponent-color codes are then interpreted as higher order neural codes that result from a certain combination of neural primary codes.

The linking proposition invoked for relating Grassmann codes and primary receptor codes is:

$$A \equiv B \Leftrightarrow \int E_A(\lambda) V_i(\lambda) \, d\lambda = \int E_B(\lambda) V_i(\lambda) \, d\lambda$$

$$i = 1, 2, 3$$

where $E_A(\lambda)$ is the spectral energy functions of the light A, and $V_i(\lambda)$ are the spectral sensitivity

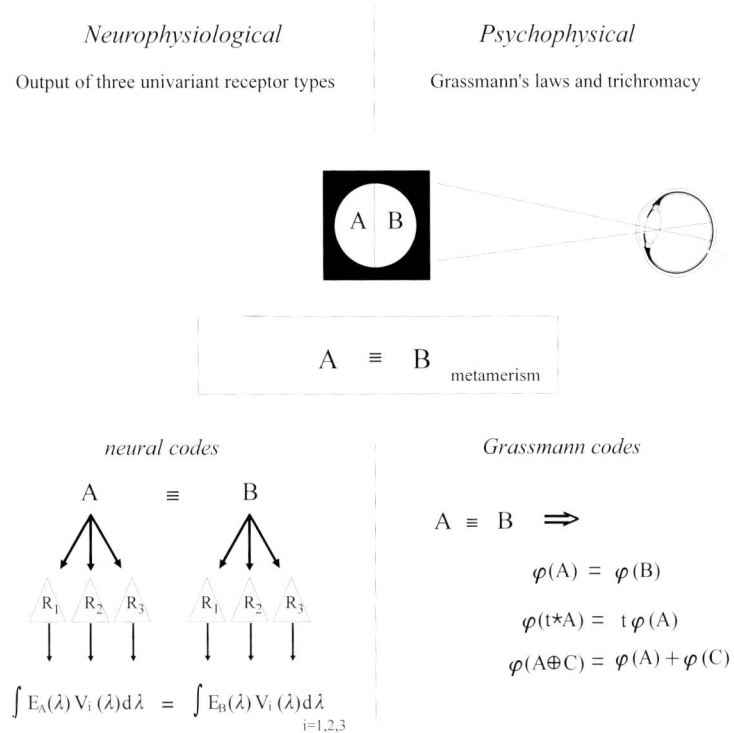

Fig. 12.2: Basic color codes.

distributions for each of the three types of receptors.

In this way $\varphi_i(A)$ can be identified with $\int E_A(\lambda) V_i(\lambda) d\lambda$, and psychophysical color space is associated with a corresponding three-dimensional sensor space. Figure 12.2 juxtaposes the basic elements of neural and psychophysical color codes in the experimental situation of a small light in an otherwise dark visual field.

Whether this linking proposition is empirically adequate, is still a matter of dispute, since there is conflicting empirical evidence from various sources, notably,
- variability within cone types,
- violations of the persistency rule (metameric lights remain metameric if both viewed in a different context; see below) for women with an additional cone type and for subjects with normal color vision.

Psychophysicists as well as neurophysiologists therefore called into question the validity of a linking proposition as simple as the one stated above. To quote two examples:

"... evidence for the variability among cones is enough to raise serious doubts as to whether trichromatic matches are determined at the receptor level: the cones probably are distinguishing reliably between the matched fields. ... it seems to me that we still do not have a satisfactory physiological basis for trichromacy; but we can say that under some conditions at least trichromacy rests on a neural (and not a receptoral) trivariance." (MacLeod, 1986, 109/111)

"Evidence is accumulating to suggest that the idea, that individuals with normal color vision have only three spectrally different cone photoreceptors, is also invalid. ... trichromacy of normal vision has its origin at a level of the visual pathway beyond that of the cone pigments, likely beyond the receptors." (Neitz et al., 1993, p. 122)

Other interesting empirical findings come from experiments with people who exhibit unilateral dichromatism. These rare cases allow dichoptic color matches and comparisons between the two eyes by color-naming techniques that – under certain assumptions (e.g., that their color sensations in the dichromatic eye are the same as those of congenital dichromats, and not due to disease) – provide insight into the relation between the two- and three-dimensional Grassmann spaces involved and their neurophysiological basis. The experimental study of unilateral dichromatism therefore has been considered of particular interest for our attempts to understand the early coding of color (von Hippel, 1880; MacLeod and Lennie, 1976; Alpern et al., 1983).

What experimental results can be expected, if there are, for instance, no shortwave receptors (tritanopia) and if thus the input φ_1 is lacking? The Young-Helmholtz theory and standard opponent-color theory assume that only some of the higher order codes depend on φ_1 and thus that the blue-yellow channel Q_{b-g} is missing. According to the standard interpretation of the Young-Helmholtz theory (which links the Grassmann theory with color appearances) one might conjecture that a unilateral tritanopic subject should, with his tritanopic eye, see the spectrum as 'red', 'green' and 'yellow' and combinations thereof; neither 'blue' nor 'white' should be seen, and there should be a green that looks more saturated than any green attainable by the normal eye. According to the standard version of opponent-color theory the loss of the 'yellow-blue' channel should result in seeing 'white', 'red' and 'green' as for the normal eye, while the mixture of red and green would be achromatic. Both predictions are in conflict with the experimental results: a unilateral tritanope sees the entire spectrum on the shortwave side of the neutral point between 440 nm and 550 nm – as blue, i.e., he matches it to 485–490 nm in his normal eye. The colors he sees in the spectrum are red, white and blue with only a small amount of yellow and no green at all. Thus it seems that central elements in the linking propositions of the Young-Helmholtz theory and opponent-color theory are utterly wrong:

"those central mechanisms which, in the normal observer, correspond to blueness (and we assume, have heavy dependence on the output of the short-wave cones) are most active indeed in the tritanope." (Alpern et al., 1983, p. 694)

This and other results support the conjecture that the psychophysically observed three-dimensionality of color matches in the 2°-paradigm cannot be attributed in a simple way to the existence of three types of photoreceptors:

> "There must be a limitation to only three degrees of freedom at the level of central mechanisms, not merely at the level of photopigments." (Alpern et al., 1983, p. 693)

Whereas a neurophysiological perspective on color deals with the neural architecture of the visual system and the minutiae of the neural coding of color, psycho-physics deals with the interplay of phenomenology and physics and with abstract 'strategies' that the visual system employs for achieving its tasks, without embarking on speculations about neural mechanisms. To reveal the underlying strategies is first and foremost a psychological or psychophysical task, since only when we have an idea of the basic 'logic' of the system can we speculate on neurophysiological implementation (which may pertain to a unit of analysis other than the level of neurons). Though there is not and cannot be a sharp boundary between psychophysical and neurophysiological work, differences in emphasis and orientation with respect to these two levels of analysis can be discerned.

Attempts to understand the relation between psychophysical codes and the neurophysiology of color coding have since the beginnings of color research been the driving forces in the field. For the psychology of color perception this situation is not without problems, since psychology faces in its history the danger of a centrifugal tendency by which certain sub-fields spin away into other disciplines. This is certainly the case with large areas of color science. Here, psychology has not yet taken on its due role and to a large extent has relinquished a field of genuine psychological interest to neurophysiology. The tendency that perceptual psychologists notoriously avail themselves of neurophysiological terms when it suits their 'explanatory' purposes and hastily call upon ad hoc pseudo-explanations for isolated psychophysical phenomena in terms of equally isolated neurophysiological findings is testimony to the higher 'epistemological dignity' they ascribe to neurophysiology. However, given the complexity now apparent both in psychophysical observations and in neurophysiological findings, claims that empirical results provide sufficient constraints to bridge the logical gap between the two levels of description seem to be based on forlorn hopes. In the light of what little is presently understood of the physics of the brain, neuroreductionism amounts to no more than a bold speculation about what might be the relevant aspects. Even worse, it rests on a misconstrued account of the development of scientific theories which almost always was due to explanatory unification rather than reduction.

12.4.5 Elementary Color Codes Accounting for Variations in Spatial and Temporal Context

So far I have only referred to experimental situations where the stimulus is a small spatially and temporally homogeneous light in an otherwise dark visual field (typically experimentally studied under so-called Maxwellian viewing conditions, shown in Figure 12.1, where the subject's head is fixed and a beam of light is projected through the pupil on the retina). Though it is assumed that the Grassmann laws and qualitative laws of color cancellation are valid over a wide range of spatial and temporal contexts, the color appearances themselves can change with variations of context. It therefore appears natural to try to accommodate the effects of context in theories of early color coding.

Several theoretical perspectives have been developed to account for spatial and temporal effects; these perspectives are intimately tied to certain phenomena and corresponding paradigmatic experimental situations; the terms 'adaptation', 'induction' and 'contrast' can – in an idealized manner – be associated with specific experimental stimulus situations. However, evaluation of the many experiments investigating spatial and temporal aspects of color perception is impeded by the poorly understood effects of the details of the experimental situations (which often involve complex interactions of spatial and temporal aspects as well as different judgmental criteria and viewing conditions). This abundant variety of different experimental setups and stimulus conditions mirrors the theoretical uncertainty about how to carve the multitude of phenomena into those which are considered as 'basic' and those which are considered as side-effects.

The Young-Maxwell-Helmholtz-Grassmann theory describes the transduction of light into a psychophysical or neural code and – together with the linking proposition proposes a receptoral mechanism that accounts for the Grassmann laws. Since metamerism is the only psychological relation involved, the theory does not refer to color appearances. However, color appearances are often tacitly associated with the equivalence classes of metameric lights. In this case the theory becomes a *locally-atomistic* account of color appearances. It then has to deal with the problem that at one location of a visual scene the *same* triple of Grassmann codes/receptor outputs can give rise to quite *different* color appearances if the temporal or spatial context is varied. The existence of a surround changes the color appearances in characteristic ways and produces new appearances, e.g., brown, that cannot be observed in a dark surround (see chapter 10).

From a locally-atomistic perspective these are secondary effects, to be treated under the heading of 'context' effects. On the other hand, they could also show that the basic mechanisms determining color appearances in natural scenes can only be tapped by 'minimal stimuli' that are richer than the 2° lights appropriate for isolating receptoral transduction.

For the elementaristic perspective on color perception (as opposed to a functional one guided by ecological physics) the effects of certain temporal and spatial variations on the local color appearance were considered an important challenge. To a surprising extent, the Young-Helmholtz tradition, however, was successful in developing an extension of the theory that could – at least in principle – incorporate an important class of these effects.

The first systematic investigations into mechanisms responsible for these variations were performed by Fechner (1840). The complementary character of afterimages led Fechner to the idea of a tiring of physiological processes (based on an analogy with a "loss of tension" – *"Verlust an Spannkraft"*) by which "all phenomena concerning afterimages and adaptation can be reduced to sensitivity processes in the eye" Fechner, 1840, p. 430)[3]. This intuition lead Helmholtz to his concept of "fatigue of receptors" (*"Ermüdungstheorie"*), which was given a more precise form by von Kries' "coefficient scheme" (*"Koeffizientensatz"*).

Because the Young-Helmholtz theory took as basic units of analysis single light spots in a dark surround, it had to postulate additional mechanisms to account for the effects of spatial and temporal context. For opponent-color theory on the other hand it was more natural to incorporate spatial and temporal effects, since its underlying intuitions were historically rooted in phenomena that depend on variations of temporal and spatial contexts (Hering attributed a much more basic role to contrast and adaptation than Helmholtz did). To theoretically deal with the situation of a single isolated light in a dark surround only became possible after the invention of the color cancellation technique which according to Brückner (1927) was already used by Hering.

In the following sections, I shall briefly outline how the Young-Helmholtz theory and a variant of opponent-color theory deal with temporal and spatial contexts in terms of appropriate codes (or code transformations).

12.4.5.1 The von Kries Coefficient Scheme

Helmholtz took up Fechner's intuitions and conjectured that "the fatiguing of the organ of vision modifies the sensation of the just-sensed light approximately in a way as if the objective intensity of the light is reduced to a certain fraction of its magnitude." (Helmholtz, 1911, Vol. 2, p. 200)[4].

This perspective allows any effects of adaptation to be translated back to physics and to describe them *as if* only the effective physical stimulus had changed.

---

[3] "durch die man die ganze Erscheinung der Nachbilder auf ein Spiel von Empfindlichkeit des Auges reduciren kann"

[4] "... die Ermüdung der Sehnervensubstanz die Empfindung neu einfallenden Lichtes ungefähr in dem Verhältnis beeinträchtigt, als wäre die objektive Intensität dieses Lichtes um einen bestimmten Bruchteil ihrer Größe vermindert."

An explicit model of this intuition to account for the effects of temporal adaptation was first proposed by von Kries (1882). Based on the hypothesis of linear sensitivity control acting on three types of primary receptors, this so-called *von Kries coefficient* scheme assumed that the effect of adaptation can, for each receptor type, (approximately) be described as multiplication of each receptor code by a real number.

Adaptation is regarded here as a differential fatiguing of the three types of receptors. The sensitivity of each type of receptor is assumed to be reduced over the spectrum by a constant factor, i.e., the spectral sensitivity curves change their amplitude but not their form, i.e.

$$V'_i(\lambda) = \rho_i \cdot V_i(\lambda) \qquad \rho_i \in (0,1)$$

Three numbers ρ_1, ρ_2, ρ_3 thus suffice to completely describe the process of adaptation.

Though it was originally intended to be a *neurophysiological* hypothesis ("fatigue of receptors"), many of the corresponding empirical investigations address its *psychophysical* counterparts.

To formulate its psychophysical counterpart, I shall use the notation of Mausfeld and Niederée (1993) for the characterization of the stimuli employed: two stimuli A and B that are presented after pre-adapting by a light S, will be written as $<A,S>$ and $<B,S>$. More generally, I shall use this notation for any temporal or spatial context S. Two such stimuli $<A,S>$ and $<B,T>$ which have the property that the testfields A and B look 'the same color' will be called *isophene*:

$$<A,S> \equiv <B,T>.$$

For the case of a dark surround (S, T = **0**, where **0** is the zero energy distribution) the concepts of metamerism and isophenism coincide, i.e., $A \equiv B$ can be identified with $<A,\mathbf{0}> \equiv <B,\mathbf{0}>$.

Now, if the linking proposition that characterizes the Young-Helmholtz theory, namely

$$A \equiv B \Leftrightarrow \int E_A(\lambda) V_i(\lambda) \, d\lambda = \int E_B(\lambda) V_i(\lambda) \, d\lambda$$

is valid for the dark-adapted eye, then the von Kries coefficient scheme amounts to the validity of the following linking proposition for the eye pre-adapted by some light S:

$$<A,S> \equiv <B,S> \Leftrightarrow \int E_A(\lambda) \, \rho_i(S) \cdot V_i(\lambda) \, d\lambda$$
$$= \int E_B(\lambda) \, \rho_i(S) \cdot V_i(\lambda) \, d\lambda$$
$$i = 1, 2, 3$$

where (ρ_i is a function of $\varphi(S)$ (or of $\varphi_i(S)$ if it is assumed to be independent of the two remaining channels). In terms of primary receptor codes this means that the effect of context S on the color appearance of a testfield A can be completely captured by a transformation $\varphi_i(A) \to \rho_i(\varphi(S)) \cdot \varphi_i(A)$.

The right equation directly shows the symmetry of the operations 'reducing receptor sensitivity by a factor' and 'reducing the effective intensity of light for this receptor by the same factor' (though there is not necessarily a physically realizable light that fulfills this symmetry condition for all three receptor types simultaneously).

From this linking proposition a number of important psychophysical consequences follow: Metameric classes of lights must be preserved under adaptation (*"Persistenzsatz"*, persistency rule):

$$A \equiv B \Rightarrow <A,S> \equiv <B,S>$$

for any pre-adapting light S

Furthermore, the Grassmann linearity laws must remain valid for any constant state of adaptation of the eye. This must be true also for the case of *asymmetric* adaptation (e.g., both eyes adapted differently, matches between both eyes):

$$<A,S> \equiv <B,T> \quad \text{and} \quad <C,S> \equiv <D,T>$$
$$\Rightarrow <A \oplus C, S> \equiv <B \oplus D, T>$$

and

$$<A,S> \equiv <B,T>$$
$$\Rightarrow <t * A, S> \equiv <t * B, T> \quad \text{proportionality rule}$$
("Proportionalitätssatz")

The transition from one state of adaptation to another can, according to this theory, be described by a linear transformation of the corresponding tristimulus values, i.e., by a 3×3 matrix M. With respect to the spectral sensitivity functions of the cones this transformation is completely described by three numbers, i.e., a diagonal matrix D. Von Kries already was aware of the fact that the validity of these laws provides another possibility for estimating the cone spectral sensitivities by transforming the 3×3 matrix M by $B^{-1}MB$ into a diagonal matrix D of reals (daß *"die Ermüdungsversuche die Möglichkeit zu einer directen Bestimmung der Componenten bieten"*, von Kries, 1882, p. 108).

The *von Kries coefficient scheme* is at the core of many approaches for dealing with mechanisms of sensitivity control, adaptation and color constancy in psychophysics, neurophysiology ('multiplicative gain control') and computational vision. In fact, 'the' psychophysical von Kries hypothesis as well as the proportionality rule split up into a variety of different hypotheses dependent on the experimental and theoretical paradigm chosen. Von Kries' original ideas of including adaptational phenomena within the Young-Helmholtz theory primarily refer to aspects of temporal adaptation ('successive contrast'), whereas the use of von Kries type transformations in computational approaches to color perception primarily refers to effects of spatial contexts that mirror changes in the prevailing illumination (a typical example is to interpret the transformation $\varphi_i(A)$ $(\varphi_i(\rho(S)) \cdot \varphi_i(A)$ as a kind of normalization of the receptor codes corresponding to a surface A under some illumination by the receptor codes of a white surface under the same illumination).

Various psychophysical investigations into the von Kries hypothesis have been carried out since, with more or less negative results (cf. Wyszecki and Stiles, 1982, p. 429 ff.). Many of the relevant experimental studies have concentrated on consequences of the von Kries hypothesis rather than on the hypothesis itself, notably the linearity laws (Wyszecki and Stiles, 1982, p. 431) and among these the *proportionality rule*. This rule has, under several experimental paradigms, been shown to fail (cf. Jameson and Hurvich, 1972). There is abundant evidence both in psychophysics and neurophysiology that there are many types and sites of adaptation in the visual system (cf. MacLeod, 1978; Walraven and Valeton, 1984; Walraven et al., 1990). For instance, Ahn and MacLeod (1993) found that chromatic adaptation had different effects on flicker photometry and unique yellow settings.

Even in cases where a multiplicative von Kries transformation is suggested by the data, the coefficients might not be easily identifiable with a certain stage of neural processing, since a single coefficient can comprise the effects of many transformations at quite different stages. Nevertheless, the failure of 'the' von Kries law/proportionality rule gave rise to search for 'additional mechanisms' (in an attempt to preserve the basic spirit of a linear coefficient law), notably 'subtractive' ones.

12.4.5.2 The "Two-Process Interpretation" of Spatial and Temporal Effects in Opponent-Color Theory

The effects on color appearance of spatial and temporal variations of context were at the origin of opponent-color theory. Hering focused on certain spatial interactions of colors and corresponding phenomena traditionally subsumed under the headings 'light induction', 'color induction', 'simultaneous contrast' etc. These phenomena offer a natural starting point for a spatially oriented relational point of view as advanced by Fechner, Mach, Hering, Katz, Bühler, Koffka, and Land, to mention only a few well-known names. According to this perspective, color is inherently determined by features of the entire visual scene. Both aspects, the preadaptational and the relational one, are often couched in the same language of adaptation, and it is, in fact, often difficult to tell them apart in experimental or theoretical work.

Within the framework of opponent-color theory an explicit mathematical model to account for the effects of adaptation and induction in terms of opponent-color processing was proposed by Jameson and Hurvich (e.g., 1972). This is the so-called *"two-process interpretation"*, whose mathematical core is a formal scheme, which, like the von Kries coefficient scheme, allows for different interpretations.

Whereas the linear version of opponent-color theory discussed in section 12.4.3 refers to a single spot of light only, the "two-process interpretation" also refers to the effect of a (spatial) context in which a test light is seen and yields an affine version of opponent-color theory. When applied to a system φ of linear primary codes, the model can, for the 'red-green system', be given the following schematic form:

$$Q_{r-g}(A;S) = \Sigma_{i=1,2,3}\, k_i(S)\cdot \varphi_i(A) - I(S)$$

where A denotes the presented lights and S the (spatially or temporally) adapting light, and $k_i(S)$ and $I(S)$ are real numbers. The Jameson-Hurvich model postulated analogous equations for the other two channels.

This model is different from the linear opponent-color model of section 12.4.3.2. that was based on color-cancellation experiments. Whereas, under suitable linearity assumptions, the opponent codes derived from color-cancellation experiments with a single homogeneous spot of light belong to the class of Grassmann codes, the opponent codes of the Jameson-Hurvich model are affine functions of the linear primary codes and are, thus, not Grassmann codes themselves.

There are several important variants of this model like Walraven's (1976) *"discounting the background"* model:

$$Q_{r-g}(A;S) = \Sigma_{i=1,2,3}\, k_i(S)\cdot (\varphi_i(A) - \varphi_i(S))$$

This model assumes that in stimuli of the kind $A = S \oplus \Delta$ only the incremental part Δ is subjected to a von Kries type sensitivity control:

$$Q_{r-g}(\Delta;S) = \Sigma_{i=1,2,3}\, k_i(S)\cdot \varphi_i(\Delta).$$

A discussion of these models can be found in Mausfeld and Niederée (1991; 1993).

In the next section I shall summarize a theoretical scheme for color codes in center-surround stimuli, put forward by Mausfeld and Niederée (1993), that is based on a contrast code of primary receptor signals and incorporates both multiplicative and subtractive mechanisms of sensitivity control. This scheme, called the *Octant Model* (because it partitions the receptor excitation space into eight regions), on the one hand allows a simple interpretation in traditional terms of front end contrast coding. On the other hand, theoretical as well as empirical observations connected with it lead in a natural way to a more sophisticated reading of this model in terms of complex perceptual achievements. I shall turn to the corresponding functionalist and ethology-inspired perspective in section 12.6.

12.4.5.3 The Octant Model and Increment-Decrement Asymmetry

There is ample evidence in color research supporting the idea that spatio-temporal transients provide the essential 'information' for the coding of color. The following model is based on corresponding theoretical ideas and empirical results and tries to specify some basic aspects of such a transient-based perspective for a 'minimal' kind of stimulus configuration that suits a relational transient-based perspective of color, according to which, at each point, color is determined by the relation between (at least) two 'lights', characterized by their spectral compositions, one pertaining to this very point and the other(s) to its neighborhood.

As above, I shall denote a stimulus consisting of a central infield A presented in a surround/background S (each characterized by the primary color codes $\varphi_i(A), \varphi_i(S), i = 1, 2, 3$) by $<A,S>$. (In the following I use the terms 'surround' and 'background' interchangably, A, B, ... always denote the absolute infields.)

Consider two such stimuli $<A,S>$ and $<B,T>$. Of course, if the two infields A and B have identical values with respect to a Grassmann code φ and if the two surrounds S and T also have identical φ-values, the two stimuli are isophene:

If $\varphi(A) = \varphi(B)$ and $\varphi(S) = \varphi(T)$,

then $<A,S> \equiv <B,T>$.

The converse, however, is not true, since different vectors in six-dimensional real vector space may result in isophene infields. Therefore, many attempts in color science have been made to find a color code Φ that captures the appearance of the infield, i.e.

$$<A,S> \equiv <B,T> \Leftrightarrow \Phi(A,S) = \Phi(B,T).$$

and that is some simple function h of the corresponding Grassmann code. More precisely, one wants to find some vector valued function on the six-dimensional real vector space such that $\Phi(A,S) = h(\varphi(A), \varphi(S))$ is a color code for the appearance of the infield.

Examples for h are linear functions in the infield for a fixed surround (e.g., von Kries, Land) and affine functions (e.g., Jameson and Hurvich, Walraven, Shevell, Larimer) that take values in the three-dimensional real vector space.

The Octant Model is an incrementally linear model consonant with several empirical and theoretical findings on color coding. It assumes a contrast code Φ_i for each channel i and predicts that between the infields of two such configurations a color match is obtained if the respective contrast codes for the two stimuli coincide (interestingly enough, neurophysiological as well as psychophysical observations suggest that the primary signals in the retina result from contrast coding, whereas absolute brightness and color must be approximately reconstructed by higher-order processes). The contrast code Φ_i is given by the difference $\phi_i(A) - \phi_i(S)$, which in turn is subjected to a multiplicative surround-dependent transformation $\rho_{i\pm}[S]$ (or, more precisely, $\rho_{i\pm}[\phi(S)]$). The distinctive feature of the Octant Model is that these transformations are allowed to be different for increments (i.e., $\phi_i(A) - \phi_i(S) \geq 0$) and decrements (i.e., $\phi_i(A) - \phi_i(S) < 0$): $\rho_{i+}[S] \neq \rho_{i-}[S]$. In neurophysiological terms, the sign of the response in each of the three color channels depends entirely on the background, and the 'ON' and 'OFF' parts of each channel are subjected to different multiplicative gain controls. The result that incremental and decremental stimuli are processed differently does not come as a surprise in view of both the phenomenological distinction between aperture and surface modes of color perception, and the functionalist distinction between illumination colors and object colors.

All incrementally linear models that assume that incremental and decremental stimuli were subjected to the same multiplicative surround-dependent transformation $\rho_i[S]$ imply a qualitative law of *increment-decrement symmetry*: let Δ be an increment superimposed on a background S and Δ' another increment on a background T such that the two infields are isophene (i.e., $<S \oplus \Delta, S> \equiv <T \oplus \Delta', T>$); then the infields of the corresponding decremental stimuli (if they are physically realizable) must also be isophene (i.e., $<S \ominus \Delta, S> \equiv <T \ominus \Delta', T>$). If, on the other hand, the principle of increment-decrement symmetry is violated for a certain viewing condition and judgmental mode, then for such a condition no incrementally linear model with $\rho_{i+}[S] = \rho_{i-}[S]$ can hold.

A simple phenomenon, called *luminance contrast phenomenon* (Niederée and Mausfeld, 1996), already qualitatively shows that increment-decrement symmetry cannot hold generally. Furthermore, quantitative experiments of ours show that the multiplicative 'gain control' coefficients differ indeed considerably for increments and decrements (Mausfeld and Niederée, 1992). This difference does not only show up between proper increments and proper decrements, but between several octant boundaries: Heyer (1996) by explicitly extending the Octant model to a subsequent stage of opponent coding – was able to show experimentally 'kinks' of unique blue lines in unique yellow surrounds at several octant boundaries.

The difference in processing between increments and decrements (or, more generally, the coding properties described by the Octant Model) could possibly be understood as resulting from the structure of the elementary perceptual categories of 'object color' and 'illumination color', which will be addressed below.

The above presentation confined itself to the abstract core of basic elementary color codes. The elementaristic perspective on color coding is, however, much more variegated and richer and incorporates for instance mechanisms related to eye-movements, filling-in processes, contrast coding etc. Nevertheless, there are many phenomena that cannot be easily accommodated in the elementaristic perspective on color coding (cf. Mausfeld and Niederée, 1993, sec. 9) and necessitate an additional and different approach to color perception.

12.5 Ecological and Computational Perspectives

The elementaristic perspective on color coding proved to be immensely fruitful for our understanding of the primary transduction and neurophysiology of early color coding. The elementaristic perspective is, however, ill-equipped to deal with problems of color perception in complex scenes. This does not mean that there are simply some lacunae to be filled in the future in the theoretical picture the elementaristic perspective draws of color perception. Rather the entire perspective is, in a pernicious way, misleading if one attempts to extend it to problems of color perception in natural scenes.

It goes without saying that this does not challenge the fact that the Grassmann theory constitutes the basis for any theory of complex color coding. In particular, almost all approaches to color perception assume that the pattern of color appearances which is evoked by a spatio-temporal array of lights A_j is a function of the corresponding tristimulus array $\varphi(A_j)$. This assumption, called *extended primary trichromacy* by Mausfeld and Niederée (1993), is equivalent to the assumption that the pattern of color appearances does not change if each light A_j is replaced by a metameric light.

When an elementaristic perspective on color vision attempts to incorporate functionalist aspects of goals of perception it succumbs to a measurement device (mis-)conception of perception. This may be exemplified by Barlow's (1982, p. 635) remark that *"For color vision, the task of the eye is to discriminate different distributions of energy over the spectrum."* In a similar vein Buchsbaum and Gottschalk (1983, p. 92) state: *"The visual system is concerned with estimating the spectral functional shape of the incoming color stimulus."*

The success of the elementaristic approach to color vision with respect to neurophysiological concerns has for many decades reduced psychophysics to an auxiliary discipline of neurophysiology. Corresponding attitudes have prevailed in psychophysics and veiled the fact that since the beginning of scientific investigations into color perception an alternative perspective has been developed that takes into account functionalist aspects of perception and starts from the idea that color perception deals with complex perceptual achievements in connection with the interplay of light and objects. This perspective had already been clearly expressed by Hering (1920, p. 13):

"Vision is not a matter of perceiving light rays as such, but the ability to see external objects by means of these rays; the eye's task is not to inform us about the respective intensity or quality of the light that comes from the external objects, but to inform us about the objects themselves."[5]

Hering's commitment to a functionalist perspective has since then been echoed and advanced by Bühler, Heider, Brunswik, Gibson, Shepard, to mention just a few well-known names. Unfortunately, the prevailing orthodoxies of elementaristic and neurophysiologically oriented psychophysics suppressed complex functionalist approaches to color perception to such an extent that it took quite some time and effort to once more attain the level of insights that one can find in the classic literature, e.g., in Gelb (1929) or Kardos (1935). These insights have been resurrected in a new guise due to the emergence of artificial intelligence research, where they have inspired various computational approaches to color vision.

We can schematically distinguish two kinds of approaches to theoretically deal with the internal coding of the color of objects under varying illuminations. The adaptational perspective emphasizes the role of simple elementary mechanisms that neutralize the effects of changes of the illumination. Of these the most prominent is a von Kries-type normalization of the receptor output by an illumination-dependent factor. Such an adaptive rescaling could in principle yield a good approximation to color constancy if reflectance and illuminant spectra are broad relative to the bandwidth of the receptors. The basic spirit of an adaptational perspective on color constancy can already be found in Hering, who considered color constancy as primarily due to elementary and primitive processing modes of the visual system.

---

[5] "Nicht um das Schauen der Strahlungen als solcher handelt es sich beim Sehen, sondern um das durch diese Strahlungen vermittelte Schauen der Außendinge; das Auge hat uns nicht über die jeweilige Intensität oder Qualität des von den Außendingen kommenden Lichtes, sondern über diese Dinge selbst zu unterrichten."

Explicit accounts from different theoretical perspectives were given by Ives (1912) and Jaensch (1914) who introduce the concept of level, and later, among others, by Helson, Judd, Land, Brill and West (e.g., West and Brill, 1982), MacLeod (1986), and Foster and Nascimento (1994).

Non-adaptational approaches to color constancy were developed by Sällström, Buchsbaum, Brill, Maloney and Wandell, and D'Zmura and Iverson. These approaches are explicitly couched in terms of the computational goal of recovering from the sensory input a function that depends only on certain physical properties of objects, viz. characteristics of surface reflectance.

In the following I shall very briefly sketch some of the basic ideas of the adaptational and non-adaptational approaches using the example of Land's Retinex scheme and of Maloney's algorithm which is based on the linear framework approach.

12.5.1 The Problem of Approximate Color Constancy from a Computational Point of View

A strong locally-atomistic perspective on color perception takes the color appearance at each location k of the visual field to be determined by the light pertaining to this very location, i.e., by the respective triple $\varphi(A_k)$ alone. This alleged point-to-point correlation of wavelength composition and color appearance is in conflict with many empirical phenomena, among them colored shadows and the phenomenon that colors of objects tend to remain fairly constant under changes of the color of the illumination.

The formal core of the problem of color constancy as viewed from a computational perspective is schematically shown in Figure 12.3. The variables involved are the spectral energy distribution $E(\lambda)$ of the illumination and the spectral reflectance function $R(x,\lambda)$ at a location x of a surface. The signal coming to the eye is the point-wise product of illumination and reflectance, as it were. It causes in each type i of photoreceptors a neural signal. In this signal the illumination component and the reflectance component are completely confounded. Nevertheless, the internal representation, i.e., the percept of the (approximately) 'true' color of the surface, requires a kind of disentangling of the two components. On the basis of local information of a single position x this is, of course, impossible, on logical grounds (analogously to the impossibility of identifying each of the factors for a given product of two numbers). Visual mechanisms that accomplish a (largely) illumination-independent perceptual assessment of the color of

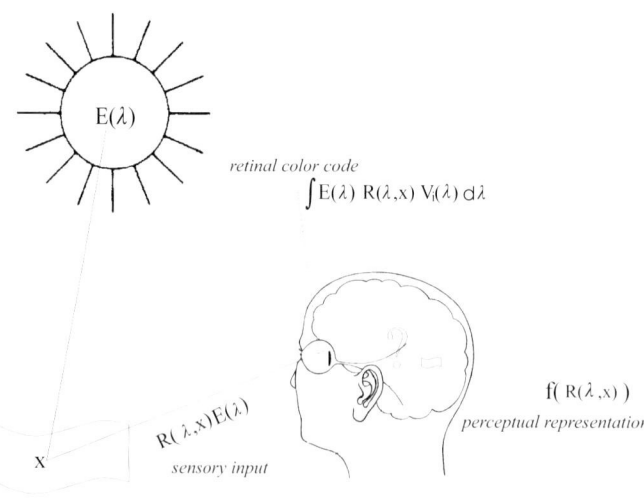

Fig. 12.3: The problem of color constancy.

objects must consequently be based on some global operations of the visual scene.

12.5.1.1 Land's Approach to Color Constancy

Investigations into the problem of color constancy underwent a revival due to the ingenious 'Mondrian' demonstrations of Edwin Land. To account for his findings Land put forward several versions of a simple computational scheme, which he called *Retinex Theory*. This scheme was motivated by the idea that the illuminant has to be completely discounted. Land's approach was to find color designators (i.e., a triple of numbers) for which the following hold:

 i) designators are invariant under changes of illumination (for a fixed configuration of surfaces)
 ii) equal designators correspond to identical color appearances.

Whereas i) is a requirement from a computational perspective, ii) ties the illumination-invariant code to perceptual relations; it assumes perfect color constancy (within one fixed scene).

In Retinex theory these color designators are obtained by a simple comparison and normalization procedure. For a given test field x of a fixed Mondrian that is illuminated homogeneously, the procedure can, in terms of Grassmann color codes, be described as follows: Let $\varphi_x = (\varphi_{1,x}, \varphi_{2,x}, \varphi_{3,x})$ be the value of the Grassmann code of the light coming from x. Correspondingly, let φ_y for all other patches y of the Mondrian denote the respective Grassmann codes. The (later version of the) Retinex algorithm basically calculates the geometric mean $G(\varphi_y)$ and normalizes the color code of the test field with respect to this geometric mean, i.e., $\varphi_x/G(\varphi_y)$. This color code $L = \varphi_x/G(\varphi_y)$ is (under strong assumptions about lights and surfaces) invariant over changes in illumination if the average spectral reflectance of the Mondrian considered corresponds to a mid-grey reflectance.

It is obvious that the Retinex algorithm is formally equivalent to a von Kries-type transformation, where the coefficients ρ_i are assumed to be inversely proportional to the geometric mean of the Grassmann codes of the Mondrian areas.

Land's computational approach to color constancy, despite being theoretically unsatisfactory and at variance with empirical observations, stimulated further theoretical and empirical research on color constancy immensely.

Several other adaptational algorithms for color constancy have been developed that are also based on a von Kries-type normalization and assume that there is either a white surface available in the scene or that the average reflectance of the scene is a mid-grey. Foster and Nascimento (1994) provided evidence that illuminant invariant codes may be achieved by a direct coding of spatial color relations, since cone excitation ratios are for natural surfaces almost invariant under changes in natural illuminants. Forsyth (1990) proposed for a Mondrian world a framework for extracting illuminant information hidden in the gamut of Grassmann codes for all possible surface reflectances under some illuminant.

12.5.1.2 The Linear Model's Framework and Maloney's Algorithm

The most prominent class of non-adaptational models of color constancy are based on the following idea: analyses of large sets of empirical surfaces and lights as well as investigations into the physical processes that determine surface spectral reflectances have led to the conjecture that the spectral energy distributions of 'natural' lights and many surface spectral reflectance functions are well approximated by a linear combination of a fixed finite set of frequency-limited basis functions. Each surface spectral reflectance is then expressed as a linear combination of n basis functions. The number n and each of the n basis functions is assumed fixed and to be independent of the surfaces considered, the weights of this linear combination can vary to generate all possible surface reflectances for this particular linear model. The residual error is remarkably small, since, for instance, eight basis functions account for over 0.99 of overall variance for large sets of natural spectral reflectances.

Based on such a finite-dimensional linear physical model for the underlying physical variables - a model that is only weakly constrained by perceptual considerations – Maloney (1985, 1992) proposed a mechanism that exploits the underlying physical regularities. Its goal is to estimate from the sensory input a function that depends only on the surface spectral reflectance function. For his algorithm, Maloney assumes that for the case of three receptor types each light can be sufficiently well approximated by a linear combination of three basic lights, and each surface reflectance by a linear combination of two basic reflectance functions, i.e., the vector space of permissible lights has the dimension 3, the vector space of permissible reflectances the dimension 2. Therefore the values of the Grassmann codes of the permissible reflectances under a fixed permissible light come to lie in a two-dimensional linear subspace of the three-dimensional Grassmann space. Maloney provided natural assumptions under which this subspace is characteristic for the illumination in the sense that the illumination can – up to scalar multiplication – be determined from the position of this subspace with respect to the Grassmann space. This in turn allows the determination – up to scalar multiplication – of the reflectances. For a set of empirical reflectances the system would have to determine (according to some distance measure) the best approximating linear subspace in sensor space (if one chooses the Euclidean distance this task is accomplished by some kind of principle component analysis).

Maloney's penetrating analyses into the mathematical structure that results from the interaction of lights, surfaces and properties of the eye (together with assumptions of the visual system's task) can be considered an important accomplishment for the conceptual clarification of the problem of color constancy. On empirical grounds, however, the general assumption that the visual systems's achievement is to obtain a function of the sensory input that depends on $R(x,\lambda)$, but not on $E(\lambda)$, which on Maloney's account is tantamount to recovering reflectances, does not seem to be appropriate. Furthermore, to account for empirical surface reflectances which require (at least) three degrees of freedom in surface reflectance functions, the algorithm requires four types of receptors. But even if the algorithm should not teach us much about the actual mechanisms of human color perception, the underlying approach is certainly a whetstone to clarify our basic concepts. Maloney's approach particularly shows in a precise mathematical way, how strong the implications are that can be derived from ecological considerations about the 'physical friendliness' of our environment.

12.5.2 Qualitative Observations on the Dialectic Relationship of Illumination and Object Color

Plausible as computational approaches of the kind mentioned above are at first sight (provided one restricts attention to appropriate 'semi-ecological' situations, such as a 'Mondrian world'), these approaches have systematic drawbacks from a psychological point of view. The most general objection is that the reduction of color perception to estimating surface reflectances is, from the point of view of perceptual psychology, nearly as misleading as the locally atomistic wavelength-based perspective. The claim that *"the goal of color vision is to recover the invariant spectral reflectance of objects (surfaces)"* (Poggio, 1990, p. 147) amounts to a distal variant of the measurement device conception of perception. Though the adaptive coupling of the organism to its environment takes strong advantage of physical regularities of physical reflectances, the claim that the estimation of spectral reflectance functions is a goal of color vision amounts to underestimating constraints derived from its internal 'semantic structure', as it were, and imputes to the visual system a goal that is not consonant with its actual achievements. What is achieved is not an estimation of spectral reflectance functions, but rather an abstractive categorial description of the 'color of a perceived object', which is more stable than can be expected on the basis of the local sensory input, i.e., the wavelength composition of the light coming from the object to the eye. In this sense, the percept 'color of an object' seems to be more strongly tied to the spectral reflectance characteristics of the object than to the wavelength composition of the local sensory input. There is, however, no color constancy in the strict sense that two locations of the same spectral reflectance 'look the same' under two different illuminations. Complex scenes rather require a notion of 'equality of color appearances' whose meaning depends on the judgmental task and the observer's 'mode of perception'. This was already stressed by Katz, who also observed that color appearances under chromatic illumination have a peculiar character of a kind that cannot be encountered under normal illumination. "Attempts to establish color appearances within a field of view in qualitatively normal illumination that in all respects are equal to color appearances that can be encountered in fields of view in chromatical illumination, are prone to fail" (Katz, 1911, p. 274)[6]. The often subtle phenomenal differences in appearance have escaped appreciation in computational perspectives. This is partly due to the fact that computational psychophysicists are often loath to admit any consideration of phenomenological appearance. Consequently, the construction of illumination independent color codes tends to be divorced from the construction of appropriate appearance codes. Another reason for this situation lies in our lack of a suitable theoretical language for the phenomenal description of the percept associated with the interplay of perceived illumination and perceived objects, since such a description has to deal with aspects of, for instance, vagueness, abstraction and categorization.

In the classic literature we find many attempts to carefully describe the phenomenal peculiarities that are characteristic for color appearances under (chromatic) illumination. Helmholtz (1911, Vol. 2, p. 243) described them as "colors that can be seen *at the same location* of the visual field one behind the other."[7] Bühler (1922, p. 40) spoke of "locating colors in perceptual space one behind the other" (*"Hintereinander von Farborten im Wahrnehmungsraum"*), "colors appear as if they were composed of the actual object color and a coating by the chromatic illumination."[8] Katz (1911, p. 274) noted "the curious lability of colors under chromatic illumination." Similar observation can be found in Hering (e.g., 1888), Fuchs (1923), or Gelb (1929).

Even everyday situations, say a white wall in a room illuminated by a reddish light, can arouse intriguing kinds of impressions in a careful observer:

– we can 'see' both the color of the object ('white' wall) and the color of the illumination (in many cases there is, through shifts of attention, some freedom in how we 'decompose' the sensory input into an 'object color component' and an 'illumination color component')
– the colors of objects in the room are less distinctive and more vague than under 'normal illumination' (though we tend to have good access to the 'colors of the objects')
– the gamut of colors tends to shrink the more the illumination deviates from a white one (which gives rise to the conjecture that the visual system might use something like the variance of Grassmann codes for an assessment of the illumination)
– a white illumination seems to be special in that we cease to have the impression of a separate illumination at all.

Furthermore, a green light, for instance, and an olive-green surface exhibit some phenomenological similarity: Though in principle these two 'worlds' of colour appearances could have been phenomenologically completely divorced from each other, the adaptive requirement of colour constancy necessitates the possibility of at least a partial compensation and continuous transition between the two.

From present-day computational perspectives, phenomenological descriptions like these more or less seem to be mere exercises in phenomenology that do not promise to provide further theoretical insights. However, if one abandons the inappropriate assumption that properties of color coding can completely be understood in terms of, or even be

---

[6] "Innerhalb eines qualitativ normal beleuchteten Gesichtsfeldes wird man vergeblich Farbeindrücke herzustellen versuchen, die denen in jeder Beziehung gleichen, welche wir in buntfarbig beleuchteten Gesichtsfeldern antreffen."
[7] "Farben, die in demselben Teil des Gesichtsfeldes vorhanden sind" und wo "eine Farbe durch die andere hindurch zu sehen ist"

[8] Farben "erscheinen, als ob sie aus der eigentlichen Objektfarbe und einem daraufliegenden Häutchen aus der farbigen Beleuchtung zusammengesetzt seien"

derived from the goal of recovering spectral reflectances, the question again arises in which way adaptive properties of the internal coding of color can be described more appropriately. Observations like the ones above may then provide strong heuristics about what the actual achievements of the visual system with respect to color perception are and about how the attribute of color is interlocked with spatial aspects that in turn are interrelated with the 'interpretation' of the scenes in terms of 'objects' and 'illumination' (one cannot overemphazise the point stressed by Koffka, 1936, p. 129, that "a general theory of color must at the same time be a general theory of space and form").

12.6 Center-Surround Configurations as Minimal Stimuli for Triggering a Dual Code for 'Object Colors' and 'Illumination Colors'

The ecological perspective on color perception heuristically starts out from a physical description of the sensory input in terms of complex achievement-related concepts such as 'surface', 'specular highlights', 'shadows', etc. It then attempts to construct complex abstract color codes backwards, as it were, from an appropriate physical description of the perceptual achievements, say color constancy. For instance, one tries to find color codes (considered as functions of the input) that are equal if the reflectances that are part of the physical input description are equivalent (i.e., equal up to multiplication). Approaches like these again amount to succumbing to the physicalistic trap, since they presuppose that the perceptual categories (e.g., of 'light' or 'surface') are constituted by the corresponding physical categories (of physical lights or surfaces). Such an assumption, however, cannot be derived from the evolutionary requirement of an adaptive coupling of perceptual categories to biologically relevant physical ones. In point of fact, the perceptual categories 'surface colors' vs. 'illumination colors' are not constituted by the corresponding categories of physics and tied to them in the sense of the latter being necessary and sufficient conditions for the former. Rather they are constituted by a set of biologically relevant features that are specific to physically contingent organism-environment relations.

A proper physical description of these relations should therefore not be couched in the vocabulary of still-to-be-identified perceptual categories. Not much is known today about the internal semantics, as it were, of the visual system, but there are good reasons to assume that basic 'semantic' units of perception are predetermined and tied to certain spatio-temporal characteristics of the incoming energy.

Approaches to deal with the problem of the internal perceptual semantics of organisms were developed by v. Uexküll, v. Frisch, Lorenz, Tinbergen, and, for situations where, like in visual perception, the unit of analysis is not the entire organism but certain (often abstractly idealized) 'mechanisms', by Lashley, Bühler, Brunswik and Barlow, to mention only a few names. Barlow (1961, p. 219) summed up this perspective under the watchword *"password hypothesis"*: "Specific classes of stimuli act as 'releasers' and evoke specific responses; these classes of stimuli are thought of as 'passwords' which have to be distinguished from all other stimuli, and it is suggested that their detection may be the important function of sensory relays."

An exposition of these ethological perspectives as applied to the problem of how elementary perceptual categories come about is beyond the scope of this paper and will be given elsewhere. In the present context only some heuristic intuitions will be addressed as to the general question whether there are critical minimal stimulus characteristics that already trigger attempts of the visual system to 'interpret' them in terms of certain perceptual categories. Are the perceptual categories of 'illumination color' and 'object color' internally constituted not by an extensive set of properties of corresponding physical entities, but rather by a few 'representative' ones? If so, these physical characteristics could be instantiated by an otherwise highly reduced stimulus, which then would suffice to trigger an internal perceptual structure whose complexity far exceeds the complexity of the triggering stimulus. The initial mapping of sensory inputs on internal codes is, on this view, innately specified in terms of an 'environmental semantics'.

According to such a perspective, the dialectic relationship of illumination and object is mirrored in a perceptual bi-segmentation of the visual field (corresponding to the fovea-extrafovea segmentation of the retina). The main function of the surrounding field is – besides detection of motion and optical flow, and orientation in space – to estimate the illumination, and not to identify objects of which this surrounding field is composed. The problem of approximate color constancy is, on this view, misrepresented by current computational accounts. If color is part of the format of 'representing' the environment, i.e., a property of the organization of the perception instinct that couples our perceptuo-motorial system *as a whole* to its environment, processes underlying phenomena of approximate color constancy are not necessarily coupled to certain invariant characteristics of physical objects, to wit spectral reflectances, but rather are part of the way the system is organized. Consequently these complex internal structures can be triggered by appropriate but highly unecological stimuli (though in evolutionary history physical properties of natural spectral reflectances played a crucial role for the development of these properties of internal organization). Once triggered they create mandatory 'interpretations' in terms of a dual code for 'illumination color' and 'object color'.

An interesting candidate for such classes of stimuli are center-surround type configurations, traditionally associated with mechanisms of early color coding (like sensitivity control and opponent processing) and exhibiting phenomena like simultaneous contrast. Already Helmholtz observed that under natural conditions simultaneous contrast rarely occurs (a phenomenon that in modern terms can be related to the important computational goal of achieving scene invariance of color designators, i.e., the color of an object should not vary with the color of neighboring objects). There seems to be something special about the geometrical configuration of small and sharply demarcated infields in large surrounds. The phenomena observed in these situations led Hering and later, in a more pronounced way, Jaensch, Gelb, Bühler, Kardos and Müller to assign a special status to center-surround stimuli and to favor a functional interpretation of the corresponding results in terms of 'higher-level' achievements. For instance K. Bühler (1922, p. 131) interpreted the phenomenon of simultaneous contrast in such situations as a degenerate marginal phenomenon attesting to the visual system's capability of preserving colors under changes of illumination.

With respect to different aspects there is strong empirical and theoretical evidence that suggests regarding center-surround type stimuli as 'minimal' stimuli for triggering mechanisms of the visual system that provide basic constituents for the perceptual categories of 'illumination color' and 'object color' and their interplay. In the next two sections I shall sketch some of the experimental indications in support of such a triggering of elementary perceptual categories by center-surround situations.

12.6.1 Laminar Segmentation and a Dual Code for 'Object Color' and 'Illumination Color'

In the Octant Model, $\phi(S)$ can be regarded as a measure of some level set by $<A,S>$ with which the infield A is to be compared in such a way that $\phi(A) - \phi(S)$ is processed and for each component subjected to a surround-dependent multiplicative transformation $\rho_i[\phi(S)]$. According to this model, the corresponding three-dimensional code for the color appearance of the infield is described formally by a contrast operator which involves taking differences of primary codes and applying contrast-dependent multiplicative transformations in each of the three components.

The idea that the dialectic relationship of object and medium, and of 'object color' and 'illumination color' is a fundamental part of the structural form of our visual world, together with an ethology-inspired perspective that considers center-surround configurations as kinds of sign stimuli for an 'object under chromatic illumination' sheds new light on the specific way – as captured in the incrementally linear color code of the Octant Model – in which in center-surround configurations 'large-disc information' and 'small-disc information' are segregated by the visual system. From this perspective, this segregation mirrors processes that are related to the segregation of object and illumination information. If the center-surround configurations contain physico-geometrical properties that already trigger the visual system's 'interpretation' in terms of small, sharply demarcated objects under chromatic illumination, one should be able to observe, under suitable conditions, phenomena like those described in section 12.5.2 also in center-surround configurations.

Indeed, in our color-cancellation experiments we found phenomena, where, again in Bühler's words, "colors appear as if they were composed of the actual object color and a coating by the chromatic illumination" and where in perceptual space one color is located behind the other.

The following example of an experiment may serve to illustrate such phenomena: We used under Maxwellian-viewing conditions – using the apparatus shown in Figure 12.1 – a red surround ($\lambda = 649$ nm, 150 td, 8–10°), where the 2°-infield was composed of a mixture of monochromatic light ($\Delta R_{649} \oplus \Delta G_{546}$). The subjects had to perform (by a two-alternative forced choice double-random staircase) reddish/greenish-judgments and to make a setting where the infield appears neither reddish nor greenish. While for most values of stimulus parameters subjects were able to satisfy this judgmental criterion (and made settings that are consonant with predictions derived from the Octant Model), they reported for certain stimulus parameters (large surrounds, contrasts not too high, predominantly in the decremental domain) seeing a reddish and a greenish component simultaneously.

Figure 12.4 shows for a typical experiment the range of dominant wavelengths of the infield (for different intensities) within which a reddish and greenish color appearance (with a, in Katz's words, "curious lability of colors") is seen simultaneously (the left curve indicates the lower bound of reddish appearances of the infield, the right curve the upper bound of greenish appearances, in between are infields that appear reddish and greenish simultaneously).

Subjects were not able to completely cancel the amount of redness at the position of the infield by increasing the green component of the infield. There seem to be two layers between which there is no complete trade-off. I consider this observation as a further indication that center-surround

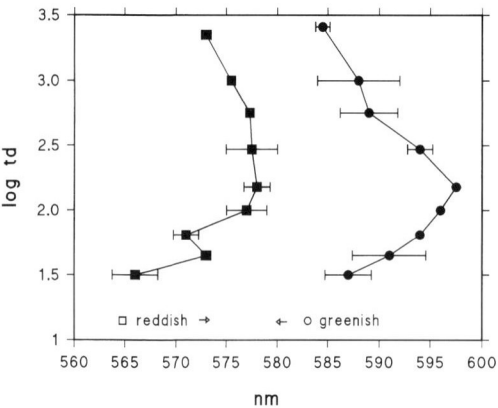

Fig. 12.4: Range of reddish/greenish appearence of infield on red background of 150 td.

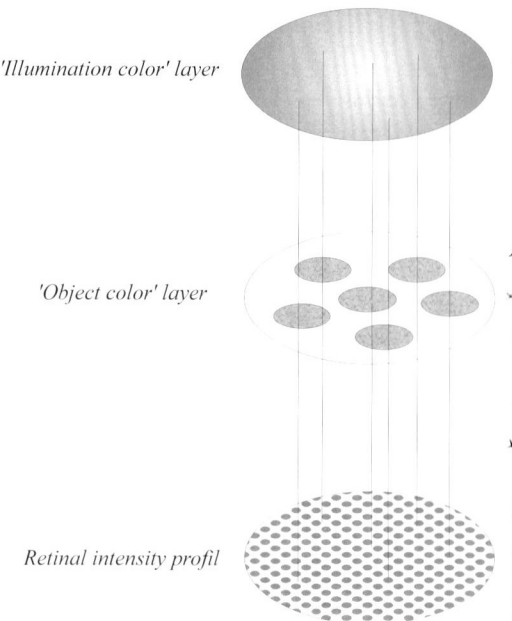

Fig. 12.5: Laminar segmentation of the retinal intensity profil.

situations already trigger a laminar segmentation of the retinal intensity profile into an 'object color' component and an 'illumination color' component – as metaphorically indicated by Figure 12.5 – and give rise to a dual color code for these two components.

12.6.2 Segregation of 'Object Color' and 'Illumination Color' in Minimal Seurat-type Configurations

So far I only referred to center-surround configurations in which the surround corresponds to an area that is spatially uniform, i.e., homogeneous in terms of spectral energy distributions. The central heuristic underlying the approach proposed here is that such homogeneous center-surround configurations can be regarded as minimal stimuli for triggering a dual code for 'object colors' and 'illumination colors'. Though the above phenomenon of laminar segmentation already can be interpreted as some indication along this line, in order to establish a more convincing case in favor of this conjecture, one has to establish a 'continuous path', as it were, that connects this minimal situation via increasingly more complex ones with semi-ecological ones, like Mondrian-type situations or three-dimensional scenes.

It is not the physico-geometrical property of being a center-surround configuration, but rather the perceptual feature of a certain figure-ground segmentation that triggers basic mechanisms subserving 'color constancy' that is of importance here. Already Rubin (1921, p. 56) observed that transformations in the direction of color constancy are stronger if a certain area is perceived as figure than if it is perceived as ground.[9] The homogeneous center-surround configuration can be considered as the prototypical situation for triggering a figure-ground segmentation, according to what

Rubin (1921, p. 79) called a "fundamental law" (*"Fundamentalregel"*): in situations where a homogeneous field of small size is surrounded by a much larger homogeneous field, there is a predominant tendency to perceive the enclosed smaller field as figure.

In a series of experiments in collaboration with Johannes Andres we attempted to bridge the gap from homogeneous center-surround configurations to Mondrian configuration by a sequence of configurations (presented on a CRT screen) of the following kind. For each homogeneous surround (characterized by the corresponding Grassmann coordinates) a family of spatially inhomogenous surrounds, which have the same space-average Grassmann coordinates (globally, and within several smaller annular regions of increasing distance from the infield), is constructed by varying the following parameters:

– bandwidth of spatial variation of spectral inhomogeneities
– spatial inhomogeneities achieved by varying the degrees of modulation along the luminance axis
– spatial inhomogeneities achieved by varying the degrees of modulation along the red-green axis

The geometrical layout of spatial variations of the surround is given by a random structure of overlapping circles (with occluding intersections) of a certain diameter (defining bandwidth of spatial variation). The infield has the same size as in the previous experiment with homogeneous center-surround configurations and consists of a mixture of red and green which has to be brought to a red-green equilibrium.

For very small diameters of the circles of the surround and if both luminance and chromatic modulations are employed, the stimulus configuration is reminiscent of the Neo-Impressionistic style of painting (see Fig. 1.20 of chapter 1). Because of this, I refer to these stimuli as Seurat-type configurations. Increasing the diameter leads to patterns that resemble, say, a piece of fruit against a background of leaves, or a flower against a background of grass or soil. For circles with very large diameters a Mondrian-type of configuration is obtained. Using these kinds of stimulus configurations we can systematically investigate continuous transitions of complexity between center-sur-

---

[9] "... daß diejenigen zentralen Faktoren, durch welche die auf einer farbigen Beleuchtung beruhende Veränderung in der Farbe der Dinge kompensiert werden, stärker wirksam sind an dem Felde, das als Figur, als an dem, welches als Grund hervortritt."

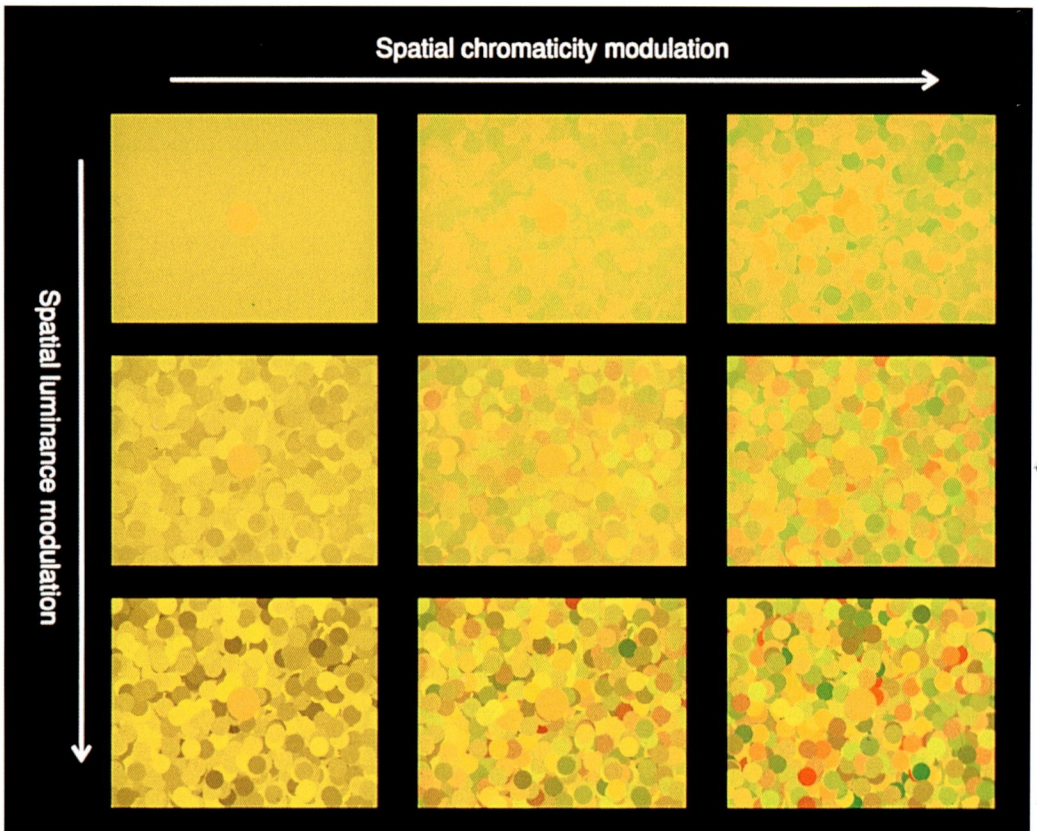

Fig. 12.6: Seurat configurations of intermediate bandwidth of spatial variation of the surround and of the same spatially-averaged chromaticities, with spatial luminance modulation increasing on the vertical axis, and chromaticity modulation increasing on the horizontal axis.

round type stimuli with a homogeneous surround and Mondrian-type configurations and thereby study those physical properties of such configurations that trigger an interpretation in terms of the elementary perceptual categories of 'object color' and 'illumination color'.

For an intermediate bandwidth of spatial variation of the surround, Figure 12.6 shows typical configurations with spatial luminance modulation increasing on the vertical axis, and chromaticity modulation increasing on the horizontal axis. For all four displays in this figure the space-average Grassmann codes of the surrounds are identical to the ones of the homogeneous surround in the display in the upper left.

According to traditional adaptational models all these stimuli are functionally equivalent, i.e., are expected to exhibit the same effect on the unique yellow settings at the location of the infield. A typical example of a simple adaptation model of a space-averaged von Kries-type sensitivity control assumes that $\Phi(A,S)$ can be understood in terms of some linear 'pooling mechanism' $\varphi_i(S) = \Sigma_j w_{ji} \varphi_i(S(y_j))$, where $S(y_j)$ denotes the spectral energy distributions of the surround at the location y_j, and $w_{ji} \in [0,1]$ are location-dependent weights (possibly decreasing with distance to the infield), summing up to 1. While our data clearly reveal that in our Seurat-type stimuli, surrounds with equal space-averaged Grassmann coordinates grossly violate any functional equivalence with respect to the unique yellow settings of the infield,

12.6 Center-Surround Configurations as Minimal Stimuli for Triggering a Dual Code

they suggest an interpretation in terms of a triggering of elementary perceptual categories related to 'object color' and 'illumination color'.

Since a detailed report of our experiments will be published separately, I shall only briefly mention some qualitative results that are of interest in the present context. If a unique yellow test spot, e.g., with a dominant wavelength of 575 nm, is surrounded by a homogeneous reddish surround (with a dominant wavelength of, say, 596 nm), the dominant wavelength for the infield needs to be shifted towards longer wavelengths, e.g., to 585 nm, in order for a red-green equilibrium to be preserved. We now kept the infield at the same luminance as the surround (L = 9 cd/m^2) and spatially modulated the surround along the red-green axis only, along the luminance axis only and simultaneously along both axes, while keeping the spatial average *fixed*.

For an isochromatic surround (Fig. 12.7 left), i.e., no red-green variation and spatial luminance variation only, the red-green equilibrium settings showed a stronger shift towards longer wavelength than the ones for the corresponding homogeneous surround. A reduced variance of color codes in the surround seems to increase the visual system's propensity to interpret the configuration as an illuminated scene. For the case of an isoluminant surround (Fig. 12.7 right) with strong spatial red-green modulation only, the opposite effect showed up, i.e. the unique yellow settings strongly tended towards the ones of a dark surround or a space-averaged achromatic surround. A qualitatively similar result for a red background field with sparse white and green dots has been obtained by Jenness & Shevell (1995). The finding for isoluminant surrounds can be related to the functional goal of achieving approximate scene invariance for the color codes of the infield. (The difference between surround configurations of isoluminant and isochromatic patches is more pronounced for reddish surrounds than for greenish ones, as is to be expected from considerations about natural illumination variations.)

These experimental phenomena can be accommodated by the general perspective outlined above according to which the surround-dependent change in appearance of an infield in a center-surround configuration is not to be understood as an elementary re-coding of channels by a simple surround-dependent gain control, but in fact mirrors the triggering of a much more complex mechanism for establishing a dual code for 'object color' and 'illumination color'. The case of isoluminant chromatic spatial modulation results in a proximal stimulus pattern that is highly improbable to result from surfaces under chromatic illumination; it is a non-generic view, as it were. Such a configuration fails to trigger a proper dual code for illumination and object colors and thus does not activate any illuminance correction (this is analogous to the observation that a non-generic view of a Necker cube fails to trigger a 3D-interpretation).

The results of our experiments support, in my view, the idea that all color processing is cast into

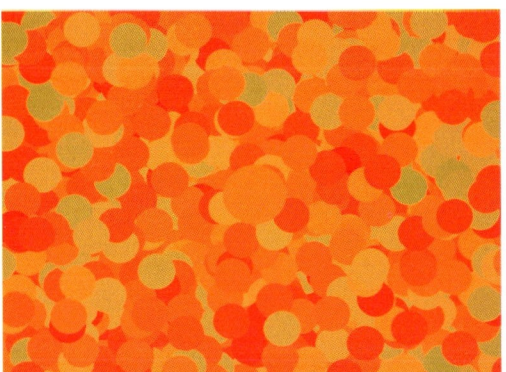 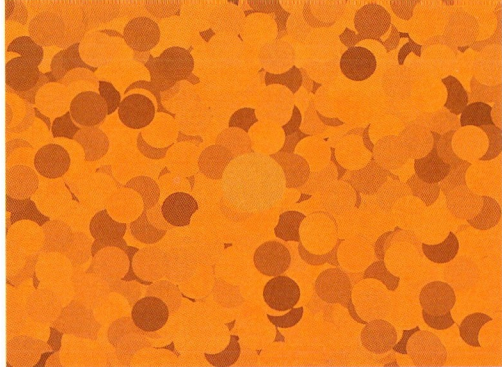

Fig. 12.7: Isochromatic (left) and isoluminant (right) Seurat configuration with same spatially averaged chromaticities.

the format of innate semantic perceptual categories of 'object color' and 'illumination color', which in turn are intimately interwoven with representations for elementary perceptual categories for the representation of surfaces, form and space. According to this view, perceptual achievements such as the segregation of object and illuminant color are brought forth by the very organization of the internal representation of color rather than being computationally derived from properties of sensory inputs. This reflects the difference between two different metaphors in perceptual theory: triggering vs. computation.

Acknowledgements

I should like to thank Johannes Andres, Don MacLeod and Larry Maloney for their valuable comments on an earlier draft of this paper.

References

Ahn, S. J. and MacLeod, D. I. A. (1993). Link-Specific Adaptation in the Luminance and Chromatic Channels. Vision Research 33, 2271–2286.
Alpern, M., Kitahara, K., and Krantz, D. H. (1983). Perception of Colour in Unilateral Tritanopia. Journal of Physiology 335, 683–697.
Barlow, H. (1961). Possible Principles Underlying the Coding of Sensory Messages. In: W. Rosenblith (Ed.), Sensory communication (pp. 217–234). Cambridge, Mass.: MIT Press.
Barlow, H. (1982). What Causes Trichromacy? A Theoretical Analysis Using Comb-Filtered Spectra. Vision Research 22, 635–643.
Brückner, A. (1927). Zur Frage der Eichung von Farbsystemen. Zeitschrift für Sinnes physiologie 58, 322–362.
Buchsbaum, G. and Gottschalk, A. (1993). Trichromacy, Opponent Colours Coding and Optimum Colour Information Transmission in the Retina. Proceedings of the Royal Society London B220, 89–113.
Bühler, K. (1922). Die Erscheinungsweisen der Farben. In: K. Bühler (Ed.), Handbuch der Psychologie. I. Teil. Die Struktur der Wahrnehmungen (pp. 1–201). Jena: Fischer.

Fechner, G. T. (1840). Über die subjective Nachbilder und Nebenbilder. Poggendorff's Annalen der Physik und Chemie 50, 193–221; 427–470.
Forsyth, D. A. (1990). Colour Constancy. In: A. Blake and T. Troscianko (Eds.), AI and the Eye (pp. 201–227). Chichester: Wiley.
Foster, D. H. and Nascimento, S. M. C. (1994). Relational Colour Constancy from Invariant Cone-Excitation Ratios. Proceedings of the Royal Society London B257, 115–121.
Frumkina, R. M. (1984). Colour, Meaning, and Similarity. Aspects of Psycholinguistic Analysis (Цвет, смысл, сходствоа). (in Russ.) Moscow: Nauka.
Fuchs, W. (1923). Experimentelle Untersuchungen über das simultane Hintereinandersehen auf derselben Sehrichtung. Zeitschrift für Psychologie 91, 145–235.
Gelb, A. (1929). Die 'Farbenkonstanz' der Sehdinge. In: A. Bethe, G. v. Bergmann, G. Embden, and A. Ellinger (Eds.), Handbuch der normalen und pathologischen Physiologie. Bd. 12, 1. Hälfte. Receptionsorgane II (pp. 594–678). Berlin: Springer.
Grassmann, H. (1853). Zur Theorie der Farbmischung. Poggendorff's Annalen der Physik und Chemie 89, 69–84.
Helmholtz, H. v. (1911). Handbuch der physiologischen Optik (3.Ed., 3 Vol., Eds. W. Nagel, A. Gullstrand, J. v. Kries). Hamburg: Voß.
Hering, E. (1888). Ueber die Theorie des simultanen Contrastes von Helmholtz. IV. Mittheilung. Die subjective 'Trennung des Lichtes in zwei complementäre Portionen.' Pflüger's Archiv für die gesammte Physiologie des Menschen und der Thiere 43, 1–21.
Hering, E. (1920). Grundzüge der Lehre vom Lichtsinn. Berlin: Springer.
Heyer, D. (1996). The Relation of Contrast Coding in the Octant Model and Opponent Processing: A theoretical and Experimental Investigation. Technical report, Institute für Psychologie, Universität Kiel.
Hippel, A. v. (1880). Ein Fall von einseitiger, congenitaler Roth-Grünblindheit bei normalem Farbensinn des anderen Auges. Gräfes Archiv für Ophtalmologie 26, 176–186.
Hochegger, R. (1884). Die geschichtliche Entwicklung des Farbensinnes. Innsbruck: Verlag der Wagner'schen Universitätsbuchhandlung.
Irwin, E. (1974). Colour Terms in Greek Poetry. Toronto: Hakkert.
Ives, H. E. (1912). The Relation Between the Color of the Illuminant and the Color of the Illuminated Object. Transactions of Illuminating Engineering Society 7, 62–72.

Jenness, J. W. and Shevell, S. K. (1995). Color Appearance with Sparse Chromatic Context. Vision Research 35, 797–805.

Jaensch, E. (1914). Über Grundfragen der Farbenpsychologie. Bericht über den VI. Kongreß für experimentelle Psychologie (pp. 45–56). Leipzig.

Jameson, D. and Hurvich, L. M. (1972). Color Adaptation: Sensitivity, Contrast, After-Images. In: D. Jameson and L. M. Hurvich (Eds.), Handbook of Sensory Physiology. Vol. VII/4. Visual Psychophysics (pp. 568–881). Heidelberg: Springer.

Kardos, L. (1934). Ding und Schatten. Eine experimentelle Untersuchung über die Grundlagen des Farbensehens. Leipzig: Barth.

Katz, D. (1911). Die Erscheinungsweisen der Farben und ihre Beeinflussung durch die individuelle Erfahrung. Leipzig: Barth.

Koffka, K. (1936). On Problems of Colour-Perception. Acta Psychologica 1, 129–134.

Krauskopf, J., Williams, D. R., and Heeley, D. W. (1982). Cardinal Directions in Color Space. Vision Research 20, 1123–1131.

Kries, J. v. (1882). Die Gesichtsempfindungen und ihre Analyse. Leipzig: Veit.

MacLeod, D. I. A. (1978). Visual Sensitivity. Annual Review of Psychology 29, 613–645.

MacLeod, D. I. A. (1986). Receptoral Constraints on Colour Appearance. In: D. Ottoson and S. Zeki (Eds.), Central and Peripheral Mechanisms of Colour Vision (pp. 103–116). London: Macmillan.

MacLeod, D.I.A. and Lennie, P. (1976). Red-Green Blindness Confined to One Eye. Vision Research 16, 691–702.

Maloney, L. T. (1985). Computational Approaches to Color Constancy. Stanford University: Technical Report 1985–01.

Maloney, L. T. (1992). Color Constancy and Color Perception: The Linear Models Framework. In: D. E. Meyer and S. Kornblum (Eds.), Attention and Performance XIV: Synergies in Experimental Psychology, Artificial Intelligence, and Cognitive Neuroscience (pp. 59–78). Cambridge, Mass.: MIT Press.

Mausfeld, R. (1993). Methodologische Grundlagen und Probleme der Psychophysik. In: Th. Herrmann and W. Tack (Hrsg.) Methodische Grundlagen der Psychologie. Enzyklopädie der Psychologie, Bereich B, Serie I, Bd. 1, (pp. 137–198). Göttingen: Hogrefe.

Mausfeld, R. (1996). "Wär' nicht das Auge sonnenhaft …" Goethes Farbenlehre nur eine Poesie des Chromatischen oder Beitrag zu einer naturwissenschaftlichen Psychologie? ZiF Report 2/1996, Zentrum für Interdisziplinäre Forschung der Universität Bielefeld.

Mausfeld, R. and Niederée, R. (1991). Scalar Invariance in Opponent Colour Theory and the Discounting the Background Principle. In: J. P. Doignon and J.-C. Falmagne (Eds.), Mathematical Psychology: Current Developments (pp. 55-69). New York: Springer.

Mausfeld, R. and Niederée, R. (1992). On Increment-Decrement Differences in Multiplicative Gain Control. In: Advances in Color Vision Technical Digest, Optical Society of America, Washington, D.C., Vol. 4, 170–171.

Mausfeld, R. and Niederée, R. (1993). Inquiries into Relational Concepts of Colour Based on an Incremental Principle of Colour Coding for Minimal Relational Stimuli, Perception 22, 427–462.

Marty, A. (1879). Die Frage nach der geschichtlichen Entwicklung des Farbensinnes. Wien.

Neitz, J., Neitz, M., and Jacobs, G. H. (1993). More Than Three Different Cone Pigments among People with Normal Color Vision. Vision Research 33, 117–122.

Niederée, R. (1996). Continuity considerations in colour perception: Why already in centresurround stimuli colour appearances cannot be coded three-dimensionally. Technical report, Institute für Psychologie, Universität Kiel.

Niederée, R. and Mausfeld, R. (1996). Increment-Decrement Asymmetry in Dichoptic Matching with Haploscopically Superimposed Displays. Vision Research 37, 613–615.

Poggio, T. (1990). Vision: The 'Other' Face of AI. In: K. A. Mohyeldin Said, W. H. Newton-Smith, R. Viale and K. V. Wilkes (Eds.), Modelling the Mind (pp. 139–154). Oxford: Clarendon Press.

Ratliff, F. (1976). On the Psychophysical Bases of Universal Color Terms. Proceedings of the Americal Philosophical Society 120, 311–330.

Rubin, E. (1921). Visuell wahrgenommene Figuren. Kopenhagen: Gyldendalske Boghandel.

Schrödinger, E. (1920). Grundlinien einer Theorie der Farbenmetrik im Tagessehen. Annalen der Physik 63, 397–426, 427–456, 481–520.

Shepard, R. N. (1992). The Perceptual Organization of Colors: An Adaptation to Regularities of the Terrestrial World? In: J. H. Barkow, L. Cosmides and J. Toby (Eds.), The Adapted Mind. Evolutionary Psychology and the Generation of Culture (pp. 495–532). New York: Oxford University Press.

Shepard, R. N. (1994). Perceptual-Cognitive Universals as Reflections of the World. Psychonomic Bulletin and Review *1*, 2–28.

Stumpf, C. (1917). Die Attribute der Gesichtsempfindungen. Abhandlungen der königlich preussischen Akademie der Wissenschaften. Philosophisch-historische Klasse, 8. Berlin: Verlag der Königl. Akademie der Wissenschaften.

Suppes, P., Krantz, D. H., Luce, R. D., and Tversky, A. (1989). Foundations of Measurement, Vol. II. New York: Academic Press.

Walraven, J. (1976) Discounting the Background - The Missing Link in the Explanation of Chromatic Induction, Vision Research *16*, 289–295.

Walraven, J., Enroth-Cugell, C., Hood, D. C., MacLeod, D. I. A., and Schnapf, J. L. (1990). The Control of Visual Sensitivity: Receptoral and Postreceptoral Processes. In: L. Spillmann and J. S. Werner (Eds.), Visual Perception. The Neurophysiological Foundations (pp. 53–101). Academic press: San Diego.

Walraven, J. and Valeton, J. M. (1984). Visual Adaptation and Response Saturation. In A. J. Van Doorn, W. A. Van de Grind and J. J. Koenderink (Eds.), Limits in perception. Utrecht: VNU Science Press.

West, G. and Brill, M. H. (1982). Necessary and Sufficient Conditions for von Kries Chromatic Adaptation to Give Colour Constancy. Journal of Mathematical Biology *15*, 249–258.

Waetzold, W. (1909). Das theoretische und praktische Problem der Farbbenennung. Zeitschrift für Ästhetik und allgemeine Kunstwissenschaft *4*, 349–399.

Wyszecki, G., and Stiles, W. S. (1982). Color Science. Concepts and Methods, Quantitative Data and Formulae. (2nd Ed.). New York: Wiley.

13. Color Contrast Gain Control

Michael D'Zmura

13.1 Introduction

Many television sets have a knob that lets one adjust the amount of picture contrast. Turning the knob in one direction causes contrast to increase and, in the other direction, to decrease. One sometimes finds three such knobs on a color television set for adjusting black-white, red-green and yellow-blue contrast, respectively. The human visual system also has a system for controlling contrast, and the aim of this chapter is to show how it works. The method will be to trace the fate of a color image through the contrast gain control circuitry of a multiresolution model of human visual processing.

13.1.1 What is Contrast Gain Control?

Contrast gain control is demonstrated in Figure 13.1. The gray levels in the central disk on the left are physically identical to those of the disk on the right. Yet most people report that the apparent contrast of the right disk is higher than that of the left disk: the dark areas appear darker and the light areas appear lighter. The disk on the left is surrounded by an annulus of high contrast. The contrast gain control of the visual system responds to high contrast by turning local contrast down. The disk on the right is surrounded by an area of zero contrast, and the contrast gain control responds by turning local contrast up. The result is the observed difference in apparent contrast.

Over what distance does contrast in one location affect apparent contrast in another location? Does color contrast of one hue (e.g., red) affect apparent color contrast for another hue (e.g., yellow)? Where does the circuitry that is responsible for the contrast gain control reside within the visual system – is this a retinal effect or a cortical one? Singer and I have studied these and related questions over the past several years (Singer and

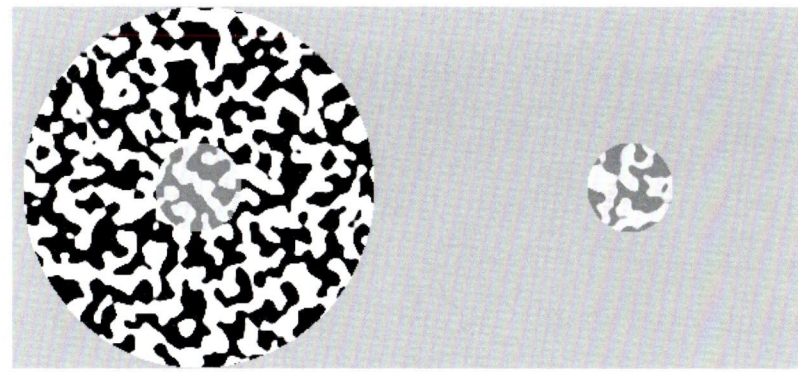

Fig. 13.1: A demonstration of contrast gain control by the human visual system. Gaze at the point midway between the central disk on the left and the disk on the right. The contrast of the disk at the right appears to be greater, although it is physically the same. (After Chubb et al., 1989).

D'Zmura, 1994, 1995; D'Zmura and Singer, 1996). We have used psychophysical experiments to measure the dependence of contrast gain control on many variables. In one experiment, observers were shown the annulus in one eye's visual field and the central disk in the other eye's visual field. The effects of contrast gain control were still visible under these circumstances, and this interocular transfer suggests strongly that the contrast gain control has a cortical locus (Blakemore and Campbell, 1969).

13.1.2 Selectivity for Spatial Frequency, Orientation and Color

Systematic studies of how contrast gain control depends on stimulus variables such as spatial frequency, orientation and color reveal a selectivity in contrast gain control that is captured well by models of visual processing with multiple channels. Chubb, Sperling and Solomon (1989) used sinusoidal patterns to show that the reduction in the apparent contrast of a central disk, found when contrast in a surrounding annulus is increased, depends on the relative spatial frequencies of center and surround. Their results are shown in Figure 13.2A. The reduction of apparent contrast is halved if the peak spatial frequency of the surround is moved to either an octave lower or an octave higher than that of the center. This selectivity can be captured by a model of visual processing that has several channels with different spatial frequency sensitivities. Contrast within a spatial frequency channel affects the gain on that channel strongly but affects the gain on channels with different sensitivities more weakly.

Solomon, Sperling and Chubb (1993) used disks and annuli filled with spatial sinusoids of varying orientation to show that the visible effects of contrast gain control depend on the relative orientation of center and surround (see Fig. 13.2B). The reduction is strongest when center and surround share the same orientation and is weakest when they have perpendicular orientations. This selectivity can be captured by a model of visual processing that has several channels with different orientation sensitivities. Contrast within a channel of specific orientation affects the gain within that channel most strongly.

Singer and I used disks and annuli of varying chromatic properties to show chromatic selectivity in contrast gain control (Singer and D'Zmura, 1994). The strongest reduction in the apparent con-

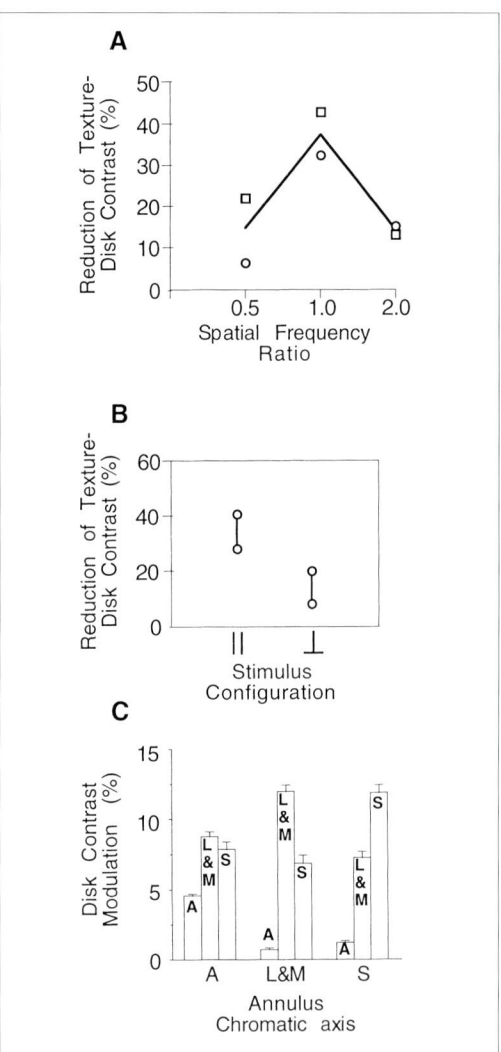

Fig. 13.2: Selectivity in contrast gain control.
A. Selectivity in spatial frequency (After Chubb et al., 1989).
B. Selectivity in orientation (After Solomon et al., 1993).
C. Selectivity in color (After Singer and D'Zmura, 1994).

trast of a central disk is found with surrounds that have identical chromatic properties (see Fig. 13.2C). Again, a multiple channel model helps to explain the result. If there are three channels that respond best to stimuli along the achromatic, L&M-cone and S-cone axes of color space, respectively (the significance of these axes is reviewed briefly just below), then the result follows if one supposes that contrast within any one channel affects the gain in that same channel most strongly.

13.1.3 Feed-Forward, Matrix-Multiplicative Circuitry

Singer and I used the results of more detailed experiments on color in contrast gain control to build a model, pictured in Figure 13.3 (Singer and D'Zmura, 1995). The first stage of the model (top) includes the three cone mechanisms L, M & S (Smith and Pokorny, 1975) and a von Kries type of adaptation that acts within each channel (von Kries, 1905). This stage is followed by a color-opponent transformation (Hurvich and Jameson, 1957) to create three channels sensitive to achromatic (A), L&M-cone and S-cone axis stimuli, respectively.

The achromatic axis in color space is the axis along which lights vary in their intensity. Lights along this axis appear to vary from white through gray to black. The L&M-cone and S-cone axes are the cardinal chromatic axes of Krauskopf (MacLeod and Boynton, 1979; Krauskopf et al., 1982; Derrington et al., 1984). Modulations among lights along the L&M-cone axis are isoluminant and are invisible to the S-cones. Lights along this

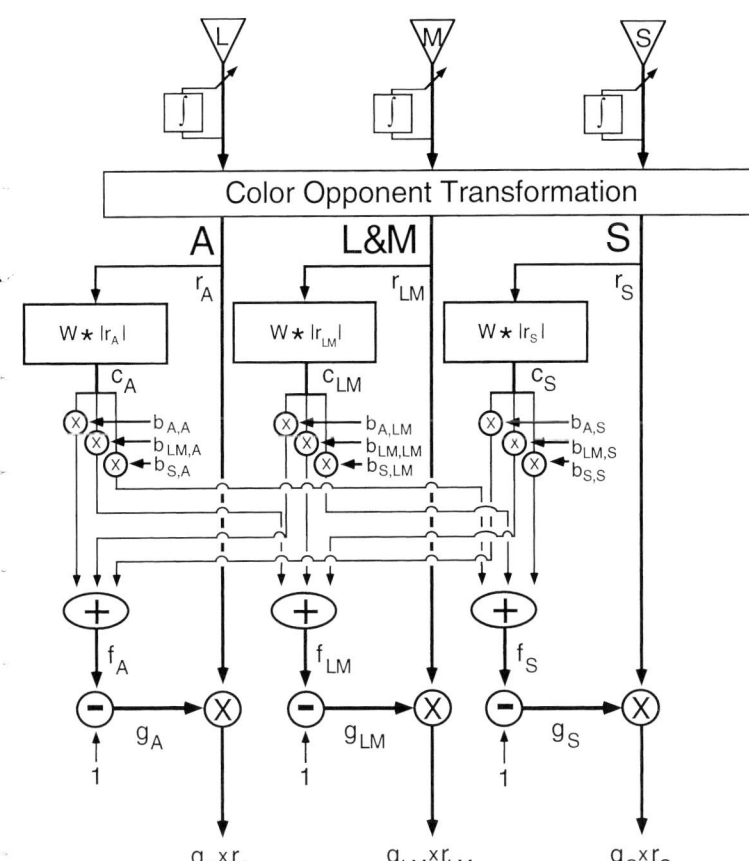

Fig. 13.3: Model of chromatic interaction in contrast gain control (after Singer and D'Zmura, 1995). The feed-forward multiplicative circuitry differs from the divisive normalization procedures proposed by Sperling (1989) and Heeger (1992). Data collected by Singer and D'Zmura (1995) on saturating nonlinearities in contrast gain control were fit well by the former but not by the latter.

axis typically range from red through gray to blue-green. Modulations among lights along the S-cone axis are isoluminant and are invisible to both the long- and medium-wavelength-sensitive (L & M) cones. Lights along this axis typically range from purple through gray to yellow-green.

Contrast is computed in each of the three second-stage channels by (1) rectifying the channel signal to create a nonnegative response at each point, and (2) determining local contrast by pooling contrast over an appropriate area. This spatial pooling is accomplished formally by convolving a spatial pooling function $W(\mathbf{x})$ with the space-varying, rectified response $|r(\mathbf{x})|$ of each channel. Such operations produce the achromatic channel's contrast $c_A = W \star |r_A|$, the L&M-cone axis channel's contrast $c_{LM} = W \star |r_{LM}|$ and the S-cone axis channel's contrast $c_S = W \star |r_S|$. The space-varying contrasts are then combined appropriately using the nine coefficients b (see Fig. 13.3), which are chosen according to empirical results on chromatic selectivity (Singer & D'Zmura, 1995). The selectively combined contrasts are used to determine gains g_A, g_{LM} and g_S on the responses of the achromatic and opponent channels. The gains act multiplicatively on the chromatic signals to produce the three outputs $g_A \times r_A$, $g_{LM} \times r_{LM}$ and $g_S \times r_S$. The contrasts c_A, c_{LM} and c_S are combined additively and then subtracted from one to determine the gains g_A, g_{LM} and g_S. In this model, the effect of increasing contrast is to reduce gain in an inhibitory fashion.

13.1.4 Spatial Pooling of Contrast

By extending the model to include second-stage channels that are selective not only for color but also for spatial frequency and orientation, we can capture the psychophysical results on selectivity in contrast gain control. One further ingredient is needed: data on the spatial pooling functions $W(\mathbf{x})$, which describe the area over which contrast is pooled by the contrast gain control. Cannon and Fullenkamp (1991) used spatial sinusoids to show that the width of the area over which contrast is pooled increases roughly linearly with spatial wavelength. Singer and I (1994) showed that pooling areas are roughly independent of stimulus

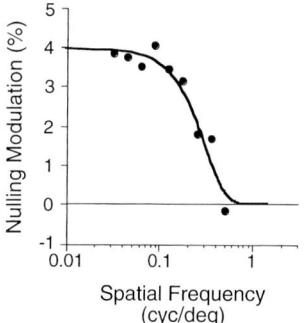

Fig. 13.4: Spatial frequency sensitivity of contrast pooling by the gain control described by a Gaussian function (after D'Zmura and Singer, 1996).

chromatic properties. More recently, Singer and I used spatially-sinusoidal modulations of contrast modulation to determine the spatial frequency sensitivity of contrast pooling (D'Zmura and Singer, 1995). The spatial frequency sensitivities were fit well by Gaussians (see Fig. 13.4). Transforming these sensitivities back to the space domain provides Gaussian receptive field profiles for contrast pooling.

13.2 Model Components

The contrast gain control model of Figure 13.3 is readily extended to (1) include results on selectivity in spatial frequency, orientation and color; (2) incorporate data on the spatial pooling of contrast, and (3) process color images. The full model has four spatial frequency bands that are octave-wide (with the exception of the lowest spatial frequency band). For each of the four spatial frequency bands, there is a Gaussian contrast pooling area with a standard deviation that is proportional to the central spatial wavelength of the band. The model has six bands of differing orientation, each of width 30 degrees. The model works with achromatic, L&M-cone and S-cone axis signals. The model has a total of 72 channels formed of the various combinations of spatial frequency, orientation and color, and these 72 channels interact selectively in contrast gain control.

Figure 13.5 shows the spatial properties of the

achromatic mechanism's channels. Along the top are six sinusoids that label channel orientation, which varies from vertical at left to horizontal in the middle and back again at right in 30° steps. Along the left side are four sinusoids that label channel spatial frequency, which varies from low at the top to high at the bottom. The spatial frequency and orientation properties of each of the 24 channels are shown in the Fourier domain. White areas in the diagrams indicate channel sensitivity.

There are also 24 L&M-cone axis channels, with spatial properties that are identical to those pictured for the achromatic mechanism. The difference is that these L&M-cone axis channels are maximally sensitive to chromatic change along the L&M-cone axis, in the red/blue-green direction, rather than to black-white change. Likewise, there are 24 S-cone axis channels with properties that are identical to those of the achromatic and the L&M-cone axis channels, except that their peak sensitivity is to chromatic change along the S-cone axis, in the yellow-green/purple direction. The model has a total of 72 channels.

The model's contrast pooling functions are shown in the right column of Figure 13.6. These are four spatially-isotropic Gaussian functions with standard deviations that increase in proportion to channel spatial wavelength. Channel spatial wavelength is labelled by the sinusoids in the three columns at left; pooling is identical for the three color channels.

The interaction in contrast gain control among the model's 72 channels is guided by the psychophysical data on selectivity (see Fig. 13.2). As discussed below, the interaction is separable; the model's selectivities in spatial frequency, orientation and color are mutually independent.

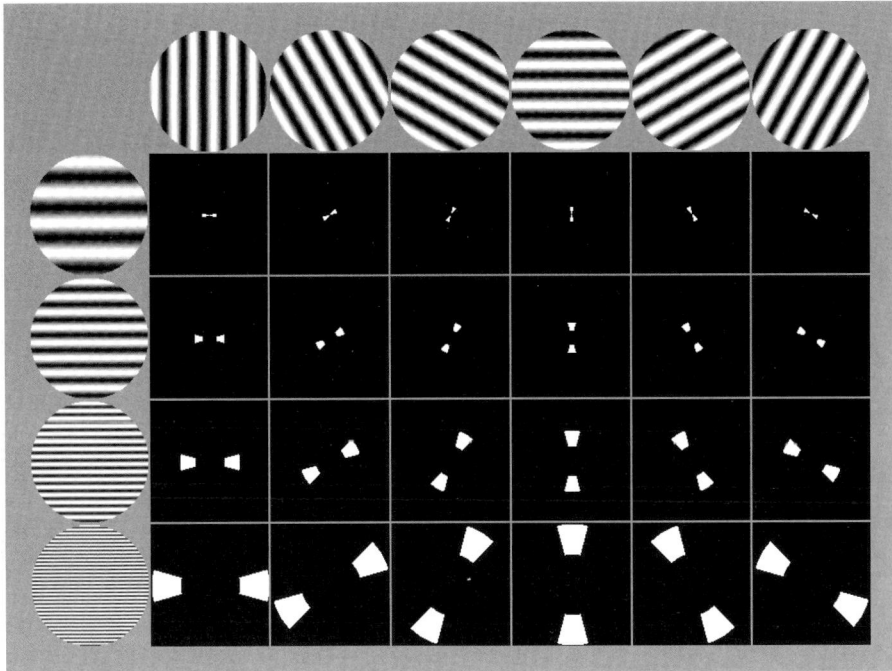

Fig. 13.5: The model's achromatic channels, tuned for spatial frequency and orientation. Each of the 24 plots of channel sensitivity is labelled by a sinusoid in the left column that indicates channel peak spatial frequency and by a sinusoid in the top row that indicates channel central orientation. Each of the 24 sensitivity plots has its origin (frequency 0) in the center; frequency increases as one moves from the center towards the edge. White areas indicate frequencies and orientations to which channels are sensitive. The L&M-cone and S-cone axis channels have identical spatial properties.

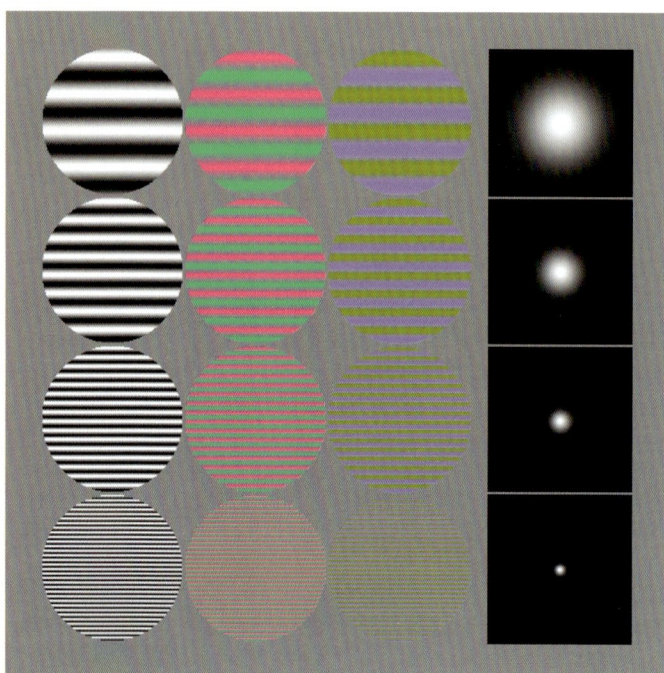

Fig. 13.6: Gaussian spatial pooling functions (right column) have standard deviations that increase linearly with channel wavelength (three leftmost columns).

13.3 Color Image Processing

Let us now illustrate the operation of the model using an actual image as input. The chosen input image is a color picture of the space shuttle "Discovery" of size 128×128 pixels. This image is shown in Figure 13.7 at the top left. In the middle row is the color decomposition of the input image along the achromatic (left), L&M-cone (center) and S-cone (right) axes. The black-white picture is readily visible. It is more difficult to make out the L&M-cone and S-cone channel images, which are presented at approximate isoluminance. In the bottom row are shown the Fourier domain spectra of the three color channels' images. Again, brighter areas signal larger values, and it is evident that much of the space shuttle image's energy lies at low frequencies, towards the centers of the three plots in the bottom row. Note also the fine horizontal and vertical lines of spectral energy that pass through the origins of the frequency-domain plots; these correspond to vertically-oriented and horizontally-oriented edges, respectively, in the original space-domain images.

13.3.1 Channel Responses

The model divides the Fourier-domain energy up into the channels described earlier (Fig. 13.5). Figure 13.8 shows the responses of each of the achromatic channels to the space shuttle image. The channels are labelled by sinusoids that indicate channel peak spatial frequency (left column) and mean orientation (top row). Most of the energy is found at low spatial frequencies (top row). The rocket, shuttle and gantry provide plenty of vertically-oriented energy (left column) at low and moderate spatial frequencies. Note also the strong, horizontally-oriented gradient at a low spatial frequency which corresponds to the gradient between the sky above and ground below in the space shuttle image.

Much the same arrangement of energy is found among L&M-cone axis channels (see Fig. 13.9), although response strength is less than that found with the achromatic mechanisms. The lighter-than-average values in these channel response images correspond to positive-valued responses by the L&M-cone channels, which code redness, while the darker-than-average values correspond

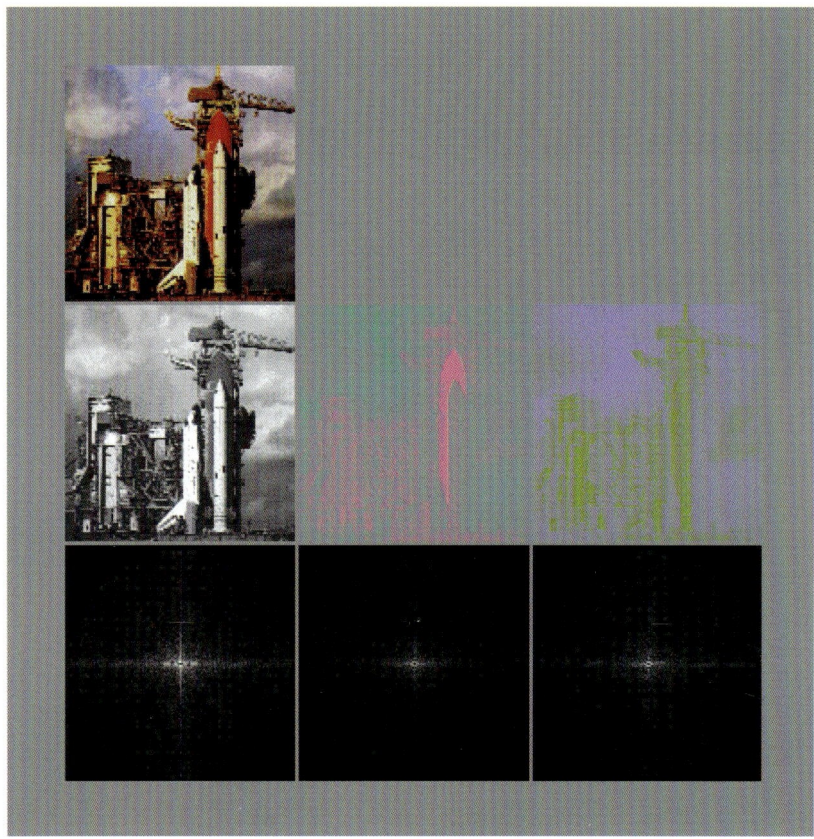

Fig. 13.7: The "Discovery" space shuttle image, input to the contrast gain control model. In the middle row are the achromatic, L&M-cone and S-cone channel images, and the Fourier amplitude spectra of these are shown in the bottom row.

to negative-valued responses, which code blue-greenness. The red rocket shows up most prominently in the low and moderate spatial frequency, vertically-oriented bands.

Figure 13.10, finally, shows the responses of the S-cone channels. The blueness of the sky is coded by positive values and shows up as a lighter region in the response image for the low-frequency, horizontally-oriented channel. Yellow areas in the input image show up as dark regions.

13.3.2 Channel Contrasts

The model's contrast gain control works by multiplying each of the 72 channel responses (Figs. 13.8–13.10) at each position by channel-specific gains. These gains are determined by taking appropriate linear combinations of local contrasts found within each of the channels. The local contrasts are computed by taking the absolute value of channel response and convolving the result with a Gaussian contrast pooling function of appropriate size. Note that if one omits the full-wave rectification (absolute value operation) and simply convolves a channel's response with a Gaussian, all that would be achieved would be a blurring that would not correspond to a calculation of contrast within the channel. The full-wave rectification causes the result of the local contrast computation to correspond to our notion of contrast as a difference between maximum and minimum values.

13. Color Contrast Gain Control

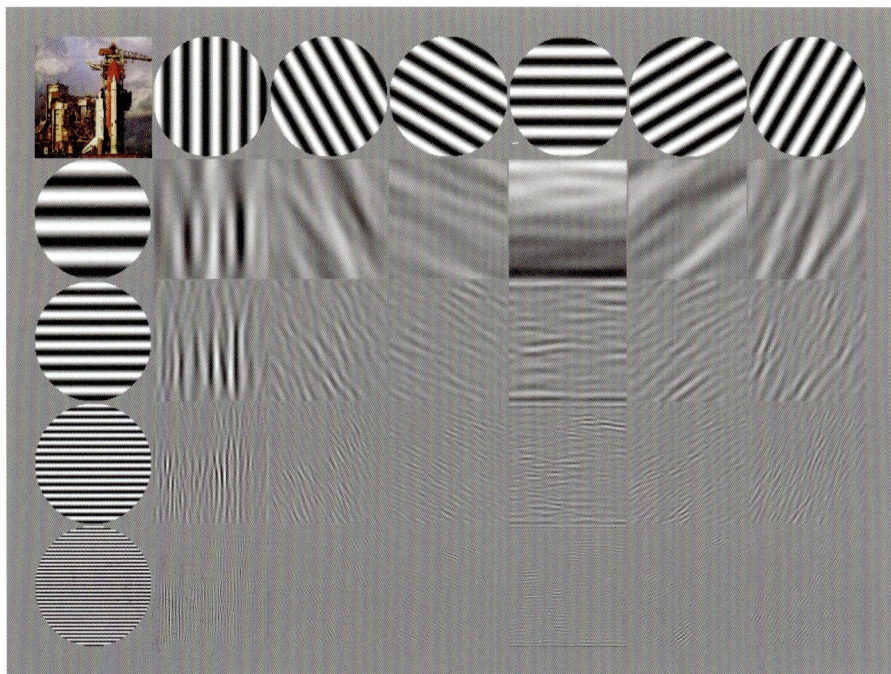

Fig. 13.8: Responses of the model's achromatic channels to the space shuttle image.

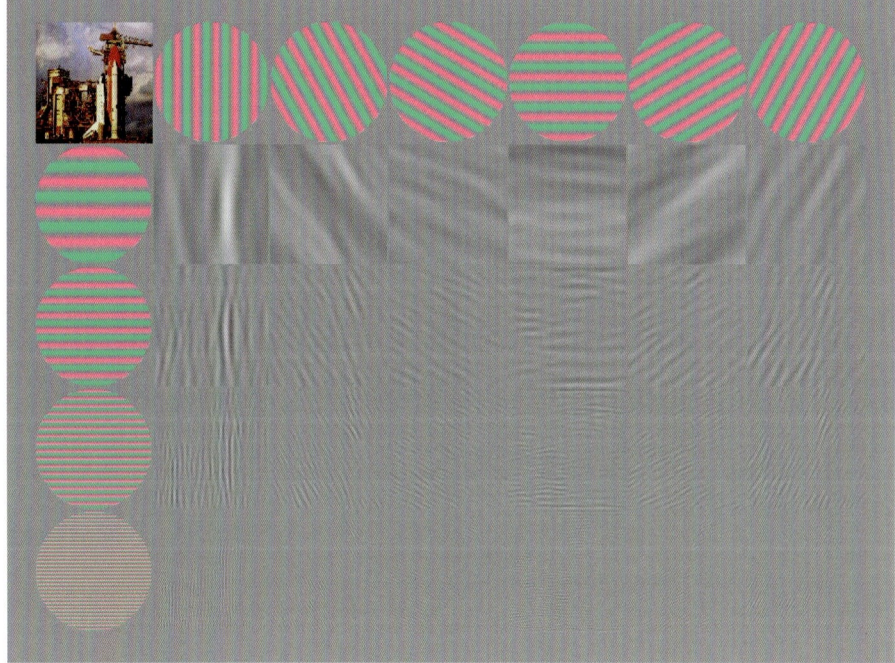

Fig. 13.9: Responses of the model's L&M-cone axis channels to the space shuttle image.

13.3 Color Image Processing

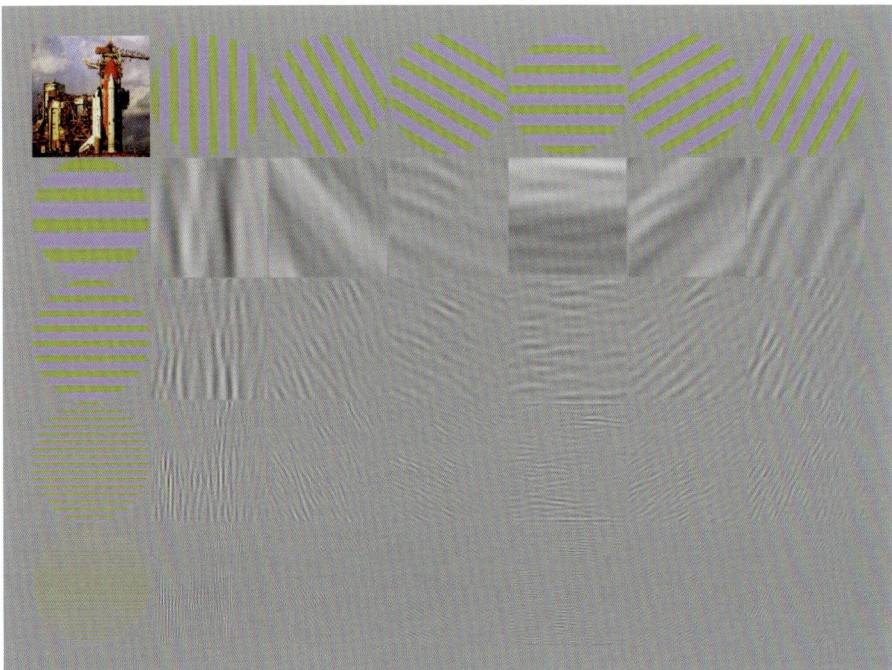

Fig. 13.10: Responses of the model's S-cone axis channels to the space shuttle image.

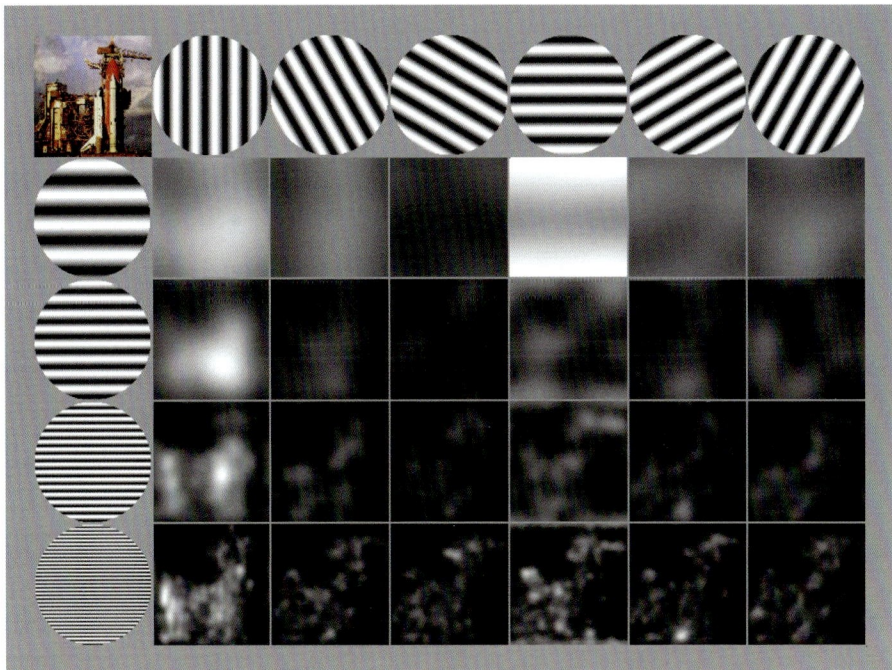

Fig. 13.11: Local contrast within the model's achromatic channels.

260   13. Color Contrast Gain Control

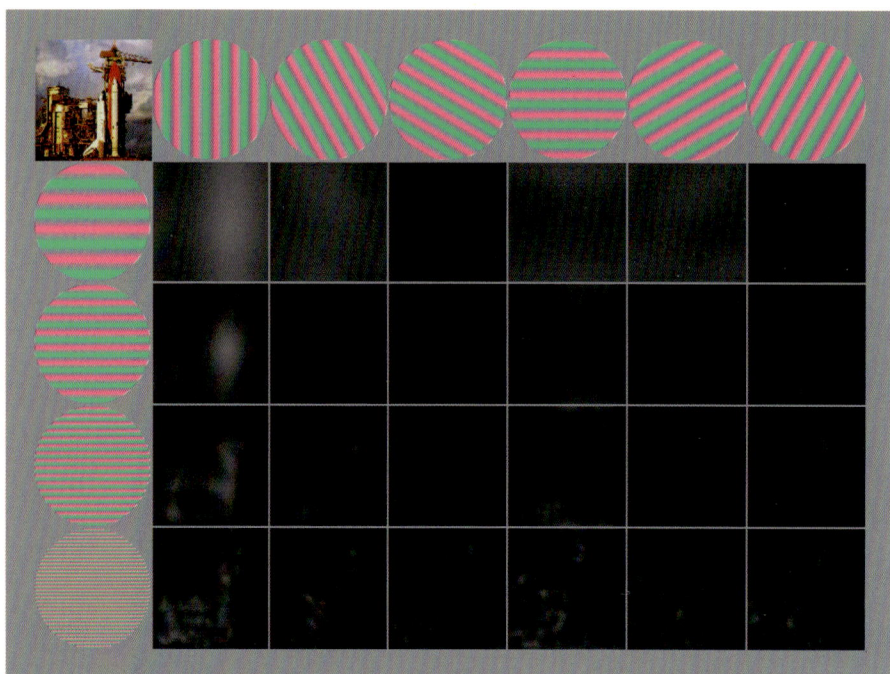

Fig. 13.12: Local contrast within the model's L&M-cone axis channels.

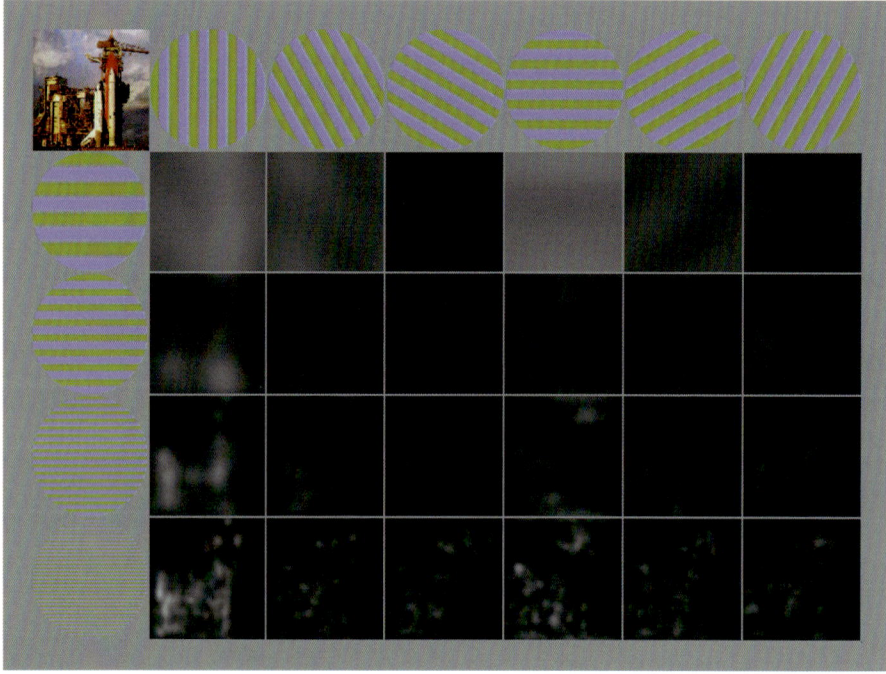

Fig. 13.13: Local contrast within the model's S-cone axis channels.

The local contrasts of the achromatic channels are shown in Figure 13.11. Higher contrasts are coded by lighter values. Most contrast is found at low frequencies and at vertical orientations. The area of the picture with the rocket and the shuttle provides vertically-oriented contrast at all frequencies, as does the gantry, especially at higher frequencies. The horizontally-oriented gradient between the sky and the ground has undergone a rectification that is clearly visible within the contrast image for the low-frequency, horizontally-oriented channel. The sky presents a contrast relative to the center of the picture; the ground also presents a contrast relative to the center.

A similar pattern for L&M-cone axis channels is shown in Figure 13.12, although there is less L&M-cone contrast than achromatic contrast in the space shuttle image. Figure 13.13 shows local contrast among the S-cone axis channels, and again the pattern is similar to that found among the achromatic channels.

13.3.3 Channel Interaction

The gain control works by forming, for each of the 72 channels, an appropriate linear combination of the local contrast responses and then using the result to inhibit channel signals. The linear combination incorporates the selectivity in spatial frequency, orientation and color that was described earlier. The model is completely separable: selectivities in spatial frequency, orientation and color are mutually independent. The coefficient that describes the contribution that one channel's contrast makes to the gain of a second channel is equal to the product of three independent factors: (1) a factor that depends on the spatial frequencies of the two channels; (2) a factor that depends on the two channels' relative orientations, and (3) a factor that depends on the two channels' chromatic properties.

The factors that are used in the model are drawn from the data of Figure 13.2. For spatial frequency (Fig. 13.2a), the factor is maximal for channels of identical spatial frequency, falls to half-maximum for channels that differ by an octave, and falls to zero for channels that differ by more than an octave. For orientation (Fig. 13.2b), the factor is maximal for channels of identical orientation, falls to half-maximum for channels that differ by 90°, and varies sinusoidally between maximum and half-maximum for the intermediate relative orientations. For color (Fig. 13.2c), the factors are nearly identical to those shown, with the exception that the contributions of isoluminant contrast to achromatic gain are taken to be zero. Achromatic contrast has strong effects on L&M-cone and S-cone channel gains, but not vice versa (Singer and D'Zmura, 1994; 1995).

13.3.4 Channel Gains

To determine a channel's gain, we combine the contrasts of each channel appropriately and then subtract the result from one, at each point. The space shuttle image gains for the achromatic channels are shown in Figure 13.14. Such a gain has a maximum possible value of one. If the value one multiplies a channel signal, then the channel signal is unchanged. These pictures use bright values to code the high gains near one. Any gain that is less than one - but greater than zero - will act to turn the contrast down. Dark values code smaller gains. The dark values mark areas in the channel response pictures where contrast will be turned down by the gain control. The minimum possible gain is zero; a negative-valued gain would reverse contrast.

The uniform gray along the top row of gains in Figure 13.14 shows that these gains will reduce contrast at low frequencies in a way that is largely independent of location. At higher frequencies, the gain control will act in a more spatially-localized manner, retaining contrast in the area of the sky and reducing contrast in the area of the shuttle, rocket, crane, and gantry.

The gains for the L&M-cone axis channels, shown in Figure 13.15, are similar to those for the achromatic channels, as are the gains for the S-cone axis channels, shown in Figure 13.16. The substantial amount of achromatic contrast in the space shuttle image, relative to chromatic contrast, and the strong influence of achromatic contrast on the gains on L&M-cone and S-cone axis signals, cause the gains on the color channels to be dominated by achromatic contrast.

262 13. Color Contrast Gain Control

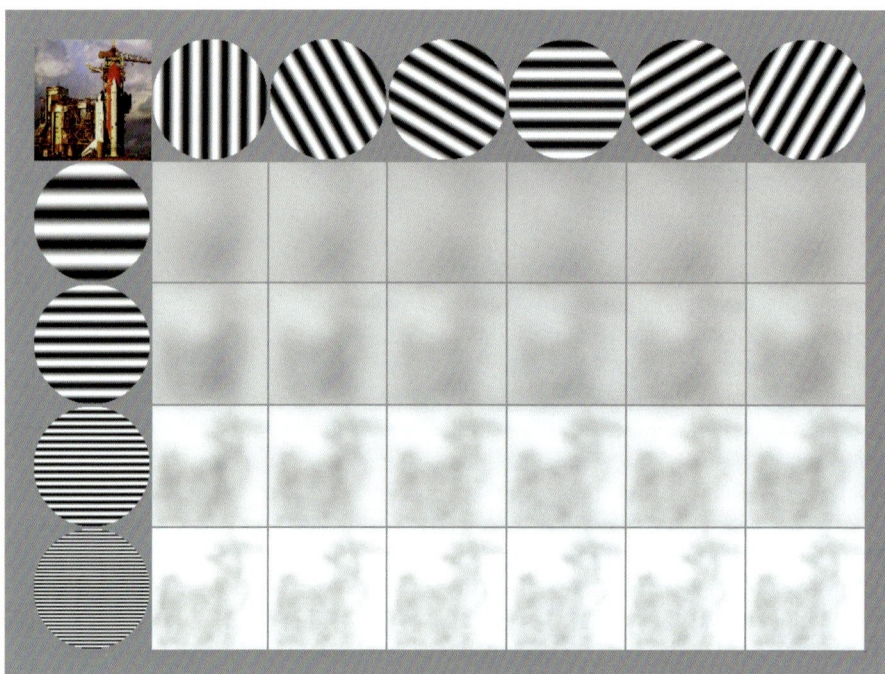

Fig. 13.14: Gains to be applied to the model's achromatic channels.

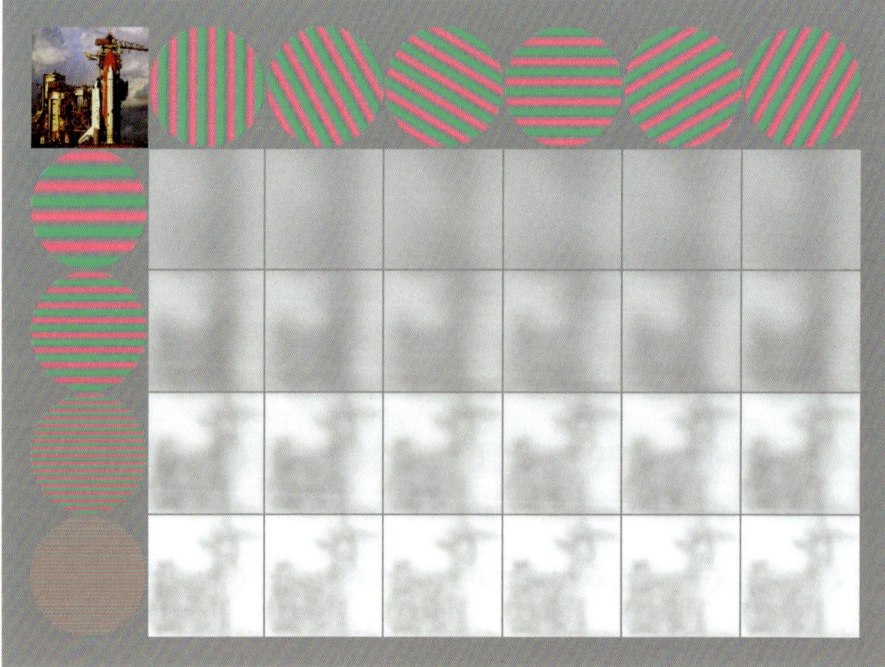

Fig. 13.15: Gains to be applied to the model's L&M-cone axis channels.

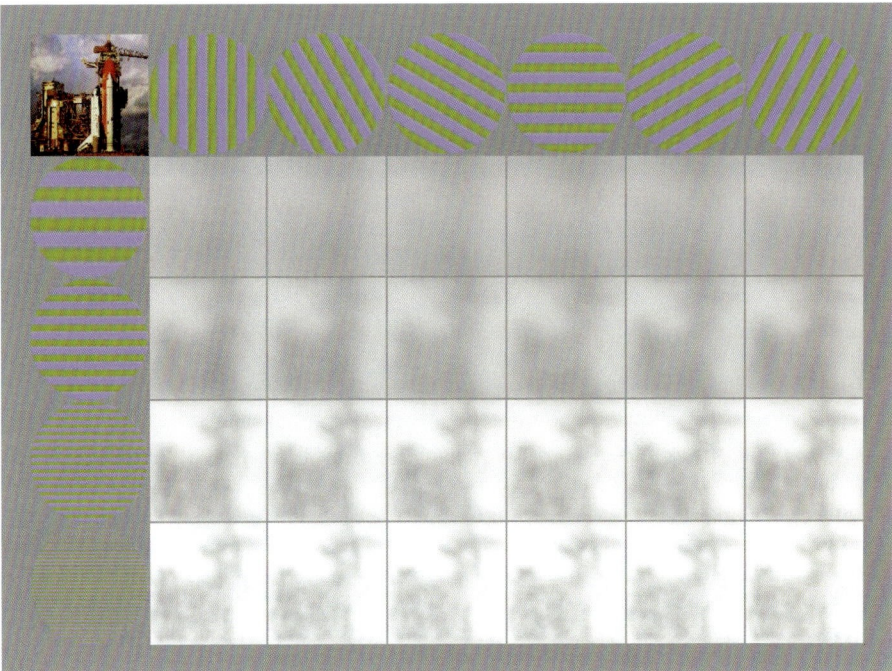

Fig. 13.16: Gains to be applied to the model's S-cone axis channels.

The gains for moderately high spatial frequency, S-cone axis channels (Fig. 13.16, next-to-bottom row) provide an example of selectivity. The crane at the top right of the space shuttle image is oriented horizontally, and it causes a reduction in gain for the horizontally-oriented channel, evident as a crane-shaped darkening, that is greater than the reduction for the vertically-oriented channel. A similar difference can be seen in Figure 13.14 for the achromatic channels and in Figure 13.15 for the L&M-cone channels. Contrast at one orientation has only half its maximum potency when determining gain at the perpendicular orientation.

13.3.5 Multichannel Contrast Gain Control

The model multiplies each channel's signal by the corresponding gain, at each picture location. One may then recombine the signals to produce an output picture. Figure 13.17 shows the model's output. At top left is the original input; immediately beside it is the output. Comparing the two pictures shows that the primary action of the contrast gain control is to turn contrast levels down. The point-by-point difference between the input image and the output image is shown immediately to the right of the output image, and this difference image shows the large change.

We can draw a more informative comparison between input and output if we match their total power levels. This procedure lets us see more clearly a result of the contrast gain control suggested by Robson (1988), which is that areas of low contrast will find their contrasts boosted relative to areas of high contrast. The power-normalized picture is shown at the top left on the right-hand side of Figure 13.17. Comparing this picture with the original input at the far left shows that the contrast of high contrast regions has been reduced substantially. The difference between the original input and the power-normalized output is shown at the right of the top row. The white of the space shuttle has been reduced, as has the red of the rocket. All other features within the image are rel-

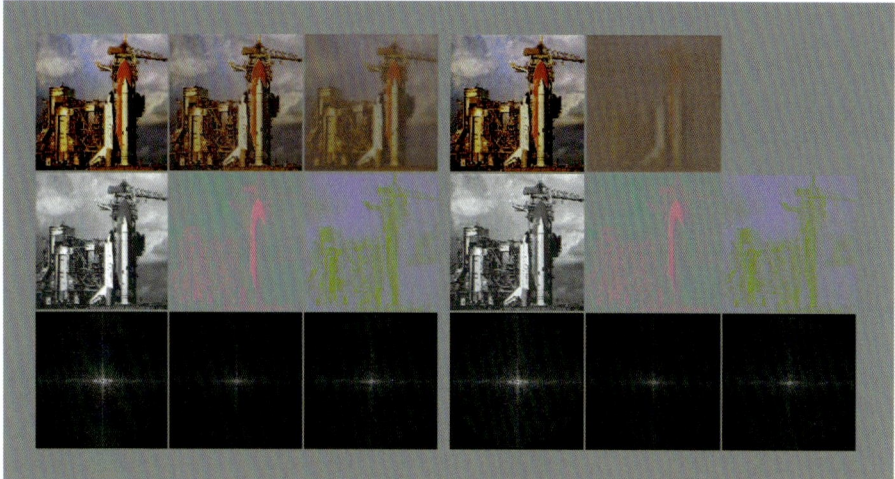

Fig. 13.17: Comparison of input (top, left, left-hand-side) and output (top, middle, left-hand-side) space shuttle images. The difference between input and output images is shown to the right of the output image (top, right, left-hand-side). The power-normalized output is shown at the top left on the right-hand-side. Immediately beside it is the difference between it and the input. The middle and bottom rows on the right-hand side show the color channel images and Fourier amplitude spectra of the power-normalized output.

atively enhanced, and it is apparent that the contrast gain control helps to equalize contrast levels across the image.

13.4 Discussion

The color contrast gain control that is presented here is simple, yet sufficiently detailed to process color images. It incorporates the results of psychophysical experiments on contrast gain control in human observers. These include findings on selectivity in spatial frequency, orientation and color and on the spatial pooling of contrast.

One element of the model's simplicity is its scale invariance. The effects of the contrast gain control on an image are roughly independent of image scale, and this is because the model works identically within all spatial frequency bands. There are several modifications that can be made to provide a model that agrees with further results on human visual processing, but that is no longer scale invariant. Such a model might prove useful in situations where images are always presented at a fixed scale to (or distance from) the visual system.

A first such modification is to eliminate the sensitivities of the L&M cone and S cone channels to signals at high spatial frequencies. The spatial frequency range of the achromatic channels is at least an octave greater than that of the two color-opponent channels (Mullen, 1985; Lennie & D'Zmura, 1988). The simplest modification would be to remove high-frequency color-opponent channels from the model.

A second modification would be to include an interaction between spatial frequency and orientation in the step where contrasts are combined linearly to produce gains. Such an interaction is suggested by the results of Solomon, Sperling and Chubb (1993), who found that orientation selectivity in contrast gain control increases as stimulus spatial frequency increases.

A third modification would be to use the pooling areas presented by Singer and me. The present model uses Gaussian functions with standard deviations that increase in proportion to spatial frequency. Our results suggest that the pooling areas are modelled better if the standard deviations increase linearly as a function of spatial frequency, not proportionately (D'Zmura and Singer, 1996). An additive constant in the relation between Gaussian standard deviation and channel spatial frequency causes the model to vary with scale, however, as do the removal of chromatic channel sensitivity to high frequencies and the inclusion of interaction in spatial-frequency and orientation selectivity.

There are other worthwhile modifications to the model that do not affect its scale invariance. Chief among these is the inclusion of saturating nonlinearities. Singer and I measured the way that the effects of contrast gain control depend on stimulus contrast and found that the effects saturate as stimulus contrast increases (Singer and D'Zmura, 1995). An important formal role of these saturating nonlinearities is to prevent gains from dropping below zero (recall that a negative gain causes an unwanted contrast reversal). Yet the present model does not include saturating nonlinearities, for the reason that natural images generally have fairly low contrast levels (Moorhead, 1985). The images that I have run through the model have never come close to giving rise to negative contrast gains.

A related modification is to use half-wave-rectified channels rather than standard second-stage channels, namely to use the six channels black, white, blue-green, red, yellow-green and purple (viz. the six halves of the achromatic, L&M cone and S cone axes). Although the model can readily be changed to accommodate such half-wave rectification, one awaits empirical evidence of independent contrast gain control – selectivity – for channel halves.

The motive for introducing half-wave rectification comes largely from the electrophysiological literature, which suggests that many cortical neurons have very low levels of maintained discharge and so cannot signal reductions in firing frequency (e.g., Lennie et al., 1990). Several pieces of evidence suggest that contrast gain control is applied by cortical neurons: (1) interocular transfer (Singer and D'Zmura, 1994); (2) orientation selectivity (Solomon et al., 1993); (3) sluggish temporal response (Singer and D'Zmura, 1994), and (4) large receptive fields (Cannon and Fullenkamp, 1991; Singer and D'Zmura, 1994; D'Zmura and Singer, 1996). Neuronal mechanisms of color contrast gain control have not yet been identified in primates, however.

13.5 Summary

I present a model for contrast gain control that is based on results from psychophysical experiments on human vision. The model pools contrast in channels that are tuned for spatial frequency, orientation and color and combines these contrasts selectively to determine channel gain. Stages in the model's processing of a color image are illustrated. The chief effect of the contrast gain control is to equalize contrast levels across space.

Acknowledgements

I thank Ben Singer, without whom this work would not have been possible. I also thank Al Ahumada and Geoff Iverson for their helpful comments. This work was supported by National Eye Institute grant EY10014 to M. D'Zmura.

References

Blakemore, C. and Campbell, F. W. (1969). On the existence of neurones in the human visual system selectively sensitive to the orientation and size of retinal images. Journal of Physiology (London) *203*, 237–260.

Cannon, M. W. and Fullenkamp, S. C. (1991). Spatial interactions in apparent contrast: inhibitory effects among grating patterns of different spatial frequencies, spatial positions and orientations. Vision Research *31*, 1985–1998.

Chubb, C., Sperling, G., and Solomon, J. A. (1989). Texture interactions determine perceived contrast. Proceedings of the National Academy of Sciences of the United States of America *86*, 9631–9635.

Derrington, A. M., Krauskopf, J., and Lennie, P. (1984). Chromatic mechanisms in lateral geniculate nucleus of macaque. Journal of Physiology (London) *357*, 241–265.

D'Zmura, M. and Singer, B. (1996). The spatial pooling of contrast in contrast gain control. Journal of the Optical Society of America A *13*, 2135–2140.

Heeger, D. J. (1992). Normalization of cell responses in cat striate cortex. Visual Neuroscience *9*, 181–197.

Hurvich, L. M. and Jameson, D. (1957). An opponent-process theory of color vision. Psychological Reviews *64*, 384–404.

Krauskopf, J., Williams, D. R., and Heeley, D. M. (1982). The cardinal directions of color space. Vision Research *22*, 1123–1131.

Kries, J. von (1905). Influence of adaptation on the effects produced by luminous stimuli. Handbuch der Physiologie des Menschen *3*, 109–282. In: D. L. MacAdam (Ed.), Sources of color vision. Cambridge, Mass.: MIT.

Lennie, P. and D'Zmura, M. (1988). Mechanisms of color vision. Critical Reviews in Neurobiology *3*, 333–400.

Lennie, P., Krauskopf, J., and Sclar, G. (1990). Chromatic mechanisms in striate cortex of macaque. Journal of Neuroscience *10*, 649–669.

MacLeod, D. I. A. and Boynton, R. M. (1979). Chromaticity diagram showing cone excitation by stimuli of equal luminance. Journal of the Optical Society of America *69*, 1183–1186.

Moorhead, I. R. (1985). Human colour vision and natural images. In: Colour in Information Technology and Information Displays, Institution of Electronic and Radio Engineers, Eds., Publication Number 61, Alderman, Ipswich, 1985, 21–35.

Mullen, K. (1985). The contrast sensitivity of human colour vision to red-green and blue-yellow chromatic gratings. Journal of Physiology (London) *359*, 381–400.

Robson, J. G. (1988). Linear and non-linear operations in the visual system. Investigative Ophthalmology and Visual Science *29*, (Supplement), 117.

Singer, B. and D'Zmura, M. (1994). Color contrast induction. Vision Research *34*, 3111–3126.

Singer, B. and D'Zmura, M. (1995). Contrast gain control: a bilinear model for chromatic selectivity. Journal of the Optical Society of America A *12*, 667–685.

Smith, V. C. and Pokorny, J. (1975). Spectral sensitivity of the foveal cone photopigments between 400 and 500 nm. Vision Research *15*, 161–171.

Solomon, J. A., Sperling, G., and Chubb, C. (1993). The lateral inhibition of perceived contrast is indifferent to on-center/off-center segregation, but specific to orientation. Vision Research *33*, 2671–2683.

Sperling, G. (1989). Three stages and two systems of visual processing. Spatial Vision *4*, 183–207.

14. Binocular Brightness Combination: A Mechanism for Combining Two Sources of Rather Similar Information

Hans Irtel

14.1 Intensity Invariance of Binocular Brightness

Our perception of the world is strongly restricted by the properties of our senses. These provide us with a rather selective view of the world where much of the potentially available information is not directly accessible. But what is accessible has been proven to be sufficient for survival, at least until now. The Ptolemaic view of the world is a nice demonstration of what is accessible by direct and unaided perception: Even if we know that the stars' distances to the earth vary greatly, they all appear to be fixed to the sky at the same distance. We are not able to discriminate their distances. So unaided perception gives us a distorted or even wrong view of the world. Nevertheless, although this is hard to quantify, it seems reasonable to say that most of our direct view of the world is correct.

For ordinary people this is an obvious fact. So obvious that, for example, it needs some really good arguments to convince new students that while perceiving generally is easy and almost effortless, studying perception and explaining perceptual phenomena is very hard. This, by the way, is a striking difference to other cognitive behavior: Playing chess for example is hard for most of us but machines have been built which do it much better than most of us will ever be able to do it. On the contrary, perceiving is easy for all of us but there is no machine which does it nearly as well as any of us.

One of the major problems with perception is that the information which is available for our senses contains a lot of noise. If we ask what is important for orientation in the world we have to concede that much of the important and accessible information is contaminated by less important information. And often information about different facts is confounded and cannot be extracted by simple means. Think about brightness or lightness perception. The light arriving in our eyes from object surfaces depends both on the reflectance properties of the surfaces and on the illumination. To recognize objects there should be a mechanism which gives us reflectance properties of the objects which are independent of illumination. However, the perceptual system should better not throw away the illumination information completely, since then it might be difficult to estimate the time of sunset which could be dangerous in a natural environment.

Problems like this are treated under the label of constancy or invariance properties of perception. These usually deal with situations where some perceptual attribute of a stimulus is invariant under certain transformations of the stimulus. A typical example is the above mentioned notion of lightness constancy under varying illumination conditions.

Lightness or perceived surface color constancy are examples for invariance properties under stimulus changes which are independent of the observer. Additional complications for the perceiving organism are created by the fact that most active behavior of the organism itself also results in certain variations of the visual stimulus. A typical example is in motion perception. Motion of the outside world and self motion of the organism are confounded in the retinal image. If the retinal image is to be used as a source of information about object motion then this confounding has to be resolved.

Before reporting an empirical analysis of some invariance properties, let me point to one common result in almost all experimental studies of constancy phenomena. All of these are invariance properties against some action or transformation in the stimulus situation. The result of the invariances are that some perceived attributes of the stimuli are constant under the respective transformation. However, I know of no case where this invariance or constancy is perfect. Very often research has concentrated on the attribute which remains nearly invariant and this usually has some obvious survival value. However, in most cases it also seems useful not to have perfect invariance. Since having perfect invariance means that the respective stimulus transformation goes unnoticed. And in most cases this would be a severe disadvantage.

The experiments to be reported here deal with binocular combination of brightness. Usually the two retinal images are rather similar. This is especially true for fused regions of the visual field and with respect to the distribution of color. For this situation one would expect that each monocular component contributes equally to the fused image. One also would expect that the brightness of a fused region of the visual field, called „binocular brightness", shows a strictly monotone dependence on the monocular stimulus intensities in this case. This is empirically confirmed.

However, the situation becomes different if the monocular stimulus components become rather different in intensity or contrast. An extreme case is the closure of one eye. We hardly notice any change in color appearance or in brightness if one eye is closed as compared to binocular viewing. Thus, the mechanism for combining the two sources of visual information works such that both components are weighted equally when the stimuli are almost equal and is dominated by a single source when this source dominates the stimulus.

The first person who investigated this problem experimentally was G. Th. Fechner in 1861 (Fechner, 1861). He looked at the sky while one of his eyes was covered with a gray filter that he could estimate the brightness of the sky for binocular viewing with one eye observing freely and the other eye getting varying amounts of light. He mostly made judgments about the change of perceived binocular brightness when closing the eye with the filter in front as compared to observation with both eyes. He found a psychophysical function which showed two special properties (Fig. 14.1):

1. The function is not monotone increasing. For zero filter transmittance the brightness corresponds to monocular viewing. Increasing the filter transmittance from zero upward first leads to a decrease in binocular brightness until a minimum is reached and only then does the brightness increase with increasing transmittance of the filter.
2. For binocular viewing without filter the brightness is approximately equal to monocular viewing, with some small advantage to binocular viewing.

The question then is how a model of the binocular fusion mechanism might look. Its general structure should contain a monocular input transformation $f(x)$ and some binocular combination rule $F(x, y)$:

$$B(x, a) = F[f(x), f(a)]$$

Questions like these are traditionally treated by goodness of fit methods. I will use a different method here which may be viewed as an experimental method to analyze the form of the psy-

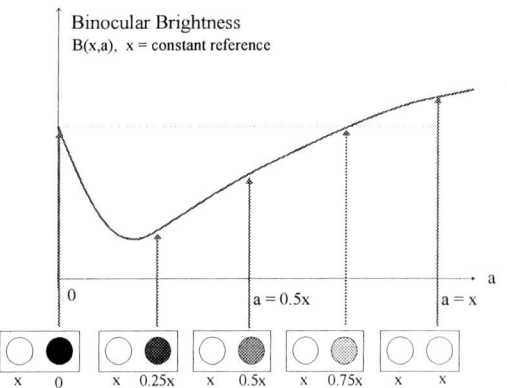

Fig. 14.1: Fechner's psychophysical function shows binocular brightness $B(x,a)$ for constant values of x and increasing filter transmittances a. Note that there is an initial decrease of binocular brightness when changing from monocular viewing to binocular viewing with one eye covered by a low transmittance filter. Monocular and binocular observation of the same stimulus results in almost the same brightness: $B(x, 0) \sim B(x, x)$.

chophysical function involved. This will allow me to experimentally test not only single models but even larger classes of models with common structural properties.

In the experiment the subject has to compare pairs of dichoptic stimuli. Each of these contains stimulus intensity components x, y, for the left and stimulus intensity components a, b, for the right eye. The stimuli are presented such that both the components x and a, and the components y and b are fused, such that we can ask the subject to compare the brightness of (x, a) and (y, b). We write $(x, a) \geq (y, b)$ iff the subject judges (x, a) to be at least as bright as (y, b). In order to analyze the structural properties of binocular fusion we can then ask what happens if we change the intensities of the stimuli involved. To derive some hypotheses about the behavior of the psychophysical function for binocular brightness we look at the following condition of *intensity invariance*: if $(x, a) \geq (y, b)$ then $(tx, ta) \geq (ty, tb)$ for all real numbers $0 < t < \infty$, where tx is the intensity x multiplied by the factor t. Fechner describes a condition which may be interpreted as intensity invariance: "… daß die Helligkeit des Himmels von keinem wesentlichen Einfluß auf die Lage des Indifferenzpunctes ist" (Fechner, 1861, p. 422).

With this condition in mind we can now look at specific points of the psychophysical function in Figure 14.1. The *equivalence point* $e(x)$ of a psychophysical function for binocular brightness is defined by $(e(x), 0) \sim (x, x)$. It is that stimulus $e(x)$ which, when viewed monocularly, looks equal to x viewed binocularly, and the *minimal point* $m(x)$ is that stimulus which, when combined with x, results in the lowest possible brightness: $(x, m(x)) \geq (x, a)$ for all a. If we combine these definitions with the intensity invariance condition we get the following two functional equations for $e(x)$ and $m(x)$:

$$e(tx) = t\, e(x),$$

$$m(tx) = t\, m(x).$$

The solutions to these functional equations are unique and rather simple (Aczél, 1966). Both functions $e(x)$ and $m(x)$ have to be linear functions of the reference intensity:

$$e(tx) = \beta\, e(x),$$

$$m(tx) = \gamma\, m(x)$$

for some non-negative real valued β and γ. The equivalence point and the minimum point thus have to move upwards in a linear fashion for increasing reference intensities (Irtel, 1991).

The previously derived behavior of the equivalence and the minimum point describe characteristic points of the psychophysical function for binocular brightness. They capture the non-monotone behavior of this function and thus actually describe their most interesting points, namely those points which are most different from the usual psychophysical functions found in psychology. These points also are those points which should be investigated experimentally. This is usually not done if data are collected for fitting some equation to them. For example, consider the data collected by de Weert and Levelt (1974). A closer look at their data set shows that they actually looked at a set of psychophysical functions at various levels of intensity for the reference stimulus. However, in their data the minimum point is constant at 10 cd/m^2 simply because they did not collect any other data between 0 and 20 cd/m^2. Such a set of data actually is not very useful for testing any model of binocular brightness fusion because the most critical part of the binocular brightness function is not tested empirically. De Weert and Levelt's model does have the intensitiy invariance condition formulated above as a necessary consequence.

Since none of the published sets of data on binocular brightness combination allows for testing the intensity invariance condition an experiment was run to explicitly test how the equivalence point and the minimum point change under varying reference intensity levels.

14.2 Methods

The experimental setup is described in full detail by Irtel (1991). It was run on a precisely calibrated monitor (BARCO CDCT 51/3) controlled by a PC with a Matrox PIP 1024 graphics controller board providing for 8 bit resolution or 256 steps per color channel. Calibration was done by an LMT 1000 photometer with high accuracy $V(\lambda)$ sensitivity function. The subject viewed the screen through a mirror haploscope such that the left part of the screen was visible for the left and the right part of the screen for the right eye only. A chinrest was used for head fixation. The display and the haploscope were adjusted for optimal fusion of the dichoptic stimuli.

The display background was black and during adaptation there was a bright 120 cd/m² ellipsoid adaptation field extending 6° vertically and 4° horizontally with a small dark fixation mark. The stimuli were bright half disks of 0.5° radius on a dark background positioned above and below the fixation mark with a 0.5° gap between the upper and the lower dichoptic stimulus. Each of the two dichoptic stimuli had a left eye and a right eye component which were fused and appeared as a single half disk for the subject. Stimulus display duration was 1.2 s and there was an adaptation period of 6 s between trials. The task was to compare the upper and the lower half disk with respect to brightness.

The first part of the experiment was used to find that stimulus component $e(x)$ which, when presented together with a zero right-eye component, appeared equal to the stimulus (x, x). x was set to 3, 6, 12, 24, 48 and 96 cd/m². The value of $e(x)$ was found by an adaptive 1-up-1-down procedure limited to 20 trials. Starting values were optimized according to preliminary data. Results were computed from the turning points only. The second part of the experiment was used to find the minimum points $m(x)$ for each of the above listed reference values x between 3 and 96 cd/m². This was done by presenting stimuli of the form (x, y) and $(x, y + \delta)$, where δ was a small luminance increment. An adaptive procedure was set up such that y was increased whenever (x, y) was chosen to be brighter than $(x, y + \delta)$ and vice versa. The increment δ was chosen according to preliminary data. The adaptive procedures were stopped after 8 turning points and the results were computed from these.

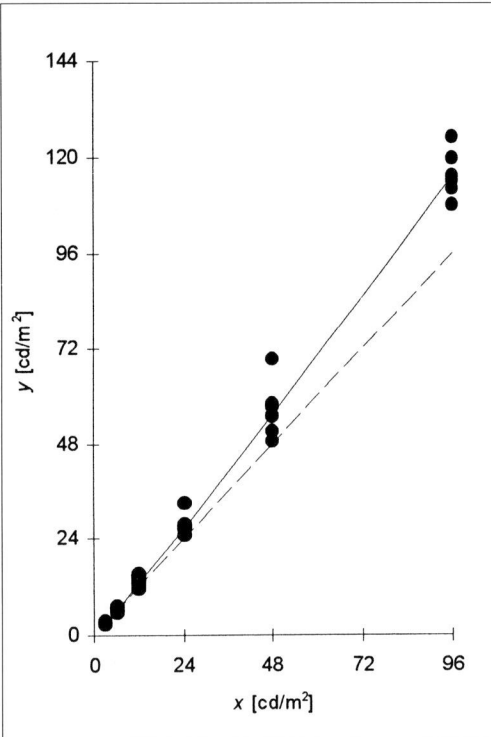

Fig. 14.2: Comparison of dichoptic stimuli of the form (x, x) which have the same binocular brightness as stimuli of the form $(y, 0)$. The data are from 3 subjects with 2 measurements for each value of x (one data point at $x = 96$ cd/m² is missing). The dashed line represents $y = x$ There is an almost constant binocular advantage of 20%. The solid line shows the predictions of the model.

14.3 Results

The results for $e(x)$ and $m(x)$ are shown in Figures 14.2 and 14.3. Figure 14.2 shows results of a comparison of stimuli of the form (x, x) and $(y, 0)$ where the first component is presented to the left eye and the second component is presented to the right eye only. It is clear that for all intensities the single-component stimulus $(y, 0)$ needs a little more intensity than the two-component stimulus (x, x). In general the factor is around 1.2 such that monocular stimuli need about 20% more intensity in order to appear equal in brightness to binocular stimuli.

The results for the minimal point are shown in Figure 14.3. Intensity invariance requires that the

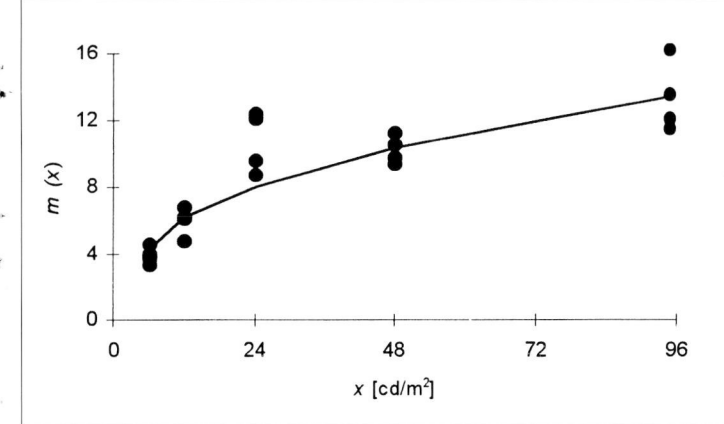

Fig. 14.3: Minimal stimuli $m(x)$ as they depend on the reference intensity x. Intensity invariance requires that $m(x)$ is linear in x. Clearly the data of 4 subjects show a strong deviation from linearity. The solid line represents predictions from the model.

minimum points increase linearly with reference intensity. This clearly is not the case. The values of $m(x)$ increase much more slowly as expected.

14.4 Discussion

Although the data of Figure 14.2 for the equivalence points indicate a linear relation between monocularly and binocularly-viewed stimuli of equal binocular brightness, the results in Figure 14.3 clearly refute intensity invariance. The minimum point of the psychophysical function for binocular brightness grows much more slowly than would be expected from intensity invariance. This refutes all models of binocular brightness which allow for a separation between the intensity dependent factor t and the fusional process $B(x, a)$:

$$B(tx, ta) = G_t[B(x, a)]$$

Thus, the fusion process $B(x, a)$ itself depends on the intensity factor t. This actually rejects almost all models of binocular brightness combination which have been suggested, including that of de Weert and Levelt (1974) and that of Curtis and Rule (1978). Both have intensity invariance as a necessary condition. The major reason that these models fail is that they assume a power function as a monocular input transformation. Note that power functions are intensity invariant: For $f(x) = x^\alpha$ we get $f(tx) = t^\alpha f(x)$ and thus the effect of t can be separated from the function itself, we have $f(tx) = G_t[f(x)]$. This also holds for a reasonable choice of binocular fusion functions $F(x, y)$ (Aczél, 1966).

An input transformation which does not have this property is the logarithmic function. MacLeod (1972) has already suggested this function as an input transformation for binocular brightness. A model for binocular fusion of color has been suggested by Schrödinger (1926) and both de Weert and Levelt's (1974) and MacLeod's (1972) models are derived from it. He suggested that each monocular component has to be weighted by a function which gives the relative intensity of each input signal. Thus Schrödinger's weight function is

$$w(x, a) = \frac{f(x)}{f(x) + f(a)}$$

where $f(x)$ is the monocular input. Note, however, that using this weight function alone is also ruled out by our data since it suggests that $w(x, 0) = 2w(x, x)$ and thus binocular and monocular observation of the same stimulus should result in the same brightness. We thus suggest a model with the following properties:

1. The monocular input transformation is a logarithmic function with an adaptation-dependent threshold parameter x_0.
2. Binocular fusion is a mixture of monocular inputs with weights that depend on relative signal strengths as suggested by Schrödinger (1926).

3. The intensity-dependent weights have a compression parameter k, such that they do not add up to 1. If this parameter is less than 1 then there is a slight advantage for dichoptic stimuli with similar intensities as compared to stimuli with strongly different intensities in both eyes.
4. There also is an eye dominance factor, δ, for giving different weights to the stimuli in the two eyes.

We thus have the following model:

$$f(x) = \begin{cases} \phi_0 + \log(x/x_0) & \text{if } x > x_0 \\ \phi_0 + & \text{if } x \leq x_0 \end{cases}$$

$$w(x, a) = \frac{f(x)}{f(x) + f(a)}$$

$$B(x, a) = \delta\, w(x, a)^k f(x) + \frac{1}{\delta}[1 - w(x, a)]^k f(a)$$

Here x_0 is the adaptation-dependent threshold parameter. Its value has been found to be between 0.03 and 12.0 cd/m², depending on adaptation stimulus level. k determines the binocular advantage for equal components in both eyes, its value is around $k = 0.92$, and δ describes individual eye dominance and should be constant for a single subject.

The solid lines in Figures 14.2 and 14.3 show the predictions of the model for the data of the experiment. The parameter δ was set equal to 1 for these data since no comparison was possible between the two eyes in this experiment. Using the data of all subjects and all tasks, k was estimated as $k = 0.919$ and x_0 was estimated as $x_0 = 4.2$ cd/m²

by least-squares minimization. Figure 14.4 contains a comparison of the data and the model's prediction for an experiment published by Irtel (1986). The major difference from the present study was that subjects were dark adapted in this case. This results in an estimate of $x_0 = 0.034$ cd/m² for the threshold value while k stays almost constant at 0.95.

Fechner had called his experiment „Paradoxer Versuch" because it showed that a stimulus can look brighter even if less light enters the eyes. In my view the non-monotone psychophysical function is a consequence of two simple invariance properties:

1. Monocular and binocular viewing results in almost the same brightness.
2. For fused dichoptic stimuli with rather similar components there is a monotone relation between stimulus luminance or contrast and brightness.

As a consequence of these two conditions one gets the non-monotone psychophysical function of binocular brightness. The function in Fig. 14.1 has to have approximately the same ordinate value $B(x, a)$ for $a = 0$ and for $a = x$ and it has to be monotone increasing at $a = x$. This implies that there is a local minimum between $a = 0$ and $a = x$.

Thus it seems that a major reason for Fechner's paradox is our ability to independently close each single eye. Since the mechanism described ensures that the world's brightness does not change significantly if we close one of the two eyes. If this is true then, contrary to the claim of Lehky (1983),

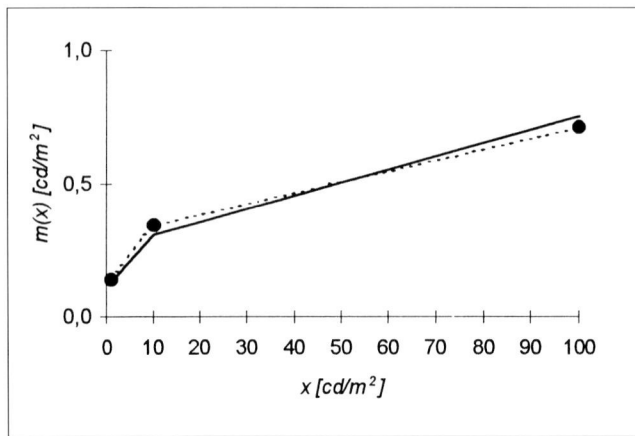

Fig. 14.4: Minimal stimuli from an experiment where the subject was dark-adapted (Irtel, 1986). Increase of minimal stimuli also is not linear. Data are connected by dotted lines, predicted points are connected by solid lines. Parameter estimation for the model results in $x_0 = 0.034$ and $k = 0.95$.

we should not have a similar non-monotone effect in binaural loudness combination, since there is no need for it there. Hübner (1991) looked for Fechner's paradox in binaural loudness combination, but could not find it. This supports the idea that Fechner's paradox is a result of approximate binocular brightness constancy under change of viewing condition.

14.5 Summary

In most natural situations binocular fusion of brightness combines two rather similar intensity components. Binocular brightness is monotone in both components for these situations. Closing one eye completely, however, leaves brightness almost invariant. A general intensity invariant fusion mechanism for brightness is proposed and qualitative conditions for its psychophysical function are derived and tested empirically. The model combines a Fechnerian, logarithmic monocular input transformation with an intensity dependent binocular mixture, where the monocular weights depend on relative intensity of the monocular inputs. It contains an adaption dependent monocular treshold parameter and an adaption independent compression of the binocular fusion weights resulting in a slightly higher efficiency of binocularly balanced stimuli as compared to monocular observation.

References

Aczél, J. (1966). Lectures on functional equations and their applications. New York: Academic Press.

Curtis, D. W. and Rule, S. J. (1978). Binocular processing of brightness information: A vector-sum model. Journal of Experimental Psychology: Human Perception and Performance 4, 132–143.

Fechner, G. T. (1861). "Uber einige Verhältnisse des binocularen Sehens". Abhandlungen der mathematisch-physikischen Classe der königlich sächsischen Gesellschaft der Wissenschaften 5, 337–564.

Hübner, R. (1991). Is there an auditory analogue to Fechner's paradox in binaural loudness perception? Archiv für Psychologie 142, 157–165.

Irtel, H. (1986). Experimente zu Fechners Paradoxon der binokularen Helligkeit. Zeitschrift für experimentelle und angewandte Psychologie 33, 413–422.

Irtel, H. (1991). Psychophysische Invarianzen in der Farb- und Helligkeitswahrnehmung. Heidelberg: Springer-Verlag.

Lehky, S. R. (1983). A model of binocular brightness and binaural loudness perception in humans with general application to nonlinear summation of sensory inputs. Biological Cybernetics 49, 89–97.

MacLeod, D. I. A. (1972). The Schrödinger equation in binocular brightness combination. Perception 1, 321–324.

Schrödinger, E. (1926). Die Gesichtsempfindungen. In Müller-Pouillets Lehrbuch der Physik. 11. Auflage, zweiter Band. Braunschweig: Vieweg.

de Weert, C. M. M. and Levelt, W. J. M. (1974). Binocular brightness combinations: additive and nonadditive aspects. Perception & Psychophysics 15, 551–562.

15. Inferences about Infant Color Vision

Kenneth Knoblauch, Michelle L. Bieber and John S. Werner

15.1 Introduction

Many early studies of infant color vision were aimed principally at elucidating the first level of visual processing (Peeples and Teller, 1975; Teller et al., 1978; Hamer et al., 1982; Packer et al., 1984; Varner et al., 1985; Volbrecht and Werner, 1987; Pulos et al., 1980; Powers et al., 1981; Werner, 1982). These studies were directed at such issues as how early can infants respond differentially to lights on the basis of wavelength differences, what is the dimension of infant color space and what photoreceptor classes mediate their responses. The evidence from these initial studies has been taken to indicate that all three cone classes and rods are functional by 8–12 weeks. In this age range, infants begin to respond differentially to pairs of monochromatic lights in the Rayleigh region of the spectrum and also to pairs that fall along tritan confusion lines. Thus, one finds statements in the literature to the effect that all three cone classes have been demonstrated to be functioning at these ages or earlier (Banks and Bennett, 1988; Morrone et al., 1993) and attention has turned to questions aimed at successive levels of visual processing. A goal of this paper will be to demonstrate that the evidence in these early studies is not conclusive on the functional status of all of the cone classes. Since three classes of functioning cones are a prerequisite to normal color vision, this evidence raises questions about the interpretation of studies on infant post-receptoral processes, as well.

15.2 Inferences from Luminosity

It has frequently been noted that estimates of infant luminosity tend to be similar to those from adults. Indeed, the spectral sensitivity for minimum heterochromatic flicker using a visual-evoked potential (VEP) response measure is well fit by the adult curve except at short wavelengths where differences are expected on the basis of age differences in pre-retinal screening factors (Bieber et al., 1995). Since the adult flicker-based luminosity curve is thought to be mediated by only middle (M) and long (L) wavelength sensitive cones (Lee et al., 1988; Eisner and MacLeod, 1980), one might think that these results support the functional presence of both M- and L-cones. This argument is valid for the L-cones, since the long wavelength limb of the flicker sensitivity curve is limited primarily by this cone class. Their absence would certainly be evident as a long wavelength luminosity loss, just as in protanopic observers. But what of the M-cones? It has often been remarked that the contribution of the M-cones to the luminosity curve is not well defined (Pitt, 1935; Hurvich, 1972; Cicerone and Nerger, 1989; Billock, 1995).

From another point of view, the similarity of infant and adult luminosity matches is surprising. On anatomical grounds, differences would be expected between infant and adult spectral sensitivities. The outer segments of foveal cones in the newborn are about forty times shorter than those in an adult (Abramov et al., 1982) If photon absorption in cones is assumed to follow the Beer-Lambert Law (Wyszecki and Stiles, 1982), then the short pathlengths of infant cones would mean that the photopigments are present in low optical density and would indicate that there is no self-screening of the visual pigment in infant eyes. The consequences of this for infant spectral sensitivity for each class of cones are illustrated in the top three panels of Figure 15.1. In each panel, the Stockman fundamentals (Stockman et al., 1993) are shown as solid lines for the L-, M- and S-cones (left to right). The dashed lines show the limiting form of the spectral sensitivity as the optical density is reduced. These calculations were performed with the assumption that the adult curves represented a density of 0.4. In addition, the lens and macular pigment absorption were reduced in accordance with estimates of their densities in infant eyes (Werner, 1982; Bone et al., 1988).

The influence of reduced photopigment optical density is evident in the narrowing of each curve on the long wavelength side. The effect of reduced pre-retinal screening is evident in the higher sensitivities in the short wavelength portion of the spectrum. The adult luminosity curve is well predicted by the formula, 0.68273 L + 0.35235 M (Stockman et al., 1993), which is shown as a solid curve

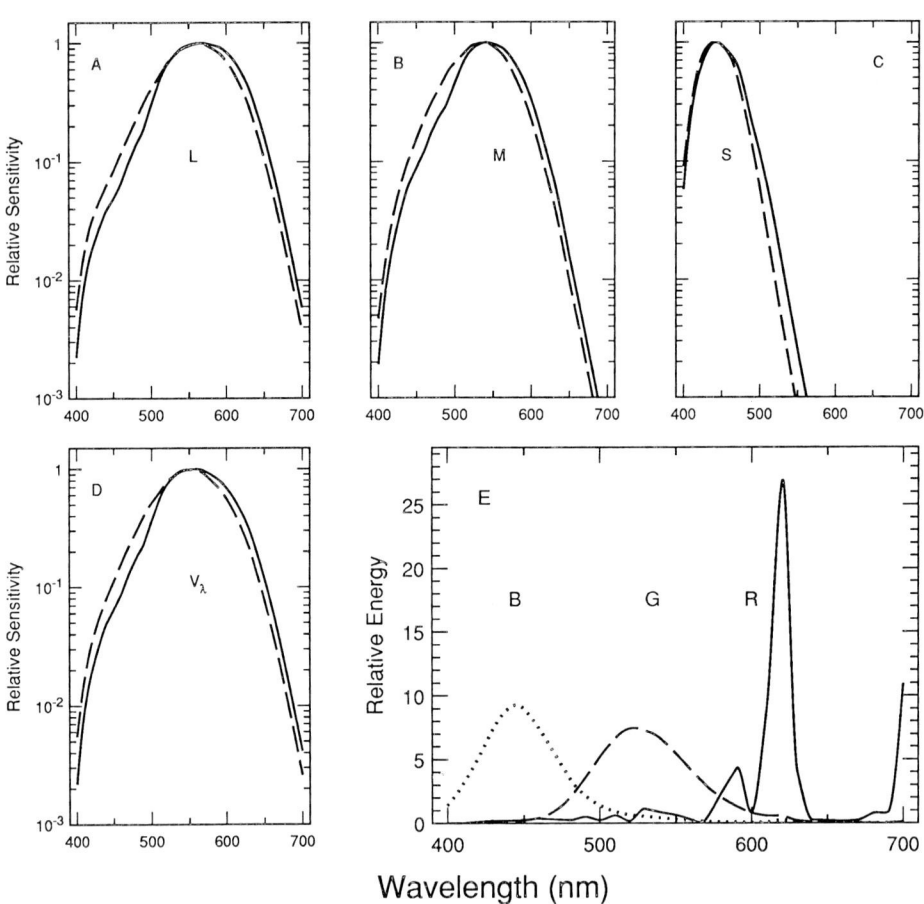

Fig. 15.1: Stockman L-cone, M-cone and S-cone fundamentals (A, B and C, respectively) for adult observer (solid) and as calculated for an infant observer (dashed) with reduced optical density and reduced lens and macular pigment screening. D. Adult (solid) and infant (dashed) luminosity functions calculated from the weighted sum, respectively, of adult and infant M- and L-cone fundamentals. E. Relative spectral energy distributions of B, G and R primaries measured from an Electrohome color display.

in the bottom left panel of Figure 15.1. Assuming low density photopigments but the same contribution of each cone class to luminosity judgments, the prediction for an infant luminosity curve is shown in the same panel as a dashed curve. The expected differences are systematic but small throughout the long wavelength portion. Nevertheless, the consequences for luminosity equations are interesting.

Consider the three curves in the bottom right panel of Figure 15.1. These are the spectral distributions of energy measured for each of the three guns, R, G and B, on an Electrohome color display. Such display systems are seeing increasing use in infant studies of color vision as they have been in vision studies in general for several years now. The curves are typical of those found on nearly all commercially available CRT-type displays. Several recent studies have investigated the responses of infants to mixtures of the G and R guns to investigate the development of sensitivity to luminance and red-green chromatic processes. Note that the G gun has a spectral distribution that extends outside of the Rayleigh region so it would be expected to stimulate S cones and rods, although this aspect is rarely emphasized (though see Dale et al., 1993).

In several studies, the G and R guns have been flickered in counterphase and the ratio of their luminances has been varied systematically to evaluate whether infants display a minimum response at a ratio that might correspond to a luminance match. The scale used is often like the one shown in Figure 15.2, in which the proportion of luminance in the R gun of the stimulus is plotted. For an observer with the adult luminosity function, the equiluminant point would fall at a value of 0.5. Arrows below the scale indicate the luminance ratios that would correspond to matches for M-cones (0.679), L-cones (0.436) and rods (0.835). An observer who only had functioning L-cones in his retina would find that the G and R primaries matched at a ratio that differs from a normal luminance match by about 15%.

We recomputed some of these matches for the infant spectral sensitivities shown in Figure 15.1 and expressed them in terms of the adult luminance scale. The values that we obtained are shown by the arrows above the scale for M-cones (0.735), L-cones (0.496) and a luminance match (0.563). The spectral sensitivities in the infant retina are all foreshortened on the long wavelength side, from which it follows that they require more of the R gun luminance for each of the predicted matches. The shift is such that the L-cone equation for an infant becomes indistinguishable from an adult luminance equation and the infant luminance equation differs from the adult by about 12%. These differences are small and would probably be difficult to detect experimentally. Nevertheless, it seems reasonable to claim that the similarity of infant luminance matches to those of an adult provides no basis for making any inferences on the status of M-cones in the infant retina.

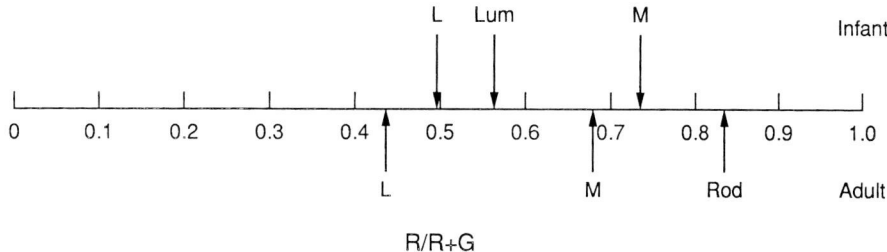

Fig. 15.2: Scale indicating the proportion of luminance of the R gun as a function of the sum of the luminances of the G and R guns. The arrows below the scale show the values at which the G and R guns would be equated for their excitation of M-cones, L-cones and rods. The arrows above the axis indicate the M-cone, L-cone and luminance matches predicted for an infant observer, but expressed in adult luminance units.

15.3 Inferences from Silent Substitution

Another line of evidence on the status of infant color vision mechanisms comes from the silent-substitution technique (Estévez and Spekreijse, 1982; Estévez et al., 1975). With this technique, stimuli are chosen to be equated for all but one of the underlying mechanisms. If there is a residual response, then it is taken as evidence that the mechanism for which the lights were not equated is functional. Care must be taken, however, that this is the only mechanism for which the lights have not been equated. A case in point is shown in Figure 15.3. The solid curve describes the type of response or sensitivity curve one might expect to counterphase flicker of the G and R primaries from Figure 15.1 for a series of luminance ratios, if an observer had only the adult luminance sensitivity or, as we have just shown, the L-cone sensitivity predicted from a newborn infant. By about eight weeks of age, most infants fail to show a null at any luminance ratio (Hamer et al., 1982; Morrone et al., 1993; Dale et al., 1993). It is argued that by this age the chromatic mechanism that differences M- and L-cone signals has begun to function and produces the residual response at equiluminance.

Consider, however, an alternate possibility. Infants are typically tested with large fields to ensure that the stimulus is sufficiently salient to attract their attention. In addition, most instrumentation used to test infants does not permit a high luminance level. Finally, fixation simply cannot be controlled to the same level of precision in infants as in adults. The first and third factors favor a contribution from the peripheral retina to infant responses. All three factors favor the contribution of rods. Under appropriate conditions, rod responses have not been difficult to demonstrate in infants (Powers et al., 1981; Werner, 1982; Brown, 1990; Hansen and Fulton, 1995; Knoblauch et al., 1996). The rod contrast of the G and R primaries is 0.671 at the adult equiluminance point. The dashed curve in Figure 15.3 shows how a rod response to equiluminant modulation could be indistinguishable from a chromatic response.

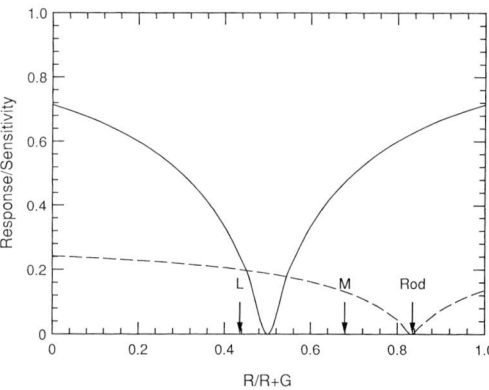

Fig. 15.3: A schematic representation of the form of response function (solid curve) one might obtain from flickering various ratios of the G and R primaries of a color display if the response was based only on the adult luminosity function. The arrows indicate the null points expected from adult M-cone, L-cone and rod spectral sensitivities. The dashed curve indicates a response function with a null consistent with a rod spectral sensitivity and illustrates how the rods could respond well at the adult equiluminance point.

15.4 Inferences about Rod Intrusion

To evaluate the possibility that rods contribute to VEP's generated by large field flicker in the Rayleigh region, we tested an adult protanope (Knoblauch et al., 1996). The stimulus consisted of a 550 nm circular field (6 deg) that was alternated in square-wave counterphase with a 590 nm light at 7.5 Hz. The ratio of the two lights was adjusted so that the modulation produced silent substitution for the M-cones. In a given trial, the mean luminance of the flickering field was smoothly increased over a 30 sec period while the fundamental frequency of the VEP signal was extracted in real time with a vector voltmeter. Given that the observer was a protanope, we expected no residual response from L-cones. The solid curve in Figure 15.4 shows the variation in VEP amplitude that we measured as a function of the mean luminance of the field. This stimulus produces a contrast of 0.57 in the rods and 0.33 in the L-cones. We suspected that the residual response was due to rods because the subject reported a strong sensation of flicker in peripheral vision probably from scattered light in his eye. Another possibility is that the observer has anomalous L-cones in his peripheral retina (Breton and Cowan, 1981) that generate a residual response to an M-cone equated modulation.

Additional evidence that this residual response is due to rods comes from the experiments in which we attempted to control for the rod modulation. Note that a flickering pair of lights permits only a single degree of freedom in the setting, the ratio of the lights, so that the lights can be equated for only one class of photoreceptors at a time. To establish a silent-substitution condition for two classes of photoreceptors simultaneously requires the introduction of an additional degree of freedom in the stimulus. To achieve this end, we flickered a 570 nm light against a mixture of 540 and 610 nm. This stimulus allows two degrees of freedom, for example, the intensity of the 570 nm light and the ratio of the 540 to the 610 nm light in the mixture. Similar to a Rayleigh equation, the lights can be adjusted to be equated for two classes of photoreceptors simultaneously. We adjusted the lights to

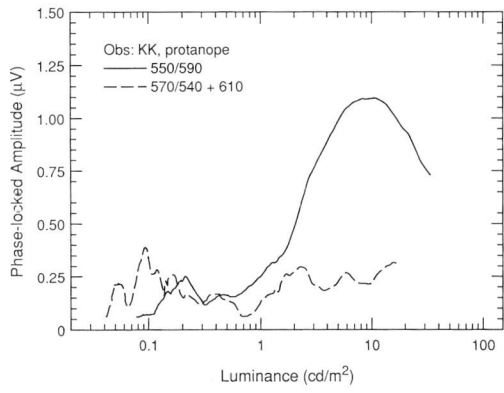

Fig. 15.4: VEP amplitude (in microvolts) at the fundamental frequency (7.5 Hz) measured from an adult protanope as a function of the mean luminance of counterphase square-wave flicker between 550 and 590 nm lights (solid) that have been equated for M-cone excitation and between 570 nm and a mixture of 540 and 610 nm lights (dashed) that have been equated for M-cone and rod excitation.

the calculated equations for M-cones and rods. The VEP response to this stimulus from the protanope is shown as the dashed curve in Figure 15.4. Now the amplitude of the fundamental remains relatively flat as the mean luminance is increased and the observer reported that the peripheral flicker was absent. This stimulus would generate a contrast of 0.37 in L-cones, if they were present, and probably somewhat less in anomalous L-cones. Thus, when the stimulus is equated for rod and M-cone excitation, no residual response remains.

15.5 Inferences about M- and L-Cones

This stimulus can also be adjusted to yield a constant response from rods and L-cones to isolate an M-cone response or from M- and L-cones to isolate a rod response. In principle, modifications of the intensities used should be necessary to isolate infant photoreceptor responses to take into account the differences in their spectral sensitivities as shown in Figure 15.1. In practice, however, we have found that such adjustments are small compared to the noise in the VEP signal and can be ignored (Knoblauch et al., 1996).

We have used these stimuli to evaluate whether or not infants respond to M- and L-cone isolating stimuli and if so, at what ages these responses can be detected (Knoblauch et al., 1994; Werner et al., 1995). Figure 15.5 shows the VEP amplitudes measured from infants at four and eight weeks. At eight weeks, there is a clear response to each of the stimuli that is qualitatively similar to the type of response that we have measured from adult observers, suggesting that both classes of cones are functioning. At four weeks, however, the responses are considerably reduced (note the difference in vertical scales). In fact, the responses are no greater than those that we find in adult dichromats to the isolating stimulus for the class of cones that they are lacking. Does this mean that M- and L-cones are not yet functioning at four weeks?

We also measured the responses to luminance modulation of the 570 nm light in each infant. We find that the responses to pure luminance modulation are also depressed at this age. If we normalize the VEP amplitudes by the mean amplitude measured for the luminance condition, in fact, the responses at four and eight weeks appear quite similar. The normalized responses of the adult dichromats remain depressed, however. In effect, the difference between these two ages can be accounted for by an overall reduction in the size of the signals generated.

While the results presented thus far support the hypothesis that M- and L-cones are functional as early as four weeks, they do not provide unequivocal evidence for this. As was mentioned above, there is reason to expect that the infant cone photoreceptor sensitivities differ systematically from those of an adult. If the isolation conditions that we calculated from adult standard curves were not adequately equated for infant cone sensitivities, then our conclusion based on the data presented above, that M- and L-cones are functional in early infancy, would not be valid. A more direct test for the presence of functional M- and L-cones in early infancy is to measure the action spectra of the isolated mechanisms. For example, the action spectra measured under L-cone isolation should correspond to the L-cone fundamental and that measured under M-cone isolation should correspond to the M-cone fundamental.

The procedure that we used to determine the action spectra of the isolated mechanisms consisted of estimating how much background light as a function of wavelength needs to be added to the receptor-isolating stimulus in order to reduce the VEP response by a criterion voltage (Bieber et al., 1996). VEP-derived action spectra so obtained from five infants (8-12 weeks) and two adults in response to both the M-cone and L-cone isolating stimuli are in reasonable agreement with the Smith and Pokorny M- and L-cone fundamentals (Smith and Pokorny, 1975). Over the range tested, these curves do not differ importantly from the Stockman fundamentals used in Figure 15.1. These results provide definitive evidence for the efficacy of our isolation conditions, and thus for the functioning of M- and L-cones as early as eight weeks. In addition, the similarity of responses found at four and eight weeks suggests that both M- and L-cones are functional as early as four weeks, though the signals appear to be of lower amplitude. These results then taken together with earlier studies that conclusively identified rod (Powers et al., 1981; Werner, 1982) and S-cone responses (Volbrecht and Werner, 1987), verify that all photoreceptor classes of the adult human retina are functioning early, perhaps within a month after birth.

The stimuli that we have developed should be useful for further explorations of infant responses

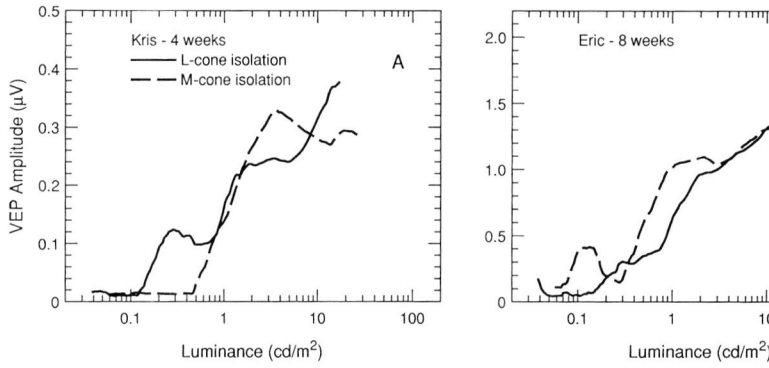

Fig. 15.5: **A.** VEP amplitude (in microvolts) at the fundamental frequency (7.5 Hz) measured from a four week old infant and **B.** an eight week old infant as a function of the mean luminance of counterphase square-wave flicker between 570 nm and a mixture of 540 and 610 nm lights that have been adjusted to isolate L-cones (solid) or M-cones (dashed). Note the difference in scaling of the ordinates between the two ages

to wavelength differences. For example, the combinations of the M- and L-cone isolating stimuli lie in a constant rod plane in the color mixture space defined by the three primary lights that we used. The demonstration of a VEP response to all such combinations would indicate that the infants can respond to chromatic differences independently of the rod response and would strengthen evidence for post-receptoral processing. The M- and L-cone isolating stimuli do not lie in an equiluminant plane, so these directions in color space are not appropriate for making inferences about chromatic responses. The responses to these stimuli could be mediated through a luminance sensitive channel. Evidence for both chromatic and luminance processing might also be obtained by varying the temporal frequency of the stimulus. In addition, it would be interesting to use these rod-equated stimuli in a behavioral paradigm, such as preferential looking, to evaluate whether infants show evidence of being able to detect modulations of these stimuli as early as the VEP responses can be detected. Finally, the rod-isolating condition, which we did not explore in this paper, should be useful for exploring the development of rod function in infants in a fashion that minimizes the contribution of cone responses.

15.6 Summary

The presence of functioning M- and L-cones in infants has sometimes been inferred from the similarity of adult and infant luminosity functions or from the presence of a residual response at equiluminance between lights that stimulate primarily the M- and L-cones. We demonstrate that neither of these criteria provide strong evidence for the functioning of M-cones in newborns. To separate the responses of M- and L-cones, we measured visual-evoked potentials and used a double silent-substitution technique to hold constant the output of one cone class and the rods. Infants at four and eight weeks are shown to respond similarly to M-cone and L-cone isolating stimuli though the amplitudes of response at four weeks are about one-fifth of those at eight weeks. Taken together with previous studies identifying S-cone and rod responses in infants, our data complete the demonstration of all cone classes in the infant retina by four weeks.

References

Abramov, I., Gordon, J., Hendrickson, A., Hainline, L., Dobson, V., and La Boissiere, E. (1982). The retina of the newborn human infant. Science *217*, 265–267.

Banks, M. S. and Bennett, P. J. (1988). Optical and photoreceptor immaturities limit the spatial and chromatic vision of human neonates. Journal of the Optical Society of America A *5*, 2059–2079.

Bieber, M. L., Knoblauch, K., and Werner, J. S. (1996). Action spectra of M- and L-cone isolated responses in early infancy. Investigative Ophthalmology and Visual Science (Suppl.) *37*, 157.

Bieber, M. L., Volbrecht, V. J., and Werner, J. S. (1995). Spectral efficiency measured by heterochromatic flicker photometry is similar in human infants and adults. Vision Research *35*, 1385–1392.

Billock, V. (1995). The spectral sensitivity of the acuity criterion: Effect of non-linear summation of isolated parvocellular receptive field centers. In: Colour Vision Deficiencies XII, B. Drum, ed. (Dordrecht, Kluwer), pp. 259–265.

Bone, R. A., Landrum, J. T., Fernandez, L., and Tarsis, S. L. (1988). Analysis of the macular pigment by HPLC: Retinal distribution and age study. Investigative Ophthalmology and Visual Science *29*, 843–849.

Breton, M. and Cowan, W. B. (1981). Deuteranomalous color matching in the deuteranopic eye. Journal of the Optical Society of America *71*, 1220–1223.

Brown, A. M. (1990). Development of visual sensitivity to light and color vision in human infants: A critical review. Vision Research *30*, 47–58.

Cicerone, C. M. and Nerger, J. L. (1989). The relative number of long-wavelength sensitive to middle-wavelength sensitive cones in the human fovea. Vision Research *29*, 115–128.

Dale, A., Banks, M. S., and Norcia, A. M. (1993). Does chromatic sensitivity develop more slowly than luminance sensitivity? Vision Research *33*, 2553–2562.

Eisner, A. and MacLeod, D. I. A. (1980). Journal of the Optical Society of America *70*, 121–123.

Estévez, O. and Spekreijse, H. (1982). The "silent substitution" method in visual research. Vision Research 22, 681–691.

Estévez, O., Spekreijse, H., Van den Berg, T.J.T.P., and Cavonius, C. R. (1975). The spectral sensitivities of isolated human color mechanisms determined from contrast evoked potential measurements. Vision Research 15, 1205–1212.

Hamer, R. D., Alexander, K. R., and Teller, D. Y. (1982). Rayleigh discriminations in young human infants. Vision Research 22, 575–587.

Hansen, R. M and Fulton, A. B. (1995). The VEP thresholds for full-field stimuli in dark-adapted infants. Visual Neuroscience 12, 223–228.

Hurvich, L. M. (1972). Color vision deficiencies. In: Handbook of Sensory Physiology, Vol. VII/4, Visual Psychophysics, D. Jameson and L. M. Hurvich, eds. (Berlin, Springer-Verlag) pp. 582–624.

Knoblauch, K., Bieber, M. L., and Werner, J. S. (1994). VEP responses to receptor-isolating stimuli in the first and second months. Infant Behavior and Development 17, Special ICIS Issue, 749.

Knoblauch, K., Bieber, M. L., and Werner, J. S. (1996). Assessing dimensionality in infant color vision. In: F. Vital-Durand, O. Braddick and J. Atkinson, eds. Infant Vision. (New York: Oxford University Press) pp. 51–61.

Lee, B. B., Martin, P. R., and Valberg, A. (1988). The physiological basis of heterochromatic photometry demonstrated in the ganglion cells of the macaque retina. Journal of Physiology 404, 323–347.

Morrone, M. C., Burr, D. C., and Fiorentini, A. (1993). Development of infant contrast sensitivity to chromatic stimuli Vision Research 33, 2535–2552.

Packer, O., Hartmann, E. E., and Teller, D. Y. (1984). Infant color vision: The effect of test field size on Rayleigh discriminations. Vision Research 24, 1247–1260.

Peeples, D. R. and Teller, D. Y. (1975). Color vision and brightness discrimination in two-month-old human infants. Science 189, 1102–1103.

Pitt, F. H. G. (1935). Characteristics of dichromatic colour vision. Spec. Rep. Sec. No. 200, Medical Research Council, London, H. M. Stationery Office.

Powers, M. K., Schneck, M., and Teller, D. Y. (1981). Spectral sensitivity of human infants at absolute threshold. Vision Research 21, 1005–1016.

Pulos, E., Teller, D. Y., and Buck, S. L. (1980). Infant color vision: A search for short-wavelength-sensitive mechanisms by means of chromatic adaptation. Vision Research 20, 485–493.

Smith, V. C. and Pokorny, J. (1975). Spectral sensitivity of the foveal cone photopigments between 400 and 500 nm. Vision Research 15, 161–171.

Stockman, A., MacLeod, D. I. A., and Johnson, N. E. (1993). Spectral sensitivities of the human cones. Journal of the Optical Society of America A 10, 2491–2521.

Teller, D. Y., Peeples, D. R., and Sekel, M. (1978). Discrimination of chromatic from white light by two-month-old human infants. Vision Research 18, 41–48.

Varner, D., Cook, J. E., Schneck, M. E., MacDonald, M. A., and Teller, D. Y. (1985). Tritan discriminations by 1- and 2-month old human infants. Vision Research 25, 821–831.

Volbrecht, V. J. and Werner, J. S. (1987). Isolation of short-wavelength-sensitive cone photoreceptors in 4-6-week-old human infants. Vision Research 27, 469–478.

Werner, J. S. (1982). Development of scotopic sensitivity and the absorption spectrum of the human ocular media. Journal of the Optical Society of America 72, 247–258.

Werner, J. S., Bieber, M. L., and Knoblauch, K. (1995). Isolated M- and L-cone responses in the VEP's of 4-week-old human infants. Investigative Ophthalmology and Visual Science (Suppl.) 36, S190.

Wyszecki, G. and Stiles, W. S. (1982). Color Science: Concepts and Methods, Quantitative Data and Formulae, 2nd edn. (New York, Wiley).

IV Color Metrics and Application

16. Dichromacy – The Simplest Type of Color Vision

Horst Scheibner

16.1 Introduction: An Initial Overview

The present contribution is an attempt to outline dichromacy – two-dimensional color vision – as a linear theory founded on visual psychophysics and embedded in a linear theory of trichromacy – three-dimensional color vision. Historical authorities in this field are Maxwell (1855), Helmholtz (1909–1911), Hering (1874), König (1893, 1903), Köllner (1912), Rosmanit (1914), Exner (1920), Schrödinger (1920, 1925), Müller (1924), Pitt (1935), Wright (1946, 1972), LeGrand (1957), Hurvich (1981), Wyszecki and Stiles (1982), and others. More recent progress is reported by, among others, Heinsius (1973), Pokorny et al. (1979), Scheibner and Wolf (1985), Marré and Marré (1986), Pokorny and Smith (1986), Vos et al. (1990), Ohta (1990), Valberg and Lee (1991), Guth (1991), Gouras (1991), Foster (1991), DeMarco et al. (1992), Stockman et al. (1993), Zeki (1993), Brainard (1995), Wandell (1995), Krastel (1995), and Kaiser and Boynton (1996).

In order to have a firm experimental basis let us start with a three-dimensional instrumental vectorial color space. It is characterized by basis vectors that represent real, physical radiation stimuli (as opposed to imaginary ones inherent, for example, in the CIE 1931 system). For measurements and for purposes of representation, we use the instrumental color space of W. D. Wright (1946), in which the basis vectors called *primaries* are realized by monochromatic radiations of wavelengths 460 nm (blue, B), 530 nm (green, G) and 650 nm (red, R). A vector equation for a color C then reads

$$C = B\boldsymbol{B} + G\boldsymbol{G} + R\boldsymbol{R}, \qquad (1)$$

where $\boldsymbol{B}, \boldsymbol{G}, \boldsymbol{R}$ are the (real) primaries and the tri-stimulus values B, G, R are the components of the color mixture. This trichromatic color space is designated in Figure 16.1 by $^3V_{BGR}$, where V stands for vector space, the superscript 3 means the dimension of the space, and the subscripts B, G, R denote the additive components.

The classical types of dichromacy are protanopia, deuteranopia and tritanopia. Here, deuteranopia has been selected as a typical representative of dichromacy. It appears in Figure 16.1 in the form of the three two-dimensional vector spaces, with the color vectors

$$C = B'\boldsymbol{B'} + R'\boldsymbol{R'} \qquad (2)$$

$$C = P\boldsymbol{P} + T\boldsymbol{T} \qquad (3)$$

$$C = K\boldsymbol{K} + L\boldsymbol{L}, \qquad (4)$$

where the letters have an analogous meaning as in eq. (1). These deuteranopic vector spaces are called the *instrumental color space*, the *fundamental color space* and the *opponent-color space*, respectively. The di-stimulus values of eqs. (2) and (3) are called the *instrumental di-stimulus values* and the *fundamental di-stimulus values*, respectively whereas the *opponent di-stimulus values* K, L of eq. (4) may be referred to as *chrominance* (K) and *luminance* (L). The fundamental color space, eq. (3), is also called the *cone excitation space* (Kaiser and Boynton, 1996).

The various spaces in Figure 16.1 are connected by arrows representing linear mappings. The double arrows mean invertible, dimension-preserving mappings, the one-sided arrows mean non-invertible, dimension-diminishing mappings.

As Figure 16.1 shows, the starting point of this linear theory is the instrumental color space $^3V_{BGR}$. The connecting mappings, then, contain the essential statements of the theory. For this reason, they

Colour spaces and their mappings

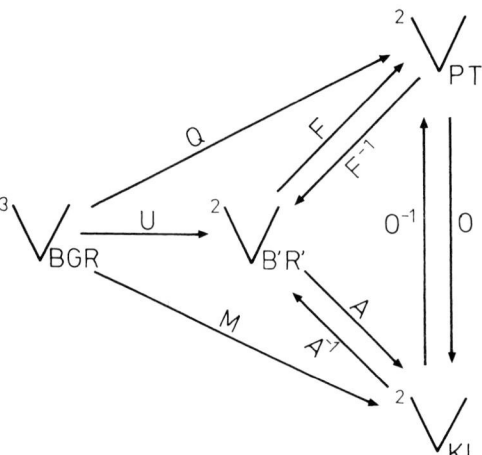

Fig. 16.1: Commutative diagram (Kostrikin and Manin, 1989) of color spaces and their mappings. $^3V_{BGR}$ trichromatic instrumental color space, $^2V_{B'R'}$ deuteranopic instrumental color space, $^2V_{PT}$ deuteranopic fundamental color space, $^2V_{KL}$ deuteranopic opponent-color space. The arrows represent linear mappings.

also offer the site of experimental attack in constructing the theory. Within the present psychophysical paradigm, the means are the following perceptual criteria: *indistinguishably equal* (i.e., the color match), *heterochromatically equally bright* (i.e., the heterochromatic brightness match) and the judgements *neither blue nor yellow* and *neither green nor red* (Scheibner and Wolf, 1985; Scheibner, 1987, 1990; Scheibner and Kremer, 1996). As a rule, these criteria determine one- or two-dimensional subspaces. They may single out such subspaces that operate as mapping kernels, i.e., subspaces that are mapped to zero (are annihilated). Examples in Figure 16.1 are the mappings U and M. Or else the criteria may single out subspaces to become subspaces of the target space, e.g., mapping Q. Comparing the cases of M and A will also illustrate that the overdimensionality 3 compared to 2 may be advantageous.

16.2 The Trichromatic Instrumental Color Space $^3V_{BGR}$

Experimentally, the instrumental color space $^3V_{BGR}$ may be given by the optical output of the visual tristimulus colorimeter used. Ours was a Guild-type colorimeter (Beck and Richter, 1958).

Figure 16.2 shows the chromaticity chart for the instrumental color space $^3V_{BGR}$ according to Wright (1946). Included are the equations for the chromaticity coordinates b, g, r; r is plotted on the abscissa and g is plotted on the ordinate. The normalization of the primaries according to Wright (1946) is also indicated.

Instrumental Primary System
$\vec{B}$(460nm), $\vec{G}$(530nm), $\vec{R}$(630nm)

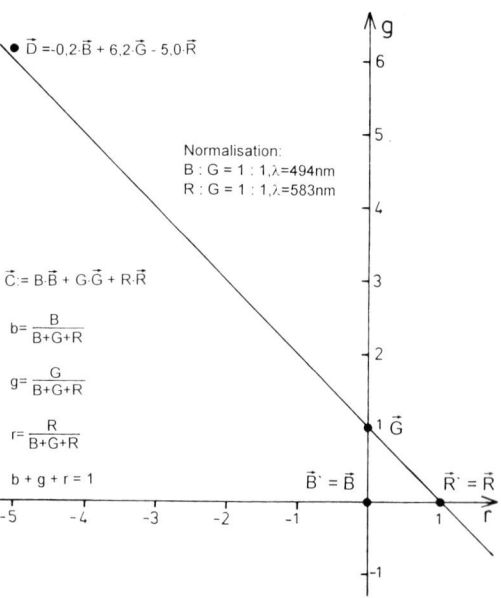

Fig. 16.2: Chromaticity chart pertaining to the instrumental color space $^3V_{BGR}$ according to W. D. Wright (1946). In the left top corner, the chromaticity locus of a typical deuteranopic missing color ***D*** is shown under the condition of the normalization indicated. (***B'***, ***R'***) is a possible set of remaining instrumental deuteranopic primaries. Here and henceforth, the primaries and other vectors are drawn with an arrow on top while in the text they are designated with bold italic letters.

16.3 Measuring the Deuteranopic Missing Color and Reducing Trichromacy to Deuteranopia

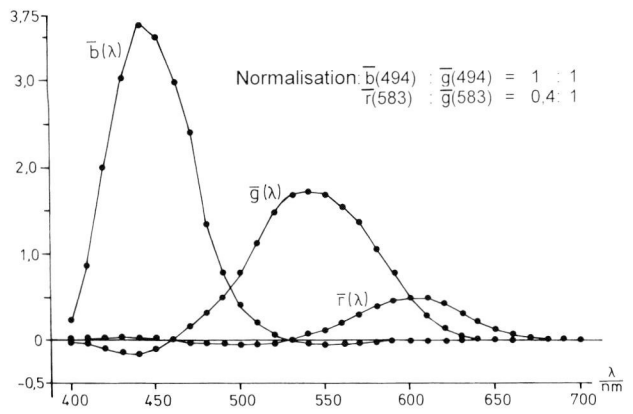

Trichromatic instrumental spectral values according to Estévez-Stiles-Burch, 2° diameter visual field

Normalisation: $\bar{b}(494) : \bar{g}(494) = 1 : 1$
$\bar{r}(583) : \bar{g}(583) = 0.4 : 1$

Fig. 16.3: Trichromatic color-matching functions with reference to the monochromatic primaries of wavelengths 460 nm, 530 nm and 650 nm (Estévez, 1982). Note the special red-green normalization.

Various sets of trichromatic color-matching functions with reference to the primaries of Figure 16.2 are known. We use the 2° functions due to Stiles and Burch as prepared by Estévez (Stiles and Burch, 1959; Estévez, 1982; cf. also Vos et al., 1990). They are shown in Figure 16.3. By definition, they show zero crossings at the wavelengths of the instrumental primaries. The ordinates of the "red" curve $\bar{r}(\lambda)$ have been depressed to 40% of the usual values due to the special red-green normalization indicated. This normalization moves the (imaginary) chromaticity locus of the deuteranopic missing color to be determined closer to the color triangle (B, G, R). The trichromatic functions $\bar{b}(\lambda)$, $\bar{g}(\lambda)$, $\bar{r}(\lambda)$ (Fig. 16.3) will be reduced, i.e., transformed under diminishing the dimension by one, to deuteranopic spectral functions (mappings Q, U and M in Fig. 16.1).

16.3 Measuring the Deuteranopic Missing Color and Reducing Trichromacy to Deuteranopia

The mapping U (Fig. 16.1) reduces the three-dimensional color space to a two-dimensional deuteranopic one by eliminating one dimension.

Because the middle or "green"-absorbing visual cone pigment is absent in the deuteranope (Rushton, 1965), one might think that it would suffice to discard the "green" instrumental primary G in Figure 16.2, thus establishing a deuteranopic instrumental color space with the two remaining primaries $B' = B$ and $R' = R$. But experiment shows that this discarding process is incorrect: the "missing color" (German: Fehlfarbe) (König and Dieterici, 1892; Schrödinger, 1920) is *not* the real color G, but an imaginary color denoted D in Figure 16.2. Because of its site quite distant from G, the usual normalization in Figure 16.2 has been changed in Figure 16.3 and subsequent figures.

The reducing mapping must be of the form

$$\begin{pmatrix} B' \\ R' \end{pmatrix} = U \begin{pmatrix} B \\ G \\ R \end{pmatrix} \quad (5)$$

where the triple on the right hand side is a trichromatic vector, the pair on the left hand side is a deuteranopic one, and U is a matrix consisting of two rows and three columns. The mapping (matrix U) is essentially determined if we know a special color vector

$$D = B_D \, B + G_D \, G + R_D \, R \quad (6)$$

for which

$$\begin{pmatrix} 0 \\ 0 \\ 0 \end{pmatrix} = U \begin{pmatrix} B_D \\ G_D \\ R_D \end{pmatrix} \qquad (7)$$

holds. This special color vector is the missing color and can be measured (Schrödinger, 1920; Nuberg and Yustova, 1957; Scheibner, 1968c, 1976; Kröger and Scheibner, 1977; Scheibner and Paulus, 1978; Paulus, 1978/79; Kröger-Paulus, 1980; Scheufens and Scheibner, 1984; Klauder, 1983/84; Scheufens, 1983/84; Scheibner and Orazem, 1997a, b).

The vector $\boldsymbol{D}$, eq. (6), spans a one-dimensional subspace

$$^1K_D = t\boldsymbol{D}, -\infty \leq t \leq +\infty, \qquad (8)$$

t being a free scalar parameter. In linear algebra (Boseck, 1984; Kostrikin and Manin, 1989) such a subspace is called the *kernel* of the mapping U,

$$\boldsymbol{D} \in {}^1K_D < {}^3V_{BGR}, \qquad (9)$$

where the symbol < is intended to mean *subspace of*. ^1K_D with $\boldsymbol{D}$ is mapped to zero, i.e., is annihilated, in agreement with eq. (7).

Figure 16.4 shows a way to measure the deuteranopic missing color. The (r,g)-chromaticity chart for our instrumental color space $^3V_{BGR}$ is shown, using the altered red-green normalization. Three sets of chromaticity loci form straight lines, so-called deuteranopic confusion lines. They were measured by means of deuteranopic color matches done within the framework of a three-dimensional color space: the green mixture component ($G_0\boldsymbol{G}$) was kept constant, the blue ($B\boldsymbol{B}$) and red ($R\boldsymbol{R}$) components were freely variable. The mixtures were matched against three spectral test stimuli of wavelengths 490 nm, 510 nm and 580 nm, respectively, indicated in Figure 16.4. The vectorial difference of two tristimulus value triples resulting from matches against an identical test stimulus, where two different green mixture components were fixed but the blue and red components were freely variable, is an individual representative $\boldsymbol{D}_{ij}$ of the missing color vector:

$$(B_i - B_j)\boldsymbol{B} + (G_{i0} - G_{j0})\boldsymbol{G} + (R_i - R_j)\boldsymbol{R} = \boldsymbol{D}_{ij}. \qquad (10)$$

Its chromaticity locus (r, g) is an individual *missing point*. The sites of such missing points were outside the triangle BGR and in the neighborhood of the dots denoted by D(490 nm), $\boldsymbol{D}$, D(580 nm) and D(510 nm) in Figure 16.4. Since a color match also implies a heterochromatic brightness match (or luminance match), a difference vector according to eq. (10) must be luminance-free. Hence, its chromaticity locus is necessarily imaginary.

The loci of the dichromatic color matches themselves are those dots which lie inside the triangle BGR including the line segment GR (Fig. 16.4). For each test stimulus, they were well approximated by a straight line, a *confusion line*.

The three confusion lines do not have a common point of intersection nor did the three sets of individual missing points pertaining to the three test stimuli coincide in a common missing point. For this reason, the individual missing points arising

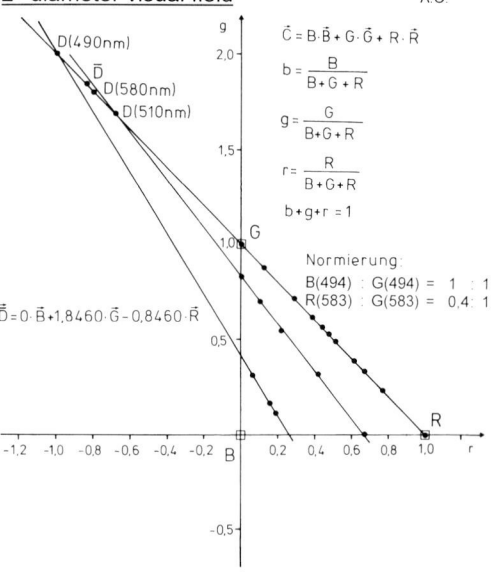

Fig. 16.4: Instrumental (r, g)-chromaticity chart. The points within the triangle BGR including the line segment GR are chromaticity loci of dichromatic color matches (see text) against spectral test stimuli of 490 nm, 510 nm and 580 nm, each test stimulus producing a confusion line. The points D(490 nm), D(580 nm) and D(510 nm) each belong to a confusion line and are (imaginary) loci of averaged missing points.

16.3 Measuring the Deuteranopic Missing Color and Reducing Trichromacy to Deuteranopia

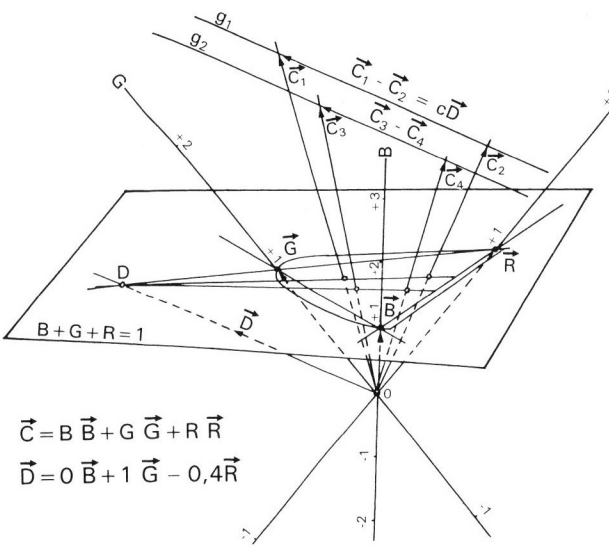

$\vec{C} = B\,\vec{B} + G\,\vec{G} + R\,\vec{R}$

$\vec{D} = 0\,\vec{B} + 1\,\vec{G} - 0{,}4\vec{R}$

Fig. 16.5: Spatial configuration of a deuteranopic missing color within $^3V_{BGR}$. The unit plane $B + G + R = 1$ is taken as the chromaticity chart containing the trichromatic spectral locus. The colors C_1 and C_2 are indistinguishably equal to a deuteranope, as are C_3 and C_4. The difference vectors $C_1 - C_2$ and $C_3 - C_4$ are equal to the missing color vector D up to a factor c. D is the missing point (from Kröger-Paulus, 1980, modified).

Deuteranopic missing colour $\vec{D}$:

$\vec{D} = B_D \cdot \vec{B} + G_D \cdot \vec{G} + R_D \cdot \vec{R}$

$\begin{pmatrix} B' \\ R' \end{pmatrix} = U \cdot \begin{pmatrix} B \\ G \\ R \end{pmatrix}$

B, G, R   tri-stimulus values
B´, R´   di-stimulus values

Missing colour as the kernel of a reduction mapping:

$\begin{pmatrix} 0 \\ 0 \end{pmatrix} = U \cdot \begin{pmatrix} B_D \\ G_D \\ R_D \end{pmatrix}$

Additionally

$\begin{pmatrix} 1 \\ 0 \end{pmatrix} = U \cdot \begin{pmatrix} 1 \\ 0 \\ 0 \end{pmatrix}$

$\begin{pmatrix} 0 \\ 1 \end{pmatrix} = U \cdot \begin{pmatrix} 0 \\ 0 \\ 1 \end{pmatrix}$

Fig. 16.6: Scheme of how to determine the $2 \cdot 3$ matrix U if the missing color D and the association with the deuteranopic primaries are known.

from a test stimulus were averaged. These averages are designated by D(490 nm), D(580 nm) and D(510 nm). Their grand average $\overline{D}$ reads

$$\overline{D} = 0\,B + 1.8460\,G - 0.8460\,R. \tag{11}$$

In this representation of the deuteranopic missing color vector, the numbers, formally tristimulus values, are normalized to chromaticity coordinates, since according to eq. (8) the normalization of vector D is free. According to eq. (9), vector $\overline{D}$ is a member of subspace ^1K_D, which, strictly speaking, is itself the deuteranopic missing color.

Expression (11) is a non-zero vector for a trichromat (non-match) but a zero vector for the deuteranope (match), in agreement with eq. (7). This vector has a certain direction within the three-dimensional color space and hence a certain chromaticity locus, namely the copunctal point through which all confusion lines ought to pass. Being a null vector with respect to the color attribute brightness, vector (11) lies within the deuteranopic null-luminance plane, the so-called deuteranopic alychne plane (see section 16.5) according to Schrödinger (1925), and its chromaticity locus and the deuteranopic alychne trace in the chromaticity chart are, therefore, incident. By the same argument, since the vector $\overline{D}$ (eq. (11)) is also a null vector with respect to the color attribute chroma, it lies coplanarly within the deuteranopic null-chrominance plane, the so-called neutral zone plane, and the chromaticity locus of $\overline{D}$ and the trace of the neutral zone in chromaticity chart are incident.

Figure 16.5 illustrates these ideas (cf. also Oleari et al. (1996) for helpful illustrations). While Figure 16.4 demonstrates the determination of a missing color within the chromaticity chart, where vector operations are not immediately discernible, Figure 16.5 shows the procedure within the vector space itself (Scheibner, 1968c; Kröger-Paulus, 1980). It may be useful to supplement the vector space by an affine (point) space (Kostrikin and Manin, 1989) such that vectors taken as differences of points are possible and a plane like the unit plane $B + G + R = 1$ can be explicitly defined. One may recognize that the difference vectors according to eq. (10) are aligned in parallel straight lines within the affine point space. The projections of these parallel straight lines from the origin O into the chromaticity chart converge to the co-punctal point D (Fig. 16.5).

Figure 16.6 gives details for determining the matrix U sought. It consists of $2 \cdot 3 = 6$ coefficients. Eq. (7), repeated in the middle of Figure 16.6, yields two coefficients of U. Associating the trichromatic primaries B and R with the deuteranopic primaries

$$B' = \begin{pmatrix} 1 \\ 0 \\ 0 \end{pmatrix} \text{ and } R' = \begin{pmatrix} 0 \\ 0 \\ 1 \end{pmatrix} \quad (12)$$

as shown in Figure 16.2, yields the four remaining coefficients of the matrix U. This is shown in the additional equations at the bottom of Figure 16.6. Fixing the deuteranopic basis vectors in this manner is not without a certain arbitrariness, but it is the simplest approach.

16.4 The Transition from the Instrumental Trichromatic Space to the Instrumental Deuteranopic Space

The measurements performed on deuteranope A.O. resulted in the deuteranopic missing color vector given by eq. (11) and shown in Figure 16.4. The resulting mapping (matrix U in Fig. 16.1) is

$$B' = B$$
$$R' = 0.4583G + R. \quad (13)$$

Applying these equations to the color-matching functions $\overline{b}(\lambda)$, $\overline{g}(\lambda)$, $\overline{r}(\lambda)$ of Figure 16.3 results

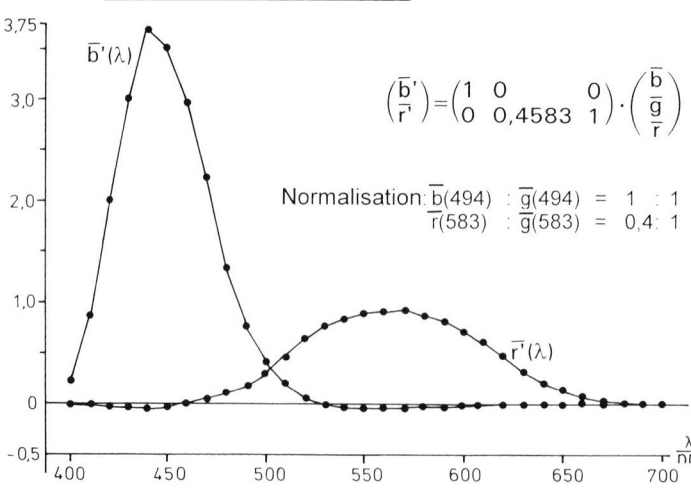

Fig. 16.7: Deuteranopic instrumental matching functions $\overline{b}'(\lambda)$ and $\overline{r}'(\lambda)$ derived from the trichromatic color-matching functions shown in Figure 16.3 using the missing color vector $\overline{D}$. Although the red-green normalization taken from Figure 16.3 does not explicitly exist any more it is still effective. The matrix is U of Figures 16.1 and 16.6.

in the deuteranopic instrumental spectral values $\bar{b}'(\lambda)$ and $\bar{r}'(\lambda)$ shown in Figure 16.7. (Note that altered red-green normalization is still effective.) Eqs. (13) are reproduced in matrix form and rewritten for color-matching functions, which, of course, are special tri-stimulus and di-stimulus values. It is apparent that the collapse of trichromacy to deuteranopia occurs in the green-red region, leaving the blue mechanism untouched.

16.5 The Transformation from the Trichromatic Instrumental Color Space to the Deuteranopic Opponent-Color Space

So far we have applied the perceptual criterion *indistinguishably equal*. As demonstrated in Figures 16.4 and 16.5, two deuteranopic color matches are sufficient to determine the kernel of the mapping U, i.e., a point locus in the chromaticity chart, and thus to reduce $\bar{b}(\lambda), \bar{g}(\lambda) \bar{r}(\lambda)$ to $\bar{b}'(\lambda), \bar{r}'(\lambda)$ (Fig. 16.7). Indeed, repeated dichromatic matches with different fixed (*green*) components result in straight lines, the so-called confusion lines. The criterion *indistinguishably equal* points to the fact that such a line describes a single dichromatic chromaticity. From a geometric point of view, these lines are elements dual to points within the chromaticity chart.

Deuteranopic *opponent*-color vision can be approached by using the two perceptual criteria *neither blue nor yellow* and *equally bright*. One could do this within the deuteranopic instrumental color space $^2V_{B'R'}$, which is characterized by eq. (2). The chromaticity chart of $^2V_{B'R'}$ is shown in Figure 16.2 as a binary color-mixture line joining the loci of the primaries B' and R', and $^2V_{B'R'}$ is connected to the trichromatic instrumental color space $^3V_{BGR}$ through eqs. (13). In view of eq. (4), one has to determine the chrominance primary K and the luminance primary L. The vector K, a luminance-free vector, is determined as the difference vector of two colors which have been equated in brightness. The vector L, a chrominance-free vector, is that sum of the primaries B' and R' which obeys the criterion *neither blue nor yellow*. (More details may be found in a paper by Bruckwilder and Scheibner, 1988/89). The result can be gathered from Figure 16.8 where K and L and their equations are shown. In Figure 16.1, this procedure corresponds to the mapping A:

$$\begin{pmatrix} K \\ L \end{pmatrix} = A \begin{pmatrix} B' \\ R' \end{pmatrix}. \qquad (14)$$

Within $^2V_{B'R'}$, however, the confusion lines with their copunctal point have been lost. In order to preserve them we decided to directly execute the mapping M instead of performing mapping A (Fig. 16.1). For that purpose, the same chromatic and achromatic criteria had to be applied by the deuteranopic observer.

For the chromatic criterion *neither blue nor yellow*, the observer adjusted various different binary color mixtures and judged these according to the criterion. This was done in the left side of the bipartite visual field of the colorimeter. When the mixture obeyed the criterion, the observer matched it to the superposition of the three instrumental primaries presented in the right half of the visual field. Thus, the colors obeying the criterion could be plotted in the (r,g)-chromaticity chart. They were well approximated by a straight, line – the so-called neutral or chrominance-free zone. In Figure 16.8, it is shown as the straight line that runs through the central area of the color triangle (***BGR***)

In applying the second, achromatic, criterion, the deuteranopic observer equated the brightness of pairs of colors, which were different in color to him. For that purpose, he applied the criterion of minimally distinct border (Boynton, 1978; Thoma, 1982). By matching the equated colors to a superposition of the three experimental primaries, the colors were specified within the B,G,R)-system. Then, pairwise vectorial differences were calculated, formally similar to eq. (10). Such difference vectors are by definition luminance-free. Their chromaticity loci lay in the imaginary region of the chromaticity chart and were well approximated by a straight line (the line to the left side of the

16. Dichromacy – The Simplest Type of Color Vision

Chromaticity charts of the spaces $^3V_{BGR}$, $^3V_{PDT}$, $^2V_{B',R'}$, $^2V_{KL}$, $^2V_{P'T'}$

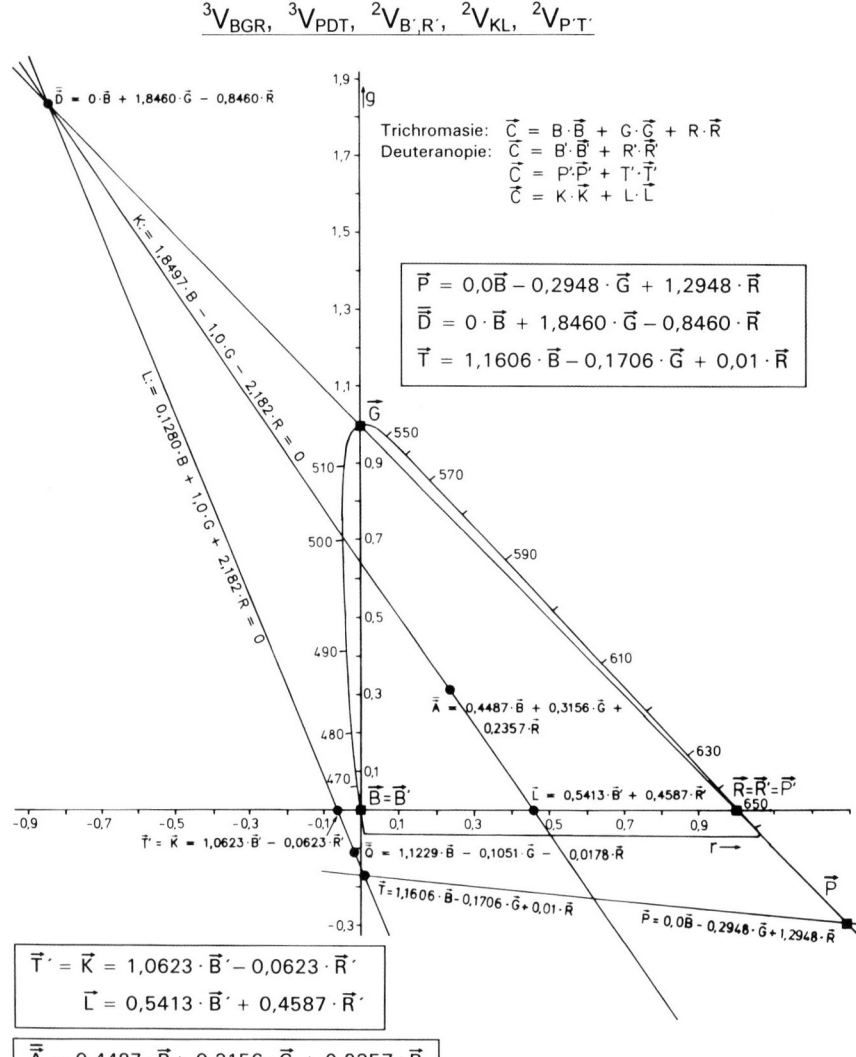

Fig. 16.8: The deuteranopic neutral zone $K = 0$ and alychne trace $L = 0$ are shown, an experimental result of observer A. O. The averaging procedure by way of the intermediate vectors A and Q took into account that the missing point of vector D in Figure 16.4 became an exact copunctal point. Additionally, the chromaticities of the fundamental primaries P, D, T, after having been adapted to observer A. O., and the chromaticities of the deuteranopic reference systems (B', R'), (P', T'), (K, L) are shown. In the boxes, the equations are repeated in a larger letter size.

16.5 Transformation from the Trichromatic Instrumental Color Space

color triangle in Fig. 16.8). It is the famous trace of the alychne (=lightless), introduced by Schrödinger (1925).

The final averaging process for constructing the neutral zone and the alychne trace took the missing point D into account such that the two lines intersected in locus D.

In deriving equations for the neutral zone and the alychne trace, we wished to express their dual character compared to point loci. Linear homogeneous forms fulfill this wish:

$$\beta B + \gamma G + \rho R = 0, \tag{15}$$

where B, G, R are tri-stimulus values and β, γ, ρ are coefficients. In a first step, the straight lines may be expressed by equations of the type

$$g = mr + h, \tag{16}$$

where the variables g and r are chromaticity coordinates pertaining to $^3V_{BGR}$, and m and h are constants. By changing from the chromaticity coordinates r, g to tristimulus values B, G, R as indicated in Figures 16.2 and 16.4, we arrive at equations of the form (15).

Eq. (15) is the general incidence condition of a point and a straight line and expresses the principle of duality (v. Staudt, 1847; Plaumann and Strambach, 1981):
a) with the triple (β, γ, ρ) constant, varying the triple (B, G, R) produces a fixed straight line;
b) with the triple (B, G, R) constant, varying the triple (β, γ, ρ), produces a pencil of straight lines through a fixed point.

For this reason, (B, G, R) are called point coordinates and (β, γ, ρ) are called line coordinates in the projective plane, which is here identified with the chromaticity chart. Eq. (15) holds only if the point described by (B, G, R) lies on the straight line described by (β, γ, ρ), i.e., if the point and the straight line are incident; if this is not the case, the left-hand side of eq. (15) takes on a non-zero value. If the point crosses the line, the left-hand side of eq. (15) changes sign, reflecting the blue-yellow color opponency present in deuteranopic color perception.

For the neutral zone, the evaluation resulted in

$$1.8497B - 1.0G - 2.182R = 0 \tag{17}$$

and for the trace of the alychne in

$$0.1280B + 1.0G + 2.182R = 0 \tag{18}$$

In both equations, the *green* coefficient γ is arbitrarily normalized to 1. In Figure 16.8, the equations are written beside the pertaining straight lines.

Eqs. (15), (17), (18) are considered to represent straight lines within the chromaticity chart, in which the tri-stimulus values B, G, R are general homogeneous coordinates (Maxwell, 1963). But we may also view the equations representing planes containing the origin, i.e., two-dimensional subspaces of $^3V_{BGR}$. In order to make the final step from these plane equations (17) and (18) to the mapping equations M of Figure 16.1 we may take advantage of the relation between incidence and non-incidence: For colors with chromaticity loci incident on the neutral zone or alychne trace, the equations (17) or (18) hold; for all other colors, the transformation M results and reads

$$\begin{aligned} K &= 1.8497B - 1.0G - 2.182R \\ L &= 0.1280B + 1.0G + 2.182R, \end{aligned} \tag{19}$$

where K and L are opponent distimulus values according to the deuteranopic color representation of eq. (4). In principle, eqs. (19) are of the type of eq. (5), eqs. (17) and (18) are of the type (7), with the difference that the target space of the mapping is the deuteranopic *opponent*-color space. Thus, the perceptual criterion *neither blue nor yellow* singles out the two-dimensional kernel ^2K_K to be annihilated:

$$^2K_K < \,^3V_{BGR}, \tag{20}$$

while the perceptual criterion *equally bright* singles out the two-dimensional kernel ^2K_L to be annihilated:

$$^2K_L < \,^3V_{BGR}, \tag{21}$$

and the two kernels intersect in the deuteranopic missing color D, (eq. (9)):

$$D \in \,^1K_D = \,^2K_K \cap \,^2K_L < \,^3V_{BGR}, \tag{22}$$

where the symbol $<$ means *subspace of*, $\cap$ means *intersection*. The two remaining, non-annihilated opponent components K and L, called *chrominance* and *luminance* build up the deuteranopic

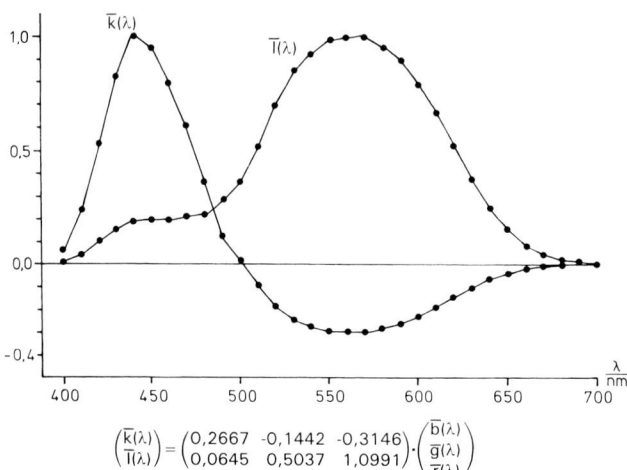

Fig. 16.9: Deuteranopic spectral opponent functions $\bar{k}(\lambda)$ and $\bar{l}(\lambda)$ are shown. They were derived from trichromatic color-matching functions $\bar{b}(\lambda)$, $\bar{g}(\lambda)$, $\bar{r}(\lambda)$ shown in Figure 16.3 by means of the 2×3 matrix M of Figure 16.1. The function $\bar{k}(\lambda)$ could be called the *spectral blue-yellow chroma sensitivity*, $\bar{l}(\lambda)$ could be called the *spectral brightness sensitivity*.

opponent-color space $^2V_{KL}$ (Fig. 16.1). Note that the kernel ^2K_K, the neutral zone, contains real colors while the kernel ^2K_L, the alychne, contains only imaginary colors.

The mapping given by eqs. (19) was applied to the color-matching functions $\bar{b}(\lambda)$, $\bar{g}(\lambda)$, $\bar{r}(\lambda)$ shown in Figure 16.3. The results are the two spectral curves $\bar{k}(\lambda)$ and $\bar{l}(\lambda)$ shown in Figure 16.9. The mapping equations have been renormalized so that the maximum of each curve assumes the value one; this leaves the ratios of the coefficients in each row of the matrix unchanged. We may call $\bar{k}(\lambda)$ the *spectral deuteranopic blue-yellow chroma sensitivity*, $\bar{l}(\lambda)$ the *spectral deuteranopic brightness sensitivity*, the terms *chroma* and *brightness* indicating sensations.

16.6 The Role of the Fundamental Color Space

The trichromatic color-matching functions (Fig. 16.3) and the dichromatic color-matching functions (Fig. 16.7) possess zero crossings and, therefore, negative curve branches, so that they are not suited to represent the spectral sensitivities of the retinal cones. The so-called fundamental color space $^3V_{PDT}$ remedies this deficit in that the pertaining spectral functions $\bar{p}(\lambda)$, $\bar{d}(\lambda)$, $\bar{t}(\lambda)$ can be interpreted as spectral cone sensitivities. According to the classical hypothesis of König (König and Dieterici, 1893), the missing colors of the three types of dichromats provide the excitations of the three cone types. By making the missing colors the basis vectors of a vectorial color space, a fundamental color space $^3V_{PDT}$, can be constructed. Within $^3V_{PDT}$, a color vector reads

$$C = P\boldsymbol{P} + D\boldsymbol{D} + T\boldsymbol{T}, \quad (22)$$

where P, D, T are fundamental tri-stimulus values, $\boldsymbol{P}$ is the *red* fundamental primary given by the protanopic missing color, $\boldsymbol{D}$ is the *green* fundamental primary given by the deuteranopic missing color and $\boldsymbol{T}$ is the *blue* fundamental primary given by the tritanopic missing color.

The space $^3V_{PDT}$ has been omitted in Figure 16.1. Its independent experimental determination would require the availability of all three types of dichromatic observers to determine their missing colors. It is interesting that an independent determination of a dichromatic fundamental color space (in our case, Figure 16.1, the deuteranopic fundamental color space $^2V_{PT}$) also requires all three types of dichromatic observers: The mapping Q (Fig. 16.1) is established by the deuteranopic missing color providing the mapping kernel, by the protanopic missing color providing the first basis vector of the target space, and by the tritanopic missing color providing the second basis vector of the target space. The procedure is similar to the determination of the mapping U delineated in Figure 16.6.

The mapping F (Fig. 16.1), which connects $^2V_{B'R'}$ with $^2V_{PT}$, does not lend itself to experimental attack, since the loss of the overdimensionality of $^2V_{B'R'}$ compared to $^3V_{BGR}$ prevents the measuring of the protanopic and tritanopic missing colors sought. The final goal is the mapping O (Fig. 16.1) which serves to describe the excitation transfer from the deuternopic retinal cones into the postreceptoral opponent-color channels (Scheibner and Wolf, 1985, 1985/86; Scheibner and Lochner, 1991).

In the following section, the data of the fundamental space $^3V_{PDT}$ are taken from the literature (reviews by Wyszecki and Stiles, 1982; Pokorny and Smith, 1986; Stockman et al., 1993; Brainard, 1995). Its primaries P, D, T were expressed within the instrumental space $^3V_{BGR}$. By means of the measured deuteranopic primary D (Fig. 16.4), it is adapted to $^2V_{PT}$. Finally, the mapping O sought (Fig. 16.1) is determined by a concatenation of the mappings F^{-1} and A.

16.7 Construction of the Fundamental Color Spaces $^3V_{PTD}$ and $^2V_{PT}$ and the Deuteranopic Opponent-Color Channels

The loci of the fundamental primaries P, D, T are taken from Bruckwilder and Scheibner (1988/89). In order to achieve coherence between our data so far and the fundamental system, the fundamental primary D of Bruckwilder and Scheibner is replaced by the missing color D of Figure 16.4. The locus of the fundamental primary T was slightly modified in that it is made incident with our deuteranope's alychne trace L = 0. This implies that our deuteranope's *blue* cones do not contribute to brightness. Figure 16.8 shows the location of the three partially modified fundamental primaries; their equations:

$$P = 0.0B - 0.2948G + 1.2948R$$
$$D = 0.0B + 1.8460G - 0.8460R \quad (23)$$
$$T = 1.1606B - 0.1706G + 0.010R.$$

These equations are normalized so that the coefficients are numerically chromaticity coordinates b, g, r (i.e., sum to unity).

From linear algebra it is known (Boseck, 1984; Kostrikin and Manin, 1989) that tristimulus values and primaries obey the following transformation scheme:

$$\begin{pmatrix} P \\ D \\ T \end{pmatrix} = W \begin{pmatrix} B \\ G \\ R \end{pmatrix}, \quad (24)$$

$$\begin{pmatrix} P \\ D \\ T \end{pmatrix} = W^{-1T} \begin{pmatrix} B \\ G \\ R \end{pmatrix}, \quad (25)$$

where the superscript T indicates the transposition of the inverted matrix W^{-1}.

Inverting and transposing the matrix of eqs. (23) makes it possible to calculate fundamental tristimulus values (P, D, T) from instrumental tristimulus values (B, G, R). In particular, this was done for the curves $\bar{b}(\lambda)$, $\bar{g}(\lambda)$, $\bar{r}(\lambda)$ shown in Figure 16.3. In the process of calculation, the matrix of eq. (24) was row-wise renormalized so that the maxima of the resulting spectral fundamental curves $\bar{p}(\lambda)$, $\bar{d}(\lambda)$, $\bar{t}(\lambda)$ assume the value 1. The result is shown in Figure 16.10. In the renormalized form, eqs. (24) read

$$\bar{p}(\lambda) = 0.0646\bar{b}(\lambda) + 0.5037\bar{g}(\lambda)$$
$$+ 1.0990\bar{r}(\lambda)$$
$$\bar{d}(\lambda) = 0.0840\bar{b}(\lambda) + 0.5792\bar{g}(\lambda) \quad (26)$$
$$+ 0.1319\bar{r}(\lambda)$$
$$\bar{t}(\lambda) = 02706\bar{b}(\lambda).$$

By virtue of the special properties of the fundamental primaries, the middle or *green* curve $\bar{d}(\lambda)$

Fundamental spectral values, 2° diameter visual field

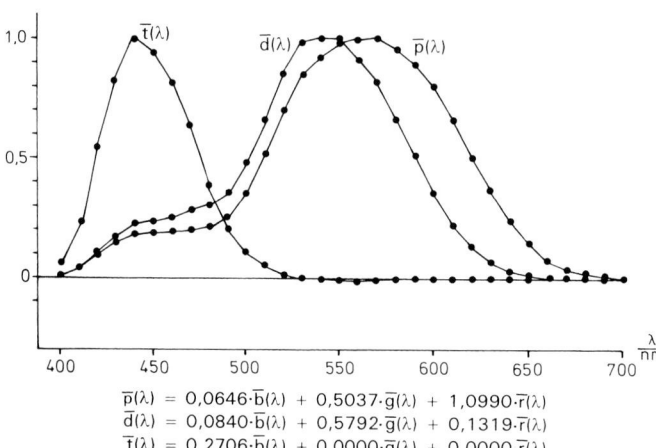

$\bar{p}(\lambda) = 0{,}0646 \cdot \bar{b}(\lambda) + 0{,}5037 \cdot \bar{g}(\lambda) + 1{,}0990 \cdot \bar{r}(\lambda)$
$\bar{d}(\lambda) = 0{,}0840 \cdot \bar{b}(\lambda) + 0{,}5792 \cdot \bar{g}(\lambda) + 0{,}1319 \cdot \bar{r}(\lambda)$
$\bar{t}(\lambda) = 0{,}2706 \cdot \bar{b}(\lambda) + 0{,}0000 \cdot \bar{g}(\lambda) + 0{,}0000 \cdot \bar{r}(\lambda)$

Fig. 16.10: Spectral fundamental functions of the normal trichromat. The equations at the bottom indicate how they have been derived from the color-matching functions shown in Figure 16.3. Since in the deuteranope the *green* or middle wavelength visual pigment is absent, the curves $\bar{t}(\lambda)$ and $\bar{p}(\lambda)$ describe the relative spectral sensitivity of the deuteranope's *blue* and *red* retinal cones.

can simply be discarded for the deuteranope. Therefore, in Figure 16.1, the mapping Q connecting $^3V_{BGR}$ with $^2V_{PT}$ is given by the first and third row of eqs. (26).

In order to exploit the transformation connections between the three deuteranopic spaces $^2V_{PT}$, $^2V_{B'R'}$ and $^2V_{KL}$ shown in Figure 16.1, the three spaces must be given within one common reference system. Here, $^2V_{B'R'}$ is chosen as the common system, the chromaticity diagram of which has shrunk to the r-axis in Figure 16.8. It may be helpful to imagine a second scale b (or b') on this axis running in the opposite direction to scale r (or r'), with its zero point located at R and the unity point located at B (Fig. 16.8). The deuteranopic chromaticity coordinates b' and r' are defined according to

$$b' = B'/(B' + R'), \qquad r' = R'/(B' + R'). \qquad (27)$$

Now, the primaries B, G, R and P, D, T must be transformed – expressed as column vectors within $^3V_{BGR}$ – into $^2V_{B'R'}$ by means of the mapping U, and the opponent primaries K and L also have to appear within $^2V_{B'R'}$. Figure 16.8 shows that the locus of K is the intersection of the alychne trace L = 0 with the r-axis, and the locus of L is the intersection of the neutral zone K = 0 with the r-axis. This constellation, moreover, demonstrates that any mapping U is equivalent to a projection starting from the projection center D, whereby any trichromatic locus is uniquely projected to a deuteranopic locus on the r-axis. The result is shown in Figure 16.8.

Besides the assumption

$$\begin{aligned} B &= B' \\ R &= R' \end{aligned} \qquad (28)$$

the equations read

$$\begin{aligned} P' &= \qquad\qquad + \quad 1R' \\ T' &= 1{,}0623B' - 0{,}0623R' \end{aligned} \qquad (29)$$

and

$$\begin{aligned} K &= 1{,}0623B' - 0{,}0623R' \\ L &= 0{,}5413B' + 0{,}4587R'. \end{aligned} \qquad (30)$$

Note that the primary $P' \in {}^2VB'R'$ is different from $P \in {}^3V_{BGR}$, as is the case with T' and T. Nevertheless, both P' and P and T' and T are of the same deuteranopic chromaticity, since they lie on the same deuteranopic confusion lines.

In view of Figure 16.1, we may identify mapping (29) with F^{-1T}, where now the deuteranopic fundamental space is denoted by $^2V_{P'T'}$ (primes added), and mapping (30) may be identified with A^{-1T}. We wish to perform the concatenation

$$\begin{pmatrix} K \\ L \end{pmatrix} = O \begin{pmatrix} P' \\ T' \end{pmatrix} = AF^{-1} \begin{pmatrix} P' \\ T' \end{pmatrix} \qquad (31)$$

16.7 Construction of the Fundamental Color Spaces $^3V_{PTD}$ and $^2V_{PT}$

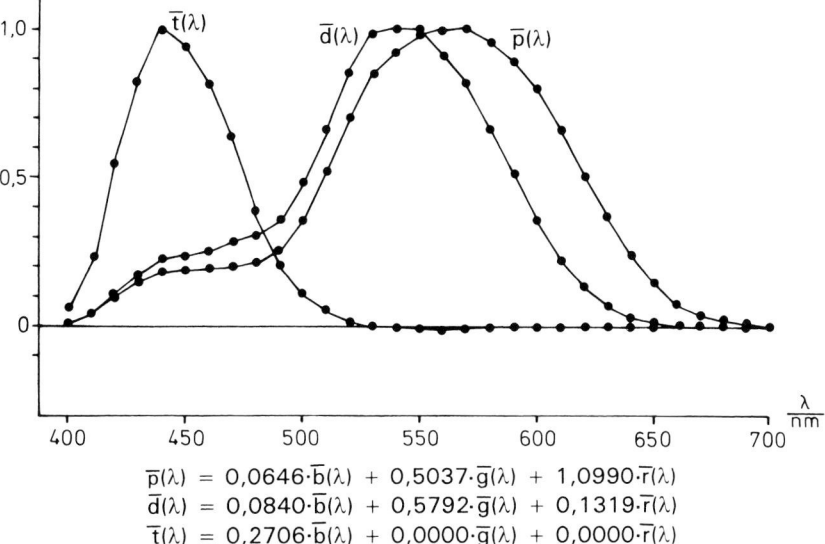

$$\bar{p}(\lambda) = 0{,}0646 \cdot \bar{b}(\lambda) + 0{,}5037 \cdot \bar{g}(\lambda) + 1{,}0990 \cdot \bar{r}(\lambda)$$
$$\bar{d}(\lambda) = 0{,}0840 \cdot \bar{b}(\lambda) + 0{,}5792 \cdot \bar{g}(\lambda) + 0{,}1319 \cdot \bar{r}(\lambda)$$
$$\bar{t}(\lambda) = 0{,}2706 \cdot \bar{b}(\lambda) + 0{,}0000 \cdot \bar{g}(\lambda) + 0{,}0000 \cdot \bar{r}(\lambda)$$

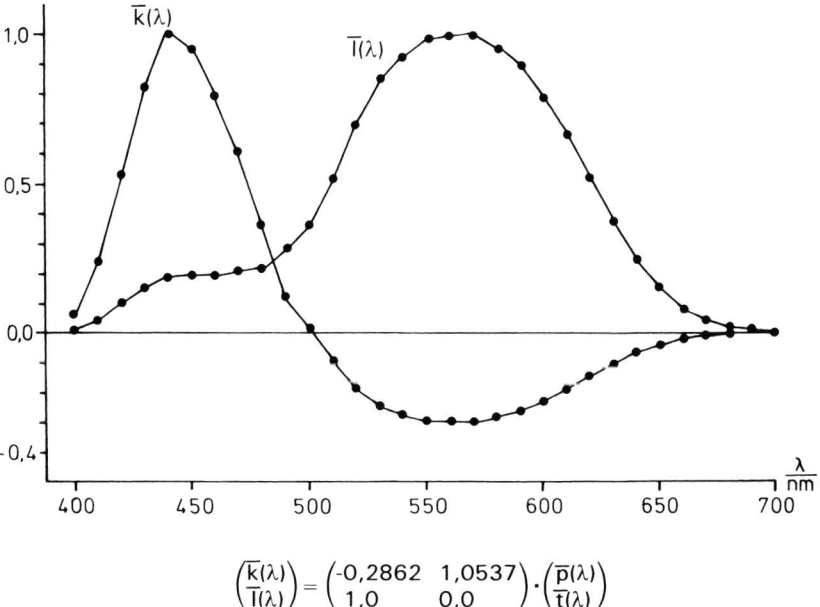

$$\begin{pmatrix} \bar{k}(\lambda) \\ \bar{l}(\lambda) \end{pmatrix} = \begin{pmatrix} -0{,}2862 & 1{,}0537 \\ 1{,}0 & 0{,}0 \end{pmatrix} \cdot \begin{pmatrix} \bar{p}(\lambda) \\ \bar{t}(\lambda) \end{pmatrix}$$

Fig. 16.11: The upper part shows the spectral fundamental functions of Figure 16.10. The lower part shows the deuteranopic spectral opponent functions of Figure 16.9. The equation at the bottom shows how the deuteranopic spectral cone sensitivities $\bar{t}(\lambda)$ and $\bar{p}(\lambda)$ are transformed by means of the 2×2 opponency matrix O (Fig. 16.1).

Therefore, the matrix F^{-1T} of eq. (29) must be transposed and, with regard to the deuteranopic spectral functions $\bar{b}'(\lambda)$, $\bar{r}'(\lambda)$, row-wise renormalized. The result is

$$\begin{pmatrix} B' \\ R' \end{pmatrix} = \begin{pmatrix} 0 & 3.6959 \\ 0.9096 & -0.2168 \end{pmatrix} \begin{pmatrix} P' \\ T' \end{pmatrix} = F^{-1} \begin{pmatrix} P' \\ T' \end{pmatrix}. \quad (32)$$

In turn, the matrix A^{-1T} of eq. (30) must be inverted and transposed and, with regard to the deuteranopic spectral opponent functions $\bar{k}(\lambda)$, $\bar{l}(\lambda)$, row-wise renormalized. This leads to

$$\begin{pmatrix} K \\ L \end{pmatrix} = \begin{pmatrix} 0.2667 & -0.3146 \\ 0.0645 & 1.0991 \end{pmatrix} \begin{pmatrix} B' \\ R' \end{pmatrix} = A \begin{pmatrix} B' \\ R' \end{pmatrix}. \quad (33)$$

The concatenation of eqs. (32) and (33) yields the transformation $O = A\,F^{-1}$:

$$\begin{pmatrix} K \\ L \end{pmatrix} = \begin{pmatrix} -0.2862 & 1.0537 \\ 1 & 0 \end{pmatrix} \begin{pmatrix} P' \\ T' \end{pmatrix} = O \begin{pmatrix} P' \\ T' \end{pmatrix}. \quad (34)$$

Equation (34) describes the excitation transfer from the deuteranopic retinal cones to the deuteranopic postreceptoral opponent-color channels. K designates the opponent distimulus value of the luminance channel, O is the opponency matrix. At the bottom of Figure 16.11, eq. (34) appears in a form written for spectral curves. The curves $\bar{k}(\lambda)$ and $\bar{l}(\lambda)$ are, of course, the same as in Figure 16.9. The curves $\bar{p}(\lambda)$, $\bar{d}(\lambda)$, $\bar{t}(\lambda)$ at the top of Figure 16.11 stand for the three trichromatic receptor sensitivities. Only the curves $\bar{p}(\lambda)$ and $\bar{t}(\lambda)$ apply to the deuteranope. Clearly, $\bar{p}'(\lambda) = \bar{p}(\lambda)$ and $\bar{t}'(\lambda) = \bar{t}(\lambda)$. Since $\bar{l}(\lambda) = \bar{p}(\lambda)$, the deuteranopic brightness is carried by the *red* cones alone.

16.8 A Synopsis of Deuteranopia

Figure 16.12 shows the commutative diagram of Figure 16.1, supplemented by the set of visible radiation stimuli, Σ. An immediate physiologically relevant meaning is present in the mappings Z and O (heavy arrows). Such a diagram may indicate ways to construct transfer paths even if some inter-

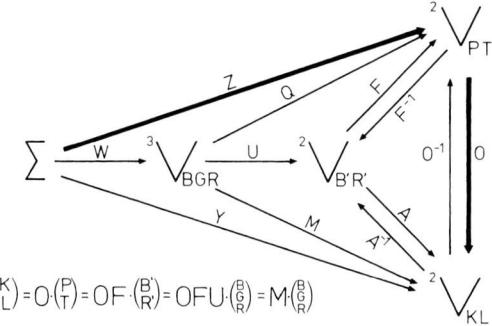

$$\begin{pmatrix} K \\ L \end{pmatrix} = O \begin{pmatrix} P \\ T \end{pmatrix} = OF \begin{pmatrix} B' \\ R' \end{pmatrix} = OFU \begin{pmatrix} B \\ G \\ R \end{pmatrix} = M \begin{pmatrix} B \\ G \\ R \end{pmatrix}$$

Fig. 16.12: The diagram of Figure 16.1 supplemented by the set of all visible radiation stimuli Σ and the mappings Z, W, Y starting from Σ. The two heavy arrows indicate the two physiologically relevant mappings Z (eqs. (36) and (37)) and O (eqs. (34) or (39)). Z symbolizes the stimulus-excitation transfer of the retinal receptors (cones); O symbolizes the excitation transfer from the retinal receptors into the postreceptoral opponent channels. The row at the bottom indicates a possible way to arrive at the deuteranopic opponent-color space via the deuteranopic fundamental space through concatenations of mappings.

mediate stages such as $^3V_{BGR}$ and $^2V_{B'R'}$ do not possess an immediate physiological meaning. An example of path shaping is the concatenation $O = AF^{-1}$ (eq. (31)).

The transfer indicated by Z and O in Figure 16.12 may run the following way. The elements of the set Σ are radiation stimuli described by a spectral power density Φ_λ, where λ means wavelength of the radiation:

$$\Phi_\lambda \, d\lambda \in \Sigma. \quad (35)$$

Such stimuli (monochromatic or composite) impinge on the retinal cones and arouse the cone excitations P (*red* cones) and T (*blue* cones):

$$P = c_p \int_S^L \bar{p}(\lambda)\,\Phi_\lambda\,d\lambda \quad (36)$$

$$T = c_t \int_S^L \bar{t}(\lambda)\,\Phi_\lambda\,d\lambda \quad (37)$$

where $p(\lambda)$ and $t(\lambda)$ are spectral sensitivities (Fig. 16.10) of the two types of deuteranopic cones; c_p and c_t are normalizing constants. Formulae of this type are well known from the fundamentals of colorimetry (Wyszecki and Stiles, 1982); historically, they first seem to have appeared with the Viennese School under Exner, around the time of the first World War (Kohlrausch, 1920).

The cone excitations represented by the vector

$$\begin{pmatrix} P \\ T \end{pmatrix} \in {}^2V_{PT} \tag{38}$$

are transferred into two postreceptoral color-opponent channels described by

$$\begin{pmatrix} K \\ L \end{pmatrix} = O \begin{pmatrix} P \\ T \end{pmatrix}, \tag{39}$$

where K is the blue-yellow chrominance and L is the luminance. The matrix O is the opponency matrix for which a numerical example is given with eq. (34), cf. Figure 16.11. K and L constitute a vector in the deuteranopic opponent-color space ${}^2V_{KL}$:

$$\begin{pmatrix} K \\ L \end{pmatrix} \in {}^2V_{KL} \tag{40}$$

The blue-yellow chrominance K correlates perceptually with an antagonistic blue-yellow chroma, the luminance L correlates perceptually with brightness. In summary, the sequence of equations (35) to (40) provides a quite complete description of deuteranopia as a representative type of dichromacy.

16.9 A Synopsis of Dichromacy

The diagrams of Figures 16.1 and 16.12 apply specifically to deuteranopia. One could repeat them for protanopia and tritanopia, but we deal here only with the physiologically relevant mappings O_i, $i = p, d, t$, which map the fundamental color spaces to the opponent-color spaces. Figure 16.13 shows all three types of dichromacy with reference to the trichromatic fundamental system (P, D, T). P stands for protanopic missing color, D for deuteranopic and T for tritanopic missing color. These loci of the *fundamental primaries* (basis vectors) are arranged in an equilateral triangle. The excitation transfer is written the following way, where fundamental and opponent di-stimulus values are used:

Protanopia
$$\begin{pmatrix} K_p \\ L_p \end{pmatrix} = O_p \begin{pmatrix} D \\ T \end{pmatrix} \tag{41}$$

Deuteranopia
$$\begin{pmatrix} K_d \\ L_d \end{pmatrix} = O_d \begin{pmatrix} P \\ T \end{pmatrix} \tag{42}$$

Tritanopia
$$\begin{pmatrix} K_t \\ L_t \end{pmatrix} = O_t \begin{pmatrix} P \\ D \end{pmatrix} \tag{43}$$

In these equations, (D, T), (P, T), (P, D) are fundamental di-stimulus values, (K_p, L_p), (K_d, L_d), (K_t, L_t) are opponent di-stimulus values, K_p, K_d meaning blue-yellow chrominance, K_t meaning green-red chrominance, L_p, L_d, L_t meaning luminance. O_i, $i = p, d, t$ are 2×2 matrices, the opponency matrices. A numerical example for eq. (42) is eq. (34), Figure 16.11.

The primaries are transformed contragrediently, as in eq. (25):

$$(\boldsymbol{D}, \boldsymbol{T}) = (\boldsymbol{K}_p, \boldsymbol{L}_p)\, O_p \tag{41a}$$

$$(\boldsymbol{P}, \boldsymbol{T}) = (\boldsymbol{K}d, \boldsymbol{L}_d)\, O_d \tag{42a}$$

$$(\boldsymbol{P}, \boldsymbol{D}) = (\boldsymbol{K}t, \boldsymbol{L}_t)\, O_t \tag{43a}$$

(These matrix equations have already been transposed, hence the left-operating rows.)

The loci of the fundamental primaries, $\boldsymbol{P}, \boldsymbol{D}, \boldsymbol{T}$ form the corners of the fundamental color triangle (Fig. 16.13). Since the missing color vectors $\boldsymbol{P}, \boldsymbol{D}, \boldsymbol{T}$ and the luminance primaries $\boldsymbol{L}_p, \boldsymbol{L}_d, \boldsymbol{L}_t$ are by definition chrominance-free, they are incident with the corresponding neutral zones n_p, n_d, n_t (e.g., $\boldsymbol{P}$ and $\boldsymbol{L}_p$ lie on n_p, etc.). Similarly, missing colors and chrominance primaries are by definition luminance-free, hence they lie on the corresponding alychne traces ($\boldsymbol{P}$ and $\boldsymbol{K}_p$ on a_p, etc.).

Such a constellation implies a direct additive decomposition of any color into chrominance and luminance, which, in technical television, is the basic principle of black-white and color compatibility (Scheibner and Wolf, 1985, 1985/86; Scheibner, 1987). The six straight lines n_p, n_d, n_t, a_p, a_d, a_t are shown in Figure 16.13 as heavy rays. In protanopia and deuteranopia, the contribution of the *blue* retinal cones (T) to luminance can be neglected, so that T and a_d are also incident. Therefore, the rays a_p and a_d become sides, K_p and K_d become corners of the fundamental triangle. These important features are missing in tritanopia: a_t is not a side and K_t is not a corner of the fundamental triangle. One reason for this tritanopic disparity may be the greater similarity of tritanopia to normal trichromacy; for the tritanopic alychne, trace a_t is close to the trichromatic alychne trace, and the tritanopic neutral zone n_t resembles the hue *yellow* of the normal trichromat.

The reduction of trichromacy to a particular type of dichromacy implies the degeneration of the fundamental color triangle to the side that is left when the missing color is removed: side DT in protanopia, side PT in deuteranopia and side PD in tritanopia (Fig. 16.13). It may appear strange that all these dichromatic *chromaticity charts* lie outside the gamut of real colors, i.e., are imaginary. It is here that the dual point of view of regarding the pencil of rays through a point as the true elements of dichromatic chromaticities reveals its strength: on this view, reducing trichromacy to dichromacy means not removing the missing primary but removing the side of the color triangle opposite the missing primary. The pencil of rays through the missing primary does pass through the region of real colors, and at the same time illustrates the collapse from trichromacy to dichromacy.

A conspicuous feature of Figure 16.13 is that the three types of alychne traces a_p, a_d, and a_t intersect in a common point, the locus T. This property may indicate both the evolutionarily old function (Mollon and Jordan, 1988/89; Mollon, 1991) and the pivotal role (Scheibner, 1987) of the blue cone mechanism in postreceptoral processing.

It is generally accepted that protanopia and deuteranopia are loss dichromacies, i.e., the respective color mechanism is absent in the human fovea. For tritanopia (Wright, 1952; Barca, 1977), the situation does not seem to be completely clarified (Mollon, 1982; Alpern et al., 1983; Foster, 1991). In the present exposition, all three types of dichromacy are treated the same way by means of the missing color. This does not necessarily mean that tritanopia is a loss dichromacy because a psychophysical finding does not permit a unique inference about detailed neurophysiological mechanisms.

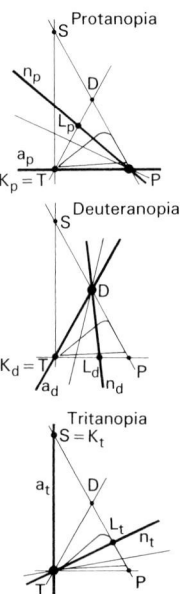

Fig. 16.13: Dichromatic vision. In each color chart, the corners of the equilateral triangle PDT are the chromaticities of the protanopic, deuteranopic, tritanopic missing colors, identified with the fundamental primaries. The rays n_p, n_d, n_t are the neutral zones, a_p, a_d, a_t are the alychne traces. K_i, i = p, d, t are the chromaticities of the dichromatic chrominance primaries (luminance-free), L_i, i = p, d, t are the chromaticities of the dichromatic luminance primaries (chrominance-free). The large filled circles are the vertices of the dichromatic chromaticity pencils. The point S may be interpreted as the copunctal point of a hypothetical fusion deuteranope exhibiting brightness sensation of the normal trichromat (and the tritanope).

16.10 A Lattice-Theoretical Classification of Dichromacy and Other Color Deficiencies

At the end of the 19th century, v. Kries (1897 a, b) reported the following interrelation between protanopia, deuteranopia and trichromacy, which according to him was already known: A trichromat accepts a color match both of a protanope and a deuteranope only if the protanope and the deuteranope accept the color match of the other. This finding and facts on classes of metameric color stimuli (*metamers*) suggest the following interpretation:

In the set Σ of color stimuli (Fig. 16.12), each type of observer induces a partition of Σ into classes of metameric stimuli by virtue of his perceptual criterion *indistinguishably equal*. This criterion works as an equivalence relation (Scheibner, 1968 a; 1968 b). The partitions of the various types of color observers form a so-called lattice (German: Verband) (Scheibner, 1968 a, 1970; cf. also Gericke, 1963; Szasz, 1963; Pracht, 1980). Making the simplest assumptions, the lattice of partitions assumes the shape shown in Figure 16.14. The partitions are designated by letters. The connecting lines and their intersections have the following lattice-theoretical meanings (Szasz, 1963):

The operation of *meet* (symbol Π) of two partitions results in the *highest* possible partition (point in the diagram) at which the lines leading *downward* meet; for example $D_p \Pi M_r = T$; $D_d \Pi T = T$.

The operation of *join* (symbol $\sqcup$) of two partitions results in the lowest possible partition at which the lines leading *upward* join; for example $D_p \sqcup M_r = \{\Sigma\}$; $T \sqcup D_d = D_d$.

The operation $M_b \Pi D_p = D_p$ implies the relation of refinement $D_p < M_b$ between the two partitions, etc.

The *lattice*-theoretical operation of *meet* rests on the *set*-theoretical intersection of classes the elements of which are metamers here. An experimental implementation are the confrontation experiments reported by v. Kries (1897a, b). According to the same procedure, attempts have been reported to establish a connection between normal trichromacy, anomalous trichromacy and dichromacy (Scheibner et al., 1972; Scheibner, 1974a, b, c; Scheibner and Boll, 1972; 1974).

The transfer of the lattice-theoretical operations and relations to the structures (spaces) of Figure 16.12 requires modifying their definition. Thus, the concepts inherent in Figures 16.12 and 16.14 may join together in a natural way and open new insights.

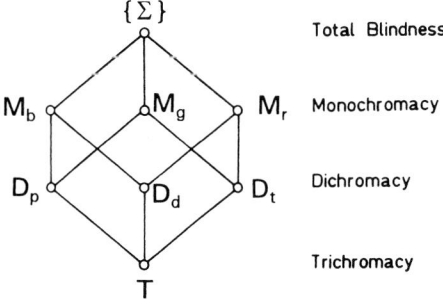

Fig. 16.14: The lattice of color stimulus partitions. Σ, set of visible radiation stimuli; $\{\Sigma\}$, coarsest partition, amaurosis; M_b, M_g, M_r, partitions of blue-cone monochromats, green-cone monochromats, red-cone monochromats; D_p, D_d, D_t, partitions of protanopes, deuteranopes, tritanopes; T, finest partition, of trichromats.

16.11 Concluding Remarks

The preceding exposition demonstrates a *linear* description of dichromacy. This certainly justifies the statement in the title of a *simple* structure. Moreover, the linearity is fulfilled quite well. This is due to the compression of the dimension of the color space from 3 to 2, which hides non-linearities. For instance, the Abney effect is hardly noticeable (Knottenberg and Scheibner, 1993).

The main statements concern dichromatic opponent-color spaces, the determination of which rests on the fact that two dichromatic color attributes, chroma and brightness, can be perceived and quantified. Embedding in a three-dimensional color space makes it possible to determine a null-chrominance plane and a null-luminance plane, both of which intersect in the missing color, a one-dimensional subspace that represents a carrier of a bundle of dual planes.

A noticeable deviation from the two-dimensional nature of dichromatic color vision may emerge if the visual field is larger than foveal, in which case an additional red-green discrimination becomes effective in protanopia and deuteranopia (Scheibner and Boynton, 1968; Orazem and Scheibner, 1995). Hence, classical requirements for a simple expression and description of dichromacy (and trichromacy) are the following: foveal visual field, unrelated and free colors (cf. Scheibner, 1990; Kaiser and Boynton, 1996), and a photopic light level.

The claim that dichromacy is the *simplest* type of color vision may have the basis that, operationally, only one chromatic perceptual criterion is applied, the other criteria being free of a predicate concerning chromaticness. It is true that the chromatic criterion captures two (antagonistic) hues. But this seems to be an inherent property of human color vision. A monochromatic color vision (Scheibner, 1968b) seems inconceivable.

The preceding exposition, in particular Figure 16.13, also demonstrates the importance of the dichromatic alychne trace: it is an imaginary confusion line. One primary of a dichromatic opponent-color space is real, the other is imaginary. The extension to a trichromatic opponent-color space adds one imaginary primary (Scheibner and Wolf, 1985).

An interesting aspect would be to develop the dual character of confusion lines further (section 16.5). Some initial attempts have been reported elsewhere (Scheibner, 1993; Scheibner and Orazem, 1997).

16.12 Summary

Dichromacy is treated as a reduced form of normal trichromacy. Experimentally, the required transformations are determined by means of three perceptual criteria, which single out the kernels of the desired mappings. The kernels are the *missing color*, the null-chrominance plane (the *neutral zone*) and the null-luminance plane (the *alychne*). Deuteranopia is discussed in detail, the perceptual criteria being *indistinguishably equal, neither blue nor yellow and equally bright*. The chain of events starts with the radiation stimulus, goes on to the excitation of retinal cones and ends with the excitation of an opponent-color channel and a luminance channel.

Acknowledgements

The experimental data of this report were taken from the thesis of Arnd Orazem. I thank him for his good cooperation. Thanks are also due to Sinclair Cleveland for critical reading and helpful suggestions.

References

Alpern, M., Kitahara, K., and Krantz, D. H. (1983). Classical tritanopia. J. Physiol. *335*, 655–681.

Barca, L. (1977). Sguardo bibliografico al problema della tritanopia. Fondazione "Giorgio Ronchi", no. XLIII, Baccini & Chiappi, Firenze, Italia.

Beck, J. and Richter, M. (1958). Neukonstruktion des Dreifarbenmeßgerätes nach Guild-Bechstein. Die Farbe *7*, 141–152.

Boynton, R. M. (1978). Ten years of research with the minimally distinct border. In: Armington, J. C., Krauskopf, J. G., and Wooten, B. R. (eds.) Visual Psychophysics and physiology. Academic Press, New York.

Boseck, H. (1984). Einführung in die Theorie der linearen Vektorräume. Deutscher Verlag der Wissenschaften, Berlin.

Brainard, D. H. (1995). Colorimetry. In: Bass, M. (Ed. in Chief) Handbook of Optics. 2nd Edition. Vol. I chapt. 26. McGraw-Hill, New York.

Bruckwilder, R. and Scheibner H. (1988/89). Spektralwerte des Protanopen, insbesondere ihre Bestimmung bei minimaler Buntsättigung. Die Farbe *35/36*, 215–258.

DeMarco, P., Pokorny, J. and Smith, V. C. (1992). Full-spectrum cone sensitivity functions for X-chromosome-linked anomalous trichromats. J. Opt. Soc. Am. A *9*, 1465–1476.

Estévez, O. (1982). A better colorimetric standard observer for color vision studies: The Stiles and

Burch 2° color matching functions. Color Res. Applic. *7*, 131–134.

Exner, F. (1920). Zur Kenntnis der Grundempfindungen im Helmholtz'schen Farbensystem, Sitzungsber. Akad. Wiss. Wien, Abt. IIa, *129*, 27–46.

Foster, D. H. (Ed.) (1991). Inherited and Acquired Colour Vision Deficiencies: Fundamental aspects and Clinical Studies. MacMillan Press, London.

Gericke, H. (1963). Theorie der Verbände. Bibliograph. Institut, Mannheim.

Gouras, P. (ed.) (1991). The Perception of Colour. CRC Press, Boca Raton, FL.

Guth, S. L. (1991). Model for color vision and light adaptation. J. Opt. Soc. Am. A *8*, 976–993.

Heinsius, E. (1973). Farbsinnstörungen und ihre Prüfung in der Praxis. Enke, Stuttgart.

Helmholtz, H. L. F. von (1909–1911). Handbuch der physiologischen Optik. 3rd Edition, 3 Vols. Voss, Hamburg.

Hering, E. (1874). Zur Lehre vom Lichtsinn. Sechste Mitteilung, Grundzüge einer Theorie des Farbensinnes. Sitzungsber. Kaiserl. Akad. Wiss. Wien (Mathem. Nat. Classe Abth. III) *70*, 169–204.

Hurvich, L. M. (1981). Color Vision. Sinauer, Sunderland Mass.

Kaiser, P. K. and Boynton, R. M. (1996). Human Color Vision. 2nd Edition. Optical Society of America, Washington D.C.

Klauder, C.-A. (1983/84). Gegenfarbensehen und Grundspektralwerte des Protanopen. Die Farbe *31*, 339–389.

Knottenberg, T. and Scheibner, H. (1993). Berücksichtigung des Abney-Effekts im Rahmen der linearen Gegenfarbentheorie. Opthalmologe *90*, 155–160.

Köllner, H. (1912). Die Störungen des Farbensinnes, ihre klinische Bedeutung und ihre Diagnose. Karger, Berlin.

König, A. (1903). Gesammelte Abhandlungen zur Physiologischen Optik. Barth, Leipzig.

König, A. and Dieterici, C. (1893). Die Grundempfindungen und ihre Intensitätsverteilung im Spectrum. Zeitschr. Psychol. Physiol. Sinnesorgane *4*, 221–347.

Kohlrausch, K. W. F. (1920). Beiträge zur Farbenlehre I. Physikal. Zeitschrift *21*, 396–403.

Kostrikin, A. I. and Manin, Y. I. (1989). Linear algebra and geometry. Gordon & Breach, New York.

Krastel, H. (1995). Farbsinn. In: Straub, W., Kroll, P., and Küchle, H. J. (eds.) Augenärztliche Untersuchungsmethoden. F. Enke, Stuttgart, pp. 537–566.

Kries, J. von (1897a). Über Farbensysteme. Z. Psychol. u. Physiol. d. Sinnesorg. *13*, 241–324.

Kries, J. von (1897b). Über die dichromatischen Farbensysteme (partielle Farbenblindheit). Zentralblatt Physiol. *10*, 148–152.

Kröger, A. and Scheibner, H. (1977). Reduktion der Deuteranopie aus der Trichromasie. Ber. Dtsch. Ophthal. Gesellsch., Verlag Bergmann, München, *75*, 515–517.

Kröger-Paulus, A. (1980). Reduktion der Deuteranopie aus der normalen Trichromasie. Die Farbe *28*, 73–116.

LeGrand, Y. (1957). Light, Colour and Vision. Chapman & Hall, London. Second French Edition: Lumière et Couleurs, Masson, Paris, 1972.

Marré, M. and Marré, E. (1986). Erworbene Störungen des Farbensehens. Fischer, Stuttgart.

Maxwell, J. C. (1855). Experiments on colour, as perceived by the eye, with remarks on colour-blindness. Trans. Roy. Soc. (Edinburgh) *21*, 275–298.

Mollon, J. D. (1982). A taxonomy of tritanopias. In: Verriest, G. (ed.) Colour Vision Deficiencies IV, Junk, The Hague NL, pp. 87–101.

Mollon, J. D. (1991). Uses and Evolutionary Origins of Primate Colour Vision. In: Cronly-Dillon, J. R. and Gregory, R. L. (eds.) Evolution of the Eye and Visual System. MacMillan Press, London, pp. 306–319.

Mollon, J. D. and Jordan, G. (1988/89). Eine evolutionäre Interpretation des menschlichen Farbensehens. Die Farbe *35/36*, 139–170.

Müller, G. E. (1924). Darstellung und Erklärung der verschiedenen Typen der Farbenblindheit. Vandenhoeck & Ruprecht, Göttingen.

Nuberg, N. D. and Yustova, E. N. (1958). Researches on dichromatic vision and the spectral sensitivity of the receptors of trichromats. In: National Physical Laboratory (ed.) Visual problems of colour. Vol. 2, Her Majesty's Stationary Office, London, pp. 477–486.

Ohta, Y. (ed.) (1990). Color Vision Deficiencies. Kugler & Ghedini, Amstelveen NL.

Oleari, C., Baratta, G., Lamedica, A., and Macaluso, C. (1996). Confusion points and constant-luminance planes for trichromats, protanopes and deuteranopes. Vision Res. *36*, 3501–3505.

Orazem, A. and Scheibner, H. (1995). Deuteranopia under conditions of a large field. In: Drum, B. (ed.) Colour Vision Deficiencies XII, Kluwer, Dordrecht NL.

Paulus, W. (1977). Fehlfarben und Alychnen von Protanopen und Protanomalen und ihre Bedeutung für das Farbensehen der normalen Trichromaten. Die Farbe *27*, 59–127.

Pitt, F. H. G. (1935). Characteristics of dichromatic

vision. With an appendix on anomalous trichromatic vision. Special Report Series, No. 200. His Majesty's Stationery Office, London.
Plaumann, P. and Strambach, K. (eds.) (1981). Geometry – von Staudt's point of view. D. Reidel, Dordrecht NL.
Pokorny, J. and Smith, V. C. (1986). Colorimetry and Color Discrimination. In: Boff, K. R., Kaufman, L., and Thomas, J. P. (eds.) Handbook of Perception and Human Performance. Vol. I, Chapt. 8, Wiley, New York.
Pokorny, J., Smith, V. C., Verriest, G., and Pinckers, A. J. L. G. (eds.) (1979). Congenital and Acquired Color Vision Defects. Grune & Stratton, New York.
Pracht, E. (1980). Algebra der Verbände. F. Schöningh, Paderborn.
Rosmanit, J. (1914). Anleitung zur Feststellung der Farbentüchtigkeit. Deuticke, Leipzig u. Wien.
Rushton, W. A. H. (1965). A foveal pigment in the deuteranope. J. Physiology 176, 24–37.
Scheibner, H. (1968a). Klasseneinteilungen von Farbreizen als Ordnungsprinzip von Farbsinnstörungen. Ber. Dtsch. Ophthal. Gesellsch., Verlag Bergmann, München 68, 281–284.
Scheibner, H. (1968b). Trichromasie, Dichromasie, Monochromasie. Optica Acta 15, 329–338.
Scheibner, H. (1968c). Dichromasie als Homomorphismus der Trichromasie. Optica Acta 15, 339–349.
Scheibner, H. (1970). A lattice-theoretical classification of normal and defective colour vision. In: AIC (ed.) Ber. Intern. Farbtag. COLOR 69, Stockholm 1969, Muster-Schmidt, Göttingen, pp. 67–73.
Scheibner, H. (1974a). Untersuchungen zur Deuteranomalie. Ber. Dtsch. Ophthal. Gesellsch, Verlag Bergmann, München 72, 290–295.
Scheibner, H. (1974b). Untersuchungen zur Protanomalie: Chrominanz und Leuchtdichte. Optica Acta 21, 375–385.
Scheibner, H. (1974c). Eine verbandstheoretische Klassifikation der Protanomalie und Deuteranomalie. Optica Acta 21, 489–496.
Scheibner, H. (1976). Missing colours (Fehlfarben) of deuteranopes and extreme deuteranomalous observers. In: Verriest, G. (ed.) Colour Vision Deficiencies III, Karger, Basel, pp. 21–26.
Scheibner, H. (1987). Opponent-colour vision in relation to perceptual criteria. Die Farbe 34, 243–252.
Scheibner, H. (1990). Was ist Farbe? Phänomenologie und Physiologie des Farbensehens. Galvanotechnik $81/5$, 3–10.
Scheibner, H. (1993). Transformation of luminance coefficients. J. Opt. Soc. Am. A 10, 1392–1395.
Scheibner, H. and Boynton, R. M. (1968). Residual Red-Green Discrimination in Dichromats. J. Opt. Soc. Am. 58, 1151–1158.
Scheibner, H., Kellermann, F.-J., and Boll, M. (1972). Untersuchungen zur Protanopie und Protanomalie. Ber. Dtsch. Ophthal. Gesellsch., Verlag Bergmann, München 71, 522–530.
Scheibner, H. and Boll, M. (1972). Untersuchungen zur Deuteranopie und Deuteranomalie. A. v. Graefes Arch. Klin. ex. Ophthal. 185, 145–150.
Scheibner, H. and Boll, M. (1974). Untersuchungen zur Protanomalie: Farbart. Optica Acta 21, 365–374.
Scheibner, H. and Paulus, W. (1978). An analysis of protanopic colour vision. In: Verriest, G. (ed.) Colour Vision Deficiencies IV, Karger, Basel, pp. 206–211.
Scheibner, H. and Wolf, E. (1985). Psychophysik und Physiologie des Farbensehens. In: Bodmann, H.-W. (ed.) Aspekte der Informationsverarbeitung, Funktion des Sehsystems und technische Bilddarbietung. Springer-Verlag, Berlin etc., pp. 1–65.
Scheibner, H. and Wolf, E. (1985/86). Grundzüge einer linearen Farbentheorie. Die Farbe $22/23$, 209–234.
Scheibner, H. and Lochner, D. (1991). Subspaces of an opponent-color space define chrominance and luminance channels. In: Blum, B. (ed.) Channels in the visual nervous system: Neuphysiology, psychophysics and models. Freund, London and Tel Aviv.
Scheibner, H. and Kremer, T. (1996). Deuteranomaly studied with four perceptual criteria. Vision Res. 36, 3157–3166.
Scheibner, H. and Orazem, A. (1997a). Features of foveal dichromacy illustrated by deuteranopia. In: Cavonius, C. R. (ed.) Colour Vision Deficiencies XIII, Kluwer, Dordrecht NL, pp. 245–259.
Scheibner, H. and Orazem, A. (1997b). Linear Models of Dichromacy. In: Dickinson, C. M., Murray, I. J., and Carden, D. (eds.) John Dalton's Colour Vision Legacy. Taylor & Francis, London.
Scheufens, P. (1983/84). Fehlfarben, Alychnen und Konvergenz-Abgleiche von Deuteranopen bei großer Reizfläche. Die Farbe 31, 257–337.
Scheufens, P. and Scheibner, H. (1984). Mesopic deuteranopic vision with a large observation field. In: Verriest, G. (ed.) Colour Vision Deficiencies VII, Dr. W. Junk Publishers, The Hague NL, pp. 311–318.
Schrödinger, E. (1920). Grundlagen einer Theorie der Farbenmetrik im Tagesehen I. Annal. Physik, $IV/63$, 397–456.

Schrödinger, E. (1925). Über das Verhältnis der Vierfarben- zur Dreifarbentheorie. Sitzungsber. Akad. Wiss. Wien (IIa) *134*, 471–490.

Staudt, K. G. C. von (1847). Geometrie der Lage. Verlag von Bauer und Raspe, Nürnberg.

Stiles, W. S. and Burch, J. M. (1959). NPL colour-matching investigation final report. Optica Acta *6*, 1–26.

Stockman, A., MacLeod, D. I. A., and Johnson, N. E. (1993). Spectral sensitivities of the human cones. J. Opt. Soc. Am. A *10*, 2491–2521.

Szasz, G. (1963). Introduction to lattice theory. Academie Press, New York, p. 33.

Thoma, W. (1982). Trennlinien-Deutlichkeit und tritanopische Buntsättigung. Die Farbe *30*, 167–197.

Valberg, A. and Lee, B. B. (eds.) (1991). From pigments to perception. Plenum Press, New York.

Vos, J. J., Estévez, O., and Walraven, P. L. (1990). Improved color fundamentals offer a new view on photometric additivity. Vision Res. *30*, 937–943.

Wandell, B. A. (1995). Foundations of Vision. Sinauer, Sunderland Mass.

Wright, W. D. (1946). Researches on normal and defective colour vision. Kimpton, London.

Wright, W. D. (1952). The Characteristics of Tritanopia. J. Opt. Soc. Am. *42*, 509–521.

Wright, W. D. (1972). Colour Mixture. In: Jameson, D. and Hurvich, L. M. (eds.) Visual Psychophysics. Handbook of Sensory Physiology, Vol. VII/4, chapt. 16. Springer-Verlag, Berlin.

Wyszecki, G. and Stiles, W. S. (1982). Color Science, 2nd Edition. Wiley, New York.

Zeki, S. (1993). A Vision of the Brain, Blackwell, London.

17. Current CIE Work to Achieve Physiologically-Correct Color Metrics

János Schanda

17.1 Introduction

Colorimetry became technically useful when in 1931 the CIE standardized the color-matching functions for the 2° observer and some illuminant spectral power distributions to be used with reflecting colored samples (Recommendation officielles de la Commission Internationale de l'Eclairage, 1931). The CIE 1931 color-matching functions have been used since then in a practically unchanged form. They have been interpolated, smoothed at one point or the other, their numeric values have been fixed to seven significant digits, but fundamentally everything stayed unchanged. This is the case, despite the fact that it has been known for a considerable time that the $\bar{y}(\lambda)$ function, which is identical with the $V(\lambda)$ function, defined in 1924 (Principales Décisions de la Commission Internationale de l'Eclairage, 1924), is in error in the blue part of the spectrum (Judd, 1951). This discrepancy in the $V(\lambda)$ function was acknowledged in 1988, when CIE published the spectral luminous efficiency function for photopic vision for the supplementary 2° observer (CIE Technical Report, 1988) often called the "Judd correction". The different observers do not produce significantly different luminous flux values for general purpose light sources (Schanda, 1989), therefore the CIE 1988 2° function is more of theoretical significance then of practical importance. It is, however, widely used by vision scientists to compare experimental results.

Unfortunately, the Judd corrections were not consequently implemented to correct also the $\bar{x}(\lambda)$ and $\bar{z}(\lambda)$ functions and no "Judd corrected" color-matching functions have been standardized. This resulted in the fact that color vision researchers, who have to apply some corrections to the 1931 standard color-matching functions, use slightly different corrections. This adds to the experimental differences encountered in all such investigations and makes the comparison of the results more complicated.

The endeavor of vision scientists and colorimetrists has been always to deduce the color-matching functions from basic photo-biological response functions. Therefore, when CIE realized above uncertainty it established in 1991 its Technical Committee TC 1-36, "Fundamental Chromaticity Diagram with Physiologically Significant Axes" and entrusted it to develop a chromaticity diagram where the coordinates correspond to physiologically-significant axes. It was hoped that by combining fundamental biological and psychophysical research results it might be possible to come up with a colorimetric system that is firmly based on fundamental research results and reflects human vision mechanisms.

One can assume that the mental response to a light stimulus will be related to the photochemical process taking place within the photoreceptors, for color vision in the cones. Thus, for our purpose the cone-excitation spectrum, assumed to be proportional to the absorption of the photopigments in the cones, is the fundamental visual process. One can assume that these processes obey the laws of physics and chemistry. CIE TC 1-36 has not intended to go beyond this point in the assessment of the visual signal by the human observer.

Psychophysical experiments can be done only with radiation reaching the outer layer of the eye, the absorption of the ocular media between the outer layer of the cornea and the photopigments will distort the spectrum of the cone-excitation spectra and this has to be determined. The spectral sensitivities traced back to this input point of the eye will be called "fundamentals".

With psychophysical measurements we perform color matches, and the functions needed to obtain such color matches are called "color-matching functions" (cmf's).

We will distinguish in the next sections of this paper between the psychophysical *color-matching functions*, their transformation into a system that reflects human processing, but at the entrance of the eye as *fundamental sensitivity spectra* (or shortly *fundamentals*) and the physico-chemico-biological photopigment absorption/photo-signal excitation process related *photopigment absorption spectra or cone-excitation spectra*.

17.2 Cone Excitation Spectra

To determine the primary physiological color vision mechanism, i.e., the cone photopigment absorption spectra, is not that easy. Microspectrophotometric measurements of human retinal tissue (Dartnall et al., 1983) have shown that there are three distinctly different photopigments in the human cones. The measurements show reasonable agreement with so-called suction electrode photoelectric measurements (Schnapf et al., 1987) obtained on monkey cone cells where the

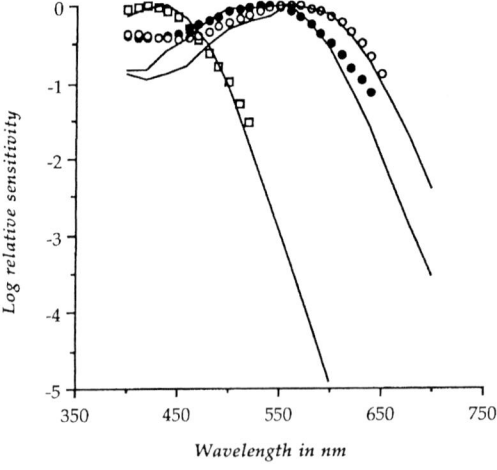

Fig. 17.1: Microspectrophotometric absorption spectra of human cones compared with suction electrode photoelectric measurements obtained on monkey cone cells.

minute electric currents produced by the illuminated cone sucked into a micropipette were investigated (see Fig. 17.1). Thus, from physiological measurements one can assume that the cones of the human retina contain three different photopigments, where two have rather similar spectral sensitivity and the third one is distinctly different. It is usual to call the three cone sensitivities as Long-Wave Sensitive (or L-) cone, Medium-Wave Sensitive (or M-) cone and Short-Wave Sensitive (or S-) cone sensitivity (see e.g., Stockman et al., 1993). (In older literature we find also the symbols R(ed), G(reen) and B(lue), or to distinguish them from real lights the symbols ρ, γ and σ are used to identify these visual sensitivities.) The precision of direct physiological investigations is not sufficient to develop from these measurements cone-excitation functions with an accuracy high enough to be used to model the visual mechanism. They serve merely for comparison with cone sensitivity functions derived from psychophysical experiments (e.g., heterochromatic brightness-matching experiments, taking Königs hypothesis into consideration, see later).

Thus, CIE TC 1-36 was faced with the problem to select those psychophysical experiments that show the highest accuracy and to derive a mechanism of transforming these data into cone excitation spectra.

17.2.1 Choice of the Color-Matching Functions

To obtain color-matching functions (cmf's) there are basically two methods; one is called Maxwell matching, where a white reference light is matched with the additive mixture of three monochromatic lights, and the wavelength of one of the lights is systematically scanned along the spectrum, setting the color matches for every selected wavelength. The other is the so-called maximum saturation method, where three, mutually independent colored lights (e.g., a red, a green and a blue one) are selected and their additive mixture is matched to a monochromatic light, which is again scanned along the spectrum. The theoretical set up for this experiment is depicted in Figure 17.2.

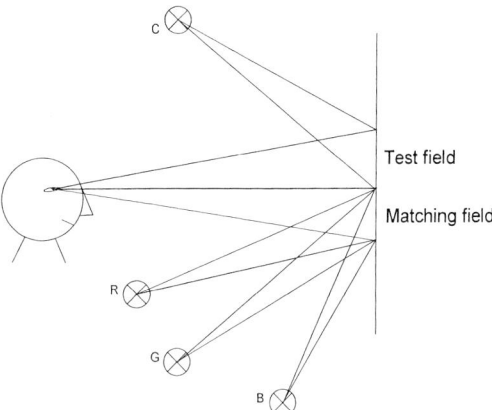

Fig. 17.2: Theoretical layout of a maximum saturation color-matching experiment.

Most of the experiments to determine cmf's have been done by this second method, and it has been shown that their results agree reasonably well with those obtained using the Maxwell match, although there are some slight, still unexplained discrepancies in some particular sections of the chromaticity diagram (for a summary see e.g., Robertson, 1993).

There are two sets of experiments to obtain cmf's with special importance: Those concerned with the original CIE standard, i.e., focused on the determination of the 2° observer and those using larger visual fields, namely field sizes of about 10° visual angle. The first ones were supposed to sample only the cones, but were individually biased due to differences in the macular pigmentation of the observer. The second ones suffered from rod intrusion, as at larger visual angles the retina contains an increasing number of rods, and if the retinal illuminance is not high enough the color match is influenced by the rod excitation as well. This leads to a tetrachromatic color match showing many complications (Trezona, 1993).

After careful check of all the published cmf's, TC 1-36 decided to start with the 10° cmf's determined by Stiles and Burch (Stiles, 1955; Stiles and Burch, 1959) as well as Speranskaya (1959). When the CIE average 10° observer cmf's were calculated, different weights were assigned to the two sets of data, depending on the number of observers used. Correction was also made for rod intrusion. The Stiles-Burch and Speranskaya data also have the advantage that they have been derived by purely radiometric and colorimetric means. In case of the CIE 1931 observer the three matching lights were measured for their luminance and thus an arbitrary photometric connection was introduced (Robertson, 1993).

It is well known that individual cmf's show considerable scatter. It was always thought that averaging these individual curves will lead to a value more representative of the average observer. Recent photo-biological research has shown that there are individual differences in the λ_{max} of the L- and M-cone pigments found in both dichromats and color-normal subjects (Neitz et al., 1991; Sanocki et al., 1993), ranging for deuteranopes about 4.3 nm and for protanopes about 3.5 nm. Thus, the L pigments should be more heterogeneous than the M pigments, causing the L-cone fundamental to be more variable than the M-cone fundamental, leading to a broader averaged L-cone response spectrum. In the comparison of the derived fundamental response curves with pigment absorption curves this should be taken into account.

17.2.2 Deriving L-, M-, S-Cone Excitation Spectra from Color-Matching Data

The measured cmf's depend on the primary lights used. Based on Grassmann's laws (1853), the cmf's determined under one set of primaries can be transformed into cmf's of another set of primaries. All sets of primaries are in this respect equally valid. Thus, from the measurement of cmf's alone the fundamental cone excitation primaries cannot be determined, only a linear transformation of them. The postulate that CIE TC 1-36 uses to derive the cone excitations from the cmf's is the assumption of the validity of König's postulate (1886), according to which dichromatic vision is a reduced form of trichromatic vision where one cone response is missing and two others are left unchanged in spectral sensitivity. Stockman et al. (1993) have grounded this postulate experimentally.

Many investigations were conducted to determine the dichromatic confusion loci. One of the most extensive evaluations and determinations of fundamentals can be found in the work of Vos and co-workers (1990), who optimized the location of the dichromatic confusion loci based on the available literature using the Stiles-Burch 2° pilot data set (Trezona, 1984).

There has been a long debate in the literature and in the committee whether S-cones contribute to the luminance sensation or not. There is evidence that luminance-like signals (flicker photometry, distinctness of border, task performance, etc.) show a spectral sensitivity similar to $V(\lambda)$, and that this spectral sensitivity is composed of the L-cone and M-cone signals (Lennie et al., 1993). These two cone types seem to be narrowly related to each other, most probably they became distinctly different only at a late stage of evolution, while the S-cones behave in a number of cases differently. All theses differences, mainly based on time-dependent variations of some effects (e.g., chromatic adaptation, flicker rate, intensity dependence), coupled with psychophysical color-matching results, help in developing experiments to derive fundamental excitation spectra.

Before we discuss the practical manipulation of the cmf's to derive cone-excitation spectra, we have to deal with the different absorption mechanisms changing the spectral power distribution of the color stimulus reaching the outer surface of the eye throughout its path to the retina.

17.2.3 Intra-Ocular Screening

Psychophysical experiments can determine the fundamental response spectra only outside the eye. The absorption of photons leading to the cone action spectra takes place at the retina. The selective absorption in the lens and macular pigment, self-screening in the outer segments of the cones (depending on the optical density of the pigments), waveguide effects, etc. have to be considered before the actual cone-excitation spectra can be derived.

17.2.3.1 Absorption by the Macular Pigment

Several investigations have been described in the literature both on the local distribution of the macular pigment and its spectral distribution. Analyzing the experiments, the committee decided to use density spectrum suggested by Vos (1972), correcting only for the maximum density. Figure 17.3 shows the wavelength dependence of the macular pigment density after Vos (1972).

Regarding the local distribution of the macular pigmentation, the committee considers a slightly modified version of the curve proposed by Moreland and Bhatt (1984), which can be described by the following equation:

$$D_{max} = 0{,}6243 \cdot 10^{(-\text{Diameter}/7{,}957)}$$

This equation can be used in the range of 1 to 10 degree diameters. Macular pigmentation seems to stay unchanged after early childhood (Werner et al., 1987; Bone et al., 1988), thus no age related function is used.

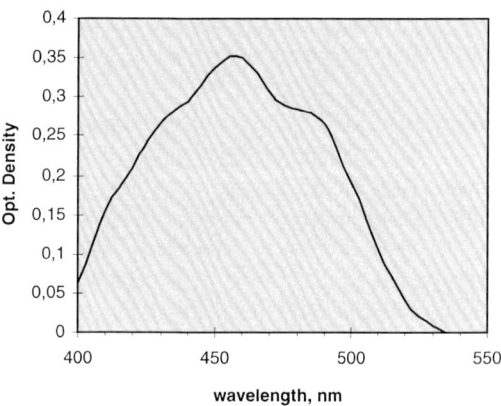

Fig. 17.3: Wavelength dependence of the macular pigment density, after Vos (1972).

17.2.3.2 Absorption of the Lens

The committee proposes to use the data as derived by Stockman et al. (1993) for considering the spectral density of the eye lens (see Fig. 17.4). This curve has a steep rise below 450 nm. It is known that the eye lens optical density increases with age (Pokorny et al., 1987; Weale, 1988;

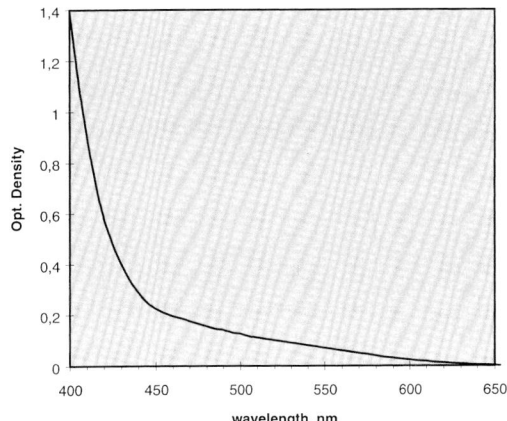

Fig. 17.4: Wavelength dependence of the lens optical density, after Stockman et al. (1993)

Werner, 1982). The committee decided to use the Pokorny et al. (1987) data. The committee has not decided yet on this age related effect (i.e., as a first recommendation the cone-excitation spectra will be calculated from experiments with young observers).

17.2.3.3 Change of the Optical Density of the Photopigments with Field Size

The effective optical density of the photopigments decreases with increasing eccentricity of the incoming radiation. It is not quite clear for the moment whether this is a real decrease of the pigment density or whether it is due to a length change of the cones. Biological investigations show that with increasing eccentricity the cones become shorter and this will lead to a decrease of the effective density. The committee has not yet reached final agreement on this eccentricity correction, although it will be important, together with the macular pigment absorption distribution in formulating cmf's for different field sizes.

A possible candidate for the visual pigment optical density distribution in the eccentricity range $30' < d < 10°$ is, according to Pokorny and Smith (1976):

For L-cones: $OD_L = 0.25 + 0.8825 \cdot e^{(-d/1.333)}$,

and

for M-cones: $OD_M = 0.15 + 0.8825 \cdot e^{(-d/1.333)}$.

17.2.4 Derivation of the Fundamental Response Curves

To get an understanding of the photochemical processes in the human retina in a form useful for practical colorimetry one has to start from two directions: From the external world by transforming the cmf's into fundamental spectral sensitivity functions, and comparing these with the fundamentals reached by folding theoretical cone absorption spectra with the transmission spectra of the ocular media as described in the previous section.

Based on Grassmann's laws, the fundamentals have to be a linear transformation of the cmf's:

$$\begin{vmatrix} L(\lambda) \\ M(\lambda) \\ S(\lambda) \end{vmatrix} = \begin{vmatrix} a_{11} & a_{12} & a_{13} \\ a_{21} & a_{22} & a_{23} \\ a_{31} & a_{32} & a_{33} \end{vmatrix} \cdot \begin{vmatrix} \bar{r}(\lambda) \\ \bar{g}(\lambda) \\ \bar{b}(\lambda) \end{vmatrix}$$

As already mentioned, according to the König postulate dichromatic vision is assumed to be identified by the loss of one of the three response systems.

A straightforward method of determining the chromaticity of the missing cone mechanism is to find the copunctual point for a class of dichromats in the chromaticity diagram (i.e., the convergence point of those straight lines that represent the confusable colors for that class of dichromats). Figure 17.5 shows according to Judd and Wyszecki's (1975) measurements the protanopic, deuteranopic and tritanopic confusion lines in a CIE 1931 chromaticity diagram. An alternate way of determining the copunctual points for protanopes and deuteranopes is a derivation from their luminosity curves.

By establishing the copunctual points for the three classes of dichromats, one obtains six of the nine coefficients required for the linear transformation from cmf's to the three fundamentals. The remaining coefficients can be obtained from considering the relative contribution of the L- and M-cones to the luminosity function. Stockman et al. (1993), (see below), constructed the luminosity function in the following way: $Y = 1.83 L + M$. CIE TC-1-36 is also considering to incorporate in the transformation equation the constraint that equal-energy white should have equal L, M, S coordinates, just as in the CIE system.

A further theoretical consideration the committee made was to apply spectral absorption templates. The most recent proposal by Lamb (1995) provides the following equation for the shape of the absorption curves:

$$S(x) = 1/[\exp a(A - x) + \exp b(B - x) + \exp c(C - x) + D]$$

where $x = v/v_{max} = \lambda_{max}/\lambda$ and $a = 70$; $b = 28.5$; $c = -14.1$; $A = 0.880$; $B = 0.924$; $C = 1.104$; $D = 0.655$.

It is anticipated that such theoretical correction

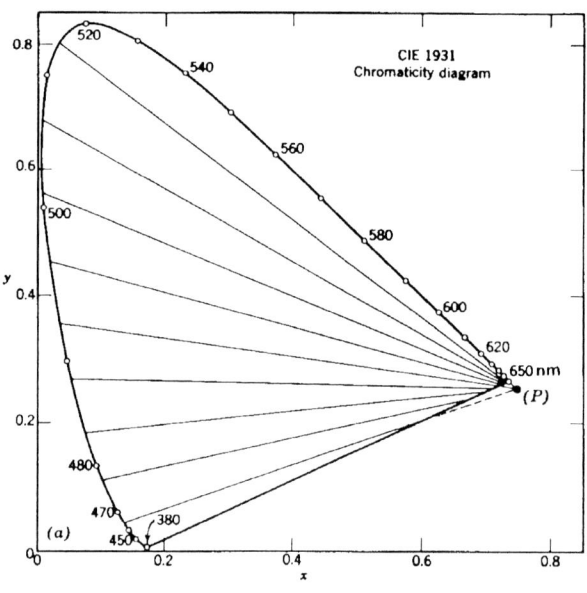

Fig. 17.5 a: Lines of constant protanopic chromaticities in the normal trichromat's chromaticity diagram.

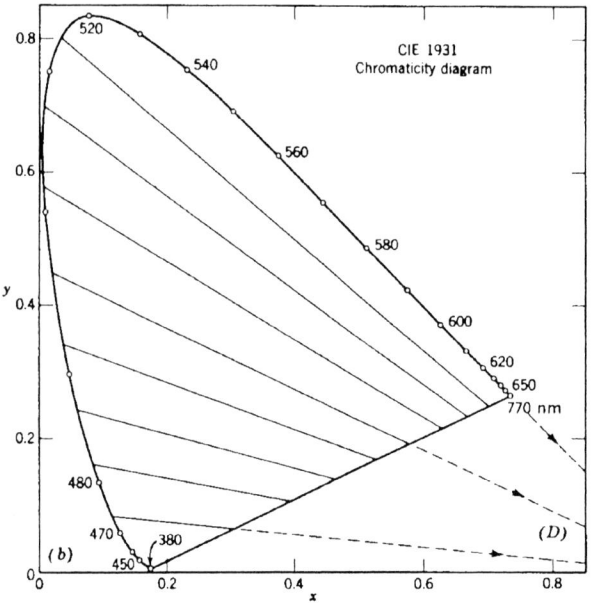

Fig. 17.5 b: Lines of constant deuteranopic chromaticities in the normal trichromat's chromaticity diagram.

17.2 Cone Excitation Spectra

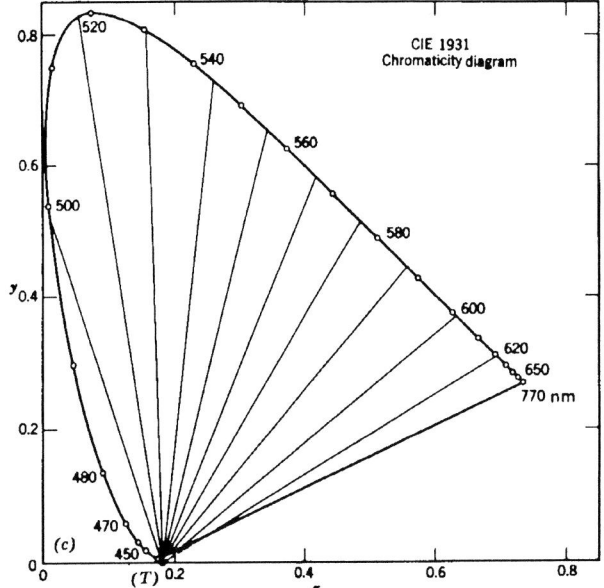

Fig. 17.5 c: Lines of constant tritanopic chromaticities in the normal trichromat's chromaticity diagram.

might be used to adjust and smooth cone-excitation spectra derived from cmf's, correcting these with the ocular media absorption and self screening.

CIE TC 1-36 contemplates to use the Stiles-Burch (1959) and Speranskaya (1959) data in the form as averaged to reach the CIE 1964 supplementary standard observer (10° observer) (Commission Internationale d'Eclairage, 1986; ISO/CIE, 1991). One possibility is to take the transformation to reach fundamentals as published by Stockman et al. (1993), based on the assumption that the S-fundamental does not contribute to luminance.

$L(\lambda) = 0.236157\, x_{10} + 0.826427\, y_{10} - 0.045710\, z_{10}$

$M(\lambda) = -0.431117\, x_{10} + 1.206922\, y_{10} + 0.090020\, z_{10}$

$S(\lambda) = 0.040557\, x_{10} - 0.019683\, y_{10} + 0.486195\, z_{10}$

for $\lambda \leq 520$ nm, and

$S(\lambda) = 10^{(10402(1/\lambda) - 21.7185)}$ for $\lambda > 520$ nm.

These spectra are shown in Figure 17.6. These functions have the draw-back that the $S(\lambda)$ curve is above 520 nm a non-linear function of the cmf's.

An alternative way would be to construct $S(\lambda)$ entirely from the $\bar{z}_{10}(\lambda)$ function. A good approximation for this is:

$S(\lambda) = 0.49326\, \bar{z}_{10}(\lambda)$

Thus, according to a private communication by Walraven, a possibility for the refinement of the matrix coefficient values based on this approximation of $S(\lambda)$ and the assumptions that only the L- and M-cones contribute to luminance $\bar{y}_{10}(\lambda)$, thus that const $\cdot L(\lambda) + M(\lambda) = \bar{y}_{10}(\lambda)$, i.e.

const $\cdot a_{11} + a_{12} = 0$

const $\cdot a_{13} + a_{22} = 0$

This enables an all linear matrix transformation and the independent derivation of the copunctual points.

After correcting for the absorption of the ocular media and the macular pigment, the L- M- S- pigment absorption curves (cone-excitation spectra) have to be derived. This will be done for different observation angles along the lines described in the previous sections. The final curves might then be further smoothed and corrected based on the theoretical estimates of the absorption curve shapes (templates).

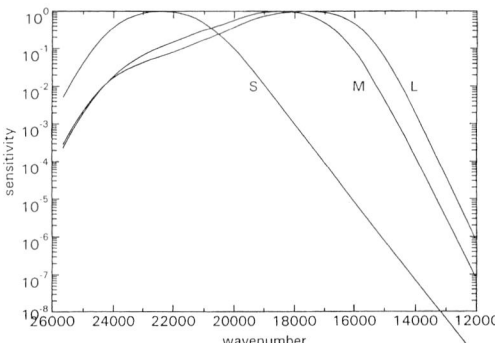

Fig. 17.6: The L- M- S-fundamentals according to Stockmann et al. (1993), as accepted temporarily by CIE TC 1-36.

There are also other good experiments from which cmf's can be deduced. Among these the 1931 Guild-Wright data are of special importance. For these the committee will study the Smith-Pokorny L- M- S- transformations (1975) as these are based on the hypothesis that the S-cones do not contribute to luminance. Stockmann et al. derived L-, M-, S- fundamentals also from the Stiles-Burch 2° data (1993). But all the 2° data will be analyzed only after completing the work on the 10° data.

17.3 Further Aspects

The committee intends to develop a new $V(\lambda)$ function, a continuous observer between 1° and 10°, based on the L- and M-fundamentals, derived by using the 10° $\bar{y}(\lambda)$ function and approximating the $V_M(\lambda)$-function.

Further on the committee wishes to develop a three dimensional LMS space, a two dimensional constant luminance diagram (i.e., constant (L + M) diagram). The system will be built in such a form that it takes into account the variation of macular pigment density, visual pigment density and assumes no change in the lens absorption.

Finally, a chromaticity diagram similar to the CIE 1931 diagram will be constructed. Preliminary calculations show that with the presently used assumptions this diagram will be very similar to the CIE-Judd 1951 diagram (1951), significant differences might occur in the 400–470 nm region.

17.3.1 Rod Intrusion

In a three-part paper Thornton (1992) described his experiments where he concluded that CIE colorimetry breaks down in the case of Maxwell matches for a 10° observer. Although the author disagrees with the assumption that the discrepancies found can, at least partly, be explained by rod intrusion, many experts were of the opinion that rod intrusion has a major influence on 10° color matches if light intensity is not high enough (Shapiro et al., 1993). Further experiments have shown discrepancies also at 2° observation.

At the time, when the CIE 1964 supplementary colorimetric observer was established, Judd and co-workers (1993) performed long calculations to correct the Stiles-Burch and Speranskaya data for rod intrusion and established real cone cmf's for the 10° observer. As the elaborations of this report are rather lengthy and not suitable for practical colorimetry, the CIE entrusted TC 1-43 to investigate the effect in more detail and come up with some further recommendations.

The committee is still working on its recommendations; the preliminary proposal claims that rod intrusion can be neglected when the following expression is larger then one:

$$\Delta R^* = \sqrt{\left(\frac{L_v'^1}{\Delta T'}\right)^2 - \left(\frac{L_v'^1}{\Delta T'}\right)^2}$$

here $L_v'^1$ and $L_v'^2$ are scotopic luminance of the metameric pair, $\Delta T'$ is calculated from retinal illuminance based on adapting field luminance.

As a general rule one can state that if task illuminance is below 1000 lux and the observation angle is larger then 4°, a trichromatic match with the 10° observer functions will contain a residual rod intrusion error that needs further correction, or more simply, 10° visual color matches should be done only if task illuminance is above 1000 lux.

17.3.2 Color Appearance

CIE colorimetry describes only color matches and cannot predict color appearance. Studies have been conducted for at least the past two decades to come up with a colorimetric description of color appearance, where chromatic adaptation and level of illumination are also considered.

The CIE started work on establishing a color appearance metric some years ago, but the committee was unable to come up with a single color appearance model. It recommended the more detailed investigation of the two most extensive models, the Hunt (1991; 1994) and the Nayatani and co-workers (Nayatani et al., 1990; 1995; Nayatani, 1995) models. Now CIE TC 1-34 is dealing with the subject, concentrating on surface colors. In its investigations some further models have been included (CIE, 1995) and the preliminary report of the chairman concluded that for most detailed tasks the Hunt model should be used, but for simpler approximate calculations the RLAB formula could be used (Fairchild and Berns, 1993).

The subject seems, however, still not ready for international agreement. The draft report produced partly major disagreement at the developers of the not recommended models, and during the time of formulating the report some new models have been put forward (Luo et al., 1996). There are also a number of experiments going on to increase the available data base that can be used to decide among the different models, e.g., Kuo et al. (1996).

Professor Hunt summarized the following principles that an agreed model should provide (1996):

1. The model should be comprehensive, so that it can be used in a variety of applications.
2. The model should cover a wide range of stimulus and adapting intensities.
3. The model should cover a wide range of viewing conditions and should be usable also in the case of unrelated colors.
4. The spectral sensitivity functions should be a linear transformation of the CIE Standard Colorimetric Observers and the Scotopic Observer.
5. There should be a possibility to include or exclude cognitive factors.
6. Model predictions should be: hue-angle and hue-quadrature, brightness, lightness, saturation, chroma and colorfulness.
7. The model should be capable of operation in a reverse mode.

None of the present day models fulfills all these requirements. But a group working on a CIE proposal is confident that by 1997 a consensus recommendation can be reached.[1]

17.3.3 Color Management Studies

One of the hot items in current colorimetric studies is the proper description of color appearance on the video display unit (VDU), cross correlation between the color appearance of an original, of its image on the VDU and the color rendering of a printed copy of the VDU image (hard-copy). CIE TC 1-27 is dealing with this question. A paper has been published (Alessi, 1995) requesting further input and defining preferred experimental situations.

The problem of cross media color fidelity is that the gamut areas of the VDU and of the printer are different; thus, not all colors that can be produced on the VDU are possible on the hard-copy and vice versa. Thus, not only must the different viewing situations be considered, but also the best colorimetric shift in color space between the color solid of the VDU and the printer has to be established.

CIE hosted an expert symposium on the subject in March 1996 in Vienna, co-sponsored by the major international standardizing organisations dealing jointly with this field (ISO, IEC, ITU), to set the course for further action in the field, both for establishing a data base to be used by model builders and for practical use by those concerned with standards in the field of graphic arts, color communication, electronic imaging and photography, as well as color facsimile transmission (CIE Expert Symposium, 1996).

---

[1] Footnote added at proof-reading: The CIE CAM97S has officially been introduced in 1997.

17.4 Summary

Colorimetry is just reaching its second phase of major development. In 1931 CIE set the direction for describing color matches. This method, based entirely on empirical observations, was able to serve well the needs of surface colors industry.

In recent years the comparison of surface color appearance and of colors produced on a VDU became more and more important. This forced the re-thinking of the fundamental principles of colorimetry and to refine the very basic tables of data and functions used in colorimetric calculations. Also new additions, mainly the introduction of color appearance analysis became necessary.

A number of CIE committees are active in the re-establishment of the rules of colorimetry and we can expect that within a few years some new guidelines will be published that will help applied colorimetry to achieve even better congruence between the visually observed and the calculated results. One has to remember, however, that color is a human perception, and as such it shows individual deviations from the mean. One can never expect that the observations of one individual will exactly be matched by the calculated results which are based on the average of results achieved by many observers. Thus, it is not possible to develop a colorimetry that describes the color perception of each individual exactly, but the mathematical descriptions will hopefully include some predictions of the deviations that can be expected.

CIE colorimetry was introduced 65 years ago to describe the colorimetric properties of colored lights and signals. Soon after establishment it turned out that it is most capable to describe the colorimetry of reflective media and is now widely applied in all branches of the coloring industries (e.g. in the textile, paper and automotive industries), where the aim is to produce as far as possible non-metameric matches i.e., matches where the standard and the test samples show similar spectral reflectance.

With the advance of modern light sources (gas discharge lamps with and without phosphors, emitting in narrow emission bands) and the use of color monitors it became important to deal with metameric matches (where only the color is the same, but the spectral power distribution is very different) and to find ways to describe not only color matches but also color appearance.

CIE TC 1-36 re-examined the fundamental spectral sensitivity functions of the human observer and is currently working on a system of colorimetry based on the very best color-matching experiments, considering the different pre-retinal filtering agents and basic vision knowledge. It is hoped that these investigations will permit a colorimetric system that can span the 1° to 10° range of observation angle.

CIE TC 1-43 extends this work by considering also light intensity effects, as at larger observation angles intensity dependent rod intrusion influences metameric color matches.

A very fundamental work on color difference evaluation has just been finished and a new color difference formula has been published, where different perturbing factors and location within the color solid can be considered.

There are several models of color appearance described in the literature, and CIE TC 1-34 is engaged in testing and comparing these models and will eventually come up with a recommendation – if not for a generally accepted model, but for methods to thoroughly learn about the performance of these models.

CIE TC 1-27 is collecting data for a specification of color appearance differences between reflective media (printed samples) and self-luminous displays (color monitors).

As seen, work is going on in many areas of colorimetry. The paper high-lights recent achievements and shows trends of current research.

References

Alessi, P. (1995). Testing colour-appearance models: Guidelines for coordinated reseach. Color Res. Appl. *20*, 262–266.

Bone, R. A., Landrum, J. T., Fernandez, L., and Tarsis, S. L. (1988). Analysis of the macular pigment by HPLC; Retinal distribution and age study. Invest. Ophthalmol. Visual Sci. *29*, 843–849.

CIE Expert Symposium '96, Colour Standards for Image Technology, Vienna (1996).

CIE TC 1-34 Testing colour appearance models, draft technical report (1995).

CIE Technical Report (1990). CIE 1988 2° spectral luminous efficiency function for photopic vision, CIE Publ. No. 86.

Commission Internationale d'Éclairage, Publ. CIE 15.2-1986 Colorimetry.

Dartnall, H. J. A., Bowmaker, J. K., and Mollon, J. D. (1983). Human visual pigments: microspectrophotometric results from the eyes of seven persons, Proc. Roy. Soc. London B 220, 115–130.

Fairchild, M. D. and Berns, R. S. (1993). Image color-appearance specification through extension of CIELAB. Color Res. Appl. 18, 178–190.

Grassmann, H. (1853). Zur Theorie der Farbenmischung. Poggendorf, Ann. Phys. 89, 69; also: Phil. Mag. (4) 7 254 (1853).

Hunt, R. G. W. (1996). The function, evolution and future of colour appearance models. CIE Expert Symposium '96. Colour Standards for Image Technology, Vienna.

Hunt, R.W.G. (1991). Revised colour appearance model for related and unrelated colours. Color Res. and Appl. 16, 146–165.

Hunt, R. W. G. (1994). An improved predictor of colourfulness in a model of colour vision. Color Res. and Appl. 19, 23–26.

ISO/CIE, CIE Standard colorimetric observers (1991). ISO 10527.

Judd's method for calculating the tristimulus values of the CIE 10° observer. In: Proc. CIE Symposium on Advanced Colorimetry, Vienna, Austria, pp. 107–114, CIE Central Bureau (1993).

Judd, D. B. (1951). Report of Secr. of TC no 7 Colorimetry and artificial daylight. In: Proc. 12th Session of the CIE, Stockholm, 2.

Judd, D. B. (1951). Report of US Secretariat Committee on Colorimetry Artificial Daylight, CIE Proceedings Stockholm, Bureau Central de la CIE, Vol. 1, Part 7, p. 11.

Judd, D. B. and Wyszecki, G. (1975). Color in Business, Science and Industry (rd. ed.). Wiley, New York.

König, A. and Dieterici, C. (1886). Die Grundemfindungen und ihre Intensitäts-Verteilung im Spektrum, J. Sitz Akad. Wiss (Berlin), 805–829.

Kuo, W.-G., Luo, M. R., and Bez, H. E. (1996). Various chromatic-adaptation transforms tested using new colour appearance data in textiles. Color Res. Appl. 20, 313–327.

Lamb, T. D. (1995). Photoreceptor spectral sensitivities common shape and in the long wavelength region. Vision Res. 35, 3083–3091.

Lennie, P., Pokorny, J., and Smith, V .C. (1993). Luminance, JOSA 10/6, 1283–1293.

Luo, M. R., Lo, M.-C., and Kuo, W.-G. (1996). The LLAB(l:c) colour model. Color Res. Appl. 21, 412–429.

Moreland, J. D. and Bhatt, P. (1984). Retinal distribution of macular pigment. In: Verriest (ed.) Colour Deficiencies VII, Junk, The Hague, 127–132.

Nayatani, Y. (1995). Revision of the chroma and hue scales of a non-linear color-appearance model. Color Res. Appl. 20, 143–155.

Nayatani, Y., Sobagaki, H., Hashimoto, K., and Yano T. (1995). Lightness dependence of chroma scales of a non-linear color-appearance model and its latest formulation. Color Res. Appl. 20, 156–167.

Nayatani, Y., Takahama, K., Sobagaki, H., and Hashimoto, K. (1990). Color-appearance model and chromatic adaptation transformation. Color Res. Appl. 15, 210–221.

Neitz, M., Neitz J., and Jacobs, G. H. (1991). Spectral tuning of pigments underlying red-green color vision. Science 252, 971–974.

Pokorny, J. and Smith, V. C. (1976). Effect of field size on red-green colour mixture equations. JOSA 66, 705–708.

Pokorny, J., Smith, V. C., and Lutze, M. (1987). Aging of the human lens. Appl. Opt. 26, 1437–1440.

Principales Décisions de la Commission Internationale de l'Eclairage (6ᵉ Session, 1924), Voeux. Compte Rendu des Séances, Genéve – 1924. pp 67–70.

Recommendation officielles de la Commission Internationale de l'Eclairage (Huitième Session, 1931), Colorimétrie. Compte Rendu des Séances Huitième Session, Cambridge – Septembre 1931 pp 19–29.

Robertson, A. R. (1993). Overview of sixty years of CIE colorimetry. In: Proc. CIE Symp. on Advanced Colorimetry, Vienna, 1993, pp. 3–6, CIE Central Bureau Publ. CIE x007.

Sanocki, E., Lindsay, D. T., Winderickx, J., Teller, D., Deeb, S. S., and Motulsky, A. F. (1993). Serine/-Alanine amino acid polymorphysm of the L and S cone pigments: effects on Rayleigh matches among deuteranopes, protanopes and color normal observers. Vision Research 15, 2139–2152.

Schanda, J. CIE Standard Observer in 1924, 1951 and now, VI Lux Europa Conf., Budapest, 3–5 Oct. 1989.

Schnapf, J. L., Kraft, T. W., and Baylor, D. A. (1987). Spectral sensitivity of human cone photoreceptors. Nature 325, 439–441.

Shapiro, A. G., Smith, V. C., and Pokorny, J. (1993). Rod activity and color matching functions. In: Proc. CIE Symposium on Advanced Colorimetry, Vienna, Austria, pp. 65–70 CIE Central Bureau.

Smith, V. C. and Pokorny, J. (1975). Spectral sensitivity of the foveal cone pigments between 400 and 500 nm. Vision Res. *15*, 161–171.

Speranskaya, N. L. (1959). Determination of spectrum color-co-ordinates for twenty-seven normal observers. Optics and Spectroscopy *7*, 424.

Stiles, W S. (1955). Interim report to the CIE, Zurich 1955. On the National Physical Laboratory's Investigation of colour matching, with an appendix by Stiles, W. S. and Burch, J. M. Optica Acta *2*, 168–181.

Stiles, W. S. and Burch, J. M. (1959). NPL colour matching investigation: final report. Optica Acta *6*, 1.

Stockman, A., MacLeod, D. I. A., and Johnson, N. E. (1993). Spectral sensitivities of the human cones. J. Opt. Soc. Am. *10A*, 2491–2521.

Stockman, A., MacLeod, D. I. A., and Johnson, N. E. (1993). Spectral sensitivities of the human cones. JOSA A *10*, 2491–2521.

Thornton, W .A. Towards a more accurate and extensible colorimetry, Part 1. (1992). Introduction, The visual colorimeter-spectroradiometer, Experimental results. Color Res. Appl. *17*, 79–122; Part 2. (1992). Discussion, Color Res. Appl. *17*, 162–186; Part 3. (1992). Discussion (continued) Color Res. Appl. *17*, 240–261.

Trezona, P. W. (1984). Individual observer data for the 1955 Stiles-Burch 2° pilot investigation. NPL Report QU 68.

Trezona, P. W. (1993). Can the tetrachromatic colour matching system solve problems of trichromatic colour matching? In: Proc. CIE Symp. on Advanced Colorimetry, Vienna, 1993, pp. 91–96, CIE Central Bureau Publ. CIE x007.

Vos, J. J. (1972). Literature review of human macular absorption in the visible and its consequences for the cone receptor primaries. Report Inst. for Perception TNO 1972-17.

Vos, J. J., Estévez O., and Walraven, P. L. (1990). Improved colour fundamentals offer a new view on photometric additivity. Vision Research *30*, 937–943.

Weale, R. A. (1988). Age and the transmittance of the human crystalline lens. J Physiol. (London) *395*, 577–587.

Werner, J. S. (1982). Development of scotopic sensitivity and the absorption spectrum of the human ocular media. J. Opt. Soc. Am. *72*, 247–258.

Werner, J. S., Donnelly, S. K., and Kliegl, R. (1987). Aging and human macular pigment density; appended with translations from the work of Max Schultze and Ewald Hering. Vision Res. *27*, 257–268.

18. Use of Computer Graphics in PostScript for Color Didactics

Klaus Richter

18.1 Introduction

The quality of image reproduction in image science is defined by the differences between the original and the reproduction. In many fields of application the reproducibility of image reproduction is important. The different reproduction systems have very different properties, e. g., use linear (scanners), square root (video-cameras) and logarithmic (film-cameras) signals as a function of luminance. The failures in reproduction must be measured and corrected. For this optimization, reference originals and measurements of their output are important. Such reference testcharts (achromatic and chromatic) are defined by the German standard organisation (DIN) in the standard DIN 33 866 for testing color-copying machines.

In the publishing industry the achromatic and chromatic colors within figures are usually defined by a special programming language called PostScript (PS). Definitions of *device-dependent* and *device-independent* colors are included in PS.

PostScript (see Adobe 1990) allows one to use *device-independent* color specifications of the Commission Internationale de l'Eclairage (CIE) (CIE, 1978) for the description of colors. The layout is then often defined by vector computer graphics, which fills different areas by different device-independent colors. The output devices, e. g., monitors or printers in combination with software-programs, use the device-independent color definitons in the PS program to match the CIE colors by device-dependent colors.

A monitor uses device-dependent phosphors emitting light which looks orange-red O, yellowish-green L and violet-blue V (color set *OLV*) and a printer uses paint reflecting light which looks cyan-blue C, magenta-red M, yellow Y, and black N (french = noir) (color set *CMYN*) for this purpose. The color set names used for reproduction are refered as *RBG* and *CMYK* in the PostScript language respectively. The color set names *OLV* and *CMYN* are more useful for educational purposes as the letters R, G, and B are reserved for elementary colors (see section 18.2).

PS was used to create the color figures in this article. The PostScript programming language will not be described. The following parts describe some basic points of color order, color mixture, color measurement, color vision, color scaling, and color thresholds. The figures and the short description are especially useful for educational purposes.

More than 500 similar color figures (with German terms) are published and printed in a book (Richter, 1996). The PostScript program code of all figures is available in the CD-ROM of the book. The CD-ROM includes the Software "Adobe Reader with Search" for MAC, WIN and UNIX and all the color figures in the data formats PostScript (PS) and Portable Document (PDF) which are about three times compressed compared to PS and includes specifications for video and sound.

All the color figures can be printed on overhead transparency in DIN A4 size. The figures can be modified, e. g., freely scaled and the (German) terms can be easily translated into other languages. The figures can be easily used in desk top publication systems (Pagemaker, Quark Express, etc.).

There are about 300 PS devices from 60 manufacturers on the market. With display-PS computer systems, e. g., NEXTSTEP or OPENSTEP on Intel-Hardware (with Microsoft Windows 3.1 or Windows NT 4.0) one can write and edit PS-code in one window and view the color figure in the other window. Most of the color figures were created that way.

Desk top publishing products with a display PostScript extension allow one to position and view the figures within the text. In the case of digital or cross media output via Internet the resolution and the color rendering dictionary of the output device is used for optimization. Using PS- or PDF-computer graphics of the figures in the book reduces file size by a factor 1000 compared to pixel graphics. This is one of the reasons why the PDF-format is often used in the Internet.

There are free PS- and PDF-printer drivers on the market which allow one to produce PS- or PDF-code from any application, e. g., Microsoft (MS) WORD in MS-Windows. The PDF-code can be viewed in Internet with the Acrobat Reader. The layout is not changed by the viewing process. The color output devices can be color calibrated. Then the visual color differences are minimized between the device-independent CIE colors defined in the PS- or PDF-program code and the mixture of the device-dependent colors of the output device, and often no visual differences occur.

Any color output device can be specified by the color output of device independent CIE test colors. The CIE has defined 14 CIE test colors for color rendering properties in 1974 and the CIELAB color space for color order and tolerance specification in 1986. The coordinates of the CIELAB color space are *lightness L**, *red-green chromaticness a**, and *yellow-blue chromaticness b**.

There are 100 steps (CIELAB units) between black and white defined in the CIELAB lightness L^* scale. One can discriminate two gray samples with about one unit CIELAB difference if the samples are located side by side. For separated samples on a gray surround about three CIELAB units can be discriminated.

The DIN testcharts (DIN 33 866) use the CIE test colors and the CIELAB $L^*a^*b^*$ color specification in the PS program code. The digital PS program code of the produced analog DIN testcharts (DIN 33 866, one achromatic and one chromatic) will be published as new digital DIN testcharts useful for color output specification and color calibration of color output devices.

These digital DIN standards can be used for the luminance and color calibration of monitors, printers and printing processes. Visual color comparison of the device output with the originals, the analog DIN testcharts, or color measurement of the device output allows one to correct the digital input. In a few steps a calibration matrix can be calculated for the output device and often an output is reached within visual tolerances of three CIELAB units for the CIE test colors and equidistant gray scales.

The digital DIN standards are very flexible. Some properties are:
– device independent $L^*a^*b^*$ color specification in PS or PDF program code,
– output on any computer platform (Mac-OS, MS-Windows, Unix),
– output of PDF code on any printer (use Adobe Reader and File: Print),
– output of PS code on any PS printer (copy PS code to PS printer),
– flexible digital correction by visual comparison with analog DIN testcharts,
– flexible digital correction by $L^*a^*b^*$ color measurement, use ColorMouse,
– "black box" optimization for:
  any color monitor justification,
  any output paper,
  any color ink,
  any reproduction process.

If no visual difference in the output occurs, than the mean color difference is less than three CIELAB units for the 14 CIE chromatic test colors and five DIN achromatic test colors (see DIN 33 866).

It is not intended to describe the PS program code nor the experimental details of experiments in this paper. More information on both areas are published (Richter, 1996). The aim of this paper is to illustrate how to use the PS program code for creating color figures with device-independent colors specified by the $L^*a^*b^*$ color coordinates in the CIELAB color space.

The possibility of color calibration and management by DIN color test charts indicate the importance of the PS program code for the area of color education and color reproduction.

Next to each figure number there is another

number, e.g., 8512-1 for Figure 18.1. These numbers are out of a list of more than 500 color figures published by Richter (1996). There is a plan to have the PS program code of the figures in different sizes (5.4 cm × 4.0 cm and A4) and figure text in different languages (German, English, French, Spanish, Italian) in Internet. More information on this project may be obtained in Internet at the address: http://www.bam-berlin.de and the BAM department VIII.3 or by email: klaus.richter@bam.de.

18.2 Multiplicity of Colors

All that we see has color. Colors form the elements of our visual sensations. Different from these sensations are the materials and processes which produce colors. According to Judd and Wyszecki (1975), people with normal color vision can distinguish about 10 million different colors. A classification by common attributes is thus necessary to order this multiplicity.

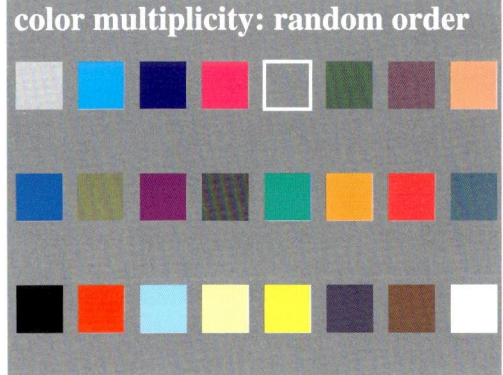

Fig. 18.1: Multiplicity of color samples in a random arrangement [8512-1].

Figure 18.1 shows a random arrangement of color samples.

Figure 18.2 shows a random arrangement of color samples which first of all can be separated into groups of achromatic and chromatic colors. In Figure 18.2 the achromatic colors are marked, the others are chromatic.

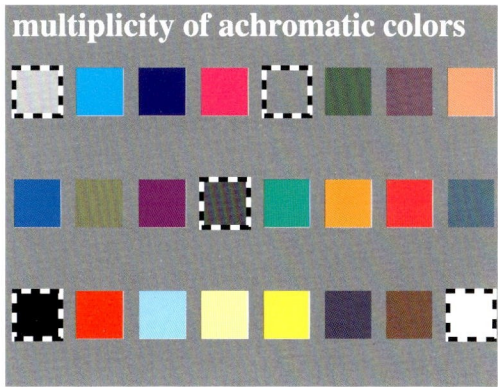

Fig. 18.2: Multiplicity of colors. The achromatic colors are marked and the others are chromatic [8512-2].

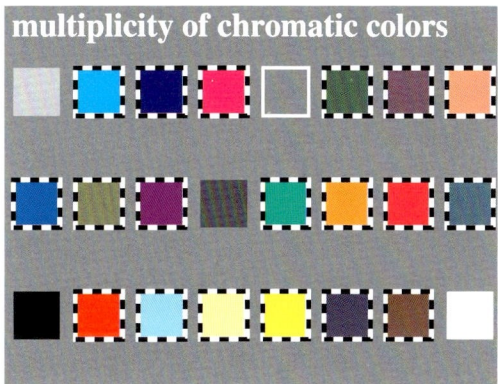

Fig. 18.3: Multiplicity of colors. The chromatic colors are marked, the others are achromatic. [8512-3].

Figure 18.3 shows a random arrangement of color samples. The marked colors are chromatic and the others are achromatic.

Figure 18.4 shows hexadecimal codes for a random arrangement of color samples. The achromatic colors show three equal hexadecimal codes and the chromatic colors show three different codes. An asterix (*) describes equally-spaced scales. A gray with the hexadecimal code 777* is located approximately in the middle between black (code 000*) and white (code FFF*). The three hexadecimal codes describe the amount of orange-red (code F00*), yellowish-green (0F0*) and violet-blue (00F*) within a color.

The hexadecimal code is *device-dependent* and especially used for color monitors. Color monitors

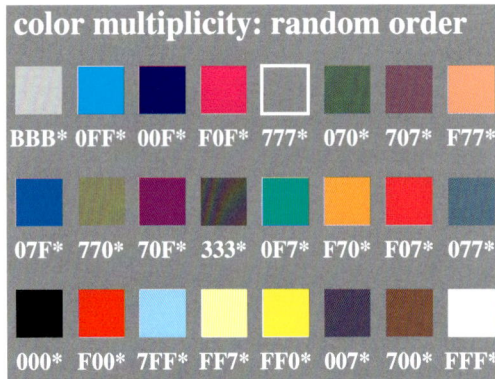

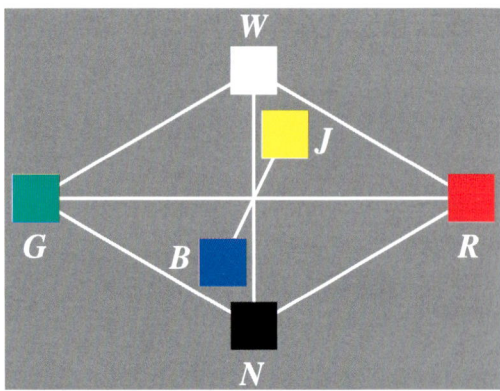

Fig. 18.4: Achromatic colors with three equal hexadecimal codes and chromatic colors with three different hexadecimal codes [8513-1].

Fig. 18.5: Double cone that illustrates the separation into achromatic and chromatic colors [8520-1].

with different phosphors and different color calibration will lead to different color outputs. A similar code for three-paint printers is in use. New printers and reproduction processes mix colors by four, five, six or seven paints and in this case the code is less useful. The only solution is to use the *device-independent* color specifications in CIELAB color space and try to mix the CIE colors by the *device-dependent* paints or phosphors.

18.3 Color Solid, Basic Colors and Color Attributes

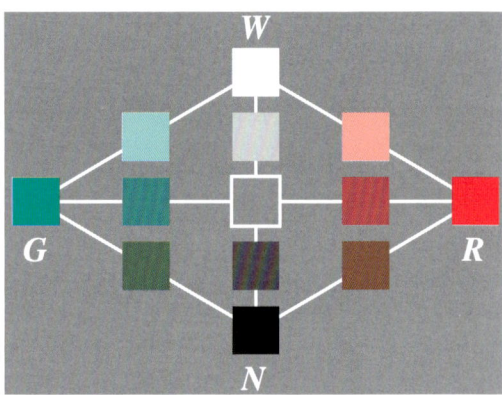

Fig. 18.6: Vertical cut through the color double cone in the red–green hue plane [8520-2].

Leonardo da Vinci (1452–1519) ordered the multitude of colors by selecting six "elementary" colors; one neutral or achromatic pair (white–black), and two chromatic pairs (red–green and yellow–blue). The double cone of Figure 18.5 serves as a simplified model to illustrate his ideas, the vertical axis corresponding to the array of neutral colors (black to white) and the circumference corresponding to the pure chromatic colors.

Figure 18.5 shows the color double cone with six "simple" colors or six "elementary" colors as they are called here. In Figure 18.5 the letters stand for:

    W white   *J* yellow   *R* red
                  (french: jaune)
    N black   *B* blue   *G* green.
      (= noir)

Figure 18.6 shows the color double cone with intermediate steps in the vertical red–green plane cut through the achromatic (white–black) axis. The same letters are used as in Figure 18.5.

Figure 18.7 shows the color double cone with intermediate steps in the vertical yellow–blue plane cut through the achromatic (white–black) axis. The same letters are used as in Figure 18.5.

In Figure 18.8 one can easily determine the elementary yellow *J* as neither reddish nor greenish. The criterion for the determination of the elementary color yellow *J* in a hue circle are given. In Figure 18.8 the letters mean:

    J yellow (french: jaunne)
    O orange-red   *L* leaf-green   *V* violet-blue.

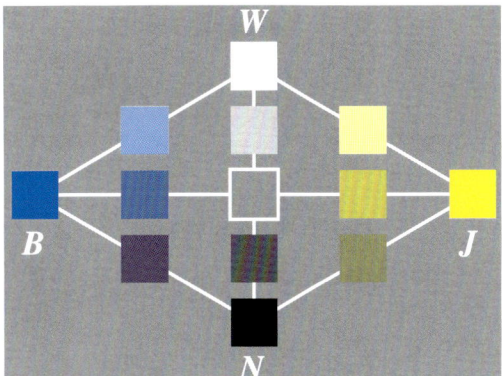

Fig. 18.7: Vertical cut through the color double cone in the yellow-blue hue plane [8520-3].

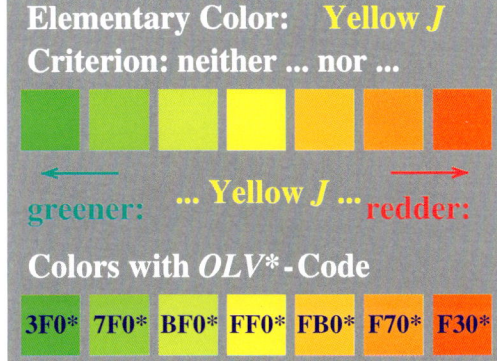

Fig. 18.8: Criterion for the determination of the elementary color J out of a hue circle in the yellow region [8522-5].

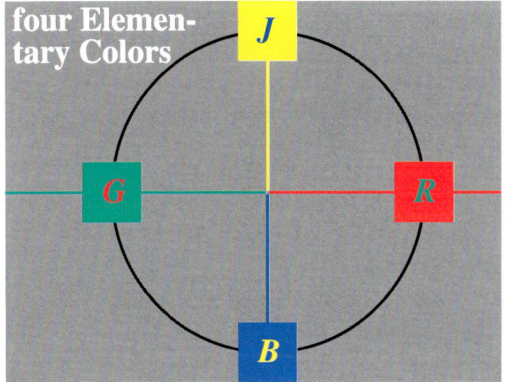

Fig. 18.9: Symmetric hue circle with four elementary colors R, J, G, and B [8522-4].

In addition, the hexadecimal OLV^*-code is shown for all color samples out of the hue circle.

In each hue circle there are four chromatic colors which are perceptually simple. We call them elementary colors and we distinguish elementary red, elementary yellow, elementary green and elementary blue. The colors on either side of the two perpendicular elementary hue axes, R–G and J–B, become increasingly yellower or bluer, redder or greener respectively, as they depart from the achromatic center.

Figure 18.9 shows a symmetric hue circle with the opposing elementary colors red–green and yellow–blue. In Figure 18.9 the designations stand for:

Elementary colors: J yellow R red
                          B blue G green

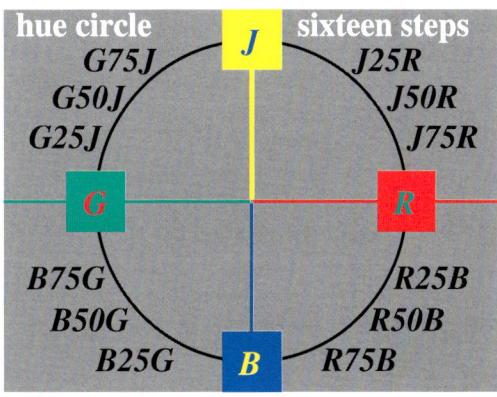

Fig. 18.10: Symmetric hue circle with sixteen chromatic colors [8672-4].

Figure 18.10 shows a hue circle with sixteen chromatic colors. The figure shows always three colors between two elementary colors and 100 steps between two elementary colors. The letters stand for:

$J25R$ visually 75% yellow and 25% red
$J50R$ visually 50% yellow and 50% red
$J75R$ visually 25% yellow and 75% red
and similarly for the other sectors R–B, B–G, and G–J of the hue circle.

Perceptually, *three* color attributes specify a color. Most of the color order systems choose *hue* as the first attribute, e. g., the Munsell System

(Newhall et al., 1943), the German DIN System (Richter, 1963), and the Swedish Natural Color System (Hard, 1981). These color systems differ in the choice of the two other attributes. The Munsell System chose the color attribute chromaticness C^* (named Chroma) and lightness L^* in a hue plane. This is also the choice in the CIELAB color space (CIE, 1978).

Figure 18.11 shows colors of constant chromaticness C^* and of different lightness L^* in a red hue plane. There are 100 lightness steps between black and white and 100 chromaticness steps between mean grey and red. In that case the colors in Figure 18.11 have the chromaticness $C^* = 25$ and the lightness is $L^* = 10, 30, 50, 70,$ and 90 for the vertical color series.

Figure 18.12 shows colors of constant lightness L^* and of different chromaticness C^* in a red hue plane. The colors in Figure 18.12 have the lightness $L^* = 50$ and the chromaticness is $C^* = 0, 25, 50, 75,$ and 100 for the horizontal color series.

18.4 Spectrum and 3-Dimensional Color Values

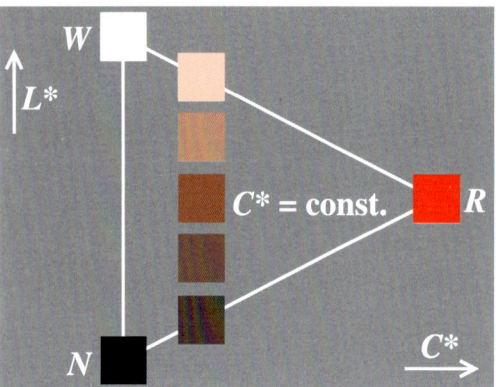

Fig. 18.11: Colors of constant chromaticness $C^* = 25$ and of different lightness ($L^* = 10, 30, 50, 70, 90$) in a red hue plane [8521-2].

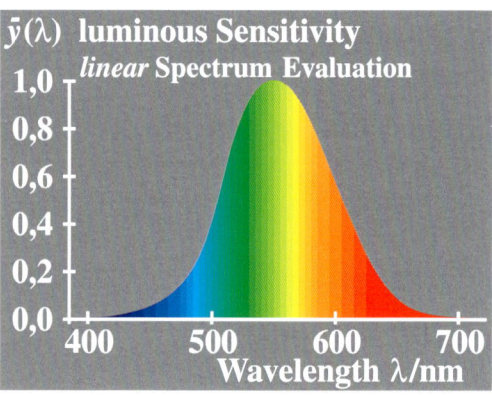

Fig. 18.13: Visible spectrum and spectral luminous sensitivity $V(\lambda) = \bar{y}(\lambda)$ between $\lambda = 380$ nm and $\lambda = 760$ nm [8532-1].

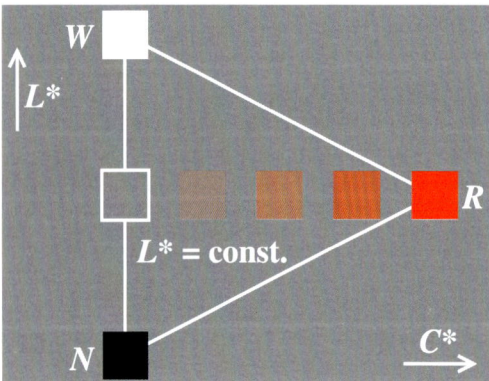

Fig. 18.12: Colors of constant lightness $L^* = 50$ and of different chromaticness ($C^* = 0, 25, 50, 75, 100$) in a red hue plane [8521-3].

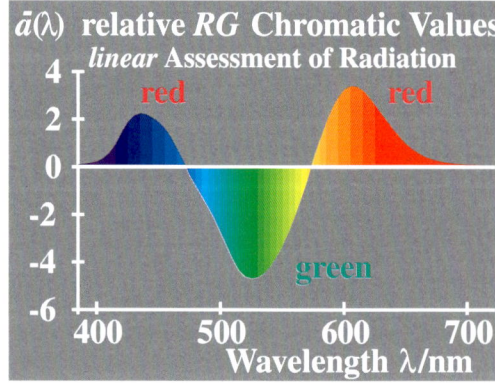

Fig. 18.14: Spectral red–green chromatic values $\bar{a}(\lambda)$ of the opponent red–green color system for spectral colors between $\lambda = 380$ nm and $\lambda = 760$ nm [8532-5].

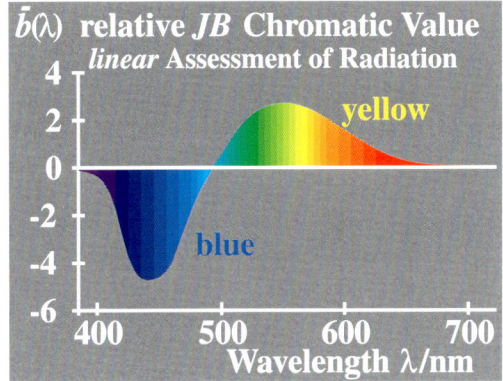

Fig. 18.15: Spectral yellow–blue chromatic values b̄(λ) of the opponent yellow–blue color system for spectral colors between λ = 380 nm and λ = 760 nm [8532-6].

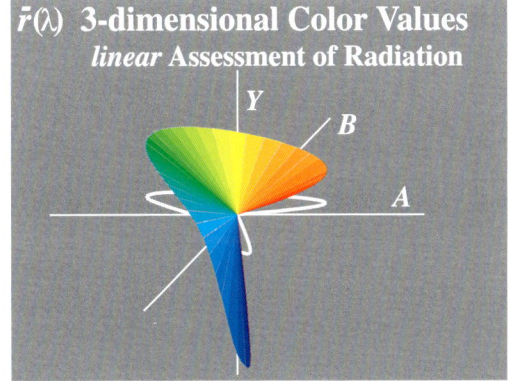

Fig.18.16: Spectral colors in a three-dimensional color space with the coordinates luminous reflectance Y, and chromatic values red-green A and yellow-blue B [8532-3].

The region of light radiation with all wavelengths (λ) in the visible spectrum between λ = 380 nm and λ = 760 nm (1 nanometer = 10^{-9}m) is shown.

Figure 18.13 shows the spectral luminous sensitivity V(λ) = ȳ(λ) between λ = 380 nm and λ = 760 nm which is the visible spectrum. According to the figure, the color spectrum appears darker from the middle yellow-green region to both ends.

Figure 18.14 shows spectral red–green chromatic values ā(λ) of the opponent red–green color system for spectral colors between λ = 380 nm and λ = 760 nm.

Figure 18.15 shows spectral yellow–blue chromatic values b̄(λ) of the opponent yellow–blue color system for spectral colors between λ = 380 nm and λ = 760 nm.

Figure 18.16 demonstrates the valences (values) of the spectral colors in the color mixture. The valences of the spectral colors are described by color vectors in a three-dimensional space with the coordinates: luminous reflectance Y, red-green chromatic value A, and yellow-blue chromatic value B.

18.5 Color Measurement, Mixture and Contrast

Figure 18.17 shows the spectral tristimulus values x̄(λ), ȳ(λ), and z̄(λ) defined by the Commision International de l'Eclairage (CIE, 1986). The three spectral tristimulus functions describe the three sensitivities of the CIE standard observer, providing the basis for color measurement. Together with the relative spectral power distribution S(λ) of an illuminant and the spectral reflectance curve R(λ) of a surface one can calculate the three tristimulus values X, Y, and Z.

The three tristimulus values X, Y, and Z are coordinates that specify a color. Beside the tristimulus values, the chromaticity coordinates x and

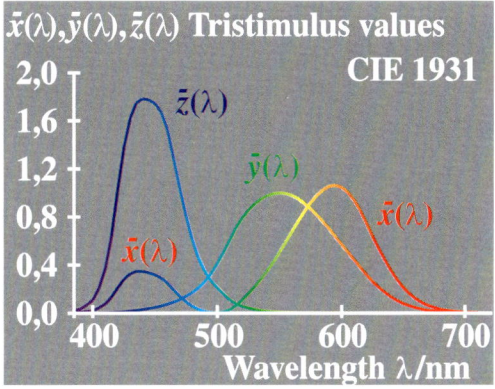

Fig. 18.17: Spectral tristimulus values x̄(λ), ȳ(λ), and z̄(λ) defined by the CIE in 1931 [8542-5].

y may be used. These can be calculated from the tristimulus values X, Y, and Z by the following equations:

$x = X / (X + Y + Z)$
$y = Y / (X + Y + Z)$

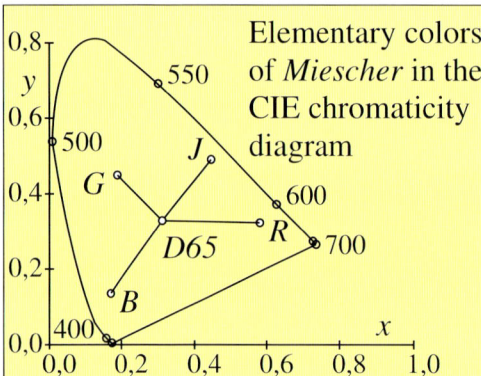

Fig. 18.18: Elementary colors of Miescher et al. (1982) in the CIE chromaticity diagram with the chromaticity coordinates x and y [8333-5].

Figure 18.18 shows the elementary colors of Miescher et al. (1982) in the CIE chromaticity diagram. The chromaticity coordinates x and y, and the luminous reflectance Y (which according to the CIE Colorimetry recommendations is expressed as a ratio relating to the value 100 for white) can be used to specify a color just as clearly as the three tristimulus values X, Y, and Z. In accordance with the recommendations of colorimetry, numer-ical values of the tristimulus values X, Y, and Z generally lie between 0 and 100. The chromaticity coordinates x and y are always smaller than 1.0. The x and y coordinates specify chromaticity points on a rectangular (x, y) diagram.

Figure 18.19 shows both the three basic colors orange-red O, leaf-green L and violet-blue V of the additive color mixture and the three mixed colors yellow Y, cyan-blue C, and magenta-red M. White is produced from the mixture of all three basic colors.

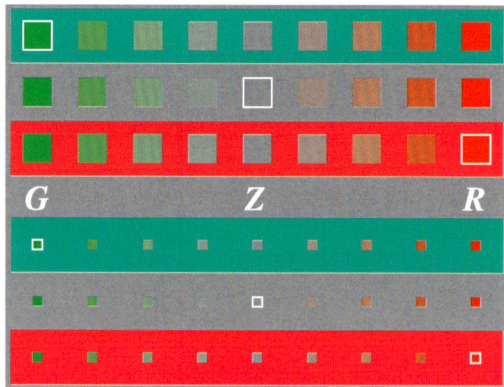

Fig. 18.20: Three identical color scales with equidistant chromaticness steps on a grey background are shown here on grey, red and green backgrounds for two central field sizes [8561-3].

Figure 18.20 shows three identical color series with equidistant chromaticness steps against a surround color of medium grey which is the reference condition and also in red and green surrounds for two central field sizes.

The red color samples on a green surround appear redder then on a red surround. The green color samples on a red surround appear greener then on a green surround. Also, the grey samples in the middle no longer appear grey, but are influenced in opposite directions by the surround.

The change of appearance of colors by the colors that surround them is conditioned by physiological processes in the visual system. Up to now models of color vision can not fully describe these contrast effects.

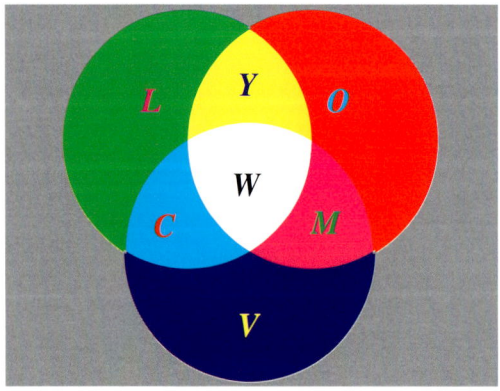

Fig. 18.19: Additive color mixture of basic colors orange-red O, leaf-green L and violet-blue V [8550-1].

18.6 Colors: Equally Spaced and Thresholds

Figure 18.21 shows a color series between a very chromatic turquoise T along grey $D65$ (daylight) to a very chromatic purple-red P which is approximately equally spaced. The experimental condition is shown in the upper left of the figure. In a white surround there is a quadratic gray field. In this grey surround to end colors purple-red P and turquoise T were shown. In the lower circle field colors of equal luminance between the two end colors T and P can be mixed continuously.

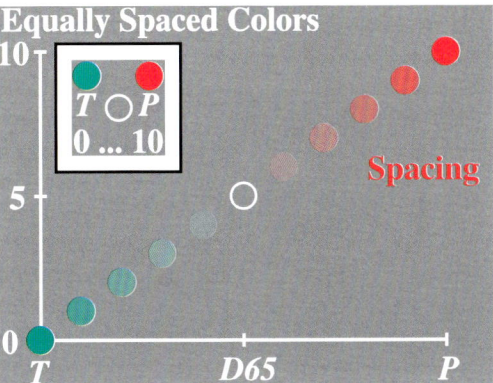

Fig. 18.21: Color spacing of a series turquoise T – grey $D65$ – purple-red P. Equal color differences of the color steps between $T – D65$ and $D65 – P$ [8762-1].

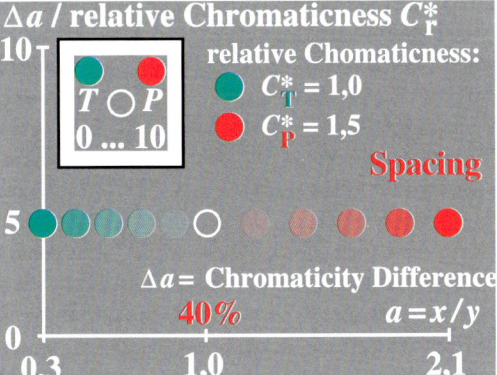

Fig. 18.22: Color spacing of the series turquoise T – grey of $D65$ – purple-red P; constant values of Δa with color measurement values $a = x / y$ [8762-6].

Figure 18.22 shows experimental results of the equidistant color spacing for series turquoise T – grey $D65$ and grey $D65$ – purple-red P as a function of the coordinate $a = x / y$. Constant geometrical difference values of Δa correspond to equal visual chromatic differences.

The description of equal chromaticness steps by equal geometrical differences of a color valence value ($a = x / y$) is here very simple. Therefore the geometrical difference Δa can be used to set color tolerances in industrial fields.

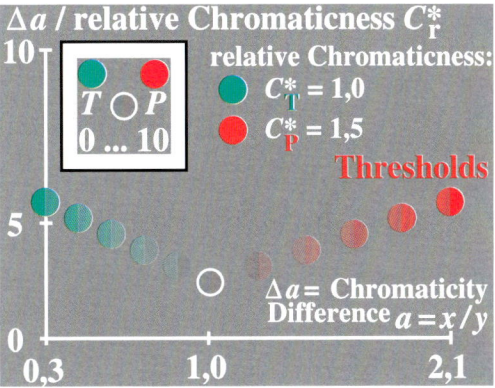

Fig. 18.23: Color thresholds within a series turquoise T – grey $D65$ – purple-red P. The smallest value of Δa is reached near acromatic central field colors [8762-7].

Figure 18.23 shows color thresholds within a series turquoise T – grey $D65$ – purple-red P. The smallest value of Δa is reached near the achromatic central field color. The experimental situation is shown in the upper left of the Figure. In a grey surround with a white border there are shown two end colors, purple-red P and turquoise T.

In the lower circle, field colors of equal luminance between the two end colors T and P could be mixed continuously. On the left and right bipartite field equal amounts of equiluminance colors T and P are projected. About one percent of luminance is necessary for seeing a color difference between the left and right bipartite field. The chromaticity difference (Δa) of this threshold perception is measured and plotted in Figure 18.23. The geometrical differences (Δa) are not constant as expected by the scaling experiments in Figure

18.22. They are smallest near the achromatic surround and increase linearly as a function of the chromaticity difference from grey both in the direction of turquoise T and in the direction of purple-red P. Near grey about 30 and near turquoise T and purple-red P about ten threshold steps correspond to a chromaticness step.

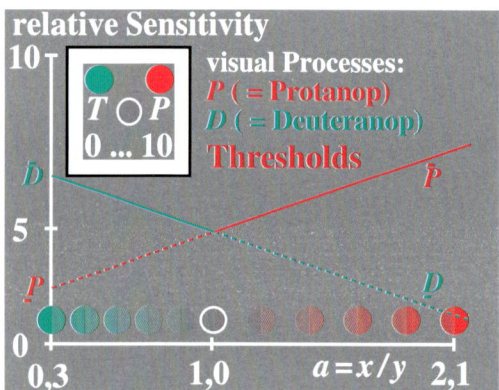

Fig. 18.24: Color thresholds within the series turquoise T – grey $D65$ – purple-red P. The variable chromaticity difference (Δa) is based on two visual processes of receptors P and D [8762-8].

Figure 18.24 shows color thresholds within the series turquoise T – grey $D65$ – purple-red P. The variable chromaticity difference (Δa) is based on two visual processes of receptors P and D.

18.7 Opponent Achromatic Color Vision

Figure 18.25 shows the luminance discrimination ($L/\Delta L$) for achromatic colors of different central field luminance (L). In experiments, five different surround field luminances L_u = 1, 10, 100, 1000, and 10000 cd/m^2 were chosen. The observer adapts to the grey surround. The two bipartite central fields were shown only for a short time (0.1 s). One can reasonably assume that during this short time no significant adaptation change of the visual system takes place.

Figure 18.26 shows luminance discrimination ($L/\Delta L$) for achromatic colors of different central

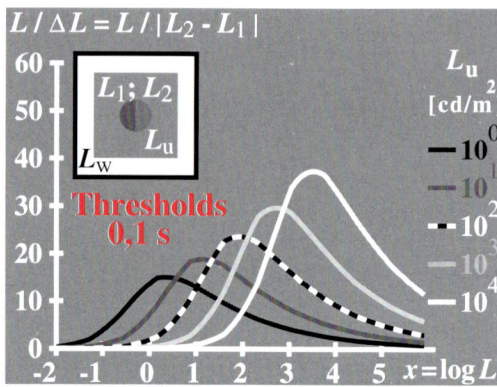

Fig. 18.25: Luminance discrimination ($L/\Delta L$) for achromatic colors of different central field luminance (L) for five different surround field luminances L_u [8753-1].

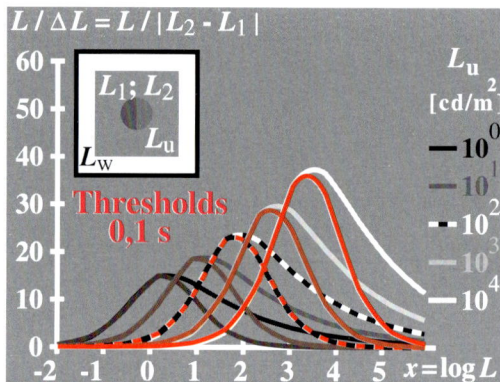

Fig. 18.26: Luminance discrimination ($L/\Delta L$) for achromatic colors of different central field luminance (L) for five different surround field luminances L_u. Approximation for five different Lu by a process black N [8753-2].

field luminance (L) for five different surround field luminances (L_u). Approximation for five different L_u by a process black N.

Figure 18.27 shows the luminance discrimination ($L/\Delta L$) for achromatic colors of different central field luminance (L) for five different surround field luminances L_u. Approximation for five different L_u by a process white W.

Figure 18.28 shows the luminance discrimination ($L/\Delta L$) for achromatic colors of different central field luminance (L) for five different surround field luminances L_u. Approximation for the mean

18.8 Sensitivity, Saturation and Chromaticity

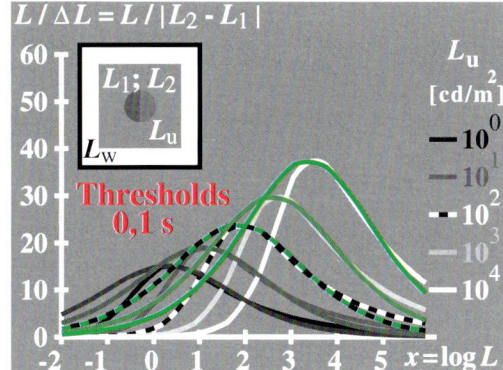

Fig. 18.27: Luminance discrimination ($\Delta L/L$) for achromatic colors of different central field luminance (L) for five different surround field luminances (L_u). Approximation for five different L_u by a process white W [8753-3].

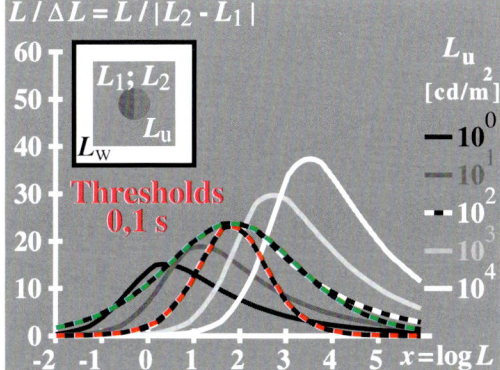

Fig. 18.28: Luminance discrimination ($\Delta L/L$) for achromatic colors of different central field luminance (L) for five different surround field luminances L_u. Approximation for the mean surround field luminance $L_u = 100$ cd/m² by a process black N and a process W [8753-4].

surround field luminance $L_u = 100$ cd/m² by a process black N and a process W.

The description of color threshold experiments by two visual processes in the red–green direction was already shown in Figures 18.23 and 18.24. Here we use two visual processes for the black–white direction. Between threshold and scaling we constructed a relationship for the red–green direction. A similar but more complex model for the black–white direction is developed elsewere (Richter, 1996).

Figure 18.29 shows the *sensitivity* of adapted receptors P'', D'' and their mean U''. The term *adapted* is used here for equal maximum sensitivity for light of equal energy within the visible spectrum. The sensivity maximum of P'' and D'' is reached for $u = -0.3$ (540 nm) and $u = 0.3$ (570 nm). The mean U'' is normalized to zero at 555 nm. This normalization is reached by multiplying factors 1.06 to compute P'' and D'' from P and D. There is no contribution of T to P (compare with Fig. 18.31).

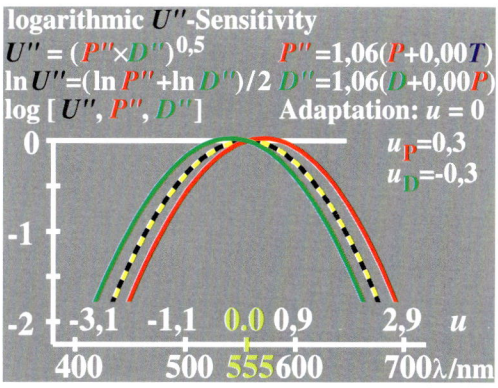

Fig. 18.29: Sensitivity of adapted receptors P'', D'' and the mean U''. Sensitivity maximum of P'' and D'' for $u = -0.3$ (540 nm) and $u = 0.3$ (570 nm). No contribution of T to P [9053-1].

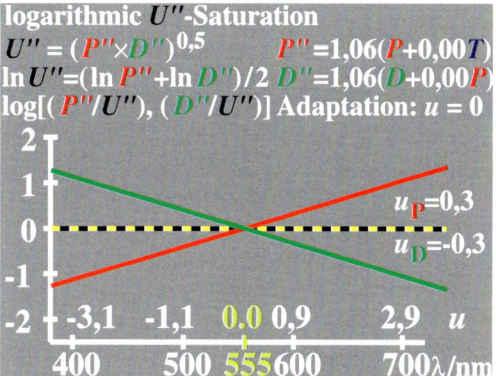

Fig. 18.30: Saturation of adapted receptors P'', D'' and the mean U''. Sensitivity maximum of P'' and D'' for $u = -0.3$ (540 nm) and $u = 0.3$ (570 nm). No contribution of T to P [9053-2].

Figure 18.30 shows the *saturation* of adapted receptors P'', D'' and their mean U'''. The sensitivity maximum of P'' and D'' is reached for $u = -0.3$ (540 nm) and $u = 0.3$ (570 nm). The mean U''' is normalized to zero at 555 nm. This normalization is reached by multiplying factors 1.06 to compute P'' and D'' from P and D. There is no contribution of T to P.

Figure 18.31 shows the *sensitivity* of adapted receptors P'', D'' and their mean U'''. The sensitivity maximum of P'' and D'' is reached for $u = -0.3$ (540 nm) and $u = 0.3$ (570 nm). The mean U''' is normalized to zero at 555 nm. This normalization is reached by multiplying factors 0.90 and 1.25 to compute P'' and D'' from P and D for a 5% contribution of T to P (compare with Fig. 18.29).

Figure 18.32 shows the *saturation* of adapted receptors P'', D'' and their mean U". The sensitivity maximum of P'' and D'' is reached for $u = -0.3$ (540 nm) and $u = 0.3$ (570 nm). The mean U''' is normalized to zero at 555 nm. This normalization is reached by multiplying factors 0.90 and 1.25 to compute P'' and D'' from P and D for a 5% contribution of T to P.

Saturation is defined by a ratio of the receptor sensitivities P'' or D'' and their mean U'''. The logarithmic ratio is either a linear function (see Fig. 18.30) or a parabolic function (see Fig. 18.32) as function of wavelength. These ratios are used to define logarithmic chromaticity diagrams.

The logarithmic chromaticity diagrams are very useful to specify chromaticness tolerances for colors of equal lightness (and luminance). Equal chromaticness steps in red–green and yellow–blue directions correspond to equal geometrical differences within the nonlinear (logarithmic or cube root) chromaticity diagrams.

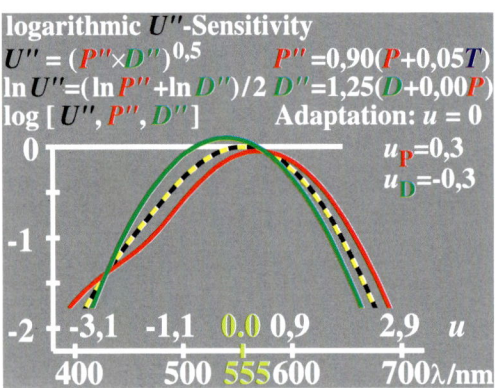

Fig. 18.31: Sensitivity of adapted receptors P'', D'' and the mean U'''. Sensitivity maximum of P'' and D'' for $u = -0.3$ (540 nm) and $u = 0.3$ (570 nm) for a 5% contribution of T to P [9063-1].

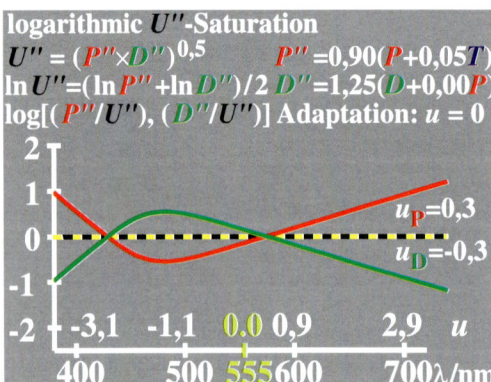

Fig. 18.32: Saturation of adapted receptors P'', D'' and the mean U'''. Sensitivity maximum of P'' and D'' for $u = -0.3$ (540 nm) and $u = 0.3$ (570 nm) for a 5% contribution of T to P [9063-2].

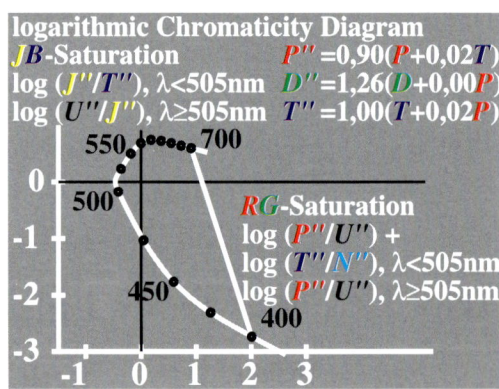

Fig. 18.33: Logarithmic chromaticity diagram with RG- and JB-saturation. The saturations are based on the ratio of receptor sensitivities P'', D'', and T'' [9472-3].

Figure 18.33 shows a logarithmic chromaticity diagram with RG- and JB-saturation. The saturations are based on the ratio of receptor sensitivities P'', D'', and T''.

Figure 18.34 shows the cube root chromaticity

18.8 Sensitivity, Saturation and Chromaticity   331

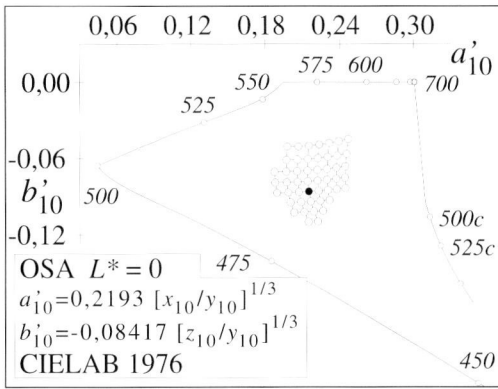

Fig. 18.34: Cube root chromaticity diagram (a'_{10}, b'_{10}) with RG- and JB-saturation. The saturations are based on the luminance ratios $a = X/Y = x/y$ and $b = -0.4 Z/Y = -0.4 z/y$ of the CIE standard observer [8220-3].

diagram (a'_{10}, b'_{10}) with RG- and JB-saturation. The saturations are based on a cube root transformation of linear luminance ratios $a = X/Y = x/y$ and $b = -0.4 Z/Y = -0.4 z/y$ of the CIE standard observer. In a first approximation the tristimulus values X, Y, and Z correspond to P'', U'', and T''. A cube root chromaticity diagram is, to a first approximation, similar to a logarithmic chromaticity diagram. This property leads to similar chromaticiy diagrams in Figures 18.33 and 18.34.

The cube root chromaticities a'_{10} and b'_{10} shown in Figure 18.34 can be used for definitions of color attributes in the CIELAB 1976 color space. The color samples of a color system defined by the Optical Society of America (OSA, see MacAdam, 1978) are plotted in the chromaticity diagram (a'_{10}, b'_{10}). The sample of equal lightness $L^*_{OSA} = 0$ (approximately $L^*_{CIELAB} = 50$) shows approxi-

---

color space CIELAB 1976, color values, attributes, chromaticities (a', b')

tristimulus values X, Y, Z -> color attributes L^*, a^*, b^*

lightness $L^* = 116 (Y/Y_n)^{1/3} - 16$

RG-chromaticness $a^* = 500 [(X/X_n)^{1/3} - (Y/Y_n)^{1/3}] = 500 [a' - a'_n] Y^{1/3}$

JB-chromaticness $b^* = 200 [(Y/Y_n)^{1/3} - (Z/Z_n)^{1/3}] = 500 [b' - b'_n] Y^{1/3}$

color attributes L^*, a^*, b^* -> tristimulus values X, Y, Z

tristimulus values $X = X_n [(L^* + 16)/116 + a^*/500]^3$

$Y = Y_n [(L^* + 16)/116]^3$

$Z = Z_n [(L^* + 16)/116 - b^*/200]^3$

chromaticities for CIELAB 1976, LABHNU 1977, LABHNU1 1979

CIELAB 1976, 2°	$a' = 0,2191 (x/y)^{1/3}$	$b' = -0,08376 (z/y)^{1/3}$
LABHNU 1977	$a' = (x/y + 1/6)^{1/3} / 4$	$b' = -(z/y + 1/6)^{1/3} / 12$
LABHNU1 1979	$a' = (x/y + 1) / 15$ linear!	$b' = -(z/y + 1/6)^{1/3} / 12$
LABHNU2 1979	$a' = (x/y + 1/6)^{2/3} / 15$	$b' = -(z/y + 1/6)^{1/3} / 12$
CIELAB 1976, 10°	$a' = 0,2193 (x_{10}/y_{10})^{1/3}$	$b' = -0,08417 (z_{10}/y_{10})^{1/3}$
chromaticity constants CIELAB, 2°,10°	$a_2 = 500 (1/X_n)^{1/3} = 0,2191$ $a_{10} = 500 (1/X_{n10})^{1/3} = 0,2193$	$b_2 = -200 (1/Z_n)^{1/3} = -0,08376$ $b_{10} = -200 (1/Z_{n10})^{1/3} = -0,08417$

Fig. 18.35: Color spaces, tristimulus values, color attributes, and chromaticities used in different applications to decribe color spacing [8192-3].

mately equal geometrical differences for equal visual differences. Therefore the geometrical tolerances can be used to define industrial color tolerances. For this purpose the CIELAB color space (CIE, 1978) is widely used.

Figure 18.35 shows the definition of color spaces, tristimulus values, color attributes, and chromaticities used in different applications to decribe color spacing (Richter, 1996). The definitions of the color attributes lightness L^*, RG–chromaticness a^*, and JB–chromaticness b^* are shown for the color spaces CIELAB 1976, 2° and 10°, LABHNU 1977, LABHNU1/2 1979. Chromaticity diagrams (a', b') are computed by chromaticity ratios x/y and z/y. An example was shown in the chromaticity diagram (a', b') of Figure 18.34.

Similar chromaticity diagrams (a'', b'') based on the chromaticity ratios x/y and z/y have been developed to decribe color thresholds (Richter, 1996). The coordinates shown in Figure 18.35 can be used in PostScript computer programs. PostScript is at present the only programming language which allows one to fill the areas in a layout with device-independent colors. About 300 PostScript devices of 60 manufacturers mix the colors of the layout by device-dependent colors within small tolerances, e. g., on monitors by the device colors orange-red O, leaf-green L and violet-blue V or within printers by the device colors cyan-blue C, magenta-red M, yellow Y, and Black N.

18.9 Summary

PostScript allows one to use device-independent CIE color spaces based on color measurement for the description of colors in computer programs. If one uses vector graphics (e. g., to describe areas and lines) the resolution of the output device describes the visual quality of images.

Some figures describe basic parts of color order, color vision and color spaces. These figures are especially useful for educational purposes. More than 500 similar color figures are published and printed in Richter (1996). The PostScript Code is available on CD-ROM. All color figures can be printed on overhead transparency in different sizes, can be modified and can be used in other publications.

References

Adobe Systems Inc. (1990). PostScript language reference Manual, Reading. Addison-Wesley.

Commission Internationale de l'Eclairage (CIE) (1978). Official recommendation on color spaces, color difference equations and metric color terms, Supplement No. 2 for CIE-Publication No. 15, Colorimetry (E-1.3.1), 1971.

Commission Internationale de l'Eclairage (CIE) (1986). Colorimetry, Colorimetrie, Farbmessung, CIE Publication No. 15,2.

Commission Internationale de l'Eclairage (CIE) (1987). Vocabulaire internationale de l'Eclairage, International lighting vocabulary. Internationales Wörterbuch der Lichttechnik. 4 edition, CIE Publication No. 17.

German standard orginisation (DIN), DIN 33 866 (draft 1997). Information technology, Office machines, Testchart for color copying machines, Beuth-Verlag, Berlin 1997.

Hard, A. and Sivik, L. (1981). NCS, Natural Color System: A Swedish Standard for Color Notation, Color Research and Application 6, *3*, 129–138.

Judd, D. B. and Wyszecki, G. (1975). Color in Business, Science and Industry, 3rd edition, Wiley, New York.

Leonardo da Vinci (1452–1519). Traktat von der Malerei; Translation into German H. Ludwig (1882), new edition of Maria Herzfeld, Diederichs, Jena 1925.

MacAdam, D. L. (1978). Colorimetric data for samples of OSA uniform color scales, J. Opt. Soc. Amer. *68*, Nr. 1, 121–130.

Miescher, K., Richter. K., and Valberg, A. (1982). Color and Color Vision. Description of experiments for color education, Farbe + Design, *23/24*, 24.

Newhall, S. M., Nickerson, D., and Judd, D. B. (1943). Final Report of the O.S.A. subcommittee on the spacing of the Munsell colors, J. Opt. Soc. Amer. *33*, 385–418.

Richter, K. (1996). Computergrafik und Farbmetrik, Farbsysteme, PostScript und geräteunabhängige CIE-Farben, VDE-Verlag, Berlin.

Richter, M. (1963). Über Entstehung, Aufbau und Anwendung der DIN-Farbenkarte DIN 6164, DIN-Mitteilungen 42, *6*, 269–275.

List of Contributors

Werner G. K. Backhaus
Theoretical and Experimental Biology
Department of Biology
Freie Universität Berlin
Thielallee 63
D-14195 Berlin
Germany
e-mail: backhaus@zedat.fu-berlin.de

Jürgen Baudewig
Department of Clinical Neurophysiology
Georg-August-University of Göttingen
Robert-Koch-Str. 40
D-37075 Göttingen
Germany
e-mail: baudewig@med.uni-goettingen.de

Michelle L. Bieber
Department of Psychology
University of Colorado
Campus Box 345
Boulder CO 80309-0345
U.S.A.
e-mail: mbieber@psych.colorado.edu

Michael D'Zmura
Department of Cognitive Sciences
University of California, Irvine
Irvine, CA 92697
U.S.A.
e-mail: mdzmura@uci.edu

Michael Finkenstaedt
Department of Neuroradiology
Georg-August-University of Göttingen
Robert-Koch-Str. 40
D-37075 Göttingen
Germany
e-mail: larafi@aol.com

Nora Freudenthaler
Department of Ophthalmology
Georg-August-University of Göttingen
Robert-Koch-Str. 40
D-37075 Göttingen
Germany
e-mail: sfreude@aol.com

Clyde L. Hardin
Department of Philosophy
Syracuse University
Syracuse, NY 13244
U.S.A.
e-mail: clhardin@syr.edu

Hans Irtel
Faculty for Social Sciences
University of Mannheim
Schloss, Ehrenhof Ost
D-68131 Mannheim
Germany
e-mail: irtel@psychologie.uni-mannheim.de

Peter G. Kevan
Department of Environmental Biology
University of Guelph,
Guelph, Ontario, N1G 2W1
Canada
e-mail: pkevan@uoguelph.ca

Reinhold Kliegl
Department
of Psychology
University of Potsdam
Postbox 601553
D-14415 Potsdam
Germany
e-mail: kliegl@rz.uni-potsdam.de

Kenneth Knoblauch
Institut de l'Ingénierie de la Vision
Université Jean Monnet
Site GIAT-Industries
3, rue Javelin-Pagnon, BP 505
42007 Saint-Etienne Cedex 01
France
e-mail: knoblauc@univ-lyon1.fr

Renate Kolle
Department of Clinical Neurophysiology
Georg-August-University of Göttingen
Robert-Koch-Str. 40
D-37075 Göttingen
Germany
e-mail: renankolle@aol.com

Jan Kremers
Department of Experimental Ophthalmology
University of Tübingen
Eye Hospital
Röntgenweg 11
D-72076 Tübingen
Germany
e-mail: jan.kremers@uni-tuebingen.de

Mathias Kunkel
Im Winkel 34
D-37077 Göttingen
Germany
e-mail: mkunkel@gwdg.de

Barry B. Lee
Neurobiology
Max-Planck-Institute for Biophysical Chemistry
Am Fassberg
D-37077 Göttingen
Germany
e-mail: lee@mike.dnet.gwdg.de

Rainer Mausfeld
Institute of Psychology
Christian-Albrecht-University of Kiel
D-24098 Kiel
Germany
e-mail: mausfeld@psychologie.uni-kiel.de

Sabine Meierkord
Department of Experimental Ophthalmology
University of Tübingen
Eye Hospital
Röntgenweg 11
D-72076 Tübingen
Germany
e-mail: sabine.meierkord@uni-tuebingen.de

Jay Neitz
Department of Cellular Biology
Medical College of Wisconsin
8701 Watertown Plank Road
Wiwaukee, WI 53226
U.S.A.
e-mail: jneitz@mcw.edu

Maureen Neitz
Department of Ophthalmology
Medical College of Wisconsin
925 N, 87th Street
Milwaukee, WI 53226-4812
U.S.A.
e-mail: mneitz@mcw.edu

Christa Neumeyer
Institute of Zoology III
Johannes-Gutenberg-University
D-55099 Mainz
Germany
e-mail: neumeyer@mzdmza.zdv.uni-mainz.de

Walter Paulus
Department of Clinical Neurophysiology
Georg-August-University of Göttingen
Robert-Koch-Str. 40
D-37075 Göttingen
Germany
e-mail: pwenig@gwdu20.gwdg.de

Klaus Richter
Federal Institute of Material
Research and Testing (BAM)
Unter den Eichen 87
D-12203 Berlin
Germany
e-mail: richter.farbe@t-online.de

Hans-Heino Rustenbeck
Department of Neuroradiology
Georg-August-University of Göttingen
Robert-Koch-Str. 40
D-37075 Göttingen
Germany

János Schanda
Image Processing and Neural Computing
University Veszprém
Egyetem u. 10.
H-8200 Veszprem
Hungary
e-mail: schanda@almos.vein.hu

Horst Scheibner
Physiological Institute of the
University of Düsseldorf
Moorenstr. 5
D-40225 Düsseldorf
Germany

Petra Stoerig
Institute of Physiological Psychology
Heinrich-Heine-University
Universitätsstr.1
D-40225 Düsseldorf
e-mail: petra.stoerig@uni-duesseldorf.de
Germany

Vicki J. Volbrecht
Department of Psychology
Colorado State University
Ft. Collins, CO 80523-1876
U.S.A.
e-mail: vicki@lamar.colostate.edu

John S. Werner
Interdisciplinary Center
of Cognitive Studies
University of Potsdam and
Department of Psychology
University of Colorado
Campus Box 345
Boulder CO 80309-0345
U.S.A.
e-mail: jwerner@clipr.colorado.edu

Stefan Weiss
Natural and Medical Science Institute NMI
Eberhardstraße 29
D-72762 Reutlingen
Germany
e-mail: Weiss@nmi.de

Eberhart Zrenner
University of Tübingen
Eye Hospital
Schleichstraße 12
D-72076 Tübingen
Germany
e-mail: ezrenner@uni-tuebingen.de

Index

Achromatic colors xiii–xiv, 45, 54, 187–202, 223, 321–322, 328
– and P-pathway 122
– see also Blackness
Achromatopsia 138, 144–145
– see also Cortical color blindness
Adaptation
– chromatic 17–21
– two-process interpretation 234–235
– see also Coefficient rule (v. Kries)
Additive light (color) mixture 9–10, 27–28, 150, 225, 326
Additivity test, see Blackness
Afterimage 14–15
– see also Successive color contrast
Aging
– and brightness 27
– and color perception 25–27
– and cone sensitivity 11–12
– and ocular media 7–8
– and unique hues 25
Alychne 289, 292–300
– see also Chromaticity diagram
Amacrine cells 6, 54
Amphibians 149, 165
Anomalous trichromacy 101, 108 117
Aperture colors 193–194
Aristotle 72, 188
Arthropods 164–165
Assimilation 19–21, 28

Basic color terms 207–215
– see also Color appearance
Bees 46, 53, 56–57, 60–74, 167–171
– see also Honeybees
– see also Solitary bees
Bezold-Brücke effect 59, 69–71, 226
Bezold spreading effect, see Assimilation
Binocular brightness combination 268–273
Bipolar cells 6, 83, 149
Birds 165
Blackness 45, 54, 187–202

– and additivity 199–201
– and color naming 195–197
– contrast effects 46
– historical 187–195
– and physiological mechanisms 201–202
– and spectral sensitivity 197–201
Blindsight 134–138, 144
Brightness
– and aging 27
– and binocular 268–273
– definition 223
– and heterochromatic matching 27, 198–199
– in honeybees 69, 167–168
Butterflies 61, 165

Carotinoid pigments 8, 172–173
Cataract 7–8, 33, 36–38
Cephalopods 164
Cézanne, P. 5
Chevreul, M. E. 17–21, 189–190
Chromatic adaptation, see Adaptation
Chromaticity diagram 58–59, 61
– alychne 289, 292–300
– center-of-gravity principle 58, 224
– CIE 325–326
– confusion lines 288–289, 310–313
– coordinates 58
– copunctal point 289, 311–313
– cube root 330–331
– dichromatic 291–294, 300
– instrumental 286–290
– logarithmic 330
– Newton's color circle 58
– physiological 307–316
– tetrachromatic 170
– turtles 153–154
CIE (Commission Internationale de l'Eclairage)
– see Chromaticity diagram
– see Color matching
– see Color spaces
– see Standard observer
Coefficient rule (v. Kries) 18, 232–234

Color appearance xiii–xiv
- attributes 222–224
- basic colors 207–215
- CIE metric 315
- definitions 223
- elementary (unique) colors xiii–xiv, 45, 71–74, 228, 189–191
- in goldfish 160
- in honeybees 71–74, 169
- unique hues (colors) 24–25, 45, 208, 227
- see also Color naming
- see also Color spaces
- see also Color vision models

Color blindness
- genetic basis of 101–116
- see also Achromatopsia
- see also Anomalous trichromacy
- see also Cortical color blindness
- see also Deuteranomaly
- see also Deuteranopia
- see also Dichromacy
- see also Monochromacy
- see also Protanomaly
- see also Protanopia
- see also Sex-linked color deficiency
- see also Tritanomaly
- see also Tritanopia

Color cancellation 24–25, 227, 244
- see also Blackness

Color constancy 21, 23, 141–143, 237–242, 245
- computational perspective 238–242
- in goldfish 155–157
- in honeybees 167
- lightness 267, 273
- retinex theory 238–239

Color contrast
- hue 19–21, 28, 33
- lightness, see Mach bands, Blackness
- simultaneous 15, 28, 30–32, 188–190, 194–195
- successive 14–15, 136, 188–190, 194–196

Color contrast gain control 251–265
- and image processing 256–263
- and multichannel model 263–264
- and spatial frequency and orientation tuning 252–253

Color difference judgment 50–51
Color discrimination (in) 51–52
- amphibians 154–155
- goldfish 150–151
- honeybees 64–71, 167
- turtles 151–152
- rod contributions 89–98, 278–279
- see also Wavelength discrimination

Color language 23–24, 207–215, 222–224
- see also Color naming

Color learning
- in honeybees 64

Color management 315
Color matching 58–60, 79
- CIE 307–314
- functions 286–287, 290–291, 307–314
- functions (dichromatic) 290–291, 301
- and macular pigment 310
- maximum saturation method 308–309
- Maxwell match 308–309, 314
- and photopigment density 311
- Rayleigh match 109, 114
- relation to photopigments 115–117, 311–314
- and rod intrusion 309, 314

Color memory 64–65
Color metrics
- see Chromaticity diagram
- see Color spaces
- see Metrics

Color mixture
- see Additive mixture
- see Color matching
- see Metamerism
- see Subtractive mixture

Color naming 24–27, 195–197, 208–215
- see also Blackness

Color reproduction 319–321
- device–dependent colors 319
- device-independent colors 319

Color science disciplines 45
Color similarity 51, 226
Color spaces
- appearance xiii–xiv, 322–323, 327
- CIE 307–315
- CIELAB 1976 320, 331–332
- color-opponent coding xiii–xiv, 26, 53–57
- – and deuteranopia 291–298
- – physiological 54–57, 61–62
- cone excitation 83–85, 253–254, 285, 308, 314
- honeybees 53, 65, 74, 168–171
- photoreceptor excitation 61
- photoreceptor sensitivity 60–61
- physiological 57–61
- psychophysical 51–54
- see also Chromaticity diagram
- see also Hering color-order system
- see also Munsell color-order system
- see also Natural color system
- see also Ostwald color-order system

Color training experiments

Index

- goldfish 150–151, 155–157
- honeybees 60, 62–64, 69
- salamanders 154–155
- see also Color vision (in)
Color vision (in)
- amphibians 149, 165
- arthropods 164–165
- birds 165
- butterflies 61, 165
- cephalopods 164
- cyprinid fishes 149
- dichromacy 89, 101–103, 285–302
- frogs 149
- goldfish 143, 150–151, 155–157
- honeybees 62–74, 167
- infants 208–209, 275–281
- insects 47
- lizards 149
- macaque monkies 142
- marmosets 89–98
- New and Old World primates 89–90
- polychromacy 51, 60–61, 65, 165, 177
- reptiles 165
- rodents 165
- salamanders 154–155
- solitary bees 61
- toads 149
- tetrachromacy 61, 116–117, 150–152, 159–160, 163–165, 170, 173, 177–178, 309
- trichromacy 51, 60–61, 65, 189, 249
- turtles 149, 151–154, 159
- wasps 61
Color vision models
- blackness 189–194, 201
- computational 220–221, 238–242, 253, 256–264
- octant model 235–236
- opponent processes 26, 72, 189–194, 201, 226–231
- trichromatic 189
- zone theories xiv, 23–27, 192–194, 201
- see also Simulations
Colorimetry 167–168
Commission Internationale de l'Eclairage (CIE)
- see Chromaticity diagram
- see Color spaces
- see Standard observer
Complementary lights (colors) 9, 17, 57, 228
Computer graphics 319–332
Cones 83–85, 253–254, 285, 308, 314
- absorption spectra 9, 17, 48, 152, 307–308
- action spectra
- – and aging 11–12, 38
- – and infants 11, 280

- oil droplets 151
- photopigment polymorphism 89, 101, 104–116, 309
- UV sensitive, 47, 150–152, 164
- see also Photopigments
- see also Spectral sensitivity
Conscious vision 71
Constancy
- floral 72, 172
- see also Color constancy
- see also Lightness constancy
Contrast colors 210, 228
- see also Blackness
Copunctal point 289, 311–313
Cornea 5–6
Cortex, see visual cortex
Cortical blindness 134–138
Cortical color blindness 72, 138–141, 141–145
Cyprinid fishes 149

Daylight 165–167
- and atmosphere 163–165
- and ultraviolet (UV) light 165
Delacroix, E. 17–21
Detection thresholds 84
- chromatic 228, 327–329
- increment–decrement asymmetry 236
Deuteranomaly 108–113
Deuteranopia 96–98, 101–103, 114–115, 285–302
- color-matching functions 290–291, 301
Dichromacy 89, 101–103, 285–302
- color-matching functions 290–291, 301
- copunctal points 289, 311–313
- genetic models 113–114
- in Marmosets 89–98
- opponent-color space 291–298
- rod contributions to discrimination 96–98
- unilateral 230
Dipole source analysis 122–124
Dischromatopsia 138
Divisionism 27–30
- see also Pointillism
Dopamine 159

Ecology and color vision 163–178
Eigengrau 188, 192
Electroencephalogram (EEG) 121–123
Ethambutol 159
Evoked potential, see Visually-evoked potential
Evolution
- and color vision 163–178
- and floral colors 171–175
- see also Ladd-Franklin

Eye 6
- camera 164
- compound 56
- dominance 272
- lens 6–8, 310–311, see also Cataract

Farnsworth-Munsell 100–hue test 139
Fechner, G. Th. 49–50, 232, 268
Fechner's law 49–50
Fechner's paradox 272–273
Film colors 193
Fishes
- see Cyprinid fishes
- see Goldfish
Floral color
- evolution 171–175
- patterns 175–177
Fovea 8
Frisch, K. v. 64, 149, 242
Frogs 149
Functional magnetic resonance imaging (fMRI) 125–127

Ganglion cells, see Retinal ganglion cells
Gelb effect 188
Genetics
- molecular 101–117
Goethe, J. W. v. 14–15, 30, 188–189, 226
Gogh, V. van 16, 27
Goldfish 143, 150–151, 155–157
Grassmann, H. 58–59, 224–226
Grassmann code (structure) 225–231, 239
Grassmann laws (rules) 61, 225–226, 309, 311
Grassmann theory 220, 225–226

Helmholtz, H. v. xiii, 9, 11, 15, 23–24, 58, 79, 187–193, 201, 223, 229, 232, 241, 243
Hering, E. xiii–xv, 15, 21, 23–25, 28, 45, 54, 80, 149, 187–195, 201, 208–209, 210–211, 223–224, 226–227, 232, 234, 237–238, 243, 285
Hering color-order system xiii–xv, 208–209, 210–211, 285
Honeybees 62–74, 155, 165
Horizontal cells 6, 83, 86
Hue
- definition of 223
- see also Color appearance
Hue contrast
- see Simultaneous color contrast
- see Successive color contrast

Image reproduction 319–321
- and contrast gain control 256–263

Image segmentation 243–248
Impressionism 3–5, 12–13, 16–23, 30–38
Insects 47, 163–167
Interocular transfer
- and contrast gain 252

Judgments
- conscious 71
- content analytical 51
- difference 50
- identity 229, 233
- similarity 51
- unconscious 71
Just noticeable difference (JND) 51, 150
- see also Color discrimination

Katz, D. 13, 191, 193, 223–224, 241, 244
Kay-McDaniel sequence/theory 211–214
König, A. 285, 287–288, 294, 309
König hypothesis 287–288, 294, 308–309, 311
Kries, J. v. xiv, 18, 25–26, 192, 223, 232–235, 253, 301

Ladd-Franklin, C. 191–192
Laminar segmentation 243–248
Lateral geniculate nucleus (LGN) 54–56, 90–98, 139
Lens (eye) 5–8, 310–311
- see also Cataract
Light
- daylight 163–167
- infrared (IR) 8
- scatter 33
- spectrum visible
- – human 6–8, 47
- – insects 47
- ultraviolet 8, 47, 165
Lightness
- constancy 267, 273
- and hue 324
Lizards 149
Luminance 285, 307, 314
- channel 81–82
- cone contributions 275–277, 310–313
- in infants 275
- see also Photometry (flicker)
- see also Spectral sensitivity

Mach, E. 45–47, 234
Mach bands 45–47
Macular pigment 8, 310
- and color matching 309
Magnetic resonance imaging (MRI) 124–125
- see also Functional magnetic resonance imaging

Magnocellular pathway 56, 80, 90–98, 121–122
Marmosets 89–98
Maximum saturation method 308–309
Maxwell, J. C. xiii, 9, 15, 24, 59, 189, 224, 285
Maxwell matching 308–309, 314
Mayer, T. 79–80
Metamerism 9, 38, 224–226, 301, 316
– see also Color matching
Method of triads, 51
Metrics
– city-block 52, 62
– Euclidean 51–52
– Minkowski 51–52
Microspectrophotometry 55, 149–150
Minimally-distinct border 198, 291
Monet, C. 3–39
Monochromacy
– cone 101
– rod 101, 103
Motion and color
– in goldfish 159
Müller, G. E. 192, 223, 227, 285
Multidmensional scaling (MDS) analysis 51, 62, 72
Munsell color-order system 52, 71–72, 207, 212, 214, 324

Natural color system (NCS) 54
Networks neuronal, see Simulations
Neurons
– see Amacrine cells
– see Bipolar cells
– see Cones
– see Horizontal cells
– see Opponent-color coding
– see Retinal ganglion cells
– see Rods
Neuroreductionism 231
Newton, I. xiii, 3, 15, 57–58, 131, 189, 224

Ocular media 7–8, 310–311
– see also Cataract
Oil droplets, colored 151
Ommatidia 56
Opponent-color coding
– double-opponent responses 149–150
– in honeybees 46, 66–68
– models 189–194, 201, 226–231
– perceptual basis of 15, 23–36, 189–194, 208–210, 226–231
– physiological basis of 24, 80–86, 149–150
– S-potentials 149
– see also Color spaces
– see also Color vision models

Opsin 105
Optic nerve 6
Optomotor response 158–159
Ostwald color-order system 54

Palmer, G. 60, 80
Parvocellular pathway 56, 80, 90–98, 121–122
Persistency rule 233
Photometry (flicker) 81–82, 197–199, 275, 307
Photopigments
– genetic code 103–116
– opsin molecule 105
– optical density 311
– optical density and spectral sensitivity 276–277
– polymorphism 89, 101, 104–116, 309
– see also Cones
– see also Rods
Photoreceptors 5–6, 47, 54, 79–80, 307–310
– see also Cones
– see also Photopigments
– see also Rods
– see also Spectral sensitivity
– see also Univariance principle
Phototransduction function (Naka-Rushton) 61
Pigments
– see Carotinoid pigments
– see Macular pigment
– see Photopigments
Pissarro, C. 5, 13, 16, 27, 29
Plexiform layer
– inner 82–84
– outer 83, 86
Pointillism 9, 27–30
Pollinators 163, 175
Polychromacy 51, 60–61, 65, 165, 177
Positron emission tomography (PET) 125, 134
PostScript 319–320
Proportionality rule 233
Protanomaly 113
Protanopia 96–98, 101–103, 113–115, 278–279
– and spectral sensitivity 199
Pseudoisochromatic plates 109, 139
Psychometric function 49–50
Pupil
– and rods 134–135
Purkinje-shift 136

Qualia 143–145

Radiation, see Light
Rayleigh color match 109, 114
Receptive fields 27–29, 55–56, 80–86, 121, 201–202
– see also Retinal ganglion cells

Renoir, P. A. 4–5, 16
Reptiles 165
Retina 6
– circuitry of 79–88
– photochemical damage 8
Retinal ganglion cells 6, 55–56, 80–86
– bistratified cells 83–86
– in fishes 149
– magno- (M-) cells 80–83, 90
– midget cells 82–84, 90
– parasol cells 80–83, 90
– parvo- (P-) cells 82–83, 90
Retinal fatigue hypothesis 190–191, 232
– see also Coefficient rule (v. Kries)
Retinex theory 238–239
Rods 6
– and color discrimination 89–98, 278–279
– and color matching 309, 314
– in infants 278–279
– photopigment absorption 131–133
– and pupil 134–135
Rod-cone interactions
– relation to retinal eccentricity 94–95
– see also Rods
Rodents 165

Salamanders 154–155
Saturation
– definition of 223
– see also Color appearance
Scaling,-
– direct, see Judgments, content analytical
– indirect 50–51
– see also Judgments
– see also Metrics
Schopenhauer, A. 188
Schrödinger, E. 61, 192, 225–226, 271, 285, 287, 289, 293
Segmentation, figure-ground 245
Sensations
– in animals 71–74
– in humans 45
Seurat, G. 27–28, 245
Sex-linked color deficiency 89, 102–117
Shadows (colored), see Simultaneous color contrast
Signac, P. 12–13, 29
Silent substitution 90, 93, 278
Simulations
– physiological 46–47, 62–74
– psychophysical 46, 62–74, 256–263
Simultaneous color contrast 15, 28, 30–32, 188–190, 194–195, 234, 243, 326
– in goldfish 157

Successive color contrast 14–15, 136, 188–190, 194–196, 232, 234
– in honeybees 70
Solitary bees 61
Spatial color contrast
– see Contrast colors
– see Simultaneous color contrast
Spectral sensitivity
– blackness process 197
– and blindsight 136–137
– brightness 198–199
– and chromatic channels 137–138
– in goldfish 150, 157–159
– in honeybees 70
– in infants 275
– photopic 131–133, 193, 197–199, 307, 325
– and photopigment optical density 276–277
– protanopic 199
– scotopic 131–133
– of photoreceptors
– – in honeybees 56–57
– – in humans 101
– see also Luminance
– see also Minimally-distinct border
– see also Photometry (flicker)
– see also Standard observer
Standard observer
– CIE 2° 307
– CIE 10° 309, 313
– CIE photopic sensitivity 307, 325
– CIE spectral tristimulus values 325–326, 331
– see also Chromaticity diagram
– see also Color matching
Stimuli 45, 47–48
– Maxwellian-view optics 221, 231
– Mondrian 123, 141–142, 239, 245
– monitors 48, 277
– see also Silent substitution
Subtractive light (color) mixture 9–10
Superior colliculus 134

Temporal color contrast
– see Successive color contrast
Test colors (CIE) 320
Tetrachromacy 61, 116–117, 150–152, 159–160, 163–165, 170, 173, 177–178, 309
Threshold
– see Color discrimination
– see Detection threshold
Thurstone's law of comparative judgment 49–50
Toads 149
Tritanomaly 103
Tritanopia 101, 103

Turner, J. M. W. 13–17, 33
Turtles 149, 151–154, 159

Unconscious inference 190–191
Unconscious vision 71–74, 143–145
Unique hues (colors), see Color appearance
Univariance principle 61, 65, 91

Visual cortex
– area V1 56, 122–126, 134
– area V2 56, 123–125
– area V3 123–125
– area V4 56, 123–125
Visually-evoked potential (VEP) 121–124
– in infants 278–281
von Kries-type normalization 237, 239, 246, 253
– see also Coefficient rule (v. Kries)
– see also Kries, J. v.

Wallace, A. R. 163–164
Wasps 61
Wavelength discrimination
– in goldfish 150–151
– in honeybees 70
– and human blindsight 137–138
– in salamanders 155
– in turtles 151–154
Weber, E. H. 49–50, 62
Weber's law 49–50, 62
World Color Survey 214–215

X-chromosome
– see Sex-linked color deficiency

Young, T. 9, 60, 79–80
Young-Helmholtz theory 189, 225, 232